Mass Cytometry: Techniques and Clinical Applications

Mass Cytometry: Techniques and Clinical Applications

Editor: Merna Corbin

AMERICAN
MEDICAL PUBLISHERS
www.americanmedicalpublishers.com

AMERICAN
MEDICAL PUBLISHERS
www.americanmedicalpublishers.com

Cataloging-in-Publication Data

Mass cytometry : techniques and clinical applications / edited by Merna Corbin.
p. cm.
Includes bibliographical references and index.
ISBN 979-8-88740-241-3
1. Cytometry. 2. Flow cytometry. 3. Flow cytometry--Diagnostic use. 4. Cytology--Technique.
5. Cellular therapy. I. Corbin, Merna.
QH585.5.F56 M37 2023
574.870 28--dc23

American Medical Publishers,
41 Flatbush Avenue,
1st Floor, New York,
NY 11217, USA

ISBN 979-8-88740-241-3 (Hardback)

Contents

Preface IX

Chapter 1 **Minimizing Batch Effects in Mass Cytometry Data** 1
Ronald P. Schuyler, Conner Jackson, Josselyn E. Garcia-Perez, Ryan M. Baxter, Sidney Ogolla, Rosemary Rochford, Debashis Ghosh, Pratyaydipta Rudra and Elena W. Y. Hsieh

Chapter 2 **Pretreatment Innate Cell Populations and CD4T Cells in Blood are Associated with Response to Immune Checkpoint Blockade in Melanoma Patients** 17
Mehdi R. Pirozyan, Helen M. McGuire, Abdullah Al Emran, Hsin-Yi Tseng, Jessamy C. Tiffen, Jenny H. Lee, Matteo S. Carlino, Alexander M. Menzies, Georgina V. Long, Richard A. Scolyer, Barbara Fazekas de St Groth and Peter Hersey

Chapter 3 **Pregnancy-Induced Alterations in NK Cell Phenotype and Function** 31
Mathieu Le Gars, Christof Seiler, Alexander W. Kay, Nicholas L. Bayless, Elina Starosvetsky, Lindsay Moore, Shai S. Shen-Orr, Natali Aziz, Purvesh Khatri, Cornelia L. Dekker, Gary E. Swan, Mark M. Davis, Susan Holmes and Catherine A. Blish

Chapter 4 **Mass Cytometry Reveals a Sustained Reduction in $CD16^+$ Natural Killer Cells Following Chemotherapy in Colorectal Cancer Patients** 43
Diana Shinko, Helen M. McGuire, Connie I. Diakos, Nick Pavlakis, Stephen J. Clarke, Scott N. Byrne and Kellie A. Charles

Chapter 5 **Validation of CyTOF Against Flow Cytometry for Immunological Studies and Monitoring of Human Cancer Clinical Trials** 55
Ramy Gadalla, Babak Noamani, Bethany L. MacLeod, Russell J. Dickson, Mengdi Guo, Wenxi Xu, Sabelo Lukhele, Heidi J. Elsaesser, Albiruni R. Abdul Razak, Naoto Hirano, Tracy L. McGaha, Ben Wang, Marcus Butler, Cynthia J. Guidos, Pam S. Ohashi, Lillian L. Siu and David G. Brooks

Chapter 6 **Mass Cytometry Imaging for the Study of Human Diseases—Applications and Data Analysis Strategies** 68
Heeva Baharlou, Nicolas P. Canete, Anthony L. Cunningham, Andrew N. Harman and Ellis Patrick

Chapter 7 **Mass Cytometry Analysis Reveals Complex Cell-State Modifications of Blood Myeloid Cells During HIV Infection** 90
Sixtine Coindre, Nicolas Tchitchek, Lamine Alaoui, Bruno Vaslin, Christine Bourgeois, Cecile Goujard, Camille Lecuroux, Pierre Bruhns, Roger Le Grand, Anne-Sophie Beignon, Olivier Lambotte and Benoit Favier

Chapter 8 **Deep Phenotyping of Urinary Leukocytes by Mass Cytometry Reveals a Leukocyte Signature for Early and Non-Invasive Prediction of Response to Treatment in Active Lupus Nephritis**......103
Martina Bertolo, Sabine Baumgart, Pawel Durek, Anette Peddinghaus, Henrik Mei, Thomas Rose, Philipp Enghard and Andreas Grützkau

Chapter 9 **Use of Mass Cytometry to Profile Human T Cell Exhaustion**......115
Frances Winkler and Bertram Bengsch

Chapter 10 **Quantitative Comparison of Conventional and t-SNE-guided Gating Analyses**......125
Shadi Toghi Eshghi, Amelia Au-Yeung, Chikara Takahashi, Christopher R. Bolen, Maclean N. Nyachienga, Sean P. Lear, Cherie Green, W. Rodney Mathews and William E. O'Gorman

Chapter 11 **Candidate Markers for Stratification and Classification in Rheumatoid Arthritis**......136
Lucius Bader, Stein-Erik Gullaksen, Nello Blaser, Morten Brun, Gerd Haga Bringeland, André Sulen, Clara Gram Gjesdal, Christian Vedeler and Sonia Gavasso

Chapter 12 **Mass Cytometry Discovers Two Discrete Subsets of CD39−Treg which Discriminate MGUS from Multiple Myeloma**......144
Felix Marsh-Wakefield, Annabel Kruzins, Helen M. McGuire, Shihong Yang, Christian Bryant, Barbara Fazekas de St. Groth, Najah Nassif, Scott N. Byrne, John Gibson, Christina Brown, Stephen Larsen, Derek McCulloch, Richard Boyle, Georgina Clark, Douglas Joshua, Phoebe Joy Ho and Slavica Vuckovic

Chapter 13 **Immunocyte Profiling Using Single-Cell Mass Cytometry Reveals EpCAM$^+$ CD4$^+$ T Cells Abnormal in Colon Cancer**......156
Ting Zhang, Junwei Lv, Ziyang Tan, Boqian Wang, Antony R. Warden, Yiyang Li, Hui Jiang, Hao Li and Xianting Ding

Chapter 14 **Characterization of Leukocytes from HIV-ART Patients Using Combined Cytometric Profiles of 72 Cell Markers**......168
Adrien Leite Pereira, Nicolas Tchitchek, Olivier Lambotte, Roger Le Grand and Antonio Cosma

Chapter 15 **Differential Dynamics of the Maternal Immune System in Healthy Pregnancy and Preeclampsia**......183
Xiaoyuan Han, Mohammad S. Ghaemi, Kazuo Ando, Laura S. Peterson, Edward A. Ganio, Amy S. Tsai, Dyani K. Gaudilliere, Ina A. Stelzer, Jakob Einhaus, Basile Bertrand, Natalie Stanley, Anthony Culos, Athena Tanada, Julien Hedou, Eileen S. Tsai, Ramin Fallahzadeh, Ronald J. Wong, Amy E. Judy, Virginia D. Winn, Maurice L. Druzin, Yair J. Blumenfeld, Mark A. Hlatky, Cecele C. Quaintance, Ronald S. Gibbs, Brendan Carvalho, Gary M. Shaw, David K. Stevenson, Martin S. Angst, Nima Aghaeepour and Brice Gaudilliere

Chapter 16 **Early-Life Compartmentalization of Immune Cells in Human Fetal Tissues Revealed by High-Dimensional Mass Cytometry**......195
Na Li, Vincent van Unen, Nannan Guo, Tamim Abdelaal, Antonios Somarakis, Jeroen Eggermont, Ahmed Mahfouz, Susana M. Chuva de Sousa Lopes, Boudewijn P. F. Lelieveldt and Frits Koning

Chapter 17 **Increased T Cell Differentiation and Cytolytic Function in Bangladeshi Compared to American Children** 208
Lisa E. Wagar, Christopher R. Bolen, Natalia Sigal, Cesar J. Lopez Angel, Leying Guan, Beth D. Kirkpatrick, Rashidul Haque, Robert J. Tibshirani, Julie Parsonnet, William A. Petri Jr. and Mark M. Davis

Permissions

List of Contributors

Index

Preface

The mass spectrometry technique, based on inductively coupled plasma mass spectrometry and time of flight mass spectrometry, used for the determination of the properties of cells, is called mass cytometry. In this method, antibodies are coupled with isotopically pure elements and are utilized to label the cellular proteins. Cells are nebulized and passed through argon plasma, which leads to the ionization of the metal-conjugated antibodies. Time of flight mass spectrometer then analyzes the metal signals. This technique overcomes the constraints of spectral overlap in flow cytometry as it makes use of distinct isotopes as reporter system in place of traditional fluorophores which have broad emission spectra. Mass cytometry has research applications in the field of medical science that includes immunology, hematology, and oncology. It is also utilized for examining hematopoiesis, cell cycle, cytokine expression, and differential signaling responses. This book is a valuable compilation of topics, ranging from the basic to the most complex advancements in the field of mass cytometry. Those in search of information to further their knowledge will be greatly assisted by it.

This book is a comprehensive compilation of works of different researchers from varied parts of the world. It includes valuable experiences of the researchers with the sole objective of providing the readers (learners) with a proper knowledge of the concerned field. This book will be beneficial in evoking inspiration and enhancing the knowledge of the interested readers.

In the end, I would like to extend my heartiest thanks to the authors who worked with great determination on their chapters. I also appreciate the publisher's support in the course of the book. I would also like to deeply acknowledge my family who stood by me as a source of inspiration during the project.

Editor

1

Minimizing Batch Effects in Mass Cytometry Data

Ronald P. Schuyler[1‡], *Conner Jackson*[1‡], *Josselyn E. Garcia-Perez*[1], *Ryan M. Baxter*[1], *Sidney Ogolla*[1†], *Rosemary Rochford*[1], *Debashis Ghosh*[2], *Pratyaydipta Rudra*[3§] and *Elena W. Y. Hsieh*[1,4*§]

[1] Department of Immunology and Microbiology, University of Colorado School of Medicine, Aurora, CO, United States, [2] Department of Biostatistics and Informatics, Colorado School of Public Health, Aurora, CO, United States, [3] Department of Statistics, Oklahoma State University, Stillwater, OK, United States, [4] Division of Allergy and Immunology, Department of Pediatrics, University of Colorado School of Medicine, Children's Hospital Colorado, Aurora, CO, United States

***Correspondence:**
Elena W. Y. Hsieh
elena.hsieh@cuanschutz.edu

† Present address:
Sidney Ogolla,
Centre for Global Health Research, Kenya Medical Research Institute (KEMRI), Kisumu, Kenya

‡ These authors have contributed equally to this work

§ These authors have contributed equally to this work and share senior authorship

Cytometry by Time-Of-Flight (CyTOF) uses antibodies conjugated to isotopically pure metals to identify and quantify a large number of cellular features with single-cell resolution. A barcoding approach allows for 20 unique samples to be pooled and processed together in one tube, reducing the intra-barcode technical variability. However, with only 20 samples per barcode, multiple barcode sets (batches) are required to address questions in robustly powered study designs. A batch adjustment procedure is required to reduce variability across batches and to facilitate direct comparison of runs performed across multiple barcodes run over weeks, months, or years. We describe a method using technical replicates that are included in each run to determine and apply an appropriate adjustment per batch without manual intervention. The use of technical replicate samples (i.e., anchors or reference samples) avoids assumptions of sample homogeneity among batches, and allows direct estimation of batch effects and appropriate adjustment parameters applicable to all samples within a batch. Quantification of cell subpopulations and mean signal intensity pre- and post-adjustment using both manual gating and unsupervised clustering demonstrate substantial mitigation of batch effects in the anchor samples used for this adjustment calculation, and in a second validation set of technical replicates.

Keywords: normalization, barcode, anchor, mass cytometry, clinical studies, human immunology

INTRODUCTION

Mass cytometry, or Cytometry by Time-Of-Flight (CyTOF), is a high-throughput single-cell analysis technology that allows simultaneous measurement of 40+ cellular parameters via detection of rare earth heavy metal isotopes conjugated to monoclonal antibodies. The high-dimensionality of mass cytometry casts a wide exploratory net to allow: (1) discovery of novel cell phenotypes, (2) quantification of differences in cell-type composition (population frequency), and (3) analysis of marker expression levels (mean signal intensity) that may reflect different activation and/or functional cellular attributes. This systems immunology approach, when applied with relevant computational strategies, has the potential to unravel the cellular diversity and heterogeneity that underlies human immune-mediated disorders, providing descriptive and mechanistic insight with translational impact. For example, mass cytometry has been used to study human B cell development in the context of healthy and abnormal progression in acute lymphoblastic leukemia, leading to improved predictive risk stratification methods (1, 2). Mass cytometry applications to understand dysregulated signaling networks and downstream cytokine production in pediatric SLE have demonstrated unique signatures that may help with diagnosis and monitoring response to therapy (3, 4). Additionally, mass cytometry has been applied to study T cell proliferation and differentiation (5), macrophage phagocytosis (6), parallel DNA, RNA, and protein biosynthesis (7), and cell cycle status in malignancy and immunotherapy (8–10), to name a few applications.

The ability of mass cytometry to address a wide variety of biological questions related to immune cellular phenotype and function illustrates a desire for the technology to be utilized in increasingly complex study designs, with increasing number of study subjects, *in vivo* therapeutic interventions, *in vitro* conditions, and different disease status/timepoints. Differences in immune cell subset abundance or functionality can be explored among multiple patient groups of different diagnosis, between patient groups receiving different therapeutic interventions, or the same interventions across therapy phases. Addressing such questions often requires multiple patients per group, and often multiple samples (accounting for *in vitro* stimulation conditions and/or incubation timepoints) per patient. Additionally, given that mass cytometry measures hundreds of cells per second, and the ideal goal data collection numbers range in the hundreds of thousands of cells per sample (or more if analyzing rare cell types), instrument run times would expand over days or weeks for well-powered studies. Inherent to human immunology studies, prospective sample collection often occurs over the course of months to years. Therefore, the combination of the need of multiple samples to be analyzed per project, the relative speed of data acquisition on the instrument, and the prospective nature of the sample collection in human studies, requires the ability to process and run samples in multiple batches. A barcoding approach allows for multiple samples to be stained together in one tube, reducing the intra-barcode technical variability, and optimizing data acquisition speed and efficiency (decreased cell loss) as it constitutes a single sample run on the instrument (11). However, at 20 samples per barcode set, multiple barcode sets (batches) are still required to address questions in robustly powered study designs. While a barcoding approach does reduce technical variability among the 20 samples within the barcode set, having multiple barcode sets adds inter-barcode variability. Variability in reagent lots, instrument maintenance and calibration (detector changes, instrument repairs), antibody concentration to cell number ratio per barcode set, and other technical issues related to sample preparation can introduce artifacts and complicate analysis of samples processed and run in different barcode sets. The antibody reagent variability issue can be potentially overcome by using lyophilized antibody cocktails (12, 13), or preparing master mixes of antibody panels that are aliquoted, frozen, and later distributed across barcode sets over time (14). Bead normalization addresses signal variation issues related to instrument changes (15), however it does not address the other factors related to batch-to-batch variability mentioned above.

To facilitate analysis of large-scale mass cytometry experiments and allow for data analysis across prospective longitudinal studies, a batch adjustment process is required to reduce variability among batches/barcode sets. Batch adjustment will allow for direct comparison of data acquired on barcode sets across time. Batch effects are ubiquitous in high-throughput experiments (e.g., RNA sequencing, proteomics, metabolomics), and methods to adjust for these effects have been developed for domain-specific application, as well as general purpose frameworks (16). Surrogate variable analysis (SVA) identifies latent factors in a data set using the singular value decomposition of a matrix. Latent factors represent coordinated modules within the data and may correspond to biological effects, batch effects, or other sources of systematic variability (16). ComBat uses a Bayesian framework to model data, including covariates for batch, and possibly latent variables identified by SVA (17, 18). These effects are then removed using regression. Remove unwanted variation (RUV) uses spike-in control samples or genes which are expected to remain relatively constant between batches to estimate technical effects (19). Combat, Surrogate Variable Analysis (SVA) and related methodologies for batch effect adjustment cannot be directly applied to mass cytometry data for the following reasons. First, they require a data matrix in which the rows correspond to genes or molecules, while the columns are samples. A single mass cytometry sample is inherently more complex, as it consists of many single cell events, each of which is represented as a vector of measurements (ion counts from each mass channel). The inherent structure of multiple batches, with multiple samples, each with many single-cell events is not naturally represented in the two-dimensional matrix format that SVA and Combat assume. It is possible to consider each single-cell event as a sample and simply concatenate all events from all samples into a single matrix, but with hundreds of thousands of cells per sample, many samples per batch, and many batches, this approach does not scale well with increasing experiment size. Second, it is important to understand the proper data distribution of mass cytometry experiments before applying batch adjustment methods. This is still an open question and needs further investigation. Higher-dimensional tensor decomposition methods have been developed (20) and could be adapted for latent variable analyses explicitly encoding batch, sample, and cell events as separate dimensions, but this has not yet been implemented for mass cytometry data.

Currently, no readily available method exists specifically for batch adjustment of mass cytometry data. As the number of cell events measured for each sample may be in the hundreds of thousands to over a million, with 20 samples per batch, and likely many batches per study, a computationally efficient method that will execute in a reasonable amount of time without specialized computing hardware is needed. Another feature incorporated into the design of this batch normalization method is a simple conceptual interpretability, in which, similarly to bead normalization, the resulting files are adjusted to address variability and the output is a ready to analyze Flow Cytometry Standard (FCS) file (21). Additionally, an optional diagnostic output allows for user-driven evaluation of the batch normalization of their dataset. Finally, a "rolling basis" capability to adjust individual batches as they become available is desirable, as it allows for inclusion of additional batches without reprocessing or changing the results for batches already completed.

To facilitate comparison across batches, it is useful to include a technical replicate in each barcode set as a biologically constant reference, or anchor sample. This anchor sample represents a single donor/cell line/tissue sample (depending on the goal of the study) that is processed in the same way as the other study samples, and distributed in aliquots to be incorporated into each barcode set. Additionally, if the study design involves *in vitro* stimulations to induce specific functional read outs, anchor samples may need to be prepared as an unstimulated and stimulated pair (or more than a pair if the study design calls for it). A "master set" of unstimulated and stimulated anchor samples can be prepared prior to the start of the project, and distributed in single aliquots to later be included in each barcode set. While this approach reduces the number of study samples per barcode set, using the same anchor sample across all batches minimizes biological differences, isolating batch effects. Rather than estimating the effects per batch based on modeling all samples, which requires assumptions such as homogeneous sample composition across batches (18, 22), batch effects for each channel (measured variable) can be directly estimated from the anchor samples, where the expectation of homogeneity in cell composition and marker expression levels is much more reasonable. Scaling or mapping parameters per channel for an anchor sample may then be applied to other samples from the same batch.

Data standardization based on location and scale adjustment are well-characterized and widely used (23). These include combinations of spread-based methods for adjusting variance (autoscaling, Pareto scaling) and magnitude-based methods such range scaling, level scaling (mean), and median or percentile matching. Here we describe a flexible method to adjust mass cytometry batches relative to a reference batch based on technical replicates, implemented in R, and available at https://github.com/CUHIMSR/CytofBatchAdjust. We implement several standard normalization options, and provide recommendations for their use. Available methods include per channel quantile normalization (QN), and location and scale methods that harmonize batches based on signal variance, mean, median, or a user-defined percentile. We note that in channels with high variability among technical replicates, particularly those with substantial variability in the fraction of zero-valued events, there may be no satisfactory adjustment to harmonize data across batches. In these cases, it may be advisable to conduct statistical testing for conditions of interest within batches, then combine results across batches using Fisher's method as recommended by others (24).

To evaluate methods and parameter settings for batch adjustment, we quantify cell subpopulations using both manual gating and unsupervised clustering, applied to multiple technical replicates run in different batches, before and after adjustment. We also quantify variability in signal intensity of cytokines measured after stimulation. As each anchor is a large random sample from the same initial population of cells, we expect the same proportions of cell types in each batch anchor. Therefore, lower variability in subpopulation frequency (percentages) and cytokine levels (signal intensity) among technical replicates after adjustment indicates successful reduction of batch effects. Decreased variability in a second set of replicate samples (i.e., stimulated samples from an anchor set) demonstrates that batch adjustment parameters based on an anchor sample are applicable to the batch that it represents.

BATCH NORMALIZATION METHOD

An example dataset of 12 barcode sets is be used to illustrate the development of this batch adjustment methodology, its validation and application. Data was acquired on a Helios CyTOF instrument (Fluidigm, San Francisco, CA) over the course of 6 months. In this data set, 38 markers (22 cell surface markers and 16 intracellular cytokines) were used to study immune dysregulation in pediatric systemic lupus erythematosus (SLE). In addition to the study samples, a pair of anchor samples was included in each barcode set (Cell-ID™ 20-plex barcoding kit, Fluidigm, San Francisco, CA). The anchor samples were generated from one single healthy donor peripheral whole blood sample, processed to include an unstimulated and a stimulated conditions (LPS + R848) to induce the 16 cytokines measured, as previously described in O'Gorman et al. (3). These samples were used to demonstrate the applicability of this adjustment methodology and validate the decrease in total variance across anchor samples post-adjustment (see **Supplementary Material** for the specific FCS files that were used, http://flowrepository.org/id/FR-FCM-Z2YR). This dataset was acquired on a Helios CyTOF instrument at Stanford University over the course of 4 months. Peripheral blood mononuclear cells (PBMCs) from a healthy control were spiked into separate barcoded samples and stained with a panel of 38 surface markers, as part of a longitudinal vaccination study. There were no stimulation conditions used in this dataset. The healthy control files (anchors/references) were not used further in the analysis of the study samples.

In Kleinsteuber et al. (25) the use of reference samples is also applied, albeit taking a different approach—CD45-barcoded anchor sample aliquots were spiked into each individual study sample, which were run sequentially (separately) across the study. This reference sample was then used to guide manual adjustment of gates. In contrast, in the approach described here, the reference sample (stimulated anchor) from each batch was then used as a representative of that batch to determine adjustment factors or mapping functions (per channel and per barcode) that bring the anchor samples into alignment. This adjustment was automated and computed for each barcode set and each channel, and independently applied to all samples from the same barcode set on a per channel basis, including the unstimulated anchor samples which served as a validation set.

Prior to batch adjustment, data was bead-normalized (15), debarcoded (11), and manually gated to remove debris and non-biological events (**Figure 1**). Alternatively, data pre-processing could be automated using FlowClean or other methods (26). For batch adjustment, a single stimulated anchor sample from a specific barcode set was designated as reference. The reference anchor may be chosen by any criterion. We recommend visual inspection of data distributions to avoid choosing an outlier batch as reference. All batches were adjusted relative to this reference, and samples from the reference batch were not modified. Importantly, signal intensity range in anchor samples used for adjustment should approximately cover the full signal range for all samples, and therefore should include experimental manipulations. We also evaluated an unstimulated anchor replicate set for validation to demonstrate that adjustments computed using the stimulated anchors are also applicable to the unstimulated samples.

Using the stimulated anchor samples from each of the 12 barcode sets, for each batch and each channel independently, an adjustment factor was computed as a function of the ratio of a descriptive summary statistic for that channel and anchor to the same value for the reference anchor sample. We implemented and tested several batch adjustment options, including scaling by mean and median [similar to bead normalization (15)], standard deviation of per event ion counts, and quantile normalization (QN), which was developed for oligonucleotide arrays and is used to normalize RNA-seq data (27, 28). Additionally, a user-defined percentile may be specified rather than median. This approach is useful in the case that any channel has more than 50% zero-valued events (from total events per file after data pre-processing steps as described in **Figure 1**), giving a median of zero and an undefined or zero-valued scaling factor. The same adjustment approach (i.e., mean, median, standard deviation, QN, percentile scaling) is applied across the entire dataset, and the same approach is applied to all channels, though each adjustment factor is tailored to each barcode set and channel. Adjustment factors may be computed and applied in an

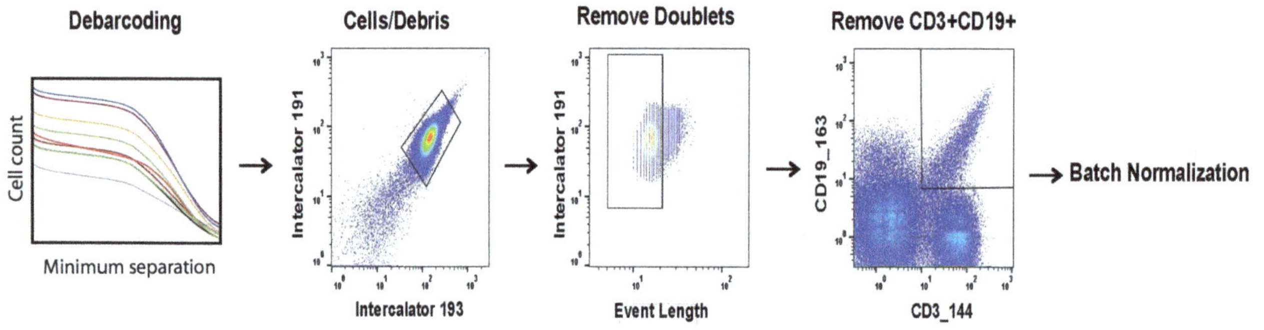

FIGURE 1 | Pre-processing of files prior to batch normalization. FCS files are bead normalized and debarcoded. A set of three consecutive gates is applied as shown prior to batch normalization.

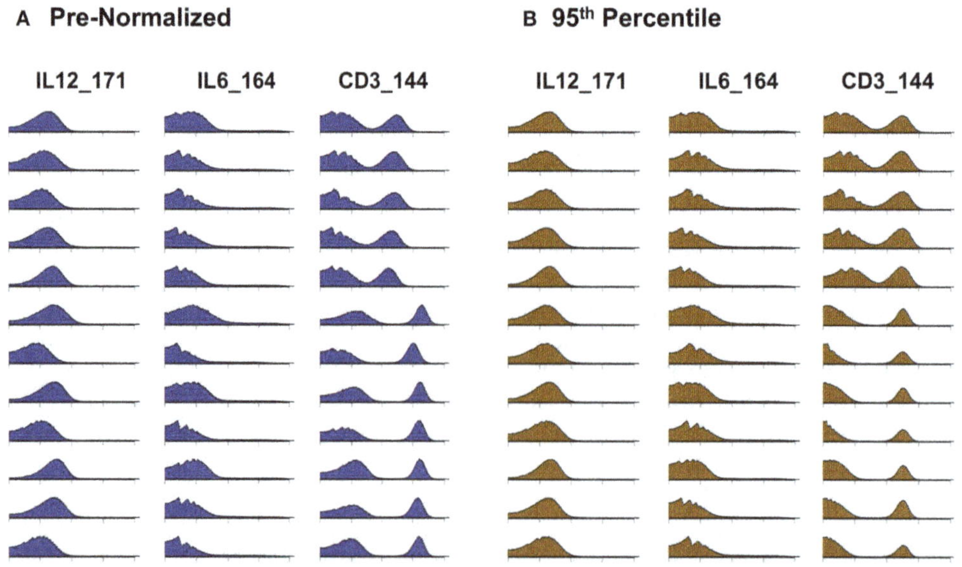

FIGURE 2 | Signal intensity distribution pre- and post-batch normalization. Density plots for all barcode anchor replicates for three representative data channels (IL12, IL6, CD3). **(A)** Before batch normalization. **(B)** After batch normalization to 95th percentile, relative to anchor 1.

arcsinh-transformed space commonly used for data visualization, or in the untransformed ion count data space. Scaling in the transformed data space effectively results in a non-linear adjustment once the inverse transformation is applied before results are written to the resulting FCS file, whereas adjustments computed in the original data space are linear.

We began by evaluating distances between distributions for all individual data channels among replicates for a set of candidate parameter combinations using the Kolmogorov–Smirnov distance metric. Using parameters that performed well in single channel consistency measurements, we then moved to evaluations considering all channels together, and finally to consistency of subpopulation frequencies simultaneously for 12 cell types in all replicates. Levine et al. scaled individual data channels to the 99.5th percentile before defining subpopulations, and Lun et al. suggested a range-based batch adjustment to linearly scale intensities between the 1st and 99th percentiles (29, 30). We used the 95th percentile as the high end for our normalization target point to avoid outliers, and 80th percentile as the low end, as up to 79% of cell events were zero-valued for some channels in this data set. Using default parameters, the adjustment factor for each channel was computed as the ratio of the 95th percentile event ion counts for each batch anchor compared to the designated reference anchor. Adjustments were made in the untransformed raw ion count data space. We found that these parameters resulted in the most stable post-adjustment population counts using the validation method described below.

Execution time scaled linearly with the number of samples. Using a Mac Mini (Apple, Cupertino, CA) with a 2.8 GHz processor requires ~8 s per sample, including time to read the input file, apply the adjustment, and write the result to disk. A log file was generated listing each batch found, each sample

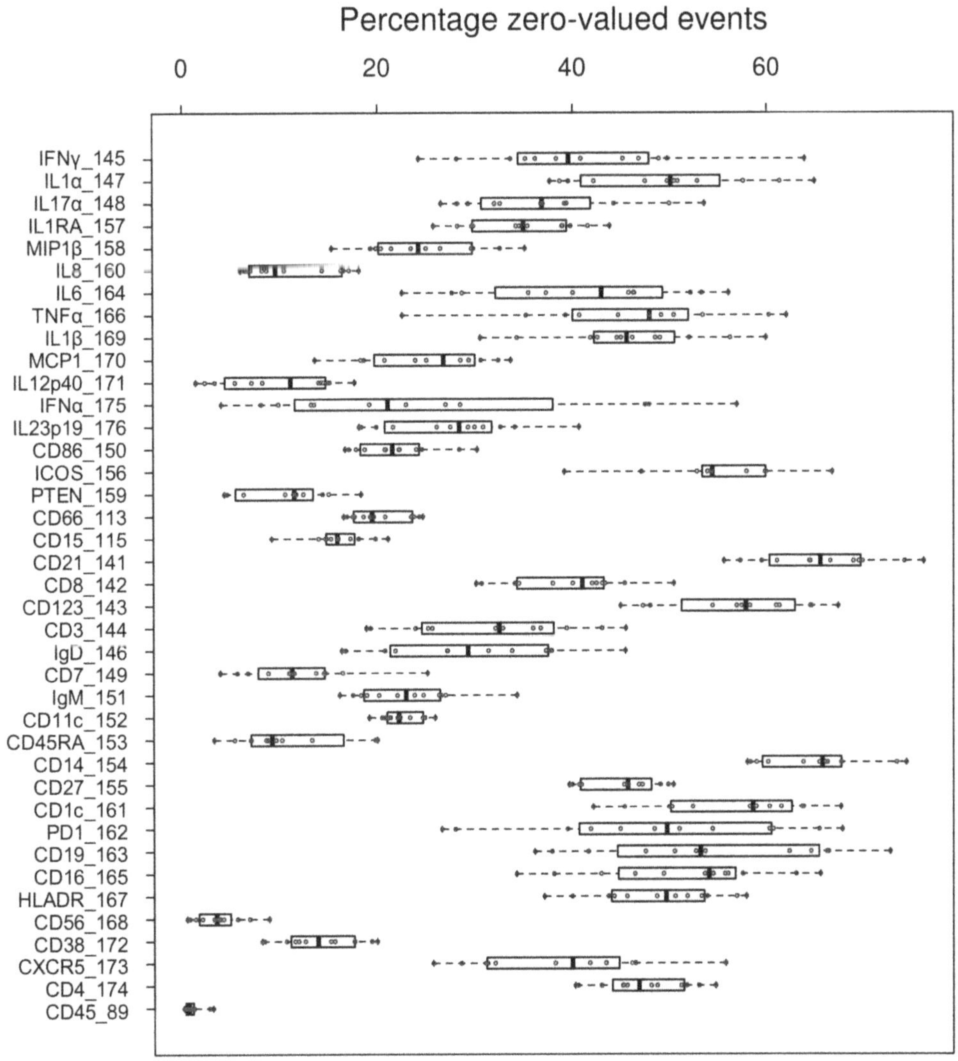

FIGURE 3 | Variability of zero-valued events among replicate anchor samples pre-normalization. The fraction of zero-valued events (X-axis) for each anchor (red dot) is shown for each channel (Y-axis).

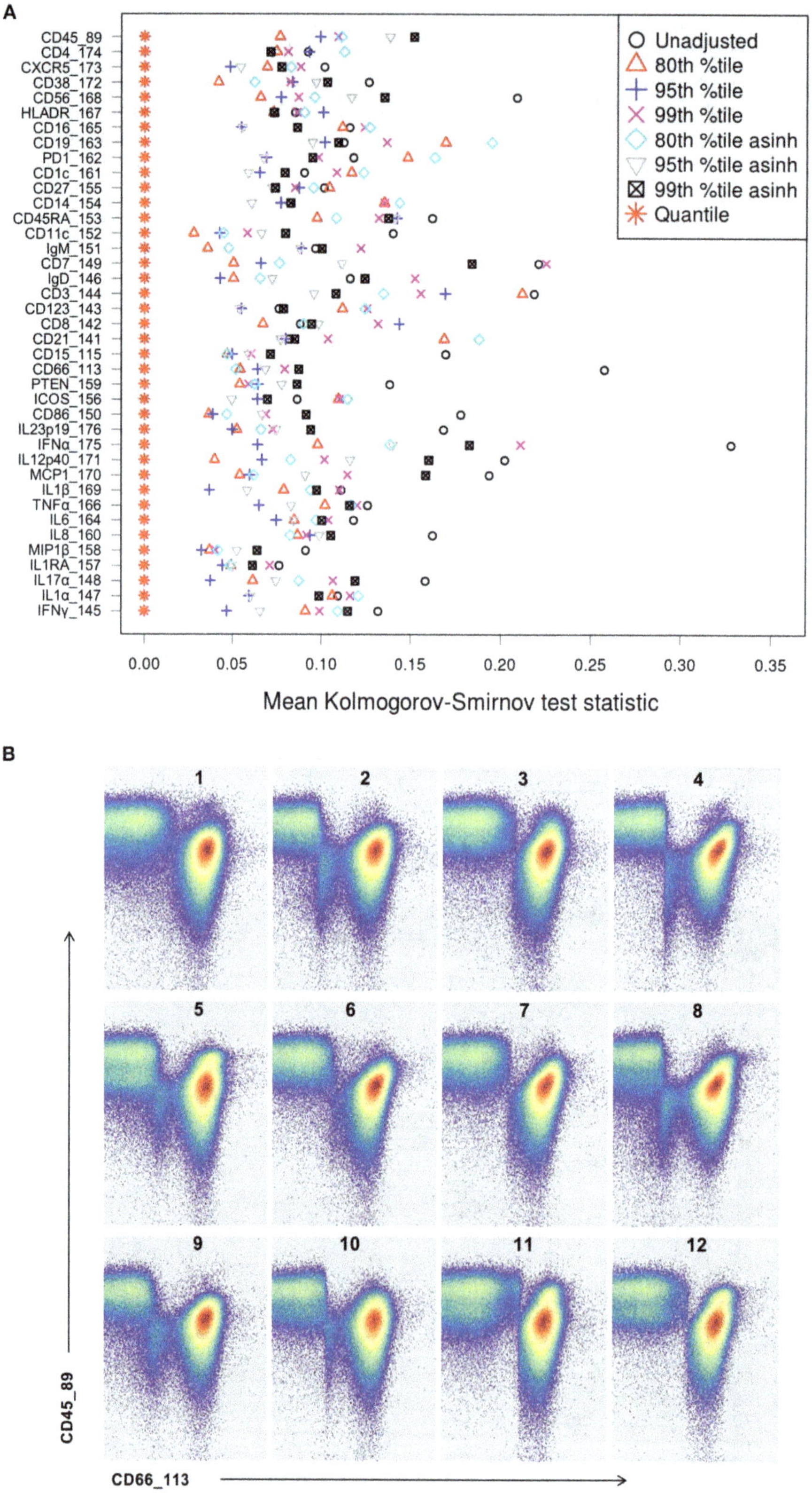

FIGURE 4 | Kolmogorov-Smirnov (KS) distance for each single channel, for each batch normalization approach examined. **(A)** Distance between distributions among replicates is computed as the average of the KS test statistic for all pairwise combinations of anchor samples, computed independently (X-axis) for each data channel (Y-axis). Smaller values indicate better consistency among replicates. **(B)** Quantile normalization artifacts in biaxial plots for each anchor replicate (numbered). Top left is the unmodified reference anchor.

processed, and additional diagnostic information, including processing time. Adjustment factors for each channel in every batch (or mapping functions in the case of QN) were saved in a .Rdata file (31). An optional diagnostic output can be generated, which includes (1) the scaling factors for every channel for each barcoded anchor that is adjusted, and (2) the signal intensity distribution for each adjusted channel for each barcoded anchor pre- and post-adjustment (from total events per file). We recommend inspecting adjustment factors, as very large values may be undesirable, and could result from outlier batches, channel labeling errors, or other issues with input data.

BATCH NORMALIZATION VALIDATION

All anchor samples, including the stimulated and unstimulated sets, were derived from aliquots of a single large sample and processed together to minimize variability. Whereas the true numbers of cells of any phenotype in the anchor samples is unknown, given the large number of cell events measured for each anchor aliquot (300–500 k events per anchor per batch), subpopulation frequencies are expected to be consistent among anchors. Therefore, variation in population frequencies among anchor samples is expected to be attributable to technical effects, and should decrease after batch adjustment. With similar reasoning, we expect the functional responses in the stimulated anchor relative the unstimulated condition to be consistent across anchor replicates.

Single Channel Consistency Measures

As an initial evaluation comparing methods and parameters, we used the Kolmogorov–Smirnov statistic to measure the distance between distributions among replicates within single channels. Within each channel, pairwise empirical distribution distances were computed between each pair of replicates and averaged, giving a single measure of consistency for each data channel across all batches of the experiment. This test was automated and less labor intensive than the manual gating evaluation

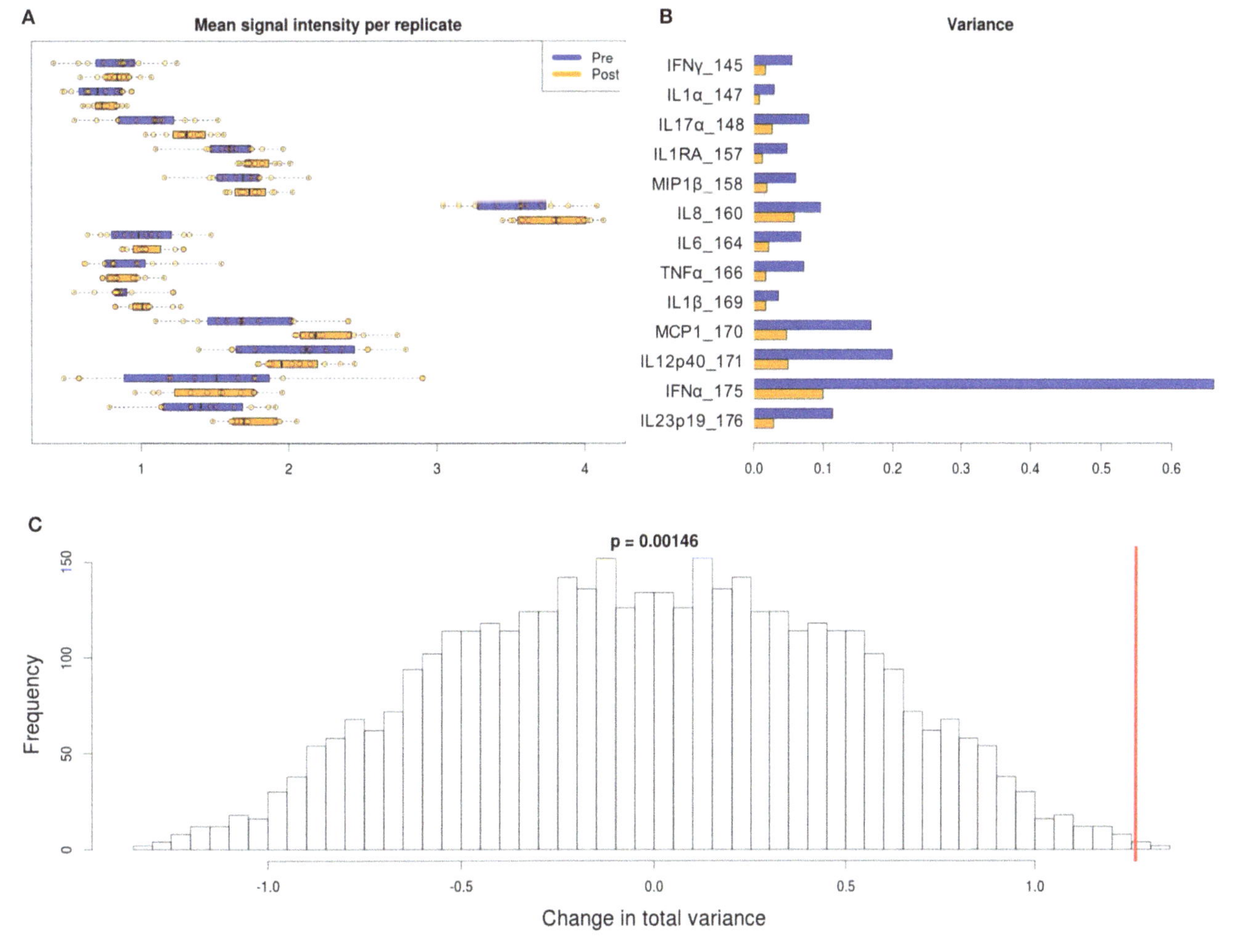

FIGURE 5 | Variability in signal intensity per channel for the 95th percentile batch normalization approach. **(A)** Mean signal intensity of each cytokine for all cell events for each anchor replicate (circles). **(B)** Variance of these mean signal intensities across replicates. **(C)** Permutation null distribution and significance of observed change in total variance (red line). *p*-value is the fraction of permutations with a change in total variance as or more extreme than that observed for unpermuted data.

described below, allowing an expedient exploration of a range of approaches and parameter settings.

For a comprehensive measure of signal variability, total variance was computed as the sum of the eigenvalues of the covariance matrix (32) of the mean signal intensity for all cell events in each channel and each replicate. The value of the total variance is equal to the sum of the diagonals of the covariance matrix, i.e., the sum of the individual variance components. The significance of the decrease in total variance due to batch adjustment was evaluated using a permutation test (33), where the labels pre- and post-adjustment were swapped for each replicate. Change in total variance was computed for all possible permutations to derive a null distribution for comparison with the observed reduction in total variance in signal intensity (**Figure S1**).

As the goal of a batch adjustment procedure is to prepare the data for further downstream analysis, a more important measure than single-channel distribution distances and mean signal intensity variability is consistency in cell subpopulation frequencies among replicates. These two evaluation approaches will not always agree because gating is hierarchical and considers multiple channels simultaneously. We show that this is the case for some parameter settings, which performed well within channels, but did not translate to better performance in cell-type classification consistency.

Cell Subpopulation Frequency Quantification Consistency Measures

Two methods to assess the consistency of cell subpopulation frequencies across anchor samples were used: a consistent manual gating strategy applied to all anchors (no tailored gates), and unsupervised population quantification via event clustering considering all anchors simultaneously. As functional read outs, cytokine production was assessed, either as percent positivity or mean signal intensity, comparing unstimulated and stimulated anchors within the relevant gated parent populations. Although the normalization procedure applied to the data did not specifically adjust pre-defined cell populations, the adjustment and subsequent reduction of variability in signal intensity

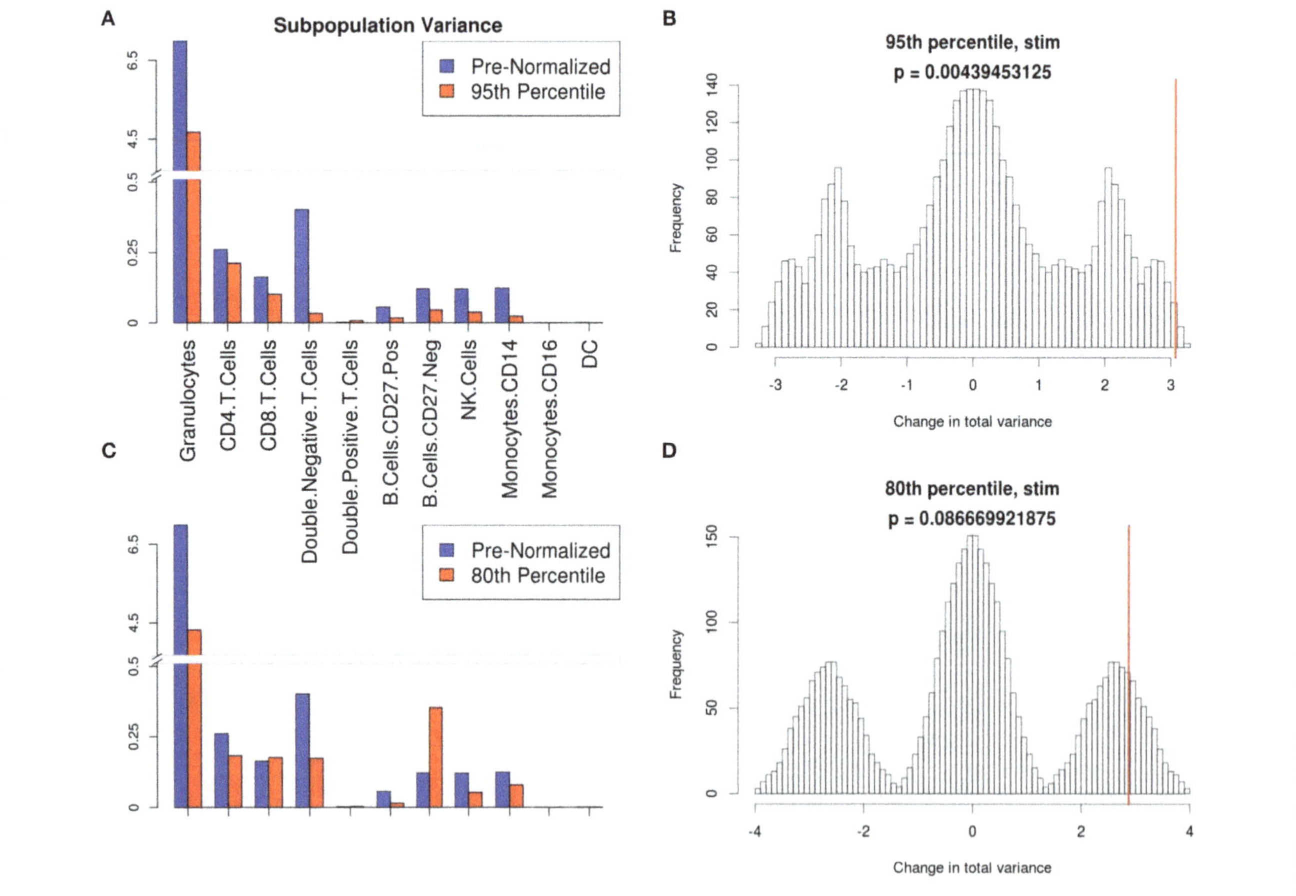

FIGURE 6 | Manual gating cell subpopulation variance post-normalization. Variance across all stimulated anchor replicates in the fraction of events assigned to each population pre- and post-normalization. Manual gates were drawn based on the reference anchor (barcode 1) and applied to all other anchor replicates. **(A,C)** Variance per subpopulation pre- (blue) and post-normalization (red) for 95th **(A)** and 80th **(C)** percentile normalization. **(B,D)** Null distribution for change in total variance for the 95th **(B)** and 80th **(D)** percentile normalization. Red bar indicates observed change in total variance. *p*-value is the fraction of permutations with a change in total variance as or more extreme than that observed for unpermuted data.

improved downstream manual gating procedures by reducing the need to manually tailor gates.

Manual Gating

The stimulated anchor sample designated as reference was manually gated using FlowJo (version 10) for the cell populations defined by the markers shown in **Table S1**. This set of gates was applied without manual adjustment to all pre- and post-normalized anchor samples separately, and each cell population frequency was quantified as the fraction of all cell events within a sample. As a further validation, unstimulated anchors were also examined. By quantifying populations in unstimulated replicates that were adjusted using the stimulated anchor samples we showed that this method is applicable to a range of samples and experimental conditions. Additionally, signal intensity for functional markers within specific manually gated populations was also compared pre- and post-batch normalization.

To quantify the magnitude of cell population frequency variability for an entire experiment we used the total variance defined as the sum of the eigenvalues of the covariance matrix of all gated subpopulation fractions in all replicates. Similar to the test of signal intensity variability described above, the difference in total subpopulation variance pre- and post-adjustment provides a measure of the effectiveness of the adjustment, and a means to compare methods and parameter settings. To assign a significance level to the change in total population fraction variance, we again used a permutation test, where labels of replicate samples were swapped between pre- and post-adjustment conditions for each replicate. The change in total variance was then recomputed for all possible permutations, giving an exact test of the probability of seeing a reduction in variance of population frequencies as or more extreme than that observed for the unpermuted data (**Figure S1**).

Unsupervised Population Quantification

Citrus version 0.8 (34) was chosen as the unsupervised clustering approach to explore differences between pre- and post-normalized files. Samples were grouped as pre- or post-normalized, with 50,000 events sampled from each file and a minimum cluster size of 2.5%. The significance analysis of microarrays (SAM) statistical model was used to examine statistical differences with a false discovery rate (FDR) below 1%. In addition to quantitative evaluation, visual inspection of data distributions per channel across anchor samples provides a qualitative assessment of pre- and post-adjustment consistency and the effectiveness of batch adjustment (**Figure 2**).

BATCH NORMALIZATION RESULTS

Signal Intensity Variability and Zero-Valued Events

Whereas some channels are quite consistent across batches, others show substantial variability (**Figure 2A**). In addition to shifts in signal density and changes in distribution shape (number of visible peaks), we observed large differences between replicates in the number of events within a mass channel with ion counts of zero (**Figure 3**, **Figure S2**). The differences in the numbers of zero-valued events are particularly troublesome for quantile normalization, which either inflates the zeros to non-zero values introducing noise, or squashes the lowest non-zero events to zero, resulting in loss of information. Further, given large initial differences among distributions, we found that adjusting each channel independently using

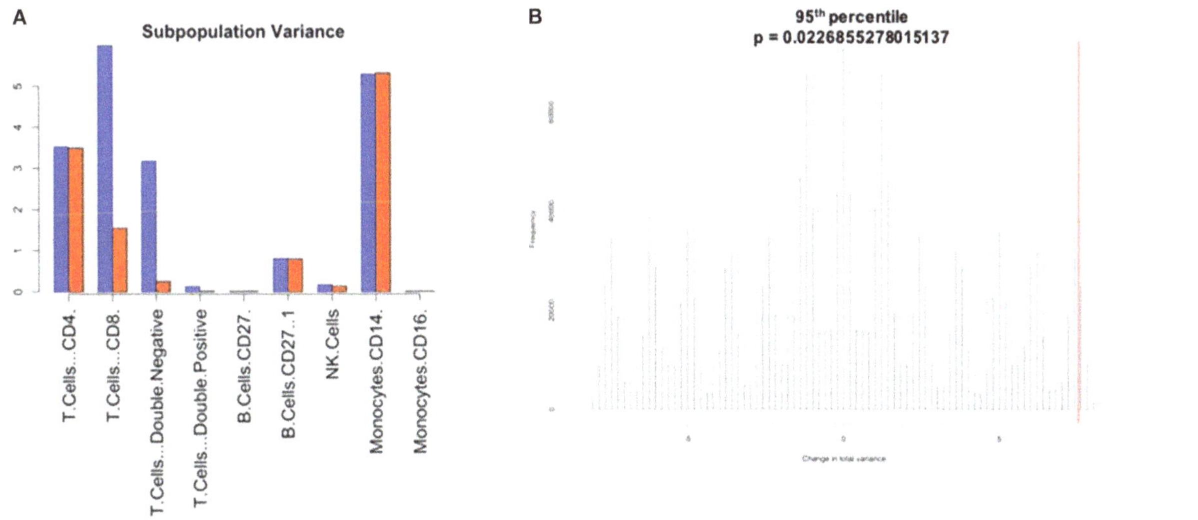

FIGURE 7 | Manual gating cell subpopulation variance post-normalization. Variance across all stimulated anchor replicates in the fraction of events assigned to each population pre- and post-normalization. Manual gates were drawn based on the reference anchor (barcode 1) and applied to all other anchor replicates. **(A)** Variance per subpopulation pre- (blue) and post-normalization (red) for 95th percentile normalization. **(B)** Null distribution for change in total variance for the 95th percentile normalization. Red bar indicates observed change in total variance. *p*-value is the fraction of permutations with a change in total variance as or more extreme than that observed for unpermuted data.

quantile normalization introduced visual artifacts when viewed as biaxial plots in the process of manual gating. Although quantile normalization can enforce identical distributions among replicates and therefore produces the most consistent results on the single-channel Kolmogorov–Smirnov test (**Figure 4A**), we excluded this option from further analysis of cell population fraction variability due to the artifacts it introduces (**Figure 4B**).

Several combinations of parameters resulted in decreased distances among empirical distributions within single channels (**Figure 4A**). Based on these results and visual inspection of distributions and gated populations, percentile-based adjustments made in the raw (untransformed) ion count data space appeared most effective, and 80th and 95th percentile scaling were chosen for further evaluation. Both options substantially reduced per-channel signal variability (**Figure 5**, **Figure S3**) and manually gated subpopulation variance (**Figure 6**, **Figure S4**), as described below.

Manual Gating Results

With a set of gates manually defined using the stimulated reference anchor and applied to all anchor samples, variance in subpopulation proportions among replicates was decreased after batch adjustment. Decrease in total variance of cell subpopulation frequencies for each of the parameter combinations above is shown in **Figure 6**. These results indicate that scaling based on the 95th percentile in the original ion count (untransformed) data space was the most effective parameter combination for batch adjustment for this dataset. This same 95th percentile scaling batch adjustment method was applied to the additional dataset from the publicly available flow repository, also demonstrating a decrease in total variance for both frequency of manually gated populations (**Figure 7**) and per-channel signal intensity variability (**Figure 8**).

Granulocytes and other lymphoid and myeloid populations of interest (T and B cell subsets, NK cells, monocytes, and dendritic cells) were examined to confirm that the batch

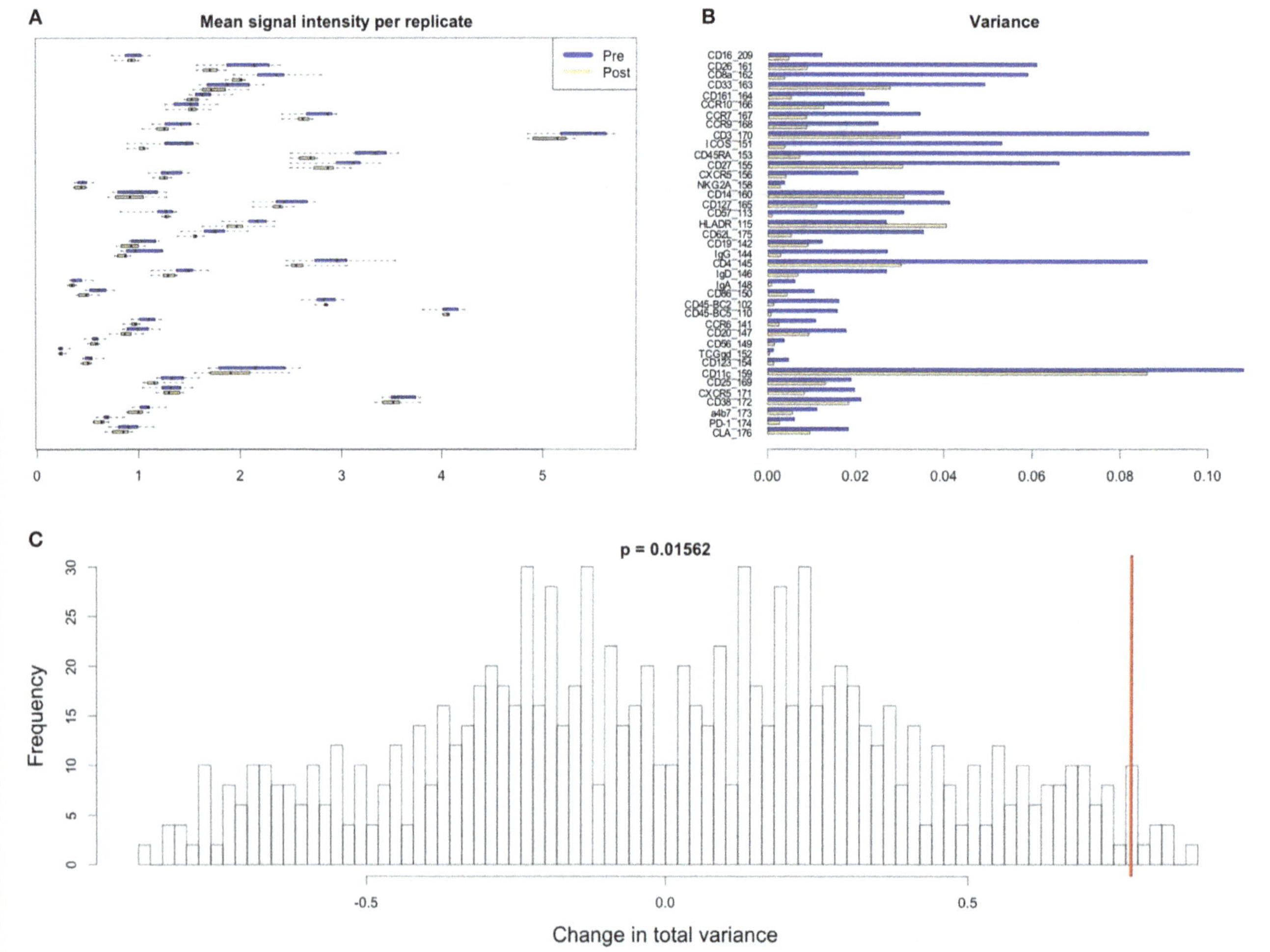

FIGURE 8 | Variability in signal intensity per channel for the 95th percentile batch normalization approach. **(A)** Mean signal intensity of each cytokine for all cell events for each anchor replicate (circles). **(B)** Variance of these mean signal intensities across replicates. **(C)** Permutation null distribution and significance of observed change in total variance (red line). *p*-value is the fraction of permutations with a change in total variance as or more extreme than that observed for unpermuted data.

normalization procedure did not alter standard manual gating and downstream analyses, and also to confirm that the procedure did not disproportionately affect certain populations relative to others. In addition to the populations examined above, gates to examine double negative (CD4–/CD8–) and double positive (CD4+/CD8+) T cells were drawn to help elucidate potential batch effects. The frequency of double negative T cells was greater in the pre-normalized group relative to the batch normalized group (p-value: 0.0005 t-test), indicating the presence of batch effects since the cells that should have been categorized as non-T cells (CD3–) were incorrectly included within the T cell gate (**Figure 9**). In addition to the decrease in variance for the batch-normalized populations, the reduced misclassification of CD3– cells further supported the conclusion that the normalization procedure reduced batch effects (**Figure 10**). Gating of the unstimulated anchors served as a secondary means of validation with similar results (**Figure S4**).

As mass cytometry is often used to address questions related to cellular functionality under stimulated conditions, intracellular cytokine markers were examined to assure the batch normalization process does not add unnecessary noise. Three functional markers (IL1RA, MIP1B, and MCP1) were examined within CD14^{hi} monocyte populations (CD45+, CD3–, CD19–, CD7–, HLADR+, CD11c+, CD14+, and CD16–) across unstimulated and stimulated anchor samples. Histograms and exported means from FlowJo indicated that the application of the batch normalization method did not eliminate the expected functional responses (i.e., cytokine production) from populations of interest, but yet adjusted the signal intensity for the mean expression values according to the adjustment factor calculated from the normalization process (**Figure 11**, **Table S2**).

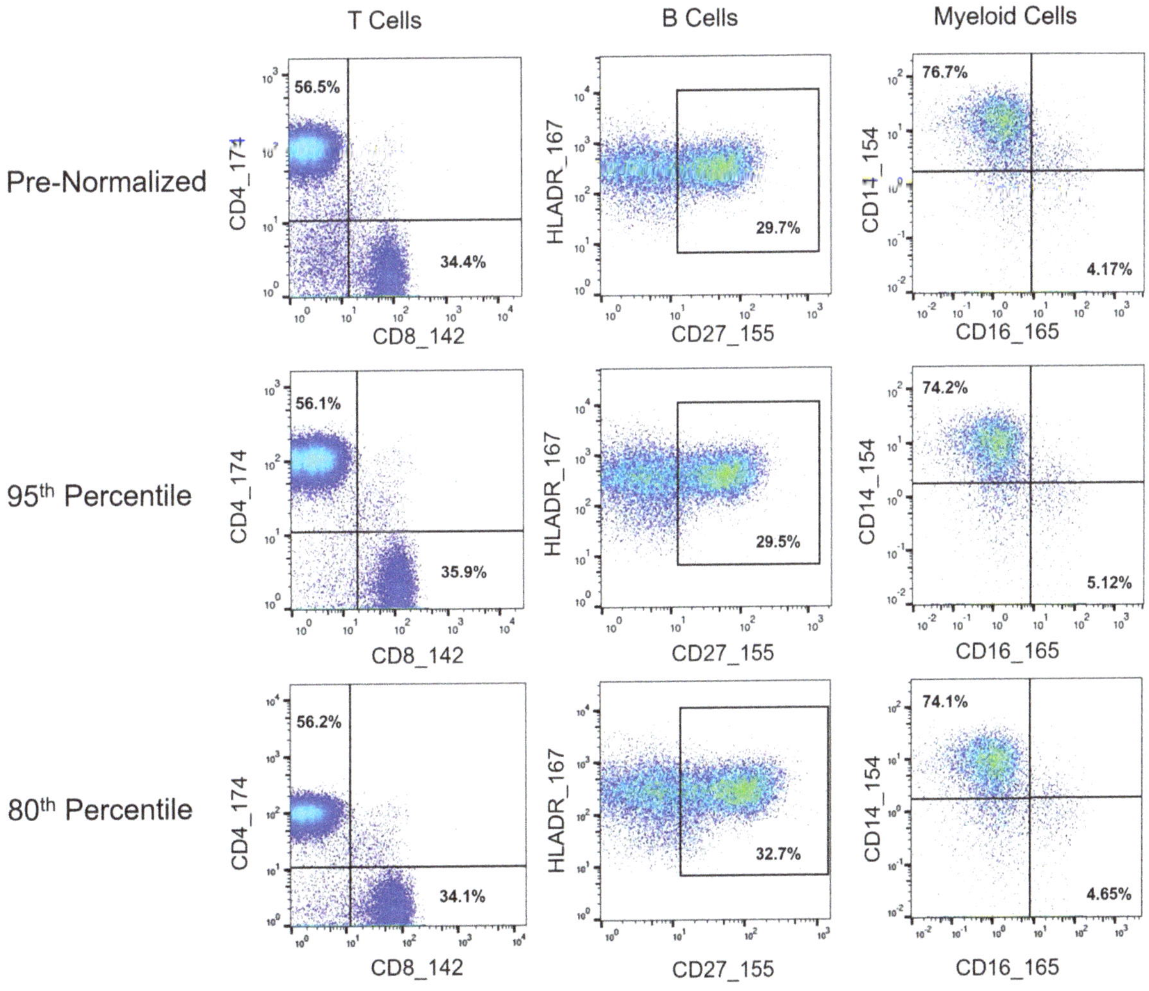

FIGURE 9 | Immune cell subset frequencies pre- and post-normalization, assessed via manual gating. Biaxial plots and population percentages (percent of parent gate) for three immune cell subsets across representative pre- and post-normalized anchor sample (80th and 95th percentile shown). Population percentages correspond to CD4 vs. CD8 T Cells (CD45+, CD3+, CD19–, and CD4+ or CD8+, respectively), CD27hi B Cells (CD45+, CD3–, CD19+, HLADR+, CD27hi), and CD14 vs. CD16 Monocytes (CD45+, CD3–, CD19–, HLADR+, CD11c+, and CD14+ or CD16+, respectively).

Clustering Results

Citrus Significance Analysis of Microarrays (SAM) analysis revealed one particular T cell subpopulation from the batch-normalized group that had significantly greater abundances relative to the pre-normalized samples (**Figure 12**). These clusters were determined to be CD4 Central Memory T Cells (CD3+, CD4+, CD27+, and CD45RA−). Of note, the variance in these clusters for the batch-normalized files was remarkably reduced relative to the pre-normalized files.

Batch Adjustment Diagnostic Output

Batch adjustment approaches and best strategies are likely to differ based on the nature/qualities of the dataset. For this reason, investigators are encouraged to explore different batch adjustment approaches available through the software package described. To facilitate this evaluation process, we have added a graphical diagnostic output for percentile-based batch adjustments depicting the relative sizes of the scaling factors used for each batch within each data channel. Investigators may quickly identify outliers from this figure and decide whether or not they wish to eliminate certain batches that are outliers (**Figure S5**). For further inspection, we have also added signal intensity distribution plots for every channel, for every anchor sample from every batch pre- and post-adjustment, with one figure generated each data channel (**Figure S6**). Using the scaling factors figures and the signal distribution figures, users may determine whether to exclude any batches from further analysis. An R data file is also saved containing scaling factors for each batch for more detailed examination.

DISCUSSION

Mass cytometry has the potential to reveal relevant differences in cell type composition and function across multiple immunological pathways, aiding in biomarker discovery and mechanistic hypothesis generation. Methods testing for differential cell subpopulation abundance or marker intensity assume that intensities are comparable across samples (30). Sample barcoding and pooling largely addresses this issue among samples within a batch, but make no adjustment for systematic differences between batches (11). Bead normalization (15) corrects for machine drift occurring over the course of a single experiment or across multiple experiments, but does not address other aforementioned technical issues contributing to batch effects—variability in reagent lots, instrument maintenance and calibration, and antibody concentration to cell number ratio per barcode amongst others.

Quantile normalization (QN) is an attractive approach to batch adjustment, as it forces all samples to fit the same target distribution regardless of the shapes (properties) of their starting distributions, and several variations have been developed for the analysis of RNA-seq data (35). Indeed, by both visual inspection and the Kolmogorov-Smirnov metric of inter-distribution distances, QN appears quite effective for single channels

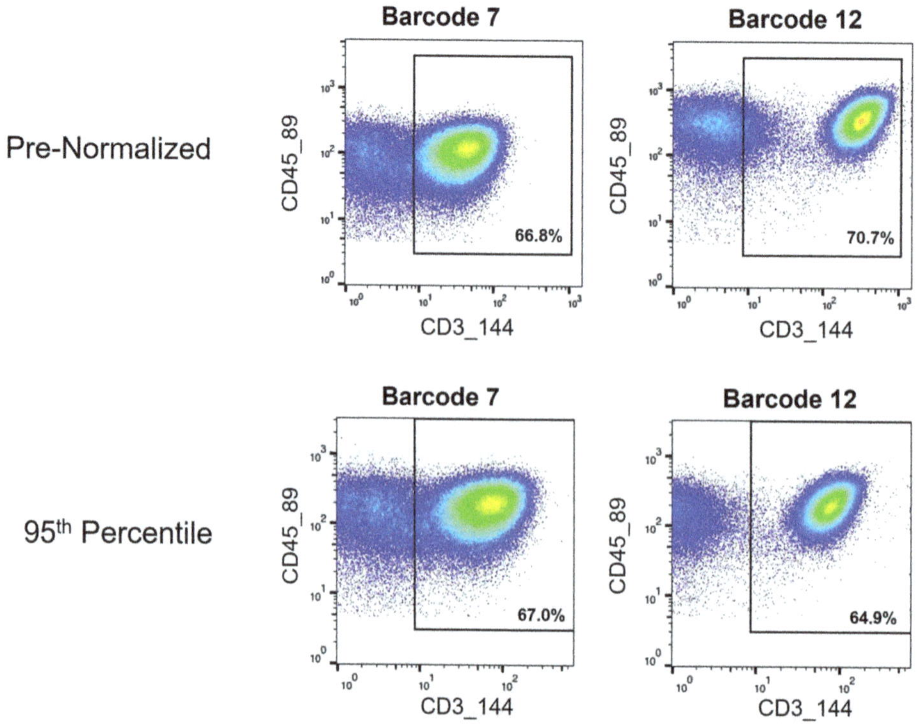

FIGURE 10 | Assignment of cell events to CD3+ T cell gate pre- and post-normalization. Biaxial plots showing cell events that fall within a CD3+ gate used for examining T cell subsets. Two pre- and post-normalized anchor samples are shown.

considered in isolation. However, here we have shown that the potentially large changes introduced by single-channel QN can introduce artifacts when viewed in two-dimensional plots. Other methods for handling batch effects rely on the assumption of sample homogeneity among batches (16). Careful experimental design requires allocating an equal number of a given condition to each batch to avoid confounding. With large enough batches (hundreds to thousands of samples, depending on the data characteristics) this assumption may be approximately valid, as outliers or variability within conditions being studied may average out with large numbers of samples. Current mass cytometry barcode sets typically consist of 20 samples. With three experimental conditions (e.g., drug, stimulation, untreated), the effective number of individuals composing a batch may drop to six, increasing the likelihood that a single outlier individual could skew a batch, violating the assumption of homogeneous composition between batches. There is substantial variability of immune system composition and function even within the healthy population, and outliers are expected in potentially heterogeneous disease conditions. This inherent variability and the small size of mass cytometry batches make assumptions of homogeneous batch composition questionable.

To address these issues, we describe the use of technical replicates included in each barcode set as reference points to anchor each batch. Adjustments are calibrated using anchor samples representing each barcode set, then applied to all samples composing a batch. This strategy avoids any batch composition assumptions, while comparing identical anchor samples eliminates biological variability and isolates the technical effects particular to each batch. For validation, we use a second set of (unstimulated) replicate samples in each batch, that are adjusted along with the other samples

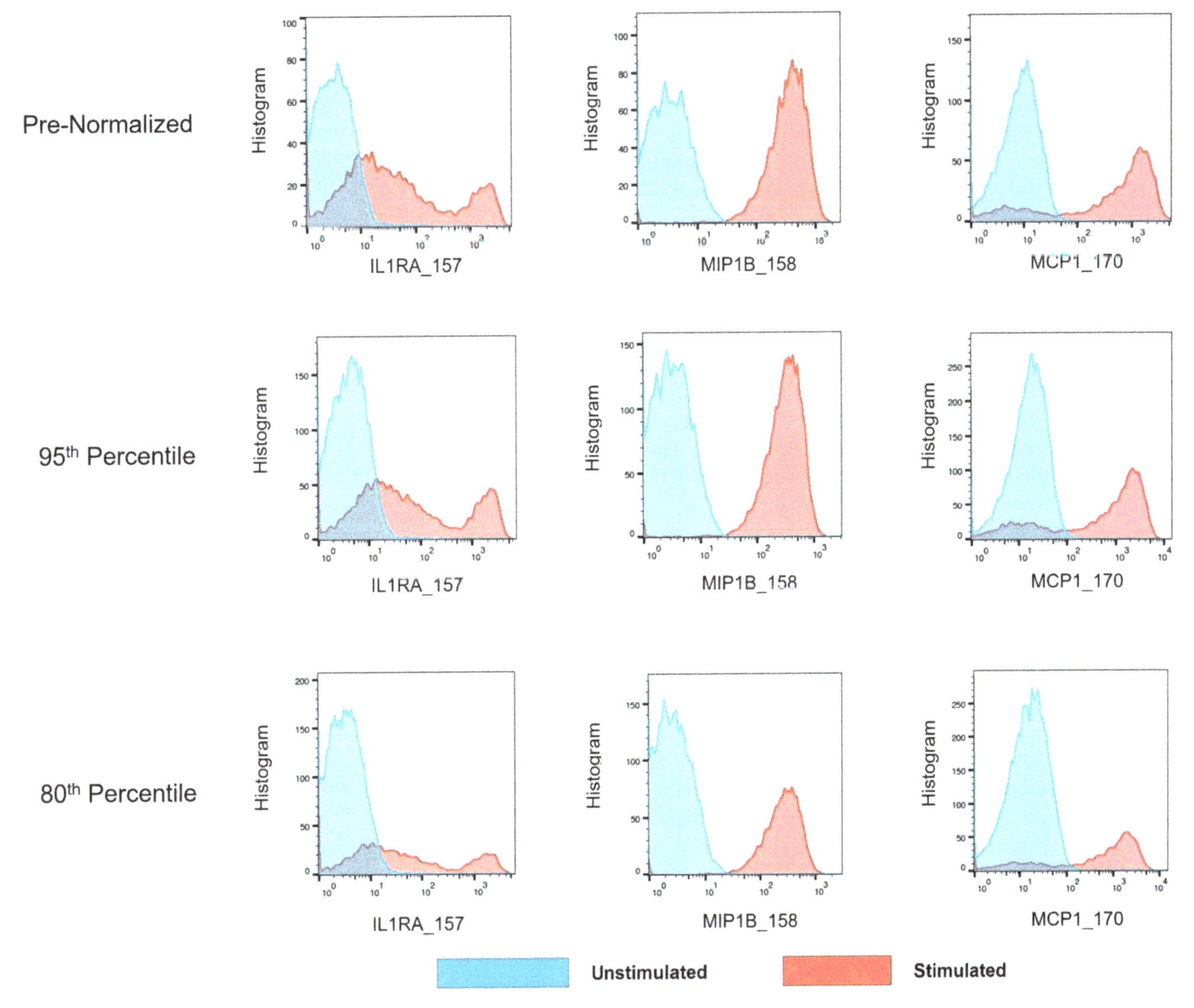

FIGURE 11 | Cytokine signal intensity distribution in unstimulated and stimulated anchor samples pre- and post-batch normalization. Histograms showing signal intensity for three cytokines for the CD14^{hi} monocytes, in paired unstimulated and stimulated anchor samples, pre- and post-normalization (95th and 80th percentile).

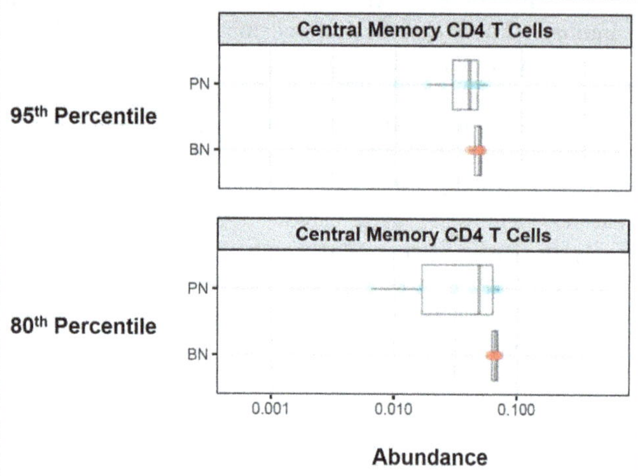

FIGURE 12 | Immune cell subset frequencies pre- and post-normalization, assessed via unsupervised citrus analysis. Citrus was applied using PAMR analysis with false discovery ratio of 0.05. Boxplots of relative abundance for central memory CD4 T cells generated from Citrus pre- (PN) and post-normalization (BN, 95th and 80th percentile).

using parameters determined with the representative anchors. Significant reductions in variability across batches in the stimulated anchor replicates, validation of this variability decrease in the unstimulated anchor samples, and the use of statistical measures to evaluate the reduction of this variability, demonstrate the feasibility and effectiveness of a normalization strategy via which an entire batch is adjusted using parameters derived from representative anchors in each barcode set.

Despite the multitude of existing mass cytometry data analysis tools, challenges in choosing the appropriate analytical strategy to answer the relevant biological question still remain—What is the appropriate algorithm to use for the study? Should one or multiple algorithms be applied to analyze the data? If more than one analytical method is used, how will results be integrated? What is the best way to go back to the raw data from the unsupervised analysis result? These questions remain a significant challenge that often discourages the application of mass cytometry analysis to human immunological studies, where single statistically meaningful outcomes are expected for clinical application. These analytical barriers are further compounded by the fact that human clinical studies often require prospective/longitudinal timeframes and multiple batches; and the lack of a batch adjustment/normalization method for mass cytometry data poses an added (if not crucial) hurdle to downstream analysis of human clinical studies. Here we describe the development, statistical validation, and application of an automated batch adjustment tool designed to minimize batch effects and allow for relevant downstream analysis. This novel tool is time efficient, incorporates flexibility for data types, investigator-driven batch adjustment approach choices, and the ability to evaluate such adjustment approaches (optional diagnostic output)—with great application potential for the analysis of large samples in human clinical studies.

MATERIALS AND METHODS

Study Approval

Human samples were obtained from the Allergy and Immunology Clinic at Children's Hospital Colorado. Age appropriate consent and assent was obtained. All human donors were enrolled under study protocol 16-0918, approved by the Institutional Review Board of the Research Compliance Office at University of Colorado. Stage III melanoma patients were recruited at the University of Colorado Cancer Center Cutaneous Oncology Clinic as part of the clinicaltrials.gov registered clinical trial NCT02403778. All patients provided a written informed consent, and the treatment protocol was approved by the Colorado Multiple Institutional Review Board (#14-0948).

Mass Cytometry Analysis

SLE patient, gender-matched control, or healthy donor (anchor) peripheral whole blood was collected into heparinized vacutainers (BD). For CyTOF analysis, blood samples were fixed with Phosflow lyse/fix buffer (BD 558049) either immediately after collection (T0); or after incubation at 37C, mixed 1:1 with RPMI 1640 (Gibco 21870076) plus protein transport inhibitor cocktail (eBioscience 00-4980-93), and with R848 (1 μg/ml; Invivogen tlrl-r848) for 6 h (T6). Lysed/fixed cells were stored at −80°C, and were thawed on the day of barcoding and staining. To decrease technical variability, palladium isotopes were used in different combinations for mass tag barcoding of separate samples, pooled in sets of 20, surface stained in a single tube with a metal-labeled antibody panel, then permeabilized with Perm/Wash buffer I (BD 558050) to facilitate intracellular staining. Barcoding methodology was adapted from Zunder et al. (11). Protocols for intracellular cytokine staining (ICS) assays were adapted from previous studies in O'Gorman et al. (3).

ETHICS STATEMENT

The studies involving human participants were reviewed and approved by Institutional Review Board of the Research Compliance Office at the University of Colorado study protocol 15-2211. The patients/participants provided their written informed consent to participate in this study.

AUTHOR CONTRIBUTIONS

RS and CJ: methodology and resources, validation, formal analysis, investigation, and writing original draft. RS, CJ, JG-P, RB, and SO: writing-review and editing. RR, DG,

PR, and EH: supervision, project administration, and funding acquisition.

ACKNOWLEDGMENTS

We thank Michael Leipold from Stanford University for his thoughtful insights.

REFERENCES

1. Bendall SC, Davis KL, Amir ED, Tadmor MD, Simonds EF, Chen TJ, et al. Single-cell trajectory detection uncovers progression and regulatory coordination in human B cell development. *Cell.* (2014) 157:714–25. doi: 10.1016/j.cell.2014.04.005
2. Good Z, Sarno J, Jager A, Samusik N, Aghaeepour N, Simonds EF, et al. Single-cell developmental classification of B cell precursor acute lymphoblastic leukemia at diagnosis reveals predictors of relapse. *Nat Med.* (2018) 24:474–83. doi: 10.1038/nm.4505
3. O'Gorman WE, Hsieh EWY, Savig ES, Gherardini PF, Hernandez JD, Hansmann L, et al. Single-cell systems-level analysis of human Toll-like receptor activation defines a chemokine signature in patients with systemic lupus erythematosus. *J Allergy Clin Immunol.* (2015) 136:132636. doi: 10.1016/j.jaci.2015.04.008
4. O'Gorman WE, Kong DS, Balboni IM, Rudra P, Bolen CR, Ghosh D, et al. Mass cytometry identifies a distinct monocyte cytokine signature shared by clinically heterogeneous pediatric SLE patients. *J Autoimmun.* (2017) 81:74–89. doi: 10.1016/j.jaut.2017.03.010
5. Good Z, Borges L, Vivanco Gonzalez N, Sahaf B, Samusik N, Tibshirani R, et al. Proliferation tracing with single-cell mass cytometry optimizes generation of stem cell memory-like T cells. *Nat Biotechnol.* (2019) 37:259–66. doi: 10.1038/s41587-019-0033-2
6. Schulz D, Severin Y, Zanotelli VRT, Bodenmiller B. In-depth characterization of monocyte-derived macrophages using a mass cytometry based phagocytosis assay. *Sci Rep.* (2019) 9:1925. doi: 10.1038/s41598-018-38127-9
7. Kimmey SC, Borges L, Baskar R, Bendall SC. Parallel analysis of tri-molecular biosynthesis with cell identity and function in single cells. *Nat Commun.* (2019) 10:1185. doi: 10.1038/s41467-019-09128-7
8. Behbehani GK, Samusik N, Bjornson ZB, Fantl WJ, Medeiros BC, Nolan GP. Mass cytometric functional profiling of acute myeloid leukemia defines cell-cycle and immunophenotypic properties that correlate with known responses to therapy. *Cancer Discov.* (2015) 5:988–1003. doi: 10.1158/2159-8290.CD-15-0298
9. Behbehani GK, Bendall SC, Clutter MR, Fantl WJ, Nolan GP. Single-cell mass cytometry adapted to measurements of the cell cycle. *Cytom Part A.* (2012) 81A:552–66. doi: 10.1002/cyto.a.22075
10. Behbehani GK, Thom C, Zunder ER, Finck R, Gaudilliere B, Fragiadakis GK, Fantl WJ, et al. Transient partial permeabilization with saponin enables cellular barcoding prior to surface marker staining. *Cytom Part A.* (2014) 85:1011–9. doi: 10.1002/cyto.a.22573
11. Zunder ER, Finck R, Behbehani GK, Amir ED, Krishnaswamy S, Gonzalez VD, et al. Palladium-based mass tag cell barcoding with a doublet-filtering scheme and single-cell deconvolution algorithm. *Nat Protoc.* (2015) 10:31633. doi: 10.1038/nprot.2015.020
12. Kronstad LM, Seiler C, Vergara R, Holmes SP, Blish CA. Differential induction of IFN-α and modulation of CD112 and CD54 expression govern the magnitude of NK cell IFN-γ response to influenza A viruses. *J Immunol.* (2018) 201:2117–31. doi: 10.4049/jimmunol.1800161
13. Gaudilliere B, Fragiadakis GK, Bruggner RV, Nicolau M, Finck R, Tingle M, et al. Clinical recovery from surgery correlates with single-cell immune signatures. *Sci Transl Med.* (2014) 6:255ra131-255ra131. doi: 10.1126/scitranslmed.3009701
14. Schulz AR, Baumgart S, Schulze J, UrbichtM, Grützkau A,Mei HE. Stabilizing antibody cocktails for mass cytometry. *Cytom Part A.* (2019) 95:910–6. doi: 10.1002/cyto.a.23781
15. Finck R, Simonds EF, Jager A, Krishnaswamy S, Sachs K, Fantl W, et al. Normalization of mass cytometry data with bead standards. *Cytometry A.* (2013) 83:483–94. doi: 10.1002/cyto.a.22271
16. Leek JT, Scharpf RB, Bravo HC, Simcha D, Langmead B, Johnson WE, et al. Tackling the widespread and critical impact of batch effects in high-throughput data. *Nat Rev Genet.* (2010) 11:733–9. doi: 10.1038/nrg2825
17. Leek JT, Johnson WE, Parker HS, Jaffe AE, Storey JD. The sva package for removing batch effects and other unwanted variation in high-throughput experiments. *Bioinformatics.* (2012) 28:882–3. doi: 10.1093/bioinformatics/bts034
18. Johnson WE, Li C, Rabinovic A. Adjusting batch effects in microarray expression data using empirical Bayes methods. *Biostatistics.* (2007) 8:118–27. doi: 10.1093/biostatistics/kxj037
19. Risso D, Ngai J, Speed TP, Dudoit S. Normalization of RNA-seq data using factor analysis of control genes or samples. *Nat Biotechnol.* (2014) 32:896–902. doi: 10.1038/nbt.2931
20. Cichocki A, Zdunek R, Amari S. *Nonnegative Matrix and Tensor Factorizations: Applications to Exploratory Multi-Way Data Analysis and Blind Source Separation.* West Sussex: John Wiley (2008). doi: 10.1002/9780470747278
21. Spidlen J, Moore W, Parks D, Goldberg M, Bray C, Bierre P, et al. Data file standard for flow cytometry, version FCS 3.1. *Cytometry A.* (2010) 77:97. doi: 10.1002/cyto.a.20825
22. Leek JT, Storey JD. Capturing heterogeneity in gene expression studies by surrogate variable analysis. *PLoS Genet.* (2007) 3:1724–35. doi: 10.1371/journal.pgen.0030161
23. van den Berg RA, Hoefsloot HCJ, Westerhuis JA, Smilde AK, van der Werf MJ. Centering, scaling, and transformations: improving the biological information content of metabolomics data. *BMC Genomics.* (2006) 7:142. doi: 10.1186/1471-2164-7-142
24. Gibbons SM, Duvallet C, Alm EJ. Correcting for batch effects in case-control microbiome studies. *PLoS Comput Biol.* (2018) 14:e1006102. doi: 10.1371/journal.pcbi.1006102
25. Kleinsteuber K, Corleis B, Rashidi N, Nchinda N, Lisanti A, Cho JL, et al. Standardization and quality control for high-dimensional mass cytometry studies of human samples. *Cytometry A.* (2016) 89:903–13. doi: 10.1002/cyto.a.22935
26. Leipold MD, Obermoser G, Fenwick C, Kleinstuber K, Rashidi N, McNevin JP, et al. Comparison of CyTOF assays across sites: results of a six-center pilot study. *J Immunol Methods.* (2018) 453:37–43. doi: 10.1016/j.jim.2017.11.008
27. Bolstad BM, Irizarry RA, Astrand M, Speed TP. A comparison of normalization methods for high density oligonucleotide array data based on variance and bias. *Bioinformatics.* (2003) 19:185–93. doi: 10.1093/bioinformatics/19.2.185
28. Dillies M-A, Rau A, Aubert J, Hennequet-Antier C, Jeanmougin M, Servant N, et al. A comprehensive evaluation of normalization methods for Illumina high-throughput RNA sequencing data analysis. *Brief Bioinform.* (2013) 14:671–83. doi: 10.1093/bib/bbs046

29. Levine JH, Simonds EF, Bendall SC, Davis KL, Amir ED, Tadmor MD, et al. Data-driven phenotypic dissection of AML reveals progenitor-like cells that correlate with prognosis. *Cell.* (2015) 162:184–97. doi: 10.1016/j.cell.2015.05.047
30. Lun ATL, Richard AC, Marioni JC. Testing for differential abundance in mass cytometry data. *Nat Methods.* (2017) 14:707–9. doi: 10.1038/nmeth.4295
31. R Development Core Team. *R: A Language and Environment for Statistical Computing.* Vienna: R Development Core Team (2014).
32. Rao CR. *Linear Statistical Inference and Its Applications.* Hoboken, NJ: Wiley (1973). doi: 10.1002/9780470316436
33. Good PI. *Permutation Tests: A Practical Guide to Resampling Methods for Testing Hypotheses.* New York, NY: Springer (2000). doi: 10.1007/978-1-4757-3235-1_3
34. Bruggner R V, Bodenmiller B, Dill DL, Tibshirani RJ, Nolan GP. Automated identification of stratifying signatures in cellular subpopulations. *Proc Natl Acad Sci USA.* (2014) 111:E2770–7. doi: 10.1073/pnas.1408792111
35. Qiu X, Wu H, Hu R. The impact of quantile and rank normalization procedures on the testing power of gene differential expression analysis. *BMC Bioinformatics.* (2013) 14:124. doi: 10.1186/1471-2105-14-124

2

Pretreatment Innate Cell Populations and CD4 T Cells in Blood are Associated with Response to Immune Checkpoint Blockade in Melanoma Patients

Mehdi R. Pirozyan[1,2,3†], *Helen M. McGuire*[4,5,6*†], *Abdullah Al Emran*[1,2,3], *Hsin-Yi Tseng*[1,2,3], *Jessamy C. Tiffen*[1,2,3], *Jenny H. Lee*[3,7], *Matteo S. Carlino*[3,8], *Alexander M. Menzies*[3,9], *Georgina V. Long*[3,9], *Richard A. Scolyer*[3,6,10,11], *Barbara Fazekas de St Groth*[4,5,6*†] and *Peter Hersey*[1,3*†]

[1] Melanoma Immunology and Oncology, Centenary Institute, Sydney, NSW, Australia, [2] Central Clinical School, The University of Sydney, Camperdown, NSW, Australia, [3] Melanoma Institute Australia, The University of Sydney, Sydney, NSW, Australia, [4] Ramaciotti Facility for Human Systems Biology, The University of Sydney, Sydney, NSW, Australia, [5] Discipline of Pathology, Sydney Medical School, The University of Sydney, Sydney, NSW, Australia, [6] Charles Perkins Centre, The University of Sydney, Sydney, NSW, Australia, [7] Biomedical Sciences, Faculty of Medicine and Health Sciences, Macquarie University, Sydney, NSW, Australia, [8] Westmead and Blacktown Hospitals, Sydney, NSW, Australia, [9] Royal North Shore Hospital, St Leonards, NSW, Australia, [10] Royal Prince Alfred Hospital, Camperdown, NSW, Australia, [11] New South Wales Health Pathology, Sydney, NSW, Australia

***Correspondence:**
Helen M. McGuire
helen.mcguire@sydney.edu.au
Barbara Fazekas de St Groth
barbara.fazekas@sydney.edu.au
Peter Hersey
peter.hersey@sydney.edu.au

† These authors have contributed equally to this work

The development of changes in T cells, referred to as T cell exhaustion, has been suggested as a cause of primary or acquired resistance to immunotherapy by immune checkpoint blockade (ICB). A limited number of studies, largely performed on tumor infiltrating lymphocytes (TILs), has provided evidence in support of this hypothesis, but whether similar changes occur in circulating blood lymphocytes has received little attention. In the present study, a comprehensive analysis of peripheral blood leukocytes from 42 patients taken over the course of treatment with anti-PD-1 was undertaken. The patients included those grouped as responders (who did not progress), primary non-responders (primary resistance) and those with acquired resistance (who initially responded then subsequently progressed). Analysis included surface markers of exhaustion, production of cytokines following *in vitro* stimulation, and assessment of transcription factor levels associated with T cell exhaustion. There were differences in innate cell populations between responders and non-responders at baseline and maintained throughout therapy. Frequencies of total and classical $CD14^{+}CD16^{-}$ monocytes were higher and the major subset of NK cells ($CD16^{hi}CD56^{+}$) was significantly smaller in the primary resistance group compared with responders. However, differences in peripheral blood expression of exhaustion markers were not evident between the treatment groups. T cell exhaustion markers were expressed in practically all patients and the major observation was an increase in CD39 on CD4 T cells during treatment. The results confirm the association of Eomes transcription factor with T cell exhaustion but levels of expression and the ratio with T-bet over Eomes did not differ between the patient groups. Thus, peripheral blood expression of T cell exhaustion markers does not distinguish between responders and non-responders to anti-PD-1 therapy. CD4 T cell expression of IFNγ also differed in pre-treatment samples, indicating that predictors of response unrelated to exhaustion may be present in peripheral blood. The association of response with innate cell populations and CD4 T cell responses requires further study.

Keywords: melanoma, cancer immunotherapy, NK cells, CyTOF, T cell exhaustion, CD4 T cells, checkpoint inhibition

INTRODUCTION

The introduction of immunotherapy based on monoclonal antibodies (mAbs) that block immune checkpoint inhibitors on T cells has been a major advance in treatment of cancers such as melanoma and lung cancer (1, 2). A number of clinical trials over the past few years have established monotherapy with anti-PD-1 or its combination with anti-CTLA-4 as the standard of care in treatment of metastatic melanoma (3–9). Resistance to these treatments is relatively common; between 40 and 60% of patients fail to respond initially, and many that initially respond subsequently progress, such that only 30-40% of patients remain progression-free at 4 years (3, 4, 10). The factors associated with primary and acquired resistance are reviewed elsewhere (5, 6) and include low or absent PD-L1 on melanoma (7) and the degree of T cell infiltration into the tumor. These factors have been used in past studies to classify patients into 4 groups that show different responses to anti-PD-1 therapy (8, 9, 11). Both primary and acquired resistance can be driven by selection of MHC loss variants of the tumor that result in failure of recognition and loss of sensitivity to killing by T cells (12, 13). Study of primary resistant melanoma cells by CRISPR/Cas9 screens revealed loss of antigen presentation as a cause of resistance to immunotherapy (14, 15). Single cell analyses of melanoma tumors prior to anti-PD-1 therapy also identified cellular programs associated with intrinsic resistance driven by CDK4/6 pathways and reversed by inhibitors of CDK4/6 (16). Similar inherent resistance pathways associated with epigenetic changes in the melanoma cells were described in resistance to targeted therapies (17).

In addition to these tumor intrinsic factors, it has been postulated that resistance to immunotherapy may result from decreased T cell function associated with a state referred to as exhaustion, which results from prolonged and repeated antigen stimulation (18, 19). Exhausted T cells are characterized by an altered transcription pattern (20) and by a loss of effector functions such as production of granzyme B and IFNγ, together with expression of multiple inhibitory receptors such as PD-1, LAG-3, TIM-3, and CD39 (21). Exhausted T cells appear to exist in 2 forms; one that is reversible by anti-PD-1 (22) and one that cannot be reversed and is believed to result from more prolonged antigen exposure (23). Recent studies have referred to cells in these 2 states as progenitor and terminally exhausted T cells (24). Single cell RNA-seq analysis on tumor-infiltrating lymphocytes (TILs) from 25 patients revealed that dysfunctional CD8 T cells often formed the majority of proliferating T cells and ranged from 3.6 to 72.1% of the TILs (25). Another single cell analysis of 48 human melanoma samples identified responses to anti-PD-1 to be associated with increased expression of genes coding for TCF7, IL7R, REL, FOXP1, and STAT4 whereas non-response was associated with genes associated with T cell exhaustion, such as CD38, PD-L1, LAG-3, TIM-3, and CTLA-4 (26). Signatures of T cell dysfunction and exclusion (TIDE) in TILs were considered accurate predictors of response to immune checkpoint blockade (ICB) (27).

The exhausted T cell state in cancers has been studied mainly in TILs, but whether this state can be detected in the circulation of cancer patients has received little attention. High dimensional flow cytometry studies on pre-treatment blood samples from 29 patients with metastatic melanoma found that these patients had higher numbers of CD4 FOXP3 T cells and Ki-67 proliferating CD8 T cells compared to normal subjects. Anti-PD-1 antibody treatment resulted in brief increases in Ki-67$^+$ CD8$^+$ T cells that expressed PD-1, CXCR5, CTLA-4, and 2B4. High Eomes transcription factors were also associated with T cell exhaustion. These changes were seen in 74% of the patients even though clinical responses were seen in only 38% (28), indicating that they are not reliable predictors of response. In another study of 20 melanoma patients treated with anti-PD-1, classical monocytes (CD14$^+$CD16$^-$) in pre-treatment peripheral blood samples were reported to be strong predictors of response to treatment (29). Similar studies using CyTOF data found that the main differences between responders vs. non-responders to anti-PD-1 were in subsets of NK cells (30, 31).

In the present study, we examined circulating peripheral blood mononuclear cells (PBMCs) for evidence of the exhaustion state by a comprehensive analysis of their expression of markers and transcription factors associated with exhaustion, as well as their production of effector molecules. Longitudinal blood samples were taken from a cohort of patients treated with anti-PD-1. Our results suggest that differences between the responders and non-responders are already evident in pre-treatment samples and undergo very few changes during treatment. They also point to limitations of published studies on PBMCs in understanding the biology of immune responses associated with clinical responses to checkpoint therapy.

MATERIALS AND METHODS

Study Subjects and Samples

The study schema is shown in **Figure 1**. Written consent was obtained from all patients at Melanoma Institute Australia, Sydney, Australia, and its affiliated hospitals, and the relevant ethical approval was obtained from Human Research Ethics Committees. Samples were collected under the biospecimen bank protocol No X15-0454 (prev. X11-0289) and HREC/11/RPAH/444. Clinical Data were collected under the MIA Melanoma Research Database protocol: Protocol No X15-0311 (previously X10-0300) and HREC/10/RPAH/530 – "Melanoma Institute Australia: Melanoma Research Database." A cohort of 42 metastatic melanoma patients treated with anti-PD-1 (Pembrolizumab or Nivolumab) therapy was retrospectively identified (**Figure 2**, **Supplementary Table 1**). Baseline bloods were collected before the first administration of anti-PD-1. Based on response evaluation criteria in solid tumors (RECIST) (32), patients were categorized into three groups - progressive disease (primary resistance), objective response (complete or partial) without subsequent progression (responder), and initial objective response followed by subsequent progression (acquired resistance). Baseline samples included 10 responders, 17 non-responders, and 9 acquired resistance. Follow up samples were obtained at ~6 weeks post treatment (range 2-9 weeks) (11 responders, 19 primary resistance, and 9 acquired resistance). However, 1 year follow up samples (range 35-85 weeks) were obtained from only 2 responder, 10 primary resistance, and 6 acquired resistance patients. For some analyses, responder and acquired resistance groups were pooled into a primary responder group equivalent to the responder groups in published studies in which progression after 3 month RECIST assessment was not used to subdivide the responder group.

All whole blood samples were processed to isolate PBMCs by density gradient centrifugation, using Lymphoprep density gradient media or SepMate isolation tubes (Stem Cell Technologies). Single-cell suspensions were then cryopreserved in fetal bovine serum (FBS) supplemented with 10% DMSO (Sigma-Aldrich), using a controlled freezing unit (Cool Cell LX) and then stored in liquid nitrogen for later use. Matched TILs

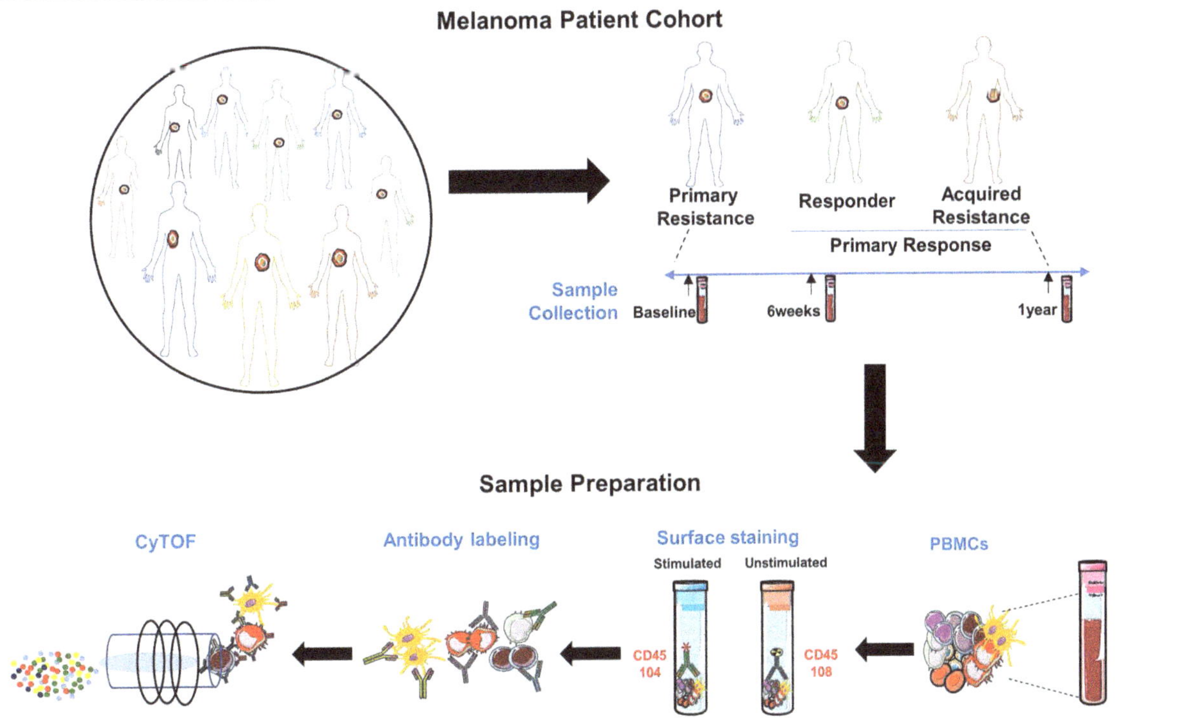

FIGURE 1 | Experimental schema. Experimental setup for processing PBMCs from matched samples before and after anti-PD-1 immunotherapy. Samples (n = 97) comprised 36 from melanoma patients prior to beginning anti-PD-1 treatment [Primary Resistance (PR) = 17, Responders (R) = 10 and Acquired Resistance (AR) = 9]; 39 from 6 weeks post-treatment (PR = 19, R = 11, and AR = 9) and 18 from the 1 year time point (PR = 10, R = 2, and AR = 6). PMA/Ionomycin stimulated cells were stained with 104Pd metal tagged anti-CD45 antibody while unstimulated cells from the same sample were stained with 108Pd metal tagged anti-CD45 antibody. Barcoded samples were washed, pooled, and subsequently stained with a panel of 39 antibodies, each conjugated to a different metal isotope, and analyzed by mass cytometry. Cells were nebulized into single-cell droplets, and an elemental mass spectrum was acquired for each. The integrated elemental reporter signals for each cell were then analyzed using a supervised gating strategy (FlowJo). For some analyses, responder and acquired resistance groups were pooled into a primary responder group equivalent to the responder groups in published studies in which progression after 3 month RECIST assessment was not used to subdivide the responder group.

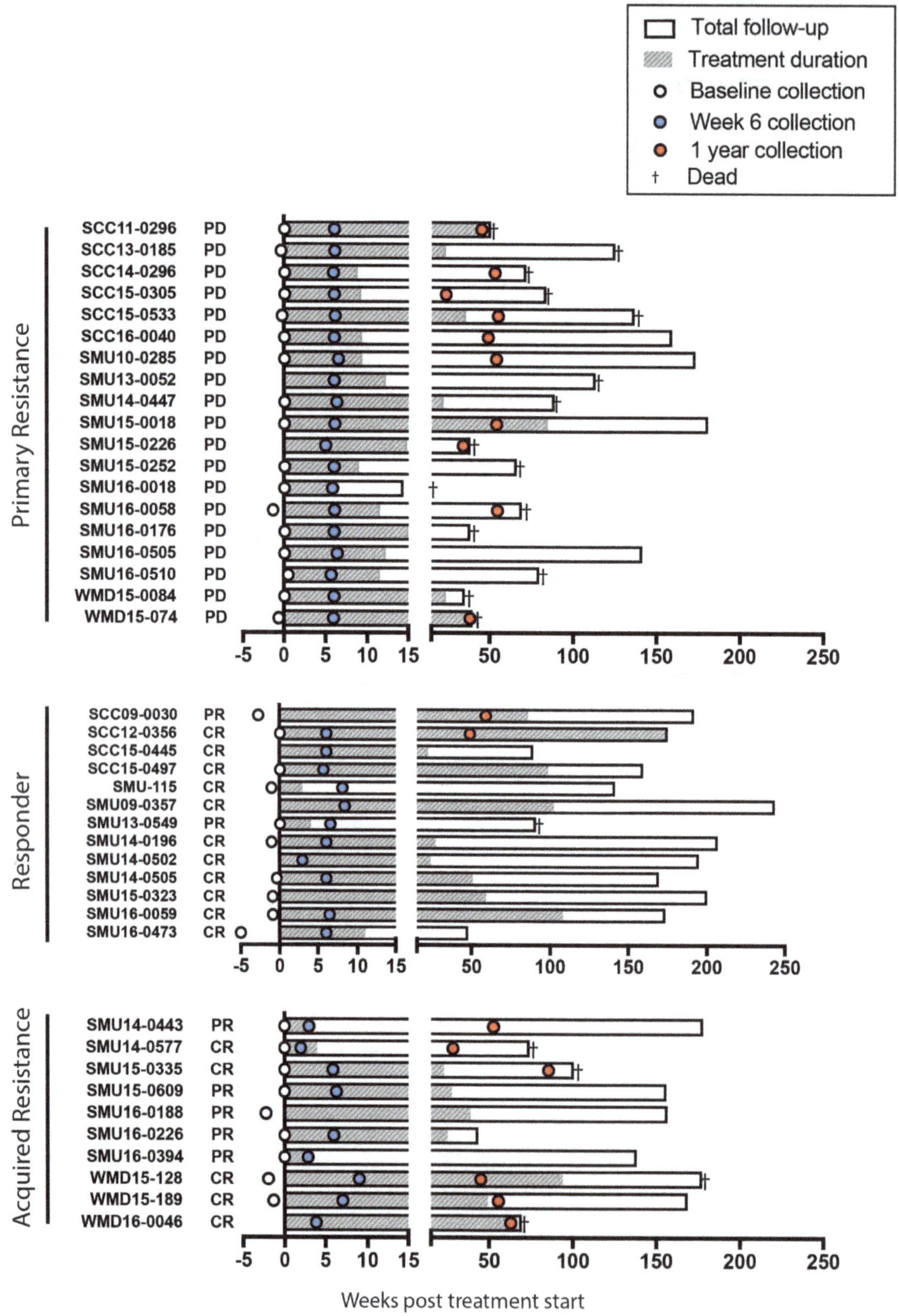

FIGURE 2 | Swimmers plot illustrates treatment duration of patients treated with anti-PD-1 (filled bars), within the study follow up period (open bars) for primary resistance, responders, and acquired resistance groups. Death is illustrated with a cross. Blood samples were obtained at baseline (open circles, range 0-5 weeks before the start of therapy), week 6 (blue filled circles, range 2-9 weeks) and 1 year (red filled circles, range 35-85 weeks) post treatment. CR, complete response; PR, partial response; PD, progressive disease, as assessed using RECIST.

from an acquired resistance patient at the 1 year time point were prepared by manual mincing followed by dissociation into single-cell suspensions using the human Tumor Dissociation Kit and gentleMACSTM Dissociator (Miltenyi Biotec), before cryopreservation as for PBMCs.

Mass Cytometry Immunophenotyping

For immunophenotyping of PBMCs, a panel of 39 metal-tagged monoclonal antibodies was optimized and employed. Antibody specificities were chosen to provide wide coverage of CD8 T cell markers (27 markers at baseline plus 3 cytokines), with much more limited coverage of markers specific to the NK and myeloid compartments. A detailed list of antibodies and corresponding metal tags is provided in **Supplementary Table 2**. All antibodies were validated, pre-titered and supplied in per-test amounts by the Ramaciotti Facility Reagent Bank. Reagent bank antibodies were either purchased from Fluidigm (Fluidigm, South San Francisco, CA) in pre-conjugated form or unlabeled antibodies were purchased in a carrier-protein-free format and conjugated at the Ramaciotti Facility with the indicated metal isotope using the MaxPAR conjugation kit (Fluidigm, South San Francisco, CA) according to the manufacturers protocol.

PBMC stimulation, staining and data acquisition by CyTOF were performed as described previously (33). Briefly, PBMC vials were thawed in a 37°C water bath for 2 min before transfer of the suspension into a 15 mL Falcon tube containing 10 mL R10 culture media RPMI-1640 (Gibco, UK) supplemented with 10% FBS and penicillin and streptomycin (Invitrogen, USA) as well as 1:10,000 universal nuclease (Thermo Fisher Waltham, MA). Cell concentration and viability were determined using a TC20 automated cell counter (Bio Rad, USA) and Trypan blue. Subsequently, a maximum of two million cells were left either untreated or stimulated for 3 h at 37°C using 100 nM of phorbol-12-myristate-13 acetate (PMA) (Sigma) and 1 μM of ionomycin in the presence of 10 μg/ml Brefeldin A (Sigma). For samples with insufficient cells, the untreated control was omitted.

Following stimulation, PBMCs were stained using 1.25 μM cisplatin in PBS for 3 min at room temperature and subsequently quenched with R10, in order to discriminate live from dead cells. Barcoding was performed by incubating cells for 30 min with CD45 antibodies conjugated with various metals. Cells were washed twice with FACs buffer (PBS, 0.02% Sodium Azide, 0.5% BSA and 2mM EDTA), differentially CD45-labeled stimulated and unstimulated samples were combined and incubated with antibodies targeting surface antigens for 30 min at 4°C. Following washing with FACS buffer, cells were fixed and permeabilized using eBiosciences FoxP3 buffer kit (San Diego, CA, USA) at 4°C for 45 min and stained with intracellular antibodies for 30 min on ice. Cells were then washed twice and fixed in 4% paraformaldehyde containing DNA intercalator (0.125μM iridium-191/193; Fluidigm) overnight. After multiple washes with FACS buffer and MilliQ water, cells were diluted to 800,000 cells/mL in MilliQ water containing 1:10 diluted EQ beads (Fluidigm) and filtered through a 35-μm nylon mesh. Cells were acquired at a rate of 200–400 cells/second using a CyTOF 2 Helios upgraded mass cytometer (Fluidigm, Toronto, Canada).

Samples were stained and run in 13 batches. When multiple samples from different timepoints were available for a patient, they were included in the same batch. Each batch also included a batch control consisting of one replicate aliquot of PBMC from a healthy donor, thawed and stimulated in parallel with the patient samples.

All .fcs files obtained from the Helios analysis were normalized using the processing function within the CyTOF acquisition software based on the concurrently run EQ four element beads.

Analysis of Mass Cytometry Data

Data analysis was performed using FlowJo version 10.4 software (FlowJo, LLC, Ashland, OR, USA). Samples were pre-gated on DNA+, live, CD45+ cells, and exported for further analysis. Manual gating was performed independently by two individuals to ensure accuracy. Major populations were gated as indicated in **Supplementary Figure 2**. Gates were adjusted on the basis of the batch-to-batch variations apparent from the batch control data. Expression of exhaustion markers and cytokines was then examined within CD4 and CD8 T cells and their subpopulations (**Figures 4–6, Supplementary Figures 3–6**).

The *t*-stochastic neighborhood embedding (*t*-SNE) algorithm was applied using the FlowJo plugin. Files containing live cells with stringent doublet exclusion were down sampled without replacement to 1,000 cells using the FlowJo DownSample plugin. Stimulated and unstimulated samples from all patients plus the 13 batch controls were concatenated separately to yield files containing ~100,000 events suitable for t-SNE analysis. The t-SNE algorithm was run on the 2 concatenated files using the 36 markers shown in **Supplementary Table 2** (excluding the cytokines IL-2, TNFα and IFNγ). Marker expression for each patient group was visualized using the tSNE global scaling script (https://github.com/sydneycytometry/tSNEplots) and is shown in **Supplementary Figures 7–10**.

Statistical Analysis

Statistical analysis and graphical representation were performed using Graphpad Prism, version 7.0 (GraphPad Software, Inc. USA, La Jolla). Group comparisons were performed as detailed in the figure legends.

RESULTS

Patients and Sample Characteristics

A summary of the study participants is presented in **Supplementary Table 1**. The overall survival of the patient groups is shown in **Supplementary Figure 1**. As expected the responder patients had a significantly longer survival than non-responders and those with acquired resistance. Blood was collected from a total of 42 patients (responder = 13, primary resistance = 19, and acquired resistance = 10). Details of the sample collection and survival of individual patients in each group are presented in **Figure 2**.

Differences in Immune Populations Between the Groups Before and After PD-1 Immunotherapy

The frequencies of the major immune populations were determined using a conventional supervised gating approach as shown in **Supplementary Figure 2**. Frequencies of B cells, CD4 and CD8 T cells and their naïve and memory subsets, $\gamma\delta$T cells, natural killer (NK) cells, and monocytes were calculated as a percentage of live cells for each of the 89 unstimulated samples. There were no significant differences in the frequencies of B cells, CD4 and CD8 T cells or their naïve and memory subsets, or $\gamma\delta$T cells between any of the three patient groups, either before or after therapy. When the responder and acquired resistance groups were pooled (as would be the usual practice in studies with shorter followup times when responder status would be determined after the 3 month RECIST assessment), no differences in B cells, CD4 and CD8 T cells or their naïve and memory subsets, or $\gamma\delta$T cells were observed.

At baseline, there was a trend toward higher frequencies of total and classical $CD14^{+}CD16^{-}$ monocytes in the primary resistance group compared to the responder group (**Figure 3A**), and this difference was statistically significant when the responder and acquired resistance groups were combined into a single primary responder group and compared with the primary resistance group. When all the timepoints were included in the comparison between responder and primary resistance groups, the increase in monocytes in the primary resistance group was no longer significant (**Figure 3B**). No difference was observed in MDSCs, identified as $CD14^{+}HLA\text{-}DR^{lo}$ cells between any of the three patient groups, either before or after therapy. There was a trend to lower NK cells in the primary resistance group at baseline, and the difference reached statistical significance in the all timepoints comparison between the combined primary responder and primary resistance groups. The major subset of NK cells ($CD16^{hi}CD56^{+}$) was smaller in the

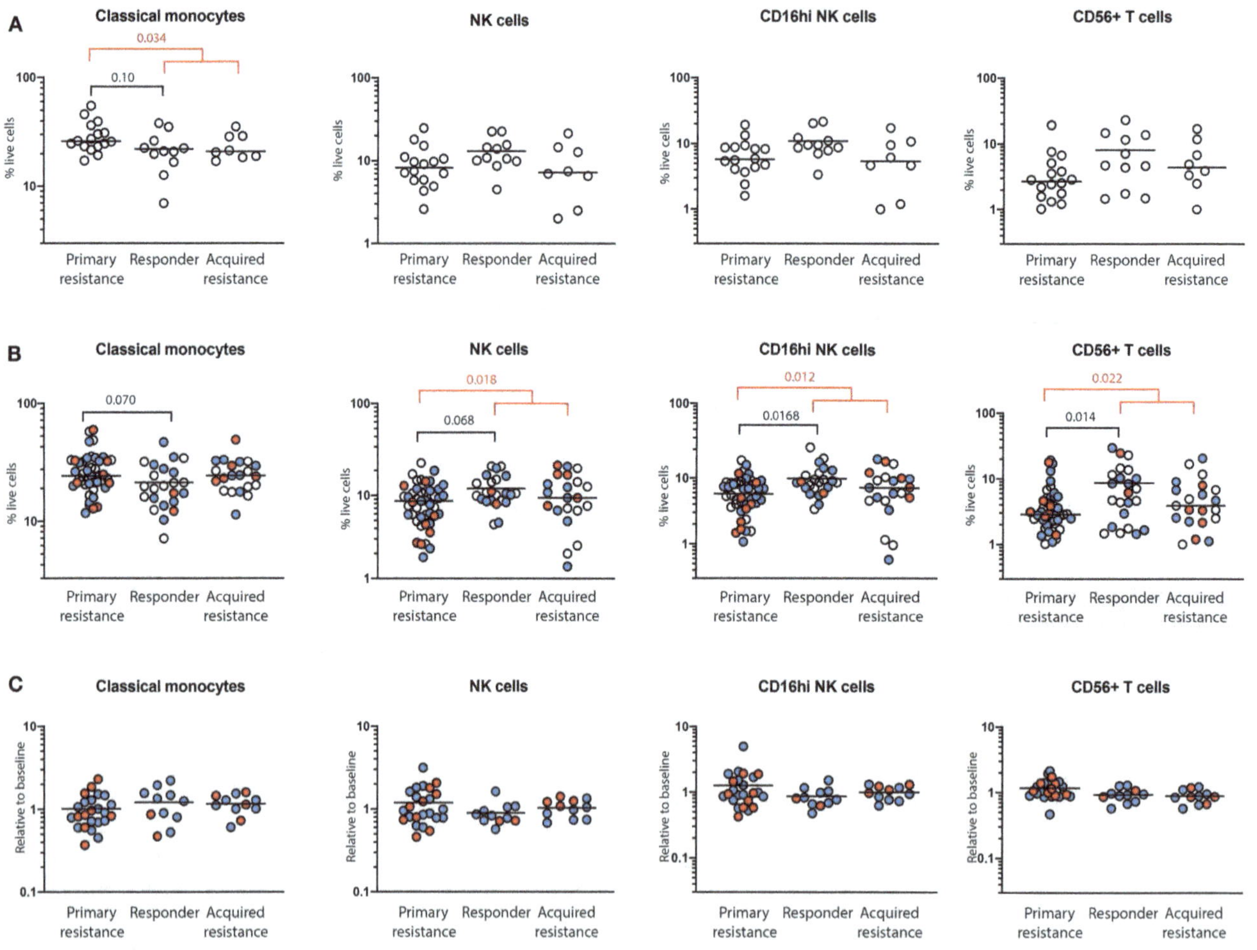

FIGURE 3 | Quantification of immune cells populations using mass cytometry. PBMCs from primary resistance, responder and acquired resistance groups were analyzed for multiple T cell, B cell, NK cell, and myeloid populations, as illustrated in **Supplementary Figures 2, 3**. Only populations that differed between groups are shown. **(A)** Frequencies of baseline cell populations in each of the groups. Each individual sample is indicated by a circle, with the group mean shown as a bar. **(B)** Frequencies of cell populations from all timepoints in each of the groups. Baseline, open circles; week 6, blue filled circles; 1 year, red filled circles. **(C)** Changes in frequencies within individual subjects over time. Values at 6 weeks, expressed as a proportion of baseline values, are indicated by blue filled circles while values at year 1, expressed as a proportion of baseline values, are indicated by red filled circles. Differences in frequencies of immune cell populations between primary resistance, responder, and acquired resistance groups were assessed using ANOVA followed by Tukey's multiple comparisons test and p-values are shown in black. Differences between primary resistance and primary responder (i.e., pooled responder and acquired resistance) groups were assessed using an unpaired t-test and p-values are indicated in red. Where no p-values are indicated, the relevant tests indicated $p > 0.05$.

primary resistance group compared with responders in the all timepoints comparison, and also in comparison with the primary responder group (**Figure 3B**). There was also a trend toward higher CD56 expression within T cells in the responder group, and this reached statistical significance in the all timepoints comparison, both between primary resistance and responder, and primary resistance and primary responder (**Figure 3B**). Pairwise comparisons revealed no significant correlation between monocyte, NK and CD56^{+} T cell numbers with subjects.

For total NK cells and the CD16^{hi}CD56^{+} NK cell subset, the variance of the primary and acquired resistance groups was higher than the responder group (**Figure 3B**). To test whether this was due to changes over time within a single individual, or to differences that pre-dated therapy and were maintained over time, we expressed the 6-week and 1-year cell subset frequencies as a proportion of baseline for those subjects where baseline values were available (**Figure 3C**). This analysis revealed that the variances of the changes in NK cell population sizes within individual patients were similar in all 3 groups, and were smaller than the variances of the patient samples within each group. Thus, the frequency of total NK cells and CD16^{hi}CD56^{+} NK cells in individual patients was relatively unaffected by therapy. The same was true for CD56^{+} T cells, but not for classical monocytes. These data indicate that patients who show primary resistance to anti-PD1 therapy have a pre-existing deficit in CD56-expressing NK and T cells that remains throughout therapy. In contrast, monocyte frequencies vary as much in individuals over time as between members of each treatment group.

Expression of Inhibitory Molecules by T Cells According to Clinical Responses

As T cells are the major targets of anti-PD-1 immunotherapy, we compared the expression of five inhibitory markers [PD-1, CD39, TIGIT, TIM-3, and killer cell lectin like receptor G1 (KLRG1)] on CD4 and CD8 T cells and assessed their potential association with clinical responses. Expression of the panel of markers examined on CD8 T cells is shown in **Supplementary Figure 3**. Some gates were set according to expression on a matched TILS sample, since PD-1, CD39, TIGIT, and TIM-3 are all expressed by a far lower proportion of PBMC than TILS (**Supplementary Figure 4**). There were no significant differences in the response group frequencies of CD4 or CD8 T cells expressing PD-1, CD39, TIGIT, TIM-3, or KLRG1 when compared at baseline, at 6 weeks or at 1 year (not shown).

Longitudinal analysis showed a reduction in expression of PD-1 within both CD8 and CD4 T cells at week 6 post treatment, as expected (**Figure 4A**). The reduction was of similar magnitude in both responder and primary resistance groups. Interestingly, PD-1 expression rebounded strongly in only 2 of the 7 primary resistance group patients whose 1-year sample was taken after cessation of therapy. There was an increase from baseline to week 6 in the frequency of CD39-expressing CD4 T cells in the

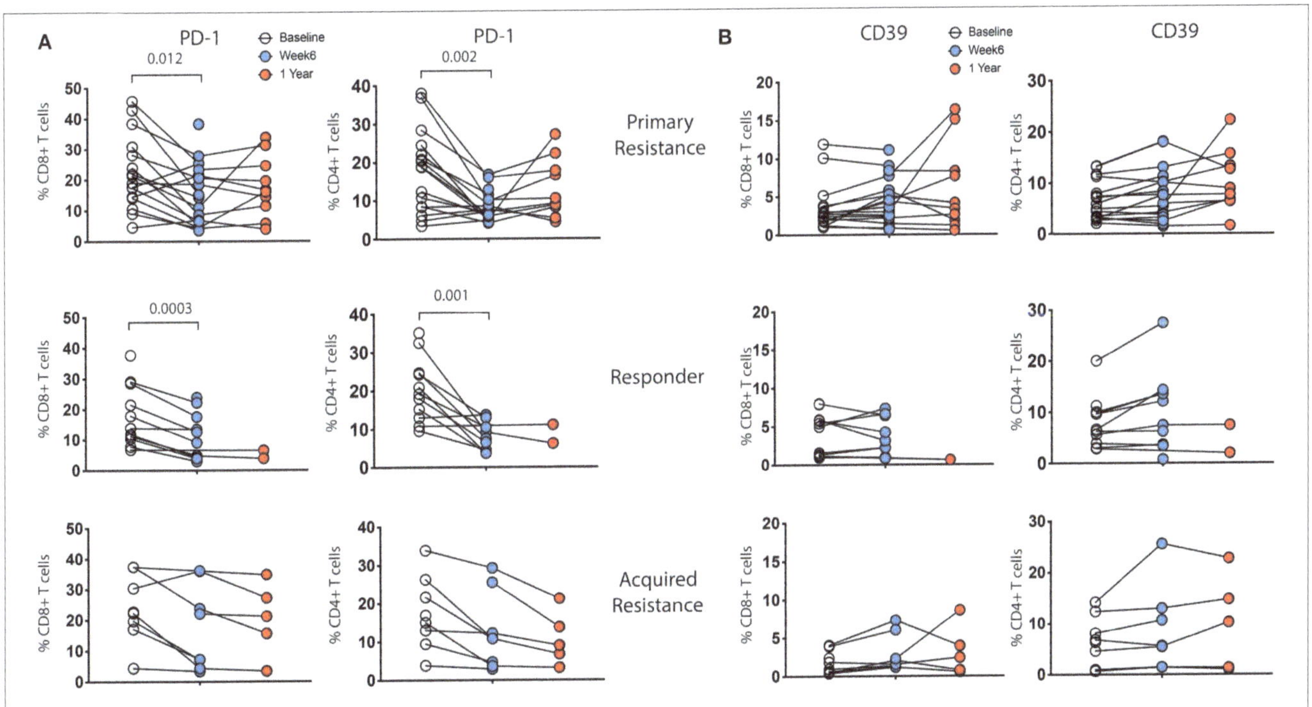

FIGURE 4 | Expression levels of inhibitory receptors on CD4 and CD8 T cells by treatment outcome. PBMCs were analyzed for expression of CD39, PD-1, TIGIT, TIM-3, and KLRG1 on CD4 and CD8 T cells. There were no significant differences in expression between the groups at any timepoint. Expression of **(A)** PD-1 and **(B)** CD39 showed changes within individual subjects over the course of therapy, while TIM-3, TIGIT, and KLRG1 did not (not shown). Baseline, open circles; week 6, blue filled circles; 1 year, red filled circles. Differences in frequencies of immune cell populations between the 3 timepoints were assessed using a repeated measures mixed effects analysis followed by Tukey's multiple comparisons test and *p*-values are indicated.

responder and primary resistance groups, but this trend did not reach statistical significance.

We analyzed the combination of expression of three inhibitory markers (CD39, PD-1, and TIM-3), using a Boolean gating approach. These markers have been recently shown to predict terminally exhausted T cells in melanoma patients (21). The major CD8 subpopulations consisted of $CD39^{-}PD\text{-}1^{-}Tim\text{-}3^{-}$ cells followed by $CD39^{-}PD\text{-}1^{+}Tim\text{-}3^{-}$ cells. Overall, we did not see significant differences in any of 8 subpopulations between responders, primary resistance and acquired resistance groups within CD4 or CD8 T cells (data not shown).

We also analyzed expression of markers recently reported to correlate with either anti-PD-1 responsiveness (28) or tumor control (34, 35) (**Supplementary Figure 3**). There was no significant difference in expression of Ki-67, TOX, or TCF1/TCF7, either between the three treatment groups or over time within each group (data not shown).

Expression of Inhibitory Receptors on CD8 T Cells According to Their Differentiation Status Over the Course of Treatment

Previous studies have shown differences in exhaustion markers according to the differentiation status of T cells (21). As shown in **Figure 5A**, four subpopulations of CD8 T cells were defined by expression of CCR7 and CD45RO: naïve ($CCR7^{+}CD45RO^{-}$), central memory (TCM, $CCR7^{+}CD45RO^{+}$), effector memory (TEM, $CCR7^{-}CD45RO^{+}$) and terminally differentiated effector memory (TEMRA, $CCR7^{-}CD45RO^{-}$) (36). We did not observe significant associations between these T cell subgroups and clinical response to immunotherapy at baseline or week 6 time points (data not shown). To test whether the CD8 T cell subpopulations showed differential reduction in PD-1 expression during therapy, we compared longitudinal patterns of expression (**Figure 5B**). PD-1 expression at baseline was highest in the TEM and TCM subpopulations in all 3 patient groups. There were drops in PD-1 expression within all 4 CD8 T cell subpopulations in the responder and primary resistance patient groups, some of which reached statistical significance, indicating that the reduction shown in **Figure 4A** was broadly present in all CD8 T cells.

The Transcription Factor Eomes in CD8 T Cells Associates With High Levels of Inhibitory Receptors and Cell Division Whereas T-Bet Associates With Cytotoxic Effector Molecules

A number of transcription factors (TFs) are known to be involved in the differentiation of T cells and to undergo changes associated with the development of T cell exhaustion. The TF T-bet was reported to regulate Th1 responses of CD4, CD8 T cells, and innate cells (37) whereas the TF Eomesodermin (Eomes) has been shown to be required to induce production of effector molecules such as granzyme B and perforin (38). In view of this, we studied expression of T-bet and Eomes in the 3 groups of patients (**Supplementary Figure 5**) and their impact on effector molecules and exhaustion markers (**Figure 6**). We did not observe any significant differences in expression of T-bet, Eomes, $T\text{-}bet^{dim}/Eomes^{hi}$, or $T\text{-}bet^{hi}/Eomes^{dim}$ populations between the three subject groups (**Supplementary Figure 5**). Furthermore, no alteration in the ratio of T-bet to Eomes expression was observed in any of the groups (**Supplementary Figure 5C**).

The expression of Eomes, however, was linked to expression of the inhibitory receptors TIGIT, KLRG1, PD-1, and CD39 in that their expression was associated with high levels of Eomes and low levels of T-bet (**Figure 6**). This also applied to Ki-67, a marker of cell division, and production of IL-2 and IFNγ. In contrast, the effector molecules perforin and granzyme B were associated with high levels of T-bet and low levels of Eomes. Taken together, these results indicate that an inverse expression pattern of T-bet and Eomes is highly associated with the up-regulation of several inhibitory receptors and cytokines as well as Ki-67 for total CD8 T cells, independently of anti-PD-1 therapy outcome in melanoma patients.

Analysis of Cytokine Production by CD4 and CD8 T Cells During Immunotherapy

Exhausted T cells have been reported to have reduced production of cytokines such as IL-2 and IFNγ and reduced expression of the effector molecules perforin and granzyme B (18). We examined CD4 and CD8 T cells for expression of granzyme B, IFNγ, IL-2, Ki-67, perforin, and TNFα as shown in **Supplementary Figure 6A**. In general, we observed higher levels of granzyme B, IFNγ, IL-2, and perforin expression by CD8 T cells compared to CD4 T cells (**Supplementary Figure 6B**). No significant differences in expression of granzyme B, IL-2, Ki-67, perforin, and TNFα by CD8 and CD4 T cells were observed between the treatment groups at any time point (**Supplementary Figure 6B**), with the exception of increased IFNγ production by CD4 T cells in baseline samples from the responder group compared with the acquired resistance group (**Figure 7**). In addition, we compared IFNγ production by NK cells and $\gamma\delta$T cells and found no significant differences between the groups at any timepoint.

Dimensionality Reduction and Visualization

Because manual gating is only rarely applied to mass cytometry data, we also applied t-SNE analysis to our dataset to check whether additional differences between response groups would become apparent (**Supplementary Figures 7–10**). For unstimulated samples, tSNE indicated a trend toward fewer NK cells and more myeloid cells (principally $CD14^{+}$ classical monocytes) in the primary resistance group compared to the responder group, with the acquired resistance group intermediate between the two (**Supplementary Figure 7**). Visualization of marker expression (**Supplementary Figure 8**) did not reveal any obvious differences between the 3 groups. The distribution of markers was consistent with the normal expression patterns that had already been revealed by our manual gating. For the stimulated samples, there was trend toward higher IFNγ expression by CD4 T cells in

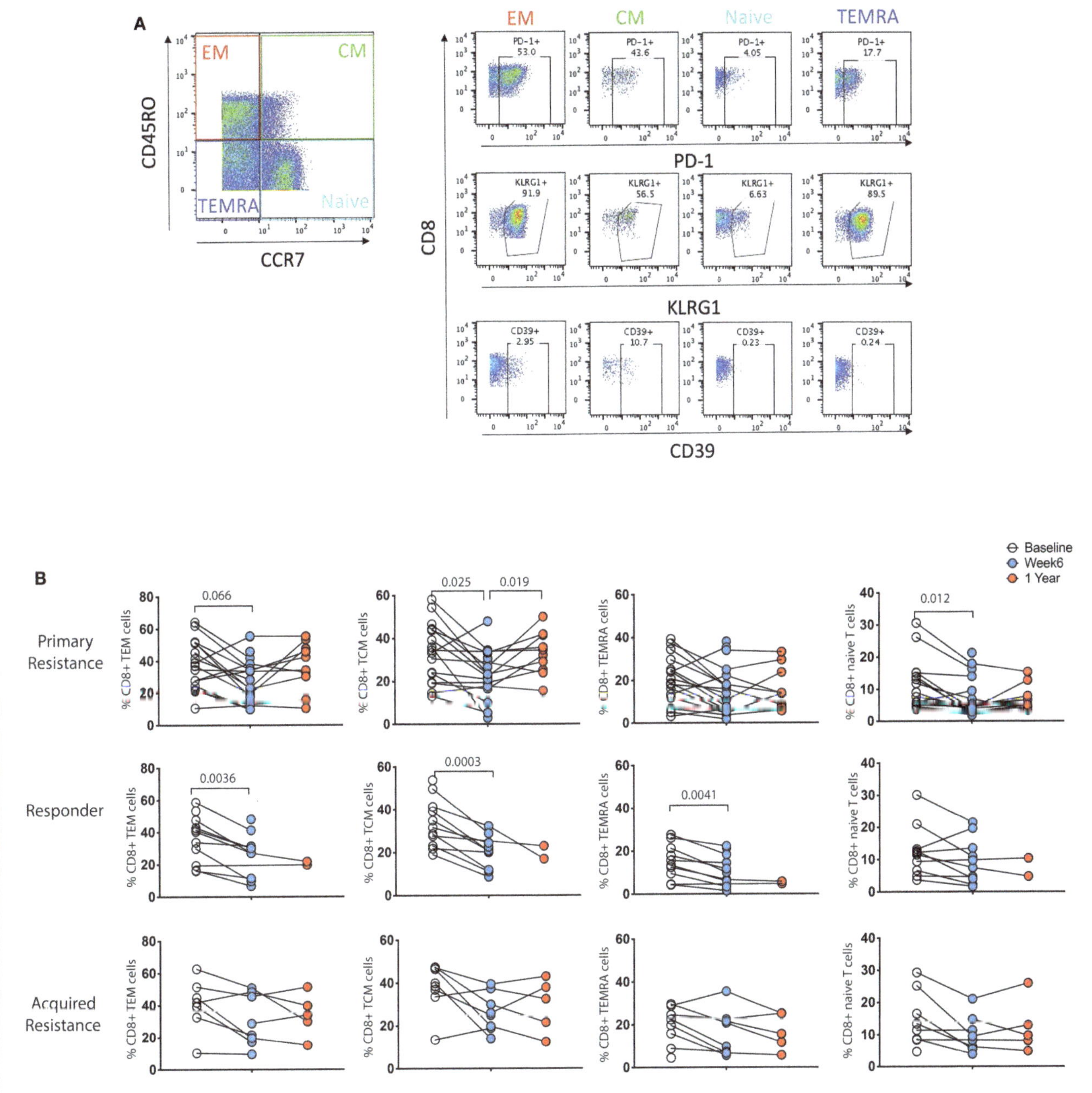

FIGURE 5 | Differential expression pattern of PD-1 within effector/memory compartments of CD8 T cells. **(A)** Gating strategy to distinguish effector memory (TEM), central memory (TCM), effector memory CD45RA (TEMRA), and naïve compartments. **(B)** Longitudinal analysis of PD-1 expression. Baseline, open circles; week 6, blue filled circles; 1 year, red filled circles. Differences in frequencies of immune cell populations between the 3 timepoints were assessed using a repeated measures mixed effects analysis followed by Tukey's multiple comparisons test and *p*-values are indicated.

the responder group, consistent with our manual gating results (**Supplementary Figures 9, 10**).

DISCUSSION

A number of studies have suggested that the development of the T cell exhaustion state may limit the effectiveness of the anti-tumor immune response. Studies on T cells infiltrating melanoma have shown that T cell exhaustion states were relatively common (25) and associated with low response rates (26). It was unknown, however, whether such states could be identified in circulating PBMCs, and whether they had the potential to serve as a more convenient measure in management of immunotherapy. This prompted the present study on a cohort of patients who had been treated by ICB and who had the expected variation in response to treatment. The study had access to highly sensitive multiparameter detection facilities. The resulting data were analyzed using expert manual gating.

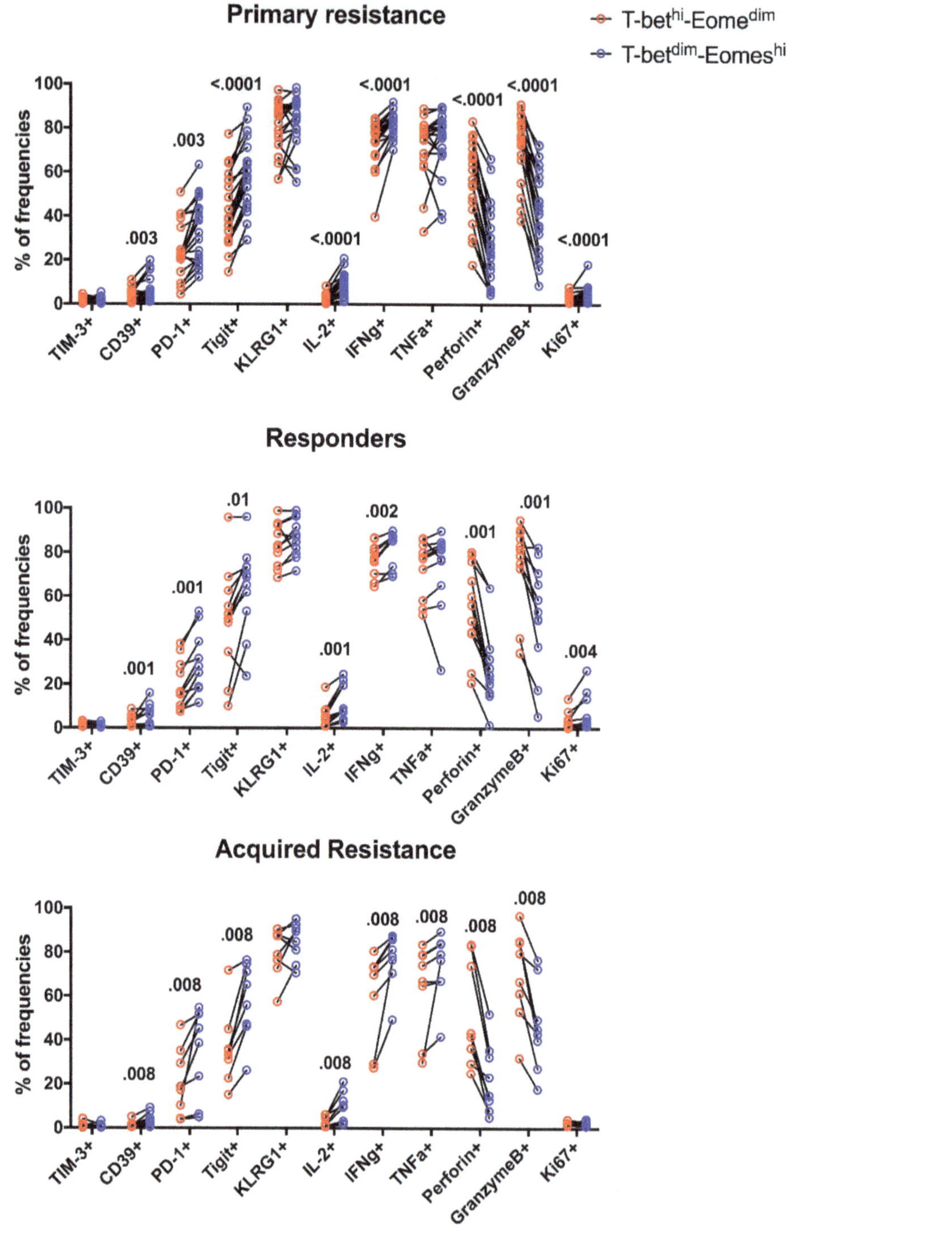

FIGURE 6 | Expression patterns of inhibitory receptors and cytokines on different subsets of CD8 T cells. The frequency of TIM-3, CD39, PD-1, TIGIT, KLRG1, IL-2, IFNγ, TNFα, Perforin, GranzymeB, and Ki-67 expressing cells within total T-bet^{dim}Eomes^{hi} (blue) and T-bet^{hi}Eomes^{dim} (red) CD8 T cells for all baseline samples. Statistical analysis was performed with a Wilcoxon matched-pairs single rank test.

Our results show that examination of different mononuclear populations reveals relatively few differences between patients who responded to treatment compared to non-responders or those failing treatment within 1 year of start of therapy. These differences were largely evident in pre-treatment samples and carried through at the 6 week and 1 year follow up timepoints. Responders had a higher frequency of NK and CD56-expressing T cells, while patients in the primary resistance group had a higher frequency of classical monocytes. Visualization of the same data using t-SNE did not reveal any additional differences

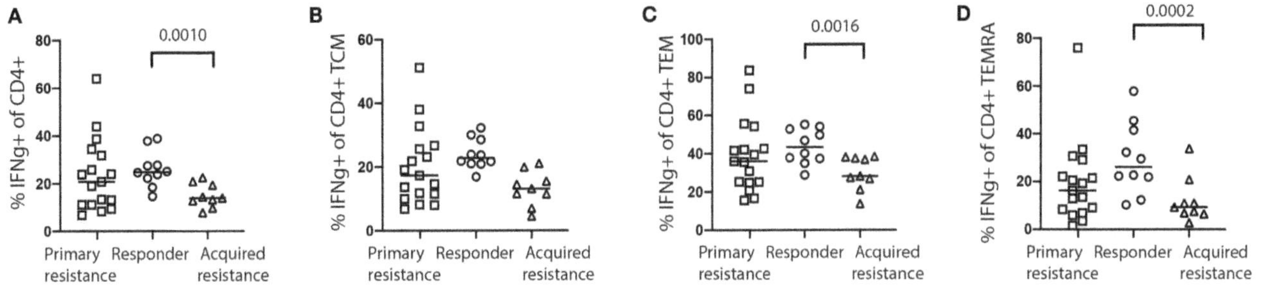

FIGURE 7 | Expression of IFNγ by stimulated baseline samples. **(A)** Comparison of primary resistance, responder, and acquired resistance groups revealed production by a significantly higher proportion of total CD4 T cells within the responder group, compared with the acquired resistance group, however not significant within the CD4 T cell CM compartments **(B)**. The difference was also statistically significant within the CD4 T cell EM **(C)** and TEMRA **(D)** compartments. The statistical differences were analyzed using a Kruskall-Wallis multiple comparisons test.

between the patient groups. A number of previous publications have reported that high circulating monocyte numbers are associated with a worse prognosis (39, 40), although a recent study of PBMCs from melanoma patients reported the opposite finding in patients treated with ICB (29). As in the latter study, we saw no significant differences in numbers of total CD4 or CD8 T cells, or in CD4 or CD8 T cell naïve and memory cell subsets between the groups prior to or during treatment. The responder group had higher IFNγ production in CD4 T cells at baseline, compared with the acquired resistance group. The exhaustion markers CD39, PD-1, TIGIT, TIM-3, and KLRG1 were detected on CD8 and CD4 T cells although TIM-3 was at low levels, consistent with so called progenitor exhausted T cells described by others (24). There were no significant differences in expression of exhaustion markers between the groups prior to treatment. At the 6 week timepoint, PD-1 was downregulated, as expected, and CD39 expression was increased in responder and primary resistance groups. Low patient numbers in the acquired resistance group limited the significance of differences seen at week 6.

It was reasoned that exhaustion markers may be expressed by relatively few T cells recirculating from the tumor, and may be restricted to certain differentiation subsets such as effector memory subsets. Variability of expression of exhaustion markers according to differentiation of T cells is well-described by others (21). In a study on TILs, exhaustion markers were found on central memory cells expressing PD-1 and the transcription factor Tcf1 (34). These cells mediated proliferative responses to immunotherapy and were detected in the blood of melanoma patients briefly in the first week after treatment. Single cell studies in TILs from melanoma patients also found that the dysfunctional T cells were the major proliferative subset, constituted up to ~70% of the TILs, and were separate to cytotoxic subsets (25). Another single cell analysis including mass cytometry of exhausted T cells from patients with viral infections or lung cancers described up to 9 different T cell exhaustion states that could be modified by therapy (21, 41).

In view of these studies we examined the expression of exhaustion markers on naïve, effector memory, central memory and terminally exhausted subsets. As expected, there were differences in expression of the markers in these subsets but importantly these did not differ between the patient groups at baseline or at the 6 week and 1 year treatment timepoints. The question remains whether particular subsets of exhausted cells as described in other diseases such as lung cancer, HIV or other infections may have differed between the subgroups (41) but a wider range interrogation would be needed to examine this.

Previous studies by Sen et al. (20) and Pauken et al. (22) have shown that the differentiation state referred to as T cell exhaustion is associated with epigenetic changes that allow interaction with transcription factors that regulate the differentiation state. Tcf1 appears to be essential in sustaining exhausted T cells and to be associated with expression of PD-1 and LAG-3 (42). A single cell analysis on TILs from 48 melanoma samples also implicated Tcf7 in positive outcomes to therapy (26). In peripheral blood, we found no difference in expression of Tcf7 in patients who did or did not respond to anti-PD-1 therapy. Eomes was identified together with other TFs as being associated with CD8 T cell dysfunction in the study by Li et al. (25). Our study on TFs implicated Eomes in T cell exhaustion in that high Eomes was associated with expression of TIGIT, PD-1, KLRG1, CD39, and Ki-67 whereas the effector molecules perforin and granzyme B were reduced. The low levels of IL-2 and reduced levels of TNFα and IFNγ are consistent with the cytokine levels shown in CD8 T cells. We reasoned that responses to ICB may be associated with T-bet driving Th1 type responses. There was a significant increase in CD4 IFNγ responses in the responders compared to the acquired resistance group, but not the primary resistance group. The reasons for this difference are not known. We examined whether the ratio of T-bet to Eomes in pre-treatment and 6 week samples would be a more sensitive measure of responses, but no differences were seen between the 3 groups. This indicated that high Eomes or T-bet:Eomes ratios could not be used as a guide to responses to ICB treatment. Eomes has been identified by others as being associated with CD8 T cell dysfunction (25). In addition, T-bet^{high}Eomes^{low} CD8 T cells have been identified as an intermediate exhausted CD8^{+} T cell population that could be reinvigorated by checkpoint inhibitors (43, 44). Further work to understand the disparate roles of T-bet and Eomes in regulating T cell function is needed.

The association of the major $CD16^{hi}CD56^{+}$ subset of NK cells with responses to ICB treatment requires further analysis. NK cells are known to express PD-1 and other checkpoint receptors (45) and their cytotoxic activity *in vitro* is increased by PD-1 blockade (46). A study on 25 melanoma patients with metastatic disease reported that patients with higher numbers of intra- and peri-tumoral NK cells had higher response rates than those with lower NK cells (47). Previous studies on 40 patients treated with anti-PD-1 also found that responders had higher numbers of $CD56^{+}CD16^{+}CD69^{+}$ NK cells in pretreatment blood samples after activation *in vitro* (30). That study also found no differences in CD4 or CD8 memory T cell subsets between responders vs. non-responders. These results need to be considered together with the inverse correlation shown between survival and $CD56^{bright}CD16^{lo}$ NK cells in blood of 29 patients with stage III/IV melanoma (48). There is also a long history of relatively low rates of response to adoptive treatment with IL-2 activated lymphokine activated killer cells that included NK cells (49). It remains possible that the $CD56^{bright}CD16^{lo}$ NK cells have an immunoregulatory role that indirectly increases adaptive responses by CD8 T cells, as described by others (50–52).

A subset of CD3 positive cells expressing CD56 was also assessed in the current study. CD56 expression on T cells is known to be associated with potent effector function in human peripheral blood (53). $CD56^{+}$ T cells were present at higher frequency in responders compared to the primary resistance group, and the differences between individuals were maintained throughout ICB therapy.

In conclusion, the intent of these studies was to identify biomarkers in blood that would be readily accessible and useful in planning treatments that may reduce T cell exhaustion states, such as treatment with epigenetic regulators (54). Although they were comprehensive in including a large number of markers associated with T cell exhaustion that had previously been validated by studies on TILs, the panel of exhaustion markers selected for this study did not distinguish patients who responded from those who did not respond to anti-PD-1 treatments. Evolving studies in other cancers and viral infections point to a number of different states of exhaustion/dysfunction that undergo dynamic changes that may not have been captured by the procedures used in this study (41). For example, it is possible that entry into the immunosuppressive tumor microenvironment may induce changes in tumor-specific T cells. In addition, the number of "bystander" T cells in blood may have also made detection of relevant small tumor-specific populations difficult and study of clonally restricted T cells that are also seen in the tumor may have identified a population more relevant to clinical outcomes, but such studies were beyond the scope of this study. Rather similar conclusions were reached in monitoring responses to hepatitis C infections where patients clearing infection had similar high PD-1 levels to those not clearing the infection (55, 56). Pre-treatment levels of NK and $CD56^{+}$ T cells and CD4 T cell IFNγ production did however appear to distinguish responders from non-responders and warrant further study.

ETHICS STATEMENT

Patient samples analyzed in the current study were obtained from The Melanoma Institute Australia biospecimen bank with written informed patient consent and institutional review board approval (Sydney Local Health District Human Research Ethics Committee, Protocol No. X15-0454 and HREC/11/RPAH/444).

AUTHOR CONTRIBUTIONS

MP, HM, BF, and PH conceived the study and served as the primary authors of the paper. MP, HM, AE, H-YT, JT, BF, and PH planned, performed, and analyzed the majority of the studies, prepared the manuscript, figures, and tables. JL, MC, AM, GL, RS, BF, HM, and PH conducted the relevant clinical trials and provided guidance clinical information and manuscript review. All authors read and approved the final manuscript.

ACKNOWLEDGMENTS

The authors would like to thank Ms. Valerie Jakrot and colleagues from Melanoma Institute Australia for assistance with sample collection and supply of patient data. We also would like to thanks all the scientific support staff of Centenary Institute, Sydney Cytometry and the Ramaciotti Facility for Human Systems Biology.

REFERENCES

1. Hersey P, Kakavand H, Wilmott J, van der Westhuizen A, Gallagher S, Gowrishankar K, et al. How anti-PD1 treatments are changing the management of melanoma. *Melanoma Manag.* (2014) 1:165-72. doi: 10.2217/mmt.14.14
2. Topalian SL, Drake CG, Pardoll DM. Immune checkpoint blockade: a common denominator approach to cancer therapy. *Cancer Cell.* (2015) 27:450–61. doi: 10.1016/j.ccell.2015.03.001
3. Robert C, Schachter J, Long GV, Arance A, Grob JJ, Mortier L, et al. Pembrolizumab versus ipilimumab in advanced melanoma. *N Engl J Med.* (2015) 372:2521–32. doi: 10.1056/NEJMoa1503093
4. Ribas A, Hamid O, Daud A, Hodi FS, Wolchok JD, Kefford R, et al. Association of pembrolizumab with tumor response and survival among patients with advanced melanoma. *JAMA.* (2016) 315:1600–9. doi: 10.1001/jama.2016.4059
5. Sharma P, Hu-Lieskovan S, Wargo JA, Ribas A. Primary, adaptive, and acquired resistance to cancer immunotherapy. *Cell.* (2017) 168:707–23. doi: 10.1016/j.cell.2017.01.017
6. Ribas A, Wolchok JD. Cancer immunotherapy using checkpoint blockade. *Science.* (2018) 359:1350–5. doi: 10.1126/science.aar4060
7. Daud AI, Wolchok JD, Robert C, Hwu WJ, Weber JS, Ribas A, et al. Programmed death-ligand 1 expression and response to the anti-programmed death 1 antibody pembrolizumab in melanoma. *J Clin Oncol.* (2016) 34:4102–9. doi: 10.1200/JCO.2016.67.2477
8. Taube JM, Klein A, Brahmer JR, Xu H, Pan X, Kim JH, et al. Association of PD-1, PD-1 ligands, and other features of the tumor immune microenvironment with response to anti-PD-1 therapy. *Clin Cancer Res.* (2014) 20:5064–74. doi: 10.1158/1078-0432.CCR-13-3271
9. Madore J, Strbenac D, Vilain R, Menzies AM, Yang JY, Thompson JF, et al. PD-L1 negative status is associated with lower mutation burden, differential expression of immune-related genes, and worse survival in stage III melanoma. *Clin Cancer Res.* (2016) 22:3915–23. doi: 10.1158/1078-0432.CCR-15-1714
10. Hodi FS, Chiarion-Sileni V, Gonzalez R, Grob JJ, Rutkowski P, Cowey CL, et al. Nivolumab plus ipilimumab or nivolumab alone versus ipilimumab alone in advanced melanoma (CheckMate 067): 4-year outcomes of a multicentre, randomised, phase 3 trial. *Lancet Oncol.* (2018) 19:1480–92. doi: 10.1016/S1470-2045(18)30700-9
11. Teng MW, Khanna R, Smyth MJ. Checkpoint immunotherapy: picking a winner. *Cancer Discov.* (2016) 6:818–20. doi: 10.1158/2159-8290.CD-16-0694
12. Sade-Feldman M, Jiao YJ, Chen JH, Rooney MS, Barzily-Rokni M, Eliane JP, et al. Resistance to checkpoint blockade therapy through inactivation of antigen presentation. *Nat Commun.* (2017) 8:1136. doi: 10.1038/s41467-017-01062-w
13. Rooney MS, Shukla SA, Wu CJ, Getz G, Hacohen N. Molecular and genetic properties of tumors associated with local immune cytolytic activity. *Cell.* (2015) 160:48-61. doi: 10.1016/j.cell.2014.12.033
14. Patel SJ, Sanjana NE, Kishton RJ, Eidizadeh A, Vodnala SK, Cam M, et al. Identification of essential genes for cancer immunotherapy. *Nature.* (2017) 548:537–42. doi: 10.1038/nature23477
15. Manguso RT, Pope HW, Zimmer MD, Brown FD, Yates KB, Miller BC, et al. *In vivo* CRISPR screening identifies Ptpn2 as a cancer immunotherapy target. *Nature.* (2017) 547:413–8. doi: 10.1038/nature23270
16. Jerby-Arnon L, Shah P, Cuoco MS, Rodman C, Su MJ, Melms JC, et al. A cancer cell program promotes T cell exclusion and resistance to checkpoint blockade. *Cell.* (2018) 175:984–97.e24. doi: 10.1016/j.cell.2018.09.006
17. Hugo W, Shi H, Sun L, Piva M, Song C, Kong X, et al. Non-genomic and immune evolution of melanoma acquiring MAPKi resistance. *Cell.* (2015) 162:1271. doi: 10.1016/j.cell.2015.07.061
18. Wherry EJ, Kurachi M. Molecular and cellular insights into T cell exhaustion. *Nat Rev Immunol.* (2015) 15:486–99. doi: 10.1038/nri3862
19. Amezquita RA, Kaech SM. Immunology: the chronicles of T-cell exhaustion. *Nature.* (2017) 543:190–1. doi: 10.1038/nature21508
20. Sen DR, Kaminski J, Barnitz RA, Kurachi M, Gerdemann U, Yates KB, et al. The epigenetic landscape of T cell exhaustion. *Science.* (2016) 354:1165–9. doi: 10.1126/science.aae0491
21. Legat A, Speiser DE, Pircher H, Zehn D, Fuertes Marraco SA. Inhibitory receptor expression depends more dominantly on differentiation and activation than "exhaustion" of human CD8 T cells. *Front Immunol.* (2013) 4:455. doi: 10.3389/fimmu.2013.00455
22. Pauken KE, Sammons MA, Odorizzi PM, Manne S, Godec J, Khan O, et al. Epigenetic stability of exhausted T cells limits durability of reinvigoration by PD-1 blockade. *Science.* (2016) 354:1160–5. doi: 10.1126/science.aaf2807
23. Philip M, Fairchild L, Sun L, Horste EL, Camara S, Shakiba M, et al. Chromatin states define tumour-specific T cell dysfunction and reprogramming. *Nature.* (2017) 545:452–6. doi: 10.1038/nature22367
24. Miller BC, Sen DR, Al Abosy R, Bi K, Virkud YV, LaFleur MW, et al. Subsets of exhausted CD8(+) T cells differentially mediate tumor control and respond to checkpoint blockade. *Nat Immunol.* (2019) 20:326–36. doi: 10.1038/s41590-019-0312-6
25. Li H, van der Leun AM, Yofe I, Lubling Y, Gelbard-Solodkin D, van Akkooi ACJ, et al. Dysfunctional CD8 T cells form a proliferative, dynamically regulated compartment within human melanoma. *Cell.* (2019) 176:775–89.e18. doi: 10.1016/j.cell.2018.11.043
26. Sade-Feldman M, Yizhak K, Bjorgaard SL, Ray JP, de Boer CG, Jenkins RW, et al. Defining T cell states associated with response to checkpoint immunotherapy in melanoma. *Cell.* (2018) 175:998–1013 e20. doi: 10.1016/j.cell.2018.10.038
27. Jiang P, Gu S, Pan D, Fu J, Sahu A, Hu X, et al. Signatures of T cell dysfunction and exclusion predict cancer immunotherapy response. *Nat Med.* (2018) 24:1550–8. doi: 10.1038/s41591-018-0136-1
28. Huang AC, Postow MA, Orlowski RJ, Mick R, Bengsch B, Manne S, et al. T-cell invigoration to tumour burden ratio associated with anti-PD-1 response. *Nature.* (2017) 545:60–5. doi: 10.1038/nature22079
29. Krieg C, Nowicka M, Guglietta S, Schindler S, Hartmann FJ, Weber LM, et al. High-dimensional single-cell analysis predicts response to anti-PD-1 immunotherapy. *Nat Med.* (2018) 24:144–53. doi: 10.1038/nm.4466
30. Subrahmanyam PB, Dong Z, Gusenleitner D, Giobbie-Hurder A, Severgnini M, Zhou J, et al. Distinct predictive biomarker candidates for response to anti-CTLA-4 and anti-PD-1 immunotherapy in melanoma patients. *J Immunother Cancer.* (2018) 6:18. doi: 10.1186/s40425-018-0328-8
31. Wistuba-Hamprecht K, Martens A, Weide B, Teng KW, Zelba H, Guffart E, et al. Establishing high dimensional immune signatures from peripheral blood via mass cytometry in a discovery cohort of stage IV melanoma patients. *J Immunol.* (2017) 198:927–36. doi: 10.4049/jimmunol.1600875
32. Eisenhauer EA. Response evaluation: beyond RECIST. *Ann Oncol.* (2007) 18(Suppl. 9):ix29-32. doi: 10.1093/annonc/mdm290
33. Norton SE, Ward-Hartstonge KA, McCall JL, Leman JKH, Taylor ES, Munro F, et al. High-dimensional mass cytometric analysis reveals an increase in effector regulatory T cells as a distinguishing feature of colorectal tumors. *J Immunol.* (2019) 202:1871–84. doi: 10.4049/jimmunol.1801368
34. Siddiqui I, Schaeuble K, Chennupati V, Fuertes Marraco SA, Calderon-Copete S, Pais Ferreira D, et al. Intratumoral Tcf1(+)PD-1(+)CD8(+) T cells with stem-like properties promote tumor control in response to vaccination and checkpoint blockade immunotherapy. *Immunity.* (2019) 50:195–211.e10. doi: 10.1016/j.immuni.2018.12.021
35. Scott AC, Dundar F, Zumbo P, Chandran SS, Klebanoff CA, Shakiba M, et al. TOX is a critical regulator of tumour-specific T cell differentiation. *Nature.* (2019) 571:270–4. doi: 10.1038/s41586-019-1324-y
36. Mahnke YD, Brodie TM, Sallusto F, Roederer M, Lugli E. The who's who of T-cell differentiation: human memory T-cell subsets. *Eur J Immunol.* (2013) 43:2797–809. doi: 10.1002/eji.201343751
37. Kallies A, Good-Jacobson KL. Transcription factor T-bet orchestrates lineage development and function in the immune system. *Trends Immunol.* (2017) 38:287–97. doi: 10.1016/j.it.2017.02.003
38. Pearce EL, Mullen AC, Martins GA, Krawczyk CM, Hutchins AS, Zediak VP, et al. Control of effector CD8+ T cell function by the transcription factor Eomesodermin. *Science.* (2003) 302:1041–3. doi: 10.1126/science.1090148
39. Schmidt H, Bastholt L, Geertsen P, Christensen IJ, Larsen S, Gehl J, et al. Elevated neutrophil and monocyte counts in peripheral blood are associated with poor survival in patients with metastatic melanoma: a prognostic model. *Br J Cancer.* (2005) 93:273–8. doi: 10.1038/sj.bjc.6602702
40. Failing JJ, Yan Y, Porrata LF, Markovic SN. Lymphocyte-to-monocyte ratio is associated with survival in pembrolizumab-treated metastatic melanoma patients. *Melanoma Res.* (2017) 27:596–600. doi: 10.1097/CMR.0000000000000404

41. Bengsch B, Ohtani T, Khan O, Setty M, Manne S, O'Brien S, et al. Epigenomic-guided mass cytometry profiling reveals disease-specific features of exhausted CD8 T cells. *Immunity.* (2018) 48:1029–45 e5. doi: 10.1016/j.immuni.2018.04.026
42. Utzschneider DT, Charmoy M, Chennupati V, Pousse L, Ferreira DP, Calderon-Copete S, et al. T cell factor 1-expressing memory-like CD8(+) T cells sustain the immune response to chronic viral infections. *Immunity.* (2016) 45:415–27. doi: 10.1016/j.immuni.2016.07.021
43. Paley MA, Kroy DC, Odorizzi PM, Johnnidis JB, Dolfi DV, Barnett BE, et al. Progenitor and terminal subsets of CD8+ T cells cooperate to contain chronic viral infection. *Science.* (2012) 338:1220–5. doi: 10.1126/science.1229620
44. Gide TN, Quek C, Menzies AM, Tasker AT, Shang P, Holst J, et al. Distinct immune cell populations define response to anti-PD-1 monotherapy and Anti-PD-1/Anti-CTLA-4 combined therapy. *Cancer Cell.* (2019) 35:238–55.e6. doi: 10.1016/j.ccell.2019.01.003
45. Beldi-Ferchiou A, Caillat-Zucman S. Control of NK cell activation by immune checkpoint molecules. *Int J Mol Sci.* (2017) 18:E2129. doi: 10.3390/ijms18102129
46. Hsu J, Hodgins JJ, Marathe M, Nicolai CJ, Bourgeois-Daigneault MC, Trevino TN, et al. Contribution of NK cells to immunotherapy mediated by PD-1/PD-L1 blockade. *J Clin Invest.* (2018) 128:4654–68. doi: 10.1172/JCI 99317
47. Lee H, Quek C, Silva I, Tasker A, Batten M, Rizos H, et al. Integrated molecular and immunophenotypic analysis of NK cells in anti-PD-1 treated metastatic melanoma patients. *Oncoimmunology.* (2019) 8:e1537581. doi: 10.1080/2162402X.2018.1537581
48. de Jonge K, Ebering A, Nassiri S, Maby-El Hajjami H, Ouertatani-Sakouhi H, Baumgaertner P, et al. Circulating CD56(bright) NK cells inversely correlate with survival of melanoma patients. *Sci Rep.* (2019) 9:4487. doi: 10.1038/s41598-019-40933-8
49. Rosenberg SA, Lotze MT, Yang JC, Topalian SL, Chang AE, Schwartzentruber DJ, et al. Prospective randomized trial of high-dose interleukin-2 alone or in conjunction with lymphokine-activated killer cells for the treatment of patients with advanced cancer. *J Natl Cancer Inst.* (1993) 85:622–32. doi: 10.1093/jnci/85.8.622
50. Vujanovic L, Chuckran C, Lin Y, Ding F, Sander CA, Santos PM, et al. CD56(dim) CD16(-) natural killer cell profiling in melanoma patients receiving a cancer vaccine and interferon-alpha. *Front Immunol.* (2019) 10:14. doi: 10.3389/fimmu.2019.00014
51. Tosello-Trampont A, Surette FA, Ewald SE, Hahn YS. Immunoregulatory role of NK cells in tissue inflammation and regeneration. *Front Immunol.* (2017) 8:301. doi: 10.3389/fimmu.2017.00301
52. Morandi B, Mortara L, Carrega P, Cantoni C, Costa G, Accolla RS, et al. NK cells provide helper signal for CD8+ T cells by inducing the expression of membrane-bound IL-15 on DCs. *Int Immunol.* (2009) 21:599–606. doi: 10.1093/intimm/dxp029
53. Guia S, Cognet C, de Beaucoudrey L, Tessmer MS, Jouanguy E, Berger C, et al. A role for interleukin-12/23 in the maturation of human natural killer and CD56+ T cells *in vivo. Blood.* (2008) 111:5008–16. doi: 10.1182/blood-2007-11-122259
54. Zhang F, Zhou X, DiSpirito JR, Wang C, Wang Y, Shen H. Epigenetic manipulation restores functions of defective CD8(+) T cells from chronic viral infection. *Mol Ther.* (2014) 22:1698–706. doi: 10.1038/mt.2 014.91
55. Kasprowicz V, Schulze Zur Wiesch J, Kuntzen T, Nolan BE, Longworth S, Berical A, et al. High level of PD-1 expression on hepatitis C virus (HCV)-specific CD8+ and CD4+ T cells during acute HCV infection, irrespective of clinical outcome. *J Virol.* (2008) 82:3154–60. doi: 10.1128/JVI.02474-07
56. Wieland D, Hofmann M, Thimme R. Overcoming CD8+ T-cell exhaustion in viral hepatitis: lessons from the mouse model and clinical perspectives. *Dig Dis.* (2017) 35:334–8. doi: 10.1159/000456584

3

Pregnancy-Induced Alterations in NK Cell Phenotype and Function

Mathieu Le Gars[1,2*], *Christof Seiler*[3], *Alexander W. Kay*[4], *Nicholas L. Bayless*[2], *Elina Starosvetsky*[5], *Lindsay Moore*[5], *Shai S. Shen-Orr*[5], *Natali Aziz*[6], *Purvesh Khatri*[1], *Cornelia L. Dekker*[3], *Gary E. Swan*[6], *Mark M. Davis*[7,8], *Susan Holmes*[4] and *Catherine A. Blish*[1,2,9*]

[1] Department of Medicine, Stanford University, Palo Alto, CA, United States, [2] Department of Stanford Immunology Program, Stanford University, Palo Alto, CA, United States, [3] Department of Statistics, Stanford University, Palo Alto, CA, United States, [4] Department of Pediatrics, Stanford University, Palo Alto, CA, United States, [5] Faculty of Medicine, Technion - Israel Institute of Technology, Haifa, Israel, [6] Department of Obstetrics and Gynecology, Stanford Prevention Research Center, Stanford University School of Medicine, Stanford University, Palo Alto, CA, United States, [7] Department of Microbiology and Immunology, Stanford University, Palo Alto, CA, United States, [8] Howard Hughes Medical Institute, Stanford University School of Medicine, Stanford, CA, United States, [9] Chan Zuckerberg Biohub, San Francisco, CA, United States

***Correspondence:**
Mathieu Le Gars
cblish@stanford.edu
Catherine A. Blish
mathieu.legars1@gmail.com

Pregnant women are particularly susceptible to complications of influenza A virus infection, which may result from pregnancy-induced changes in the function of immune cells, including natural killer (NK) cells. To better understand NK cell function during pregnancy, we assessed the ability of the two main subsets of NK cells, CD56^{dim}, and CD56^{bright} NK cells, to respond to influenza-virus infected cells and tumor cells. During pregnancy, CD56^{dim} and CD56^{bright} NK cells displayed enhanced functional responses to both infected and tumor cells, with increased expression of degranulation markers and elevated frequency of NK cells producing IFN-γ. To better understand the mechanisms driving this enhanced function, we profiled CD56^{dim} and CD56^{bright} NK cells from pregnant and non-pregnant women using mass cytometry. NK cells from pregnant women displayed significantly increased expression of several functional and activation markers such as CD38 on both subsets and NKp46 on CD56^{dim} NK cells. NK cells also displayed diminished expression of the chemokine receptor CXCR3 during pregnancy. Overall, these data demonstrate that functional and phenotypic shifts occur in NK cells during pregnancy that can influence the magnitude of the immune response to both infections and tumors.

Keywords: NK cells, pregnancy, influenza virus, cancer cells, NK repertoire

INTRODUCTION

During pregnancy, the immune system has to finely balance its activity in order to tolerate the semi-allogeneic fetus, while maintaining the ability to fight microbial challenges (1–4). These immune alterations may be at least partially responsible for the increased susceptibility of pregnant women to complications from influenza virus infection (5–9). Recent studies have demonstrated enhanced responses to influenza virus by several innate immune cell subsets during pregnancy, including monocytes, plasmacytoid dendritic cells and natural killer (NK) cells (2, 10–14). It remains unclear whether such changes could contribute to the enhanced pathogenesis of influenza virus during pregnancy because the role of NK cells in the pathogenesis of influenza virus remains controversial. Several mouse studies have shown that NK cell depletion or the use of mice deficient in NK cells improved the outcome of influenza infection (15, 16), suggesting that NK cell activity may be pathogenic in the setting of influenza infection. On the contrary, NK cells reduced influenza virus burden and promoted clearance of the virus in mice deficient in NKp46, a major NK cell receptor thought to play a role in influenza recognition (17), suggesting that NK cells may contribute to protection from influenza. Controversy remains as another mouse strain deficient in NKp46 expression is resistant to viral infection (18). In humans, NK cells were found in abundance in the lungs of fatally infected patients with the 2009 H1N1 pandemic strain of influenza virus (19). This NK cell recruitment correlated with severity of lung inflammation and poor patient outcome, but the causality in the relation between infiltration of NK cells and viral clearance and pathogenesis is unproven.

NK cells mediate their response to influenza and other pathogens using an array of germline receptors. Inhibitory receptors serve to protect healthy cells from NK cells and include the killer-cell immunoglobulin-like receptors (KIRs) and the heterodimer NKG2A-CD94. NK cell activating receptors signal 'altered self' and include NKp46, NKp30, NKp44, NKG2C, and NKG2D, among others. Together, the activating and inhibitory receptors define the degree of NK cell maturation and responsiveness to stimuli (20, 21). In response to virus-infected or cancerous cells, NK cells can kill cells via release of cytolytic molecules or through engagement of death receptors. They can also produce cytokines, such as IFN-γ, which limit viral replication and tumor proliferation (21). $CD56^{dim}$ and $CD56^{bright}$ NK cells are two major NK cell subsets identified in the peripheral blood that tend to differ in their responsiveness. $CD56^{dim}$ NK cells are more cytotoxic and $CD56^{bright}$ are better at secreting cytokines (22, 23). Due to their robust cytotoxic capabilities and immune regulatory potential, NK cell activation is tightly regulated to limit tissue damage at the site of infection. Here, we sought to better understand how NK cell activity is regulated during pregnancy and gain insight into the unusual susceptibility of pregnant women to complications from influenza virus and other infections. We used mass cytometry and *ex vivo* influenza infection to profile the expression of NK cell activating and inhibitory receptors during this critical period of development.

MATERIALS AND METHODS

Study Design

Pregnant women in their second and third trimester and control non-pregnant women were enrolled in two cohorts in separate years. In the discovery cohort, twenty-one healthy pregnant women were recruited between October 2013 and March 2014 from the Obstetrics Clinic at Lucile Packard Children's Hospital at Stanford University. Twenty-one non-pregnant (control) women were recruited for Stanford influenza vaccine studies (NCT numbers: NCT03020537, NCT03022422, and NCT02141581). In the validation cohort, 32 non-pregnant (control) women were recruited for Stanford vaccine studies (NCT numbers: NCT01827462 and NCT03022422) and 21 healthy pregnant women were recruited between October 2012 and March 2013 from the Obstetrics Clinic at Lucile Packard Children's Hospital at Stanford. Venous blood was collected from all participants at baseline; pregnant women also provided a sample at 6 weeks post-partum. Exclusion criteria included concomitant illnesses, immunosuppressive medications, or receipt of blood products within the previous year. Pregnant women were also excluded for known fetal abnormalities and morbid obesity (pre-pregnancy body mass index >40). This study was performed in accordance with the Declaration of Helsinki and approved by the Stanford University Institutional Review Board (IRB-25182); written informed consent was obtained from all participants. Blood from anonymous healthy donors at the Stanford blood bank center was obtained for confirmatory functional assays.

PBMC Isolation, Cryopreservation, and Cell Purification for Functional Assays

PBMCs from healthy donors were isolated from whole blood by Ficoll-Paque (GE Healthcare) and cryopreserved in 90% fetal bovine serum (Thermo Scientific)/10% dimethyl sulfoxide (Sigma-Aldrich). Cryopreserved PBMCs were thawed and washed with complete RP10 media [RPMI 1640 (Invitrogen) supplemented with 10% fetal bovine serum (FBS), 2 mM L-glutamine, 100 U/ml penicillin, 100 mg/ml streptomycin (Life Technologies)] and 50 U/mL benzonase (EMD Millipore). NK cells and/or monocytes were sorted using Sony sorter SH800 (Sony) with the following antibodies: CD3-Allophycocyanine (clone OKT3; BioLegend), CD14-Brilliant Violet 421 (clone HCD14; BioLegend), CD19-Alexa Fluor 488 (clone HIB19; Biolegend), and CD56-Phycoerythrin Cyanine 7 (clone NCAM; BioLegend).

NK Cell: Infected Monocyte Co-culture

A/California/7/2009 influenza (pH1N1) wild-type influenza A virus obtained from Kanta Subbarao at the National Institutes of Health was propagated in embryonated chicken eggs. Monocytes were washed and re-suspended in serum-free RPMI media at 1×10^5 per 100 μL and infected at a multiplicity of infection (MOI) of 3 for 1 h at 37°C with 5% carbon dioxide. One-hour post-infection, viral inoculum was removed and cells were resuspended in 100 μL of complete RP10. Autologous NK cells were then exposed to pH1N1-infected monocytes at a effector:target (E:T) ratio 1:1. After a further 2-h incubation, 2 μM monensin, 3 μg/mL brefeldin A (eBiosciences), and anti-CD107a-allophycocyanin-H7 (BD Pharmingen) were added to the co-culture for 4 h, followed by cell staining for flow cytometry analysis.

K562 Cell Assay

Following purification, NK cells were exposed to K562 tumor cells (ATCC) at an effector:target (E:T) ratio of 1:1. Immediately following co-incubation, 2 μM monensin, 3 μg/mL brefeldin A, and anti-CD107a-allophycocyanin-H7 were added to the co-culture for 4 h, followed by cell staining for flow cytometry analysis.

Cell Staining and Flow-Cytometry Analysis

Cells were stained with LIVE/DEAD fixable Aqua Stain (Life Technologies), followed by surface staining and then fixed and permeabilized with FACS Lyse and FACS Perm II (BD Pharmingen) according to the manufacturer's instructions. Cells were stained with anti-CD3-PE or -APC, anti-CD16-PerCPCy5.5 (clone 3G8; BioLegend), anti-IFNγ-FITC or V450 (clone B27; BD Biosciences), anti-CD56-PEcy7, or anti-CD14-APC or -APC-H7 and fixed using 1% paraformaldehyde. Uncompensated data were collected using a three-laser MACSQuant® Analyser (Miltenyi). Analysis and compensation were performed using FlowJo flow-cytometric analysis software, version 9.9.4 (Tree Star).

Antibody Labeling for CyTOF

Purified antibodies (lacking carrier proteins) were labeled 100 μg at a time according to instructions provided by DVS Sciences with heavy metal-preloaded maleimide-coupled MAXPAR chelating polymers and as previously described (24, 25). Qdot antibodies purchased from Invitrogen were used for Cd112 and were not conjugated. In115, Gd155, and Gd157 were ordered from Trace Sciences and conjugated with exactly as with metals purchased from DVS Sciences. Following labeling, antibodies were diluted in PBS to a concentration between 0.1 and 0.3 mg/mL. Each antibody clone and lot was titrated to optimal staining concentrations using cell lines and primary human samples. The gating shown in **Figures S2, S4, S6, S8** displays one individual as an example. Gates were set based on both positive and negative controls known to express markers, and all stains were validated by comparison to conventional flow cytometry, as described in our prior studies (20, 26). Cell subsets known to not express markers were used as negative controls in many cases (for instance, B cells do not express many NK cell markers). For some stains such as NKG2C, as new antibody conjugations and panels were used for the second cohort, the gating strategy modified if better ability to distinguish populations was possible. Gating was not used as part of the GLM analysis.

PBMC Staining for CyTOF Acquisition

Cryopreserved PBMCs from non-pregnant and pregnant women in discovery and validation cohort were thawed and cells were transferred to 96-well deep-well-plates, resuspended in 25 μM cisplatin (Enzo Life Sciences) for 1 min and quenched with 100% serum. Cells were stained for 30 min, fixed (BD FACS Lyse), permeabilized (BD FACS Perm II), and stained with intracellular antibodies for 45 min on ice. Staining panels are described in **Tables S3, S4**. All antibodies were conjugated using MaxPar X8 labeling kits (DVS Sciences). Cells were suspended overnight in iridium intercalator (DVS Sciences) in 2% paraformaldehyde in phosphate-buffered saline (PBS) and washed 1× in PBS and 2× in H_2O immediately before acquisition on a CyTOF-1 (Fluidigm).

Modeling of Predictors of Pregnancy in Mass Cytometry Data

To identify markers that were consistently changed during pregnancy, we used a generalized linear model (GLM) with bootstrap resampling to account for the donor-specific heterogeneity. We implemented the GLM approach and other regression models in an open source R package *CytoGLMM* (27) available here: https://christofseiler.github.io/CytoGLMM/.

Statistical Analysis

Linear discriminant analyses were implemented in R using the package MASS (28, 29). Statistical analyses for functional experiments were performed using GraphPad Prism, version 6.0d (GraphPad Software). A Mann-Whitney U-test was used to compare control to pregnant women and a Wilcoxon signed-rank was used to compare the paired data in women between pregnancy and the post-partum period.

Data Availability

Mass cytometry data supporting this publication is available at ImmPort (https://www.immport.org) under study accession SDY1537.

RESULTS

NK Cell Immune Response to Influenza Virus During Pregnancy

To investigate how pregnancy alters NK cell phenotype and function, we recruited two cohorts of pregnant and non-pregnant (control) women in subsequent years (**Tables S1, S2**). We assessed NK cell antiviral function during pregnancy by flow cytometry after exposing sorted NK cells to autologous infected monocytes [**Figure 1A**; (12, 30)]. We observed that the frequency of $CD56^{dim}$ NK cells expressing CD107a, a marker of cytolytic activity, and IFN-γ was significantly greater in pregnant women than in controls or in post-partum women (**Figures 1B,C** and **Figure S1A**). Similarly, the frequency of $CD56^{bright}$ NK cells expressing CD107a and IFN-γ was also significantly greater during pregnancy than in controls and post-partum (**Figures 1D,E** and **Figure S1A**). Bulk NK cells from pregnant women displayed enhanced killing of influenza-infected monocytes (**Figure 1F** and **Figure S1B**). These data demonstrate that the two major NK cell subsets have enhanced responses to influenza-virus infected cells during pregnancy.

NK Cell Immune Response to Cancer Cells During Pregnancy

During pregnancy, monocytes respond more robustly to influenza virus (11) which could activate NK cells through inflammatory cytokine production, potentially explaining enhanced NK cell responses. We hypothesized that if NK cell function was intrinsically elevated during pregnancy, we should observe enhanced anti-tumor responses as well. We therefore exposed sorted total NK cells from controls and pregnant women to the K562 tumor cell line (**Figure 1A**), which represents a homogenous, identical target for NK cells from controls and pregnant women. $CD56^{dim}$ NK cells from pregnant women had 1.6-fold greater expression of CD107a than $CD56^{dim}$ NK cells from non-pregnant women in response to K562 cells (**Figure 1G** and **Figure S1C**), though IFN-γ responses were not significantly different (**Figure 1H** and **Figure S1C**). $CD56^{bright}$ NK cells also displayed enhanced degranulation (**Figure 1I** and **Figure S1C**) but no difference in IFN-γ production (**Figure 1J**

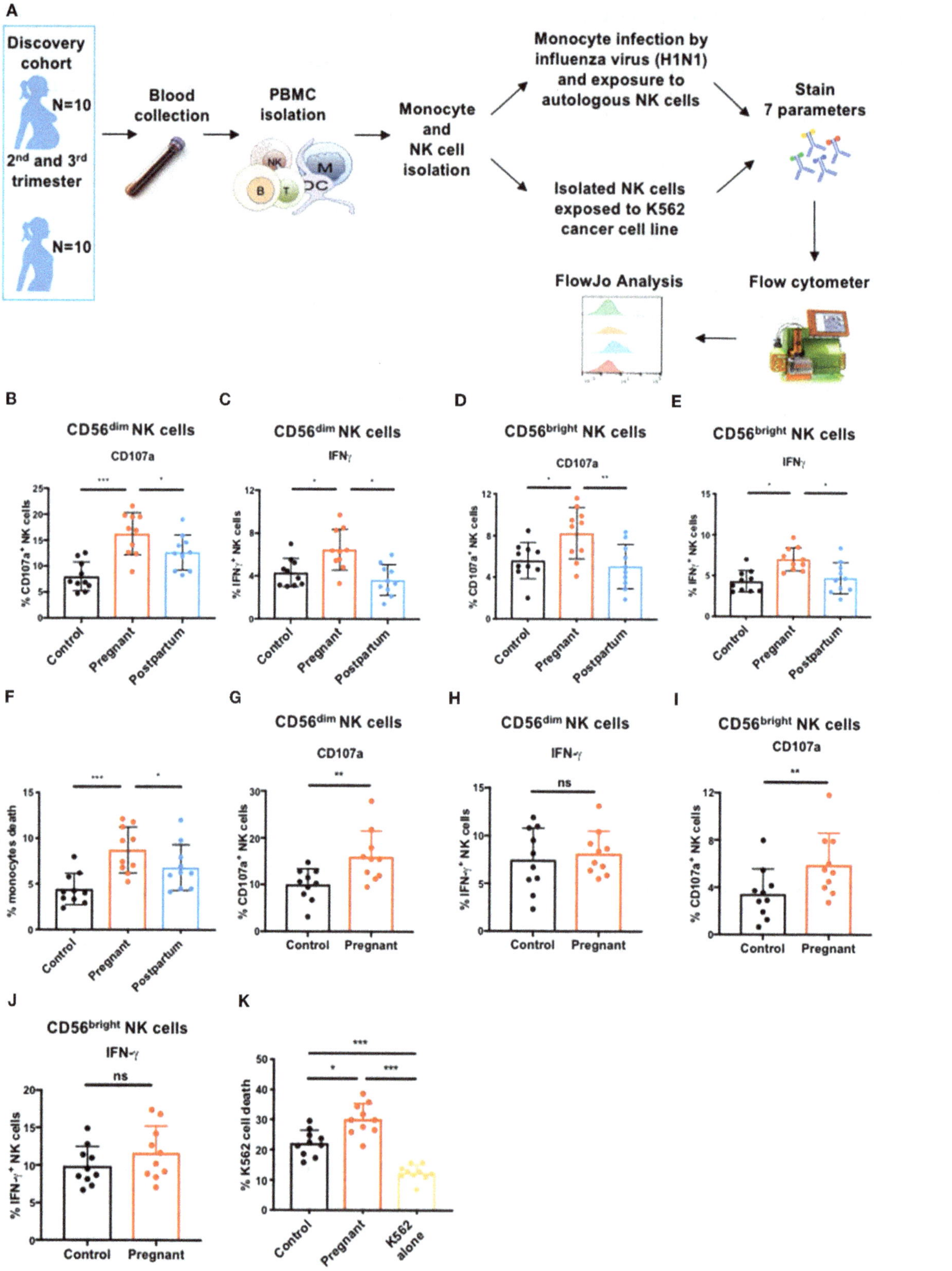

FIGURE 1 | CD56^{dim} and CD56^{bright} NK cell immune response to influenza infected and tumor cells during pregnancy. **(A)** PBMCs from controls ($N = 10$), pregnant women ($N = 10$), and post-partum women ($N = 10$) in discovery cohort were isolated from blood samples. Monocytes and total NK cells were sorted and monocytes

(Continued)

FIGURE 1 | were infected with the H1N1 influenza virus strain. NK cells were either exposed to H1N1-infected monocytes or to K562 tumor cells for 7 or 4 h, respectively. **(B–I)** CD56^{dim} and CD56^{bright} NK cell immune response was then determined by flow cytometry. The frequency of **(B)** CD107a- and **(C)** IFN-γ-expressing CD56^{dim} NK cells in response to influenza-infected monocytes is represented. The frequency of **(D)** CD107a- and **(E)** IFN-γ-expressing CD56^{bright} NK cells in response to influenza-infected monocytes is represented. **(F)** The frequency of dead or dying monocytes based on staining with viability dye in NK cell co-culture. The frequency of CD107a **(G)** and IFN-γ-production **(H)** by CD56^{dim} NK cells in response to K562 cells is represented. The frequency of CD107a **(I)** and IFN-γ-production **(J)** by CD56^{bright} NK cells in response to K562 cells. **(K)** The frequency of dead or dying K562 tumor cells based on staining with viability dye in NK cell co-culture. $^{*}P < 0.05$, $^{**}P < 0.01$, and $^{***}P < 0.001$ (Mann–Whitney *U*-Tests to compare controls vs. pregnant; Wilcoxon matched-paired test to compare pregnant vs. post-partum).

and **Figure S1C**). This increased degranulation by both NK cell subsets from pregnant women resulted in enhanced killing of K562 cells by bulk NK cells (**Figure 1K** and **Figure S1D**). These data indicate that NK cells have an intrinsically enhanced ability to kill both infected and tumor targets during pregnancy.

Deep Profiling of CD56^{dim} and CD56^{bright} NK Cells During Pregnancy in the Discovery Cohort

To understand potential drivers of this enhanced NK cell function during pregnancy, we profiled the expression patterns of inhibitory and activating surface receptors on NK cells in control non-pregnant women, pregnant women, and post-partum women (including the 10 individuals per group tested in **Figure 1**). PBMCs in both cohorts were evaluated by mass cytometry as outlined in **Figure 2A** and **Tables S3, S4**. NK cells were identified as CD3^{-} CD19^{-}CD20^{-}CD14^{-}CD56$^{dim/bright}$CD16$^{+/-}$ cells (**Figure S2A**). The frequency of NK cells did not significantly differ between pregnant and control women, nor in pregnant vs. post-partum women in either cohort (**Figures S2B,C**). To identify NK cell markers predictive of pregnancy, we used a Generalized Linear Model (GLM) with bootstrap resampling to account for correlations between cells and inter-individual variability [**Figure 2A**; (27)].

Expression of several markers such as CD38, NKp46, PD-1, and CD27 were predictive of pregnancy on CD56^{dim} NK cells, while NKp30 was more likely to predict control (**Figure 2B**). When comparing the same women during pregnancy and post-partum, CD38, NKp46, NKG2C, NKG2D, and NKp44 were predictive of pregnancy on CD56^{dim} NK cells (**Figure 2C**). Manual gating confirmed elevated expression of CD38 and NKp46 on CD56^{dim} NK cells during pregnancy (**Figures S3, S4**). To further define the markers that distinguish pregnancy, a linear discriminant analysis (LDA) was performed, revealing that CD38 and NKp46 best separate the CD56^{dim} NK cell population of pregnant women from that of control and post-partum women (**Figure 2D**). Together, our data indicate that there are differences in NK receptor expression patterns during pregnancy, and that CD38 and NKp46 expression are major drivers of these pregnancy-related changes.

As CD56^{bright} NK cells differ from CD56^{dim} NK cells in their maturation and receptor expression patterns, we analyzed them separately. CD38 and NKp46 expression levels are also predictive of pregnancy on CD56^{bright} NK cells, as is the inhibitory receptor NKG2A, which is highly expressed on CD56^{bright} NK cells (**Figure 2E** and **Figures S5, S6**). Expression of the chemokine receptor, CXCR3, and activating receptor, NKp44, were associated with non-pregnant state. Similar differences were seen when comparing pregnant and post-partum samples (**Figure 2F** and **Figures S5, S6**). LDA reveals that CD38, NKp46, NKG2A, and NKG2D best separate CD56^{bright} NK cells of pregnant women from that of control and post-partum women (**Figure 2G**). Together, these data suggest that during pregnancy, both CD56^{dim} and CD56^{bright} NK cell subsets have the potential for greater activation through an increased expression of CD38 and NKp46.

Deep Profiling of CD56^{dim} and CD56^{bright} NK Cells in the Validation Cohort

We performed a deeper profiling of NK cells in the validation cohort, using an antibody panel including an increased number of specific NK cell receptors such as KIRs (**Figure 2A** and **Table S4**). Similar to the discovery cohort, CD38 and NKp46 are predictive of pregnancy on CD56^{dim} NK cells compared to controls (**Figure 3A**). CD56^{dim} NK cells from pregnant women also display an increased expression of NKG2C, LILRB1, and KIR2DL3 compared to control, while NKG2D and CD11b expression predicted control. CD38, NKG2A, and CD244 expression are also predictive of pregnancy when compared with post-partum conditions, while several markers including KIRs predicted the post-partum state (**Figure 3B**). NKp46 predicted the post-partum state among CD56^{dim} NK cells in the validation cohort (**Figure 3B**). Manual gating confirmed the results of the GLM for this cohort (**Figures S7, S8**). LDA performed on these data showed that CD38 and NKG2A best explained the separation between CD56^{dim} NK cells from pregnant women with controls and post-partum in the validation cohort (**Figure 3C**).

For CD56^{bright} NK cells, CD11b, CD38, LILRB1, CD25, KIR2DL3, NKG2A, and NKG2C are predictive of pregnancy, while several markers predict the post-partum state (**Figures 3D,E**). These data were confirmed by manual gating (**Figures S9, S10**). LDA separation showed that CD38, NKp30, CD94, and CD244 most contribute to the separation of CD56^{bright} NK cells from pregnant women compared to controls and post-partum (**Figure 3F**). Several markers differed in their predictions between the discovery and validation cohorts. For instance, NKG2C was predictive of pregnancy in comparison to control among both CD56^{dim} and CD56^{bright} NK cells in the validation cohort, but not in the discovery cohort. This raises the possibility that there are differences in CMV status between cohorts driving the effect. Unfortunately, CMV serologies were not available; however, there were no significant differences in the frequency of "adaptive" NKG2C^{+}CD57^{+} NK cells between the control, pregnant, or post-partum women in either cohort,

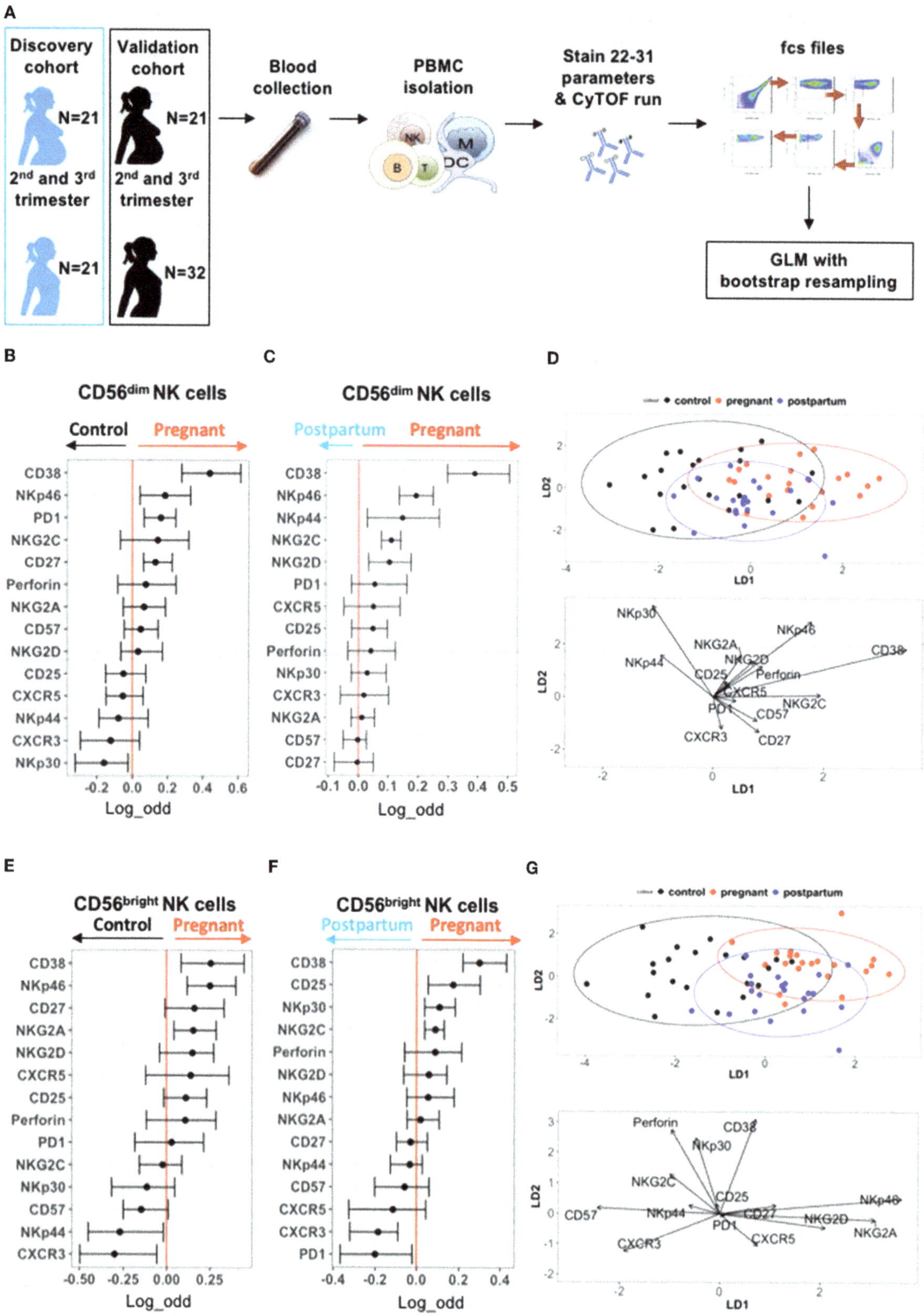

FIGURE 2 | Deep profiling of CD56^{dim} and CD56^{bright} NK cells in non-pregnant and pregnant women from discovery cohort. **(A)** PBMCs from controls (N = 21), pregnant women (N = 21), and post-partum women (N = 21) in discovery cohort were isolated from blood samples. PBMCs were isolated and stained for mass

(Continued)

FIGURE 2 | cytometry. Data obtained were analyzed using a linear regression model, GLM. **(B,C)** Markers predictive of CD56^{dim} NK cells in control vs. pregnant women in discovery cohort were assessed by GLM with bootstrap resampling. The markers are listed on the y-axis and the x-axis represents the log-odds that the marker expression levels predict the outcome (control on the left vs. pregnancy on the right). Summary data are depicted, showing the 95% confidence interval. Markers in which the bar does not cross zero are significantly predictive of one state vs. the other. **(D)** Represents the linear discriminant analysis (LDA) for CD56^{dim} NK cells between non-pregnant, pregnant, and post-partum samples from discovery cohort. **(E,F)** Markers predictive of CD56^{bright} NK cells in control vs. pregnant women in discovery cohort were assessed by GLM with bootstrap resampling. The markers are listed on the y-axis and the x-axis represents the log-odds that the marker expression levels predict the outcome (control on the left vs. pregnancy on the right). Summary data are depicted, showing the 95% confidence interval. Markers in which the bar does not cross zero are significantly predictive of one state vs. the other. **(G)** Represents the linear discriminant analysis (LDA) for CD56^{bright} NK cells between non-pregnant, pregnant, and post-partum samples from discovery cohort.

making it less likely that differences in CMV status were driving the differences in NK cell phenotype (**Figure S11**). Overall, the most consistent finding in pregnancy is the increased expression of CD38 on both CD56^{dim} and CD56^{bright} NK cells. There is significant variation in the expression patterns of activating and inhibitory NK cell receptors during pregnancy, but pregnancy is associated with a higher activation status and enhanced CD38 expression.

Co-expression of CD38 and NKp46

As the most consistently observed difference was enhanced expression of CD38 and NKp46 on CD56^{dim} NK cells during pregnancy, we examined the frequency of CD56^{dim} NK cells co-expressing these markers (**Figure 4**). CD38 and NKp46 were co-expressed on a greater frequency of NK cells both the discovery (**Figures 4A,B**) and validation cohorts during pregnancy (**Figures 4C,D**). In the discovery cohort, the frequency of CD38^{high}NKp46^{+} NK cells returned to levels found in controls during the post-partum period, but in the validation cohort, the frequency of CD38^{high}NKp46^{+} NK cells remained high in the post-partum period. There was no significant association between the frequency of CD38^{high}NKp46^{+} NK cells and "adaptive" NKG2C^{+}CD57^{+} NK cells (**Figure S11**).

DISCUSSION

During pregnancy, the maternal immune system is engaged in a fine balance: tolerance is required to preserve the fetus while defenses must be maintained to protect mother and baby from microbial challenges. NK cells play a critical role in this balance as their job is to patrol the body for "altered self" (31). NK cell activity had been thought to be suppressed during pregnancy to protect the fetus, but recent studies have suggested a more nuanced view (2). NK cells from pregnant women display diminished responses to stimulation with cytokines and phorbol-myristate acetate and ionomycin, yet NK cell responses to influenza-infected cells are enhanced (12–14, 32). Here we show that both CD56^{dim} and CD56^{bright} NK cell subsets have enhanced responses to both the influenza virus and to cancer cells, indicating a cell-intrinsic enhancement in their response to threats. Profiling CD56^{dim} and CD56^{bright} NK cells from pregnant and non-pregnant women showed that during pregnancy, both subsets are characterized by increased expression of the activation marker, CD38. CD38 is expressed on a large proportion of NK cells even in non-pregnant individuals and is significantly increased in cell surface density during pregnancy. CD56^{dim} NK cells also demonstrate increased expression of the activating receptor NKp46 during pregnancy (though it is even higher in the post-partum period in one study); this receptor may play a role in recognition of influenza-infected cells (33, 34). These observations indicate that NK cells have an enhanced expression of receptors that mark NK cell activation and contribute to the response to influenza virus and cancer cells.

Pregnant women are significantly more likely to suffer adverse consequences from influenza infection than are the general population. During the 1918 influenza pandemic, the case fatality rate for influenza infection was estimated to be 27–75% among pregnant women but only 2–3% among the general population (35). Even with improved supportive care, the case-fatality rate among pregnant women was twice that of the general population during the 2009 pandemic (36). Thus, an understanding of the mechanisms driving this enhanced susceptibility to influenza infection during pregnancy represents an important challenge for the scientific community. During influenza virus infection, the recruitment of peripheral NK cells into the lungs represents one of the first lines of defense following influenza infection (37). Though isolated NK cells stimulated with cytokines or chemicals have suppressed responses during pregnancy, our data here confirm earlier findings that NK cell responses to autologous influenza-infected cells are enhanced during pregnancy (12). This enhanced responsiveness could be deleterious to lung integrity and drive pathogenesis. Consistent with this idea, Kim et al. demonstrated that pregnant mice infected by influenza virus have increased lung inflammation and damage compared to non-pregnant mice (38). Further, Littauer et al. suggested that innate immune responses play a role in the initiation of pregnancy complications such as preterm birth and stillbirth following influenza virus infection (5). Finally, the idea that enhanced NK cell responses could be detrimental in pregnant women is consistent with observations that hyperinflammatory responses are a driving force behind severe influenza disease in humans (39–41).

To deepen our understanding of the effect of pregnancy on NK cell responses, we turned to mass cytometry to profile the expression of NK cell surface receptors. We were surprised to discover that both CD56^{dim} and CD56^{bright} NK cell subsets had a consistent and significant increase in CD38 expression during pregnancy compared to non-pregnant and post-partum samples. While CD38 is commonly viewed as an activation marker on T cells, it is more highly expressed on NK cells and has several important functions. First, CD38 confers lymphocytes with the ability to adhere to endothelial cells through its binding to

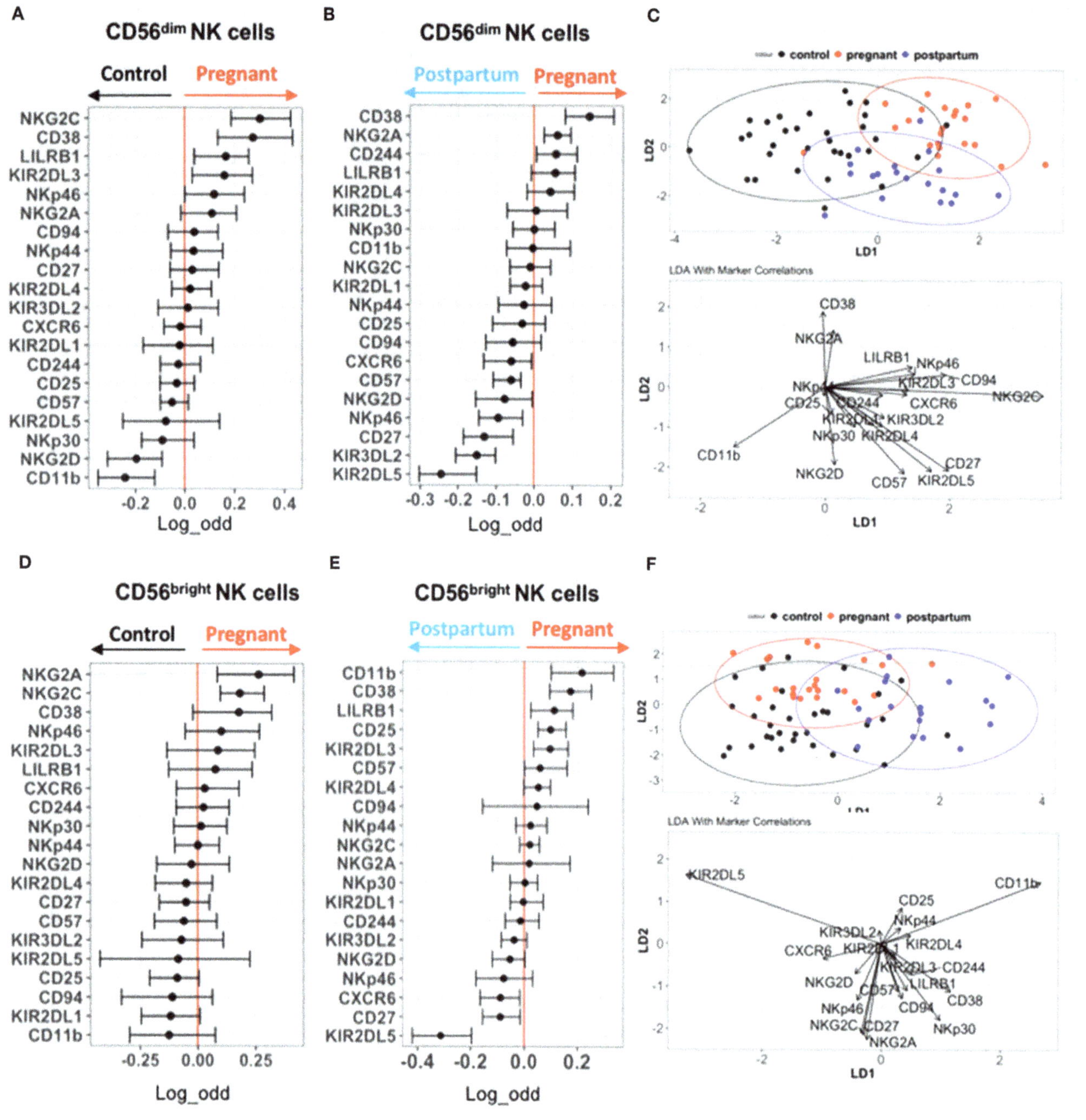

FIGURE 3 | Deep profiling of CD56^{dim} and CD56^{bright} NK cells in non-pregnant and pregnant women from validation cohort. **(A,B)** Markers predictive of CD56^{dim} NK cells in control vs. pregnant women in validation cohort were assessed by GLM with bootstrap resampling. The markers are listed on the y-axis and the x-axis represents the log-odds that the marker expression levels predict the outcome (control on the left vs. pregnancy on the right). Summary data are depicted, showing the 95% confidence interval. Markers in which the bar does not cross zero are significantly predictive of one state vs. the other. **(C)** Represents the linear discriminant analysis (LDA) for CD56^{dim} NK cells between non-pregnant, pregnant and post-partum samples from validation cohort. **(D,E)** Markers predictive of CD56^{bright} NK cells in control vs. pregnant women in validation cohort were assessed by GLM with bootstrap resampling. The markers are listed on the y-axis and the x-axis represents the log-odds that the marker expression levels predict the outcome (control on the left vs. pregnancy on the right). Summary data are depicted, showing the 95% confidence interval. Markers in which the bar does not cross zero are significantly predictive of one state vs. the other. **(F)** Represents the linear discriminant analysis (LDA) for CD56^{bright} NK cells between non-pregnant, pregnant and post-partum samples from validation cohort.

CD31, a necessary step in extravasation. CD38 also functions as an ectoenzyme, converting extracellular NAD$^+$ to cADPR through its cyclase activity or cADPR to Adenosyl-di-phosphate ribose through its hydrolase activity (42). These molecules in turn can diffuse into the cell and promote its activation by driving intracellular calcium increase, phosphorylation of

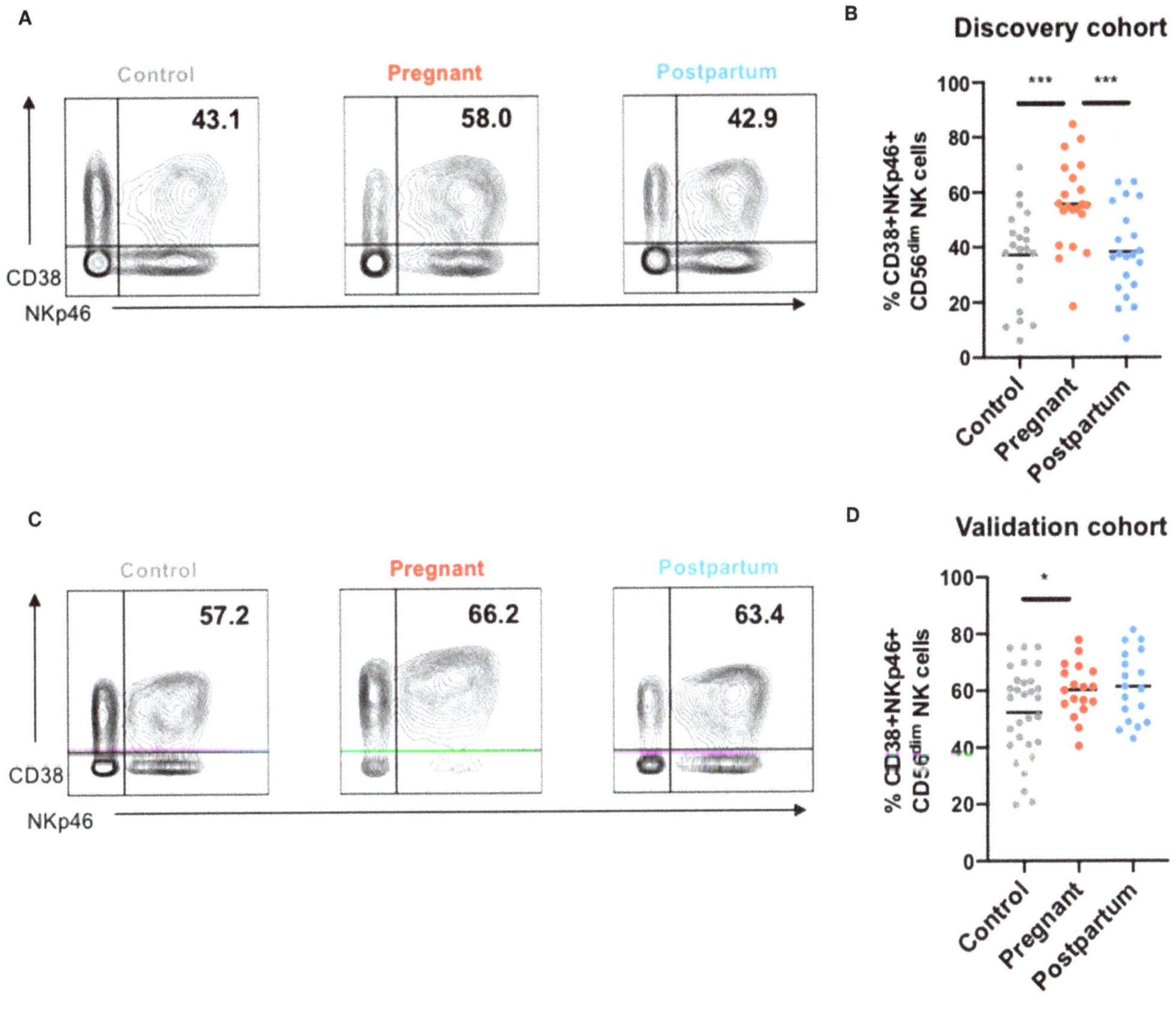

FIGURE 4 | NKp46 and CD38 co-expression in NK cells from controls, pregnant and post-partum women in the discovery and validation cohort. **(A)** Representative mass cytometry plots showing the co-expression of NKp46 and CD38 in peripheral NK cells from a control, pregnant or post-partum women in the discovery cohort. **(B)** Frequency of $CD38^+NKp46^+$ NK cells from controls, pregnant and post-partum individuals in the discovery cohort. ***$P < 0.001$ (Mann–Whitney *U*-Tests to compare controls vs. pregnant; Wilcoxon matched-paired test to compare pregnant vs. post-partum). **(C)** Representative mass cytometry plots showing the co-expression of NKp46 and CD38 in peripheral NK cells from a control, pregnant, or post-partum women in the validation cohort. **(D)** Frequency of $CD38^+NKp46^+$ NK cells from controls, pregnant and post-partum individuals in the validation cohort. *$P < 0.05$ (Mann–Whitney *U*-Tests to compare controls vs. pregnant; Wilcoxon matched-paired test to compare pregnant vs. post-partum).

signaling molecules, production of cytokines, and vesicular transport (43). CD38 crosslinking can enhance the cytotoxic activity of cytokine-activated NK cells (44–46) and plays a role in immune synapse formation in T cells (47) and NK cells (Le Gars et al., unpublished data). Thus, this increased CD38 expression during pregnancy might explain the enhanced responses of NK cells to influenza and tumor cells. Interestingly, decidual NK cells express high levels of CD38 compared to peripheral NK cells, yet their origin is still unclear (48). It has been proposed that subsets of NK cells can migrate from the maternal blood to the decidua and acquire the unique features of decidual NK cells upon exposure to decidual environment (49, 50). Our data suggest that the overall environment during pregnancy could enhance CD38 expression. Several studies suggest that KIR2DL4 could play a significant role in regulating IFN-γ production by decidual NK cells (51–53). Further, an NK cell population found in repeated pregnancies, which has a unique transcriptome and epigenetic signature, is characterized by high expression of the receptors NKG2C and LILRB1 (54). This NK cell population has open chromatin around the enhancers of IFNG and VEGF genes, which leads to an increased production of IFN-γ and VEGF upon activation. This is consistent with our finding that NKG2C and LILRB1 expression is increased in our validation cohort, and could explain the increased activation of peripheral NK cells upon encounter with infected or tumor cells during pregnancy.

Another interesting finding is the consistent increased expression of NKp46 on CD56^{dim} NK cells during pregnancy. Intriguingly, in the validation cohort, NKp46 levels were even higher on CD56^{dim} NK cells during the post-partum period. NKp46 has been shown to contribute to NK cell influenza virus responses through binding of influenza hemagglutinin (34). Signaling mediated by NKp46 following influenza sensing leads to the production of IFN-γ (33, 55). Therefore, an increased expression of NKp46 during pregnancy could make NK cells more responsive to influenza virus. Further, more elevated expression of NKp46 facilitates the control of lung cancer in mice (56) and NKp46 alteration is associated with tumor progression in human gastric cancer (57). Thus, the increased expression of NKp46 on CD56^{dim} NK cells, together with CD38, could explain the enhanced response to cancer cells during pregnancy. Two factors limited our ability to directly attribute the enhanced expression of CD38 and NKp46 to NK cell hyperresponsiveness during pregnancy. First, we did not have sufficient PBMC samples from pregnant women to perform blocking experiments. Second, even with enough material, CD38 and NKp46 are expressed on NK cells from non-pregnant women as well, albeit at lower levels, thus blocking would be expected to diminish responses in both pregnant and non-pregnant women.

Several markers differed in their expression pattern during pregnancy in only one cohort, and there was significant variation in the expression patterns of some markers between cohorts. For instance, NKG2D cells was predictive of pregnancy in the discovery cohort and predictive of post-partum/control in the validation cohort. This may reflect the substantial differences in NK cell phenotype between individuals. In earlier work we noted that NK cell receptor expression profiles, particularly those of activating receptors, differed dramatically between identical twins and based on maturation status, suggesting that these expression patterns are influenced by the environment (20, 26). This high variation between individuals may also explain our failure to observe consistent pregnancy-related changes in NKp30 or NKp44 expression. Other changes associated with pregnancy, including expression patterns of LILRB1, KIR3DL2, and KIR2DL5 were only evaluated in the validation cohort and warrant follow-up in future studies. Changes in NKG2C expression observed on CD56^{dim} NK cells between the pregnant and control subjects could reflect differences in the CMV status between the cohorts in the cross-sectional analyses; unfortunately, CMV status is not known for the cohorts. An additional feature that was observed in the discovery cohort, but unfortunately not evaluated in the validation cohort, was decreased expression of CXCR3 on CD56^{bright} NK cells during pregnancy. CXCR3, through the binding to its ligand IP-10, is an important receptor responsible for the recruitment of NK cells to the site of infection or inflammation. The CXCR3/IP-10 axis has been shown to enhance acute respiratory distress syndrome (ARDS) by the increased systemic presence of IP-10 (58). Thus, decreased level of CXCR3 on NK cells fails to explain their enhanced responses during pregnancy but could represent a mechanism of protection to avoid an excessive recruitment of CD56^{bright} NK cells to the lung of influenza-infected pregnant women and to restrain lung damage.

Why does NK cell phenotype undergo such changes during pregnancy? The answer remains unclear. The presence of fetal antigens in maternal blood could explain the increased activation state of NK cells. Monocytes and dendritic cells exert a pro-inflammatory phenotype during pregnancy (2, 11, 14) and this could be in part due to parental antigens present in the fetus. In turn, monocytes and pDCs could produce several cytokines such as IL-15,−18, or IFN-type I to promote increased NK cell receptor expression and activate NK cells (59). Another possibility to explain the observed phenotypic changes of NK cells during pregnancy is hormonal variation. These fluctuations could promote transcriptomic and epigenetic modifications driving alteration of NK cell phenotype and response to influenza virus and tumor cells. However, several studies suggest that progesterone and estrogen dampen NK cell cytotoxic activities (60, 61). A deep analysis of the transcriptomic and epigenetic landscape of NK cells during pregnancy could lead to a better understanding of these NK cell changes.

There are several limitations of our study, including the fact that our mass cytometry panels differed between the two cohorts and remain limited to ~40 markers. Thus, we may have excluded other molecules involved in NK cell immune responses during pregnancy, including critical NK cell surface molecules such as DNAM-1, TIGIT, and Siglec-7. We also did not follow-up on other differences that were seen in only one cohort. Further, here we studied peripheral blood NK cells and were not able to sample lung resident NK cells or uterine NK cells. Finally, we had limited data reflecting the history of the pregnant and control women in terms of their prior vaccination status, prior influenza infection status, cigarette and drug use, and others. We cannot exclude that unmeasured factors could influence the NK cell phenotype and the quality of the NK cell responses to influenza and cancer cells.

Here, our goal was to refine current understanding of NK cell biology and activity in the context of pregnancy and influenza virus infection. Our work reveals enhanced activity of both CD56^{dim} and CD56^{bright} NK cell subsets to influenza-infected cells and tumor cells during pregnancy. These enhanced responses are associated with a more robust expression of CD38, a receptor that plays a role in activation and cytotoxicity, and NKp46, a receptor associated with a better response to influenza virus and certain cancers. Together, our data provide a more complete view of the immune changes mediated by pregnancy and enhances our understanding of the susceptibility of pregnant women to influenza virus.

ETHICS STATEMENT

The studies involving human participants were reviewed and approved by Stanford University Institutional Review Board. The patients/participants provided their written informed consent to participate in this study. Written informed consent was obtained from the individual(s) for the publication of any potentially identifiable images or data included in this article.

AUTHOR CONTRIBUTIONS

ML, AK, NB, and CB designed experiments. ML, AK, and NB, and CS analyzed the data. LM, SS-O, and PK collaborated and provided advice in the analysis of the data. MD, CD, GS, and NA coordinated and provided human samples. ML and CB wrote the manuscript. All authors contributed revisions and edits.

ACKNOWLEDGMENTS

We thank our study volunteers for their participation, Sally Mackey for regulatory and data management, Sue Swope for consenting and conducting study visits, and the staff of the Stanford Vaccine Program for overall study coordination. This manuscript has been released as a Pre-Print at Biorxiv (62).

REFERENCES

1. Erlebacher A. Immunology of the maternal-fetal interface. *Ann Rev Immunol.* (2013) 31:387–411. doi: 10.1146/annurev-immunol-032712-100003
2. Kourtis AP, Read JS, Jamieson DJ. Pregnancy and infection. *N Engl J Med.* (2014) 370:2211–8. doi: 10.1056/NEJMra1213566
3. Periolo N, Avaro M, Czech A, Russo M, Benedetti E, Pontoriero A, et al. Pregnant women infected with pandemic influenza A(H1N1)pdm09 virus showed differential immune response correlated with disease severity. *J Clin Virol.* (2015) 64:52–8. doi: 10.1016/j.jcv.2015.01.009
4. PrabhuDas M, Bonney E, Caron K, Dey S, Erlebacher A, Fazleabas A, et al. Immune mechanisms at the maternal-fetal interface: perspectives and challenges. *Nat Immunol.* (2015) 16:328–34. doi: 10.1038/ni.3131
5. Littauer EQ, Esser ES, Antao OQ, Vassilieva EV, Compans RW, Skountzou I. H1N1 influenza virus infection results in adverse pregnancy outcomes by disrupting tissue-specific hormonal regulation. *PLoS Pathogens.* (2017) 13:e1006757. doi: 10.1371/journal.ppat.1006757
6. Pazos M, Sperling RS, Moran TM, Kraus TA. The influence of pregnancy on systemic immunity. *Immunol Res.* (2012) 54:254–61. doi: 10.1007/s12026-012-8303-9
7. Omer SB, Bednarczyk R, Madhi SA, Klugman KP. Benefits to mother and child of influenza vaccination during pregnancy. *Hum Vacc Immunother.* (2012) 8:130–7. doi: 10.4161/hv.8.1.18601
8. Raj RS, Bonney EA, Phillippe M. Influenza, immune system, and pregnancy. *Reprod Sci.* (2014) 21:1434–51. doi: 10.1177/1933719114537720
9. Siston AM, Rasmussen SA, Honein MA, Fry AM, Seib K, Callaghan WM, et al. Pandemic 2009 influenza A(H1N1) virus illness among pregnant women in the United States. *JAMA.* (2010) 303:1517–25. doi: 10.1001/jama.2010.479
10. Aghaeepour N, Ganio EA, Mcilwain D, Tsai AS, Tingle M, Van Gassen S, et al. An immune clock of human pregnancy. *Sci Immunol.* (2017) 2:eaan2946. doi: 10.1126/sciimmunol.aan2946
11. Gars ML, Le Gars M, Kay AW, Bayless NL, Aziz N, Dekker CL, et al. Increased proinflammatory responses of monocytes and plasmacytoid dendritic cells to influenza A virus infection during pregnancy. *J Infect Dis.* (2016) 214:1666–71. doi: 10.1093/infdis/jiw448
12. Kay AW, Fukuyama J, Aziz N, Dekker CL, Mackey S, Swan GE, et al. Enhanced natural killer-cell and T-cell responses to influenza A virus during pregnancy. *Proc Natl Acad Sci USA.* (2014) 111:14506–11. doi: 10.1073/pnas.1416569111
13. Kraus TA, Engel SM, Sperling RS, Kellerman L, Lo Y, Wallenstein S, et al. Characterizing the pregnancy immune phenotype: results of the viral immunity and pregnancy (VIP) study. *J Clin Immunol.* (2012) 32:300–11. doi: 10.1007/s10875-011-9627-2
14. Kraus TA, Sperling RS, Engel SM, Lo Y, Kellerman L, Singh T, et al. Peripheral blood cytokine profiling during pregnancy and post-partum periods. *Am J Reprod Immunol.* (2010) 64:411–26. doi: 10.1111/j.1600-0897.2010.00889.x
15. Abdul-Careem MF, Mian MF, Yue G, Gillgrass A, Chenoweth MJ, Barra NG, et al. Critical role of natural killer cells in lung immunopathology during influenza infection in mice. *J Infect Dis.* (2012) 206:167–77. doi: 10.1093/infdis/jis340
16. Zhou G, Juang SWW, Kane KP. NK cells exacerbate the pathology of influenza virus infection in mice. *Eur J Immunol.* (2013) 43:929–38. doi: 10.1002/eji.201242620
17. Gazit R, Gruda R, Elboim M, Arnon TI, Katz G, Achdout H, et al. Lethal influenza infection in the absence of the natural killer cell receptor gene Ncr1. *Nat Immunol.* (2006) 7:517–23. doi: 10.1038/ni1322
18. Narni-Mancinelli E, Jaeger BN, Bernat C, Fenis A, Kung S, De Gassart A, et al. Tuning of natural killer cell reactivity by NKp46 and Helios calibrates T cell responses. *Science.* (2012) 335:344–8. doi: 10.1126/science.1215621
19. Mauad T, Hajjar LA, Callegari GD, da Silva LFF, Schout D, Galas FRBG, et al. Lung pathology in fatal novel human influenza A (H1N1) infection. *Am J Respirat Critic Care Med.* (2010) 181:72–9. doi: 10.1164/rccm.200909-1420OC
20. Strauss-Albee DM, Horowitz A, Parham P, Blish CA. Coordinated regulation of NK receptor expression in the maturing human immune system. *J Immunol.* (2014) 193:4871–9. doi: 10.4049/jimmunol.1401821
21. Vivier E, Tomasello E, Baratin M, Walzer T, Ugolini S. Functions of natural killer cells. *Nat Immunol.* (2008) 9:503–10. doi: 10.1038/ni1582
22. Cooper MA, Fehniger TA, Turner SC, Chen KS, Ghaheri BA, Ghayur T, et al. Human natural killer cells: a unique innate immunoregulatory role for the CD56bright subset. *Blood.* (2001) 97:3146–51. doi: 10.1182/blood.V97.10.3146
23. Nagler A, Lanier LL, Cwirla S, Phillips JH. Comparative studies of human FcRIII-positive and negative natural killer cells. *J Immunol.* (1989) 143:3183–91.
24. Kay AW, Strauss-Albee DM, Blish CA. Application of mass cytometry (CyTOF) for functional and phenotypic analysis of natural killer cells. *Methods Mol Biol.* (2016) 1441:13–26. doi: 10.1007/978-1-4939-3684-7_2
25. Strauss-Albee DM, Blish CA. CyTOF: single cell mass cytometry for evaluation of complex innate cellular phenotypes. In: Montgomery R, Bucala R, editors. *Experimental Approaches for the Investigation of Innate Immunity.* World Scientific; Yale University School of Medicine (2015). p. 27–39. doi: 10.1142/9789814678735_0003
26. Horowitz A, Strauss-Albee DM, Leipold M, Kubo J, Nemat-Gorgani N, Dogan OC, et al. Genetic and environmental determinants of human NK cell diversity revealed by mass cytometry. *Sci Transl Med.* (2013) 5:208ra145. doi: 10.1126/scitranslmed.3006702
27. Seiler C, Kronstad LM, Simpson LJ, Le Gars M, Vendrame E, Blish CA, et al. *Uncertainty Quantification in Multivariate Mixed Models for Mass Cytometry Data.* (2019). Retrieved from: http://arxiv.org/abs/1903.07976 (accessed October 15, 2019).
28. Gentleman R, Carey V, Huber W, Irizarry R, Dudoit S. *Bioinformatics and Computational Biology Solutions Using R and Bioconductor.* Springer Science & Business Media (2006). doi: 10.1007/0-387-29362-0
29. Ripley B, Venables B, Bates DM, Hornik K, Gebhardt A, Firth D. *MASS: Support Functions and Datasets for Venables and Ripley's MASS.* R Package Version 7-3. (2011).

30. Kronstad LM, Seiler C, Vergara R, Holmes SP, Blish CA. Differential induction of IFN-α and modulation of CD112 and CD54 expression govern the magnitude of NK cell IFN-γ response to influenza A viruses. *J Immunol.* (2018) 201:2117–31. doi: 10.4049/jimmunol.1800161
31. Hilton HG, Parham P. Missing or altered self: human NK cell receptors that recognize HLA-C. *Immunogenetics.* (2017) 69:567–79. doi: 10.1007/s00251-017-1001-y
32. Veenstra van Nieuwenhoven AL, Bouman A, Moes H, Heineman MJ, de Leij LFMH, Santema J, et al. Cytokine production in natural killer cells and lymphocytes in pregnant women compared with women in the follicular phase of the ovarian cycle. *Fertil Steril.* (2002) 77:1032–7. doi: 10.1016/S0015-0282(02)02976-X
33. Glasner A, Zurunic A, Meningher T, Lenac Rovis T, Tsukerman P, Bar-On Y, et al. Elucidating the mechanisms of influenza virus recognition by Ncr1. *PLoS ONE.* (2012) 7:e36837. doi: 10.1371/journal.pone.0036837
34. Mandelboim O, Lieberman N, Lev M, Paul L, Arnon TI, Bushkin Y, et al. Recognition of haemagglutinins on virus-infected cells by NKp46 activates lysis by human NK cells. *Nature.* (2001) 409:1055–60. doi: 10.1038/35059110
35. Rasmussen SA, Jamieson DJ, Bresee JS. Pandemic influenza and pregnant women. *Emerg Infect Dis.* (2008) 14:95–100. doi: 10.3201/eid1401.070667
36. Centers for Disease Control and Prevention (CDC). Estimates of deaths associated with seasonal influenza — United States, 1976-2007. MMWR. *MMWR Morb Mortal Wkly Rep.* (2010) 59:1057–62.
37. Carlin LE, Hemann EA, Zacharias ZR, Heusel JW, Legge KL. Natural killer cell recruitment to the lung during influenza A virus infection is dependent on CXCR3, CCR5, and virus exposure dose. *Front Immunol.* (2018) 9:781. doi: 10.3389/fimmu.2018.00781
38. Kim HM, Kang YM, Song BM, Kim HS, Seo SH. The 2009 pandemic H1N1 influenza virus is more pathogenic in pregnant mice than seasonal H1N1 influenza virus. *Viral Immunol.* (2012) 25:402–10. doi: 10.1089/vim.2012.0007
39. Cheung CY, Poon LLM, Lau AS, Luk W, Lau YL, Shortridge KF, et al. Induction of proinflammatory cytokines in human macrophages by influenza A (H5N1) viruses: a mechanism for the unusual severity of human disease? *Lancet.* (2002) 360:1831–7. doi: 10.1016/S0140-6736(02)11772-7
40. de Jong MD, Simmons CP, Thanh TT, Hien VM, Smith GJD, Chau TNB, et al. Fatal outcome of human influenza A (H5N1) is associated with high viral load and hypercytokinemia. *Nat Med.* (2006) 12:1203–7. doi: 10.1038/nm1477
41. Kobasa D, Jones SM, Shinya K, Kash JC, Copps J, Ebihara H, et al. Aberrant innate immune response in lethal infection of macaques with the 1918 influenza virus. *Nature.* (2007) 445:319–23. doi: 10.1038/nature05495
42. Deaglio S, Mallone R, Baj G, Arnulfo A, Surico N, Dianzani U, et al. CD38/CD31, a receptor/ligand system ruling adhesion and signaling in human leukocytes. *Chem Immunol.* (2000) 75:99–120. doi: 10.1159/000058765
43. Lee HC. Structure and enzymatic functions of human CD38. *Mol Med.* (2006) 12:317–23. doi: 10.2119/2006-00086.Lee
44. Deaglio S, Zubiaur M, Gregorini A, Bottarel F, Ausiello CM, Dianzani U, et al. Human CD38 and CD16 are functionally dependent and physically associated in natural killer cells. *Blood.* (2002) 99:2490–8. doi: 10.1182/blood.V99.7.2490
45. Mallone R, Funaro A, Zubiaur M, Baj G, Ausiello CM, Tacchetti C, et al. Signaling through CD38 induces NK cell activation. *Int Immunol.* (2001) 13:397–409. doi: 10.1093/intimm/13.4.397
46. Sconocchia G, Titus JA, Mazzoni A, Visintin A, Pericle F, Hicks SW, et al. CD38 triggers cytotoxic responses in activated human natural killer cells. *Blood.* (1999) 94:3864–71.
47. Muñoz P, Mittelbrunn M, de la Fuente H, Pérez-Martínez M, García-Pérez A, Ariza-Veguillas A, et al. Antigen-induced clustering of surface CD38 and recruitment of intracellular CD38 to the immunologic synapse. *Blood.* (2008) 111:3653–64. doi: 10.1182/blood-2007-07-101600
48. Koopman LA, Kopcow HD, Rybalov B, Boyson JE, Orange JS, Schatz F, et al. Human decidual natural killer cells are a unique NK cell subset with immunomodulatory potential. *J Exp Med.* (2003) 198:1201–12. doi: 10.1084/jem.20030305
49. Carlino C, Stabile H, Morrone S, Bulla R, Soriani A, Agostinis C, et al. Recruitment of circulating NK cells through decidual tissues: a possible mechanism controlling NK cell accumulation in the uterus during early pregnancy. *Blood.* (2008) 111:3108–15. doi: 10.1182/blood-2007-08-105965
50. Keskin DB, Allan DSJ, Rybalov B, Andzelm MM, Stern JNH, Kopcow HD, et al. TGFβ promotes conversion of CD16+ peripheral blood NK cells into CD16− NK cells with similarities to decidual NK cells. *Proc Natl Acad Sci USA.* (2007) 104:3378–83. doi: 10.1073/pnas.0611098104
51. Goodridge JP, Lathbury LJ, John E, Charles AK, Christiansen FT, Witt CS. The genotype of the NK cell receptor, KIR2DL4, influences INF secretion by decidual natural killer cells. *Mol Hum Reproduct.* (2009) 15:489–97. doi: 10.1093/molehr/gap039
52. Li C, Houser BL, Nicotra ML, Strominger JL. HLA-G homodimer-induced cytokine secretion through HLA-G receptors on human decidual macrophages and natural killer cells. *Proc Natl Acad Sci USA.* (2009) 106:5767–72. doi: 10.1073/pnas.0901173106
53. Rajagopalan S, Bryceson YT, Kuppusamy SP, Geraghty DE, van der Meer A, Joosten I, et al. Activation of NK cells by an endocytosed receptor for soluble HLA-G. *PLoS Biol.* (2005) 4:e9. doi: 10.1371/journal.pbio.0040009
54. Gamliel M, Goldman-Wohl D, Isaacson B, Gur C, Stein N, Yamin R, et al. Trained memory of human uterine NK cells enhances their function in subsequent pregnancies. *Immunity.* (2018) 48:951–62.e5. doi: 10.1016/j.immuni.2018.03.030
55. Glasner A, Isaacson B, Viukov S, Neuman T, Friedman N, Mandelboim M, et al. Increased NK cell immunity in a transgenic mouse model of NKp46 overexpression. *Sci Rep.* (2017) 7:13090. doi: 10.1038/s41598-017-12998-w
56. Shi L, Li K, Guo Y, Banerjee A, Wang Q, Lorenz UM, et al. Modulation of NKG2D, NKp46, and Ly49C/I facilitates natural killer cell-mediated control of lung cancer. *Proc Natl Acad Sci USA.* (2018) 115:11808–13. doi: 10.1073/pnas.1804931115
57. Han B, Mao F-Y, Zhao Y-L, Lv Y-P, Teng Y-S, Duan M, et al. Altered NKp30, NKp46, NKG2D, and DNAM-1 expression on circulating NK cells is associated with tumor progression in human gastric cancer. *J Immunol Res.* (2018) 2018:6248590. doi: 10.1155/2018/6248590
58. Ichikawa A, Kuba K, Morita M, Chida S, Tezuka H, Hara H, et al. CXCL10-CXCR3 enhances the development of neutrophil-mediated fulminant lung injury of viral and nonviral origin. *Am J Respirat Critic Care Med.* (2013) 187:65–77. doi: 10.1164/rccm.201203-0508OC
59. Soudja SM, Ruiz AL, Marie JC, Lauvau G. Inflammatory monocytes activate memory CD8 T and innate NK lymphocytes independent of cognate antigen during microbial pathogen invasion. *Immunity.* (2012) 37:549–62. doi: 10.1016/j.immuni.2012.05.029
60. Arruvito L, Giulianelli S, Flores AC, Paladino N, Barboza M, Lanari C, et al. NK cells expressing a progesterone receptor are susceptible to progesterone-induced apoptosis. *J Immunol.* (2008) 180:5746–53. doi: 10.4049/jimmunol.180.8.5746
61. Nilsson N, Carlsten H. Estrogen induces suppression of natural killer cell cytotoxicity and augmentation of polyclonal B cell activation. *Cell Immunol.* (1994) 158:131–9. doi: 10.1006/cimm.1994.1262
62. Le Gars M, Seiler C, Kay AW, Bayless NL, Starosvetsky E, Moore L, et al. CD38 contributes to human natural killer cell responses through a role in immune synapse formation. *bioRxiv [Preprint].* doi: 10.1101/349084

4

Mass Cytometry Reveals a Sustained Reduction in CD16+ Natural Killer Cells Following Chemotherapy in Colorectal Cancer Patients

Diana Shinko[1], *Helen M. McGuire*[2,3], *Connie I. Diakos*[4,5,6], *Nick Pavlakis*[4,5,6], *Stephen J. Clarke*[4,5,6], *Scott N. Byrne*[7,8] *and Kellie A. Charles*[1*]

[1] Discipline of Pharmacology, Faculty of Medicine and Health, The University of Sydney, Sydney, NSW, Australia, [2] Discipline of Pathology, Faculty of Medicine and Health, The University of Sydney, Sydney, NSW, Australia, [3] Ramaciotti Facility for Human Systems Biology, The University of Sydney, Sydney, NSW, Australia, [4] Northern Sydney Cancer Centre, Royal North Shore Hospital, St Leonards, NSW, Australia, [5] Faculty of Medicine and Health, Northern Clinical School, The University of Sydney, Sydney, NSW, Australia, [6] Bill Walsh Translational Research Laboratories, Kolling Institute of Medical Research, St Leonards, NSW, Australia, [7] Discipline of Infectious Diseases and Immunology, Faculty of Medicine and Health, The University of Sydney, Sydney, NSW, Australia, [8] Westmead Institute for Medical Research, Centre for Immunology and Allergy Research, Westmead, NSW, Australia

***Correspondence:**
Kellie A. Charles
kellie.charles@sydney.edu.au

The immune system and inflammation plays a significant role in tumour immune evasion enhancing disease progression and reducing survival in colorectal cancer (CRC). Patients with advanced stages of colorectal cancer will all undergo treatment with cytotoxic chemotherapy which may alter the complexity of immune cell populations. This study used mass cytometry to investigate the circulating immune cell profile of advanced CRC patients following acute and chronic doses of standard cytotoxic chemotherapy and analysed seven major immune cell populations and over 20 subpopulations. Unsupervised clustering analysis of the mass cytometry data revealed a decrease in NK cells following one cycle of cytotoxic chemotherapy. Investigation into the NK sub-population revealed a decline in the $CD56^{dim}$ $CD16^{+}$ NK cell population following acute and chronic chemotherapy treatment. Further analysis into the frequency of the NK cell sub-populations during the long-term chemotherapy treatment revealed a shift in the sub-populations, with a decrease in the mature, cytotoxic $CD56^{dim}$ $CD16^{+}$ accompanied by a significant increase in the less mature $CD56^{dim}$ $CD16^{-}$ and $CD56^{bright}$ NK cell populations. Furthermore, analysis of the phosphorylation status of signalling responses in the NK cells found significant differences in pERK, pP38, pSTAT3, and pSTAT5 between the patients and healthy volunteers and remained unchanged throughout the chemotherapy. Results from this study reveals that there is a sustained decrease in the mature $CD16^{+}$ NK cell sub-population frequency following long-term chemotherapy which may have clinical implications in therapeutic decision making.

Keywords: mass cytometry, colorectal cancer, NK cells, chemotherapy, signalling pathways

INTRODUCTION

An estimated 1.4 million people are annually diagnosed with colorectal cancer (CRC) making it the third most common cancer in the world (1). Despite many nations operating screening programs, over half the people present with advanced or metastatic disease requiring chemotherapy (1). Therapeutic decisions for CRC patients are highly dependent on the staging and the site of the tumour. For people with locally advanced or metastatic CRC, combination cytotoxic chemotherapy is the backbone to all chemotherapy regimens, which primarily involves 5-fluorouracil (5-FU), folinic acid (leucovorin), and either oxaliplatin (FOLFOX) or irinotecan (FOLFIRI) (2, 3). With the advances in molecular targeted therapies, metastatic CRC has benefited from the addition of molecular targeted drugs, such as EGFR or VEGF inhibitors, cetuximab and bevacuzimab, respectively (4, 5). These targeted agents have extended the median long-term survival to almost 3 years for people with metastatic CRC (4). Further improvements in survival will require new drug targets to be identified.

A growing understanding of the various hallmarks of cancer has meant that new drivers of carcinogenesis can be identified and exploited (6). A characteristic feature of colorectal cancer is the complex role that the immune system and inflammation plays in tumour immune evasion and tumour progression (7). Interactions between inflammatory cytokines, immune cells, angiogenesis and malignant epithelial tumour cells may provide novel drug targets for cancer treatment (8, 9). While targeting the immune system with immune checkpoint inhibitors has had a staggering impact on some cancers, immunotherapy has not been as effective in the treatment of CRC (10). Indeed, check point inhibitors appear only to be effective in people with CRC tumours that contain a mismatch-repair deficiency (~15% of all CRC tumours) (11, 12). The development of new immunotherapies for CRC will require a more detailed understanding of the immune cells involved in CRC carcinogenesis, particularly during standard cytotoxic chemotherapy.

Mass cytometry is a multi-parametric technique that offers unparalleled insight into functional and biological systems, including immune cells, at the single cell level (13). Mass cytometry overcomes some of the deficiencies of fluorescence flow cytometry by utilising stable, heavy metal isotopes as tags that can be conjugated to over 100 membrane and intracellular targets on single cells in the same sample (13, 14). Newly developed unsupervised clustering algorithms have enabled users to move away from directed analysis of this high-dimensional data towards identification of underappreciated sub-populations (15).

This study used mass cytometry to investigate the circulating immune cell profile of advanced CRC patients undergoing chemotherapy. Our mass cytometry analysis revealed a distinct phenotypic shift in Natural Killer (NK) cell phenotype following chemotherapy treatment, with a significant decrease in $CD56^{dim}$ $CD16^{+}$ cells and a significant increase in $CD56^{dim}$ $CD16^{-}$ and $CD56^{bright}$ cells. Furthermore, the use of mass cytometry allowed the examination of the phosphorylation status of signalling responses in the NK cells and found significant differences in pERK, pP38, pSTAT3, and pSTAT5 between the CRC patients and the healthy volunteers.

TABLE 1 | Patient demographics.

	Number	Percentage
CRC patients	10	
Gender:		
Male: Female	6:4	60:40
Age:		
Median (range)	66 (40–81)	
Tumour site:		
Colon, rectum, other	5, 2, 1	50:20:10
Stage of cancer:		
III, IV	6, 4	60:40
Mismatch repair		
Deficient, proficient	1, 9	10:90
Treatment		
FOLFOX, other	10, 0	100:0

MATERIALS AND METHODS

Patient Samples

Ten patients with stage III or IV colorectal cancer (CRC) undergoing chemotherapy between 2015 and 2017 at Northern Cancer Institute (St Leonards, NSW, Australia) were recruited to this study (**Table 1**). Nine age and gender matched healthy volunteers were also recruited. This study was approved by Northern Sydney Local Health District and North Shore Private Hospital Human Ethics Committees, and written, informed consent was obtained from all patients prior to participation in the study.

Chemotherapy Treatment and Sample Collection

All patients in this study were treated with the 3 day FOLFOX regimen consisting of 5-FU, oxaliplatin and leucovorin. On day 1, a patient is administered 85 mg/m^2 oxaliplatin as an intravenous (i.v.) infusion, 50 mg calcium folinate (leucovorin) as i.v. bolus injection, 400 mg/m^2 of 5-FU as i.v. bolus injection, and 2,400 mg/m^2 5-FU as a continuous i.v. infusion via a pump over 46 h (16). Twenty millilitres of blood was collected from patients in K_2 EDTA-lavender top tubes (BD Bioscience) on day 1 (pre-treatment), day 3, and day 15 (pre-cycle 2 treatment) (**Figure 1A**). Full blood counts were collected within 24 hours of the research blood collection. Blood samples prior to the start of chemotherapy in cycles 4, 6, 8, 10 of the treatment were also collected while participants remained on active chemotherapy (**Figure 1A**). Age and gender matched blood samples from a Healthy Volunteer study, approved by the Sydney Local Health District at Royal Prince Alfred Hospital, Camperdown were utilised to compare immune cell phenotypes with the pre-chemotherapy blood samples from the patient cohort.

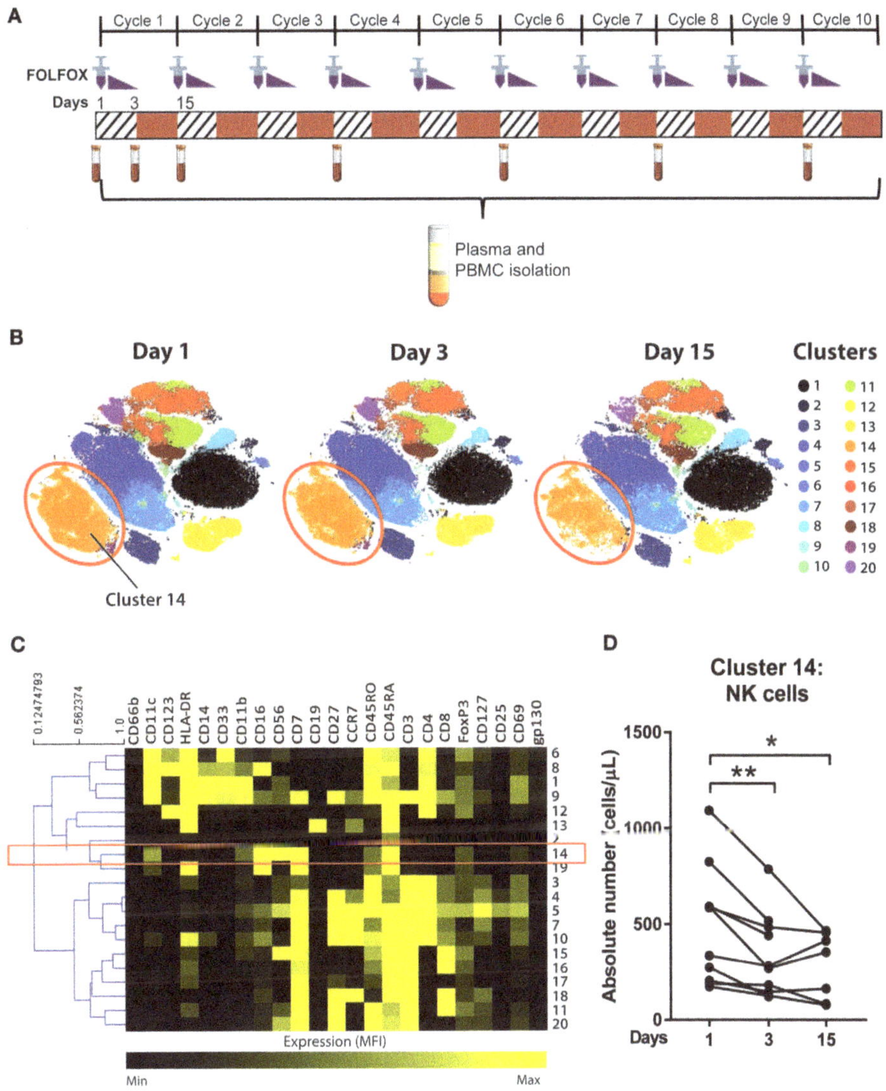

FIGURE 1 | Unsupervised clustering algorithm revealed a decline in NK cell numbers in CRC patients following acute chemotherapy. **(A)** Blood samples were collected from CRC patients undergoing FOLFOX chemotherapy on day 1 (pre-treatment), day 3, and day 15 (pre-cycle 2) of the first cycle of chemotherapy and throughout the later cycles of chemotherapy (cycles 4, 6, 8, and 10). PBMCs were isolated and stained with a 35-antibody mass cytometry panel and ran on the mass cytometer, Helios^{TM}. **(B)** Data from samples taken on the first cycle of chemotherapy (days 1, 3, and 15) was analysed using an unsupervised clustering algorithm, FlowSOM, and the 20 clusters were visualised using tSNE plots. **(C)** A heatmap was generated to show expression of the median fluorescence intensity (MFI) of each surface marker for the clusters. **(D)** The absolute number of cluster 14 throughout days 1, 3, and 15 of the chemotherapy was statistically analysed using Wilcoxon test. $^{*}p < 0.05$, $^{**}p < 0.01$. $n = 10$.

Isolation of PBMCs

Peripheral blood mononuclear cells (PBMCs) were isolated using Ficoll-paque density gradient separation (density 1.077 ± 0.003 g/dL; GE healthcare life sciences). Blood was mixed with phosphate buffer saline (PBS), added to a layer of Ficoll-paque reagent and centrifuged at 550 g for 20 min at 22°C, brake off. The layer of PBMCs is then removed and washed twice in PBS through centrifugation (550 g for 5 min at 22°C). PBMCs were resuspended in freezing media (90% foetal bovine serum; FBS and 10% dimethyl sulfoxide; DMSO) and frozen in liquid nitrogen for long term storage.

Mass Cytometry

The isolated PBMCs were labelled with metal-conjugated antibodies for mass cytometry using an optimised and established protocol (17). The antibodies used were either purchased pre-conjugated from Fluidigm, conjugated and validated in-house or provided by the Ramaciotti Facility for Human Systems Biology (RFHSB) at the University of Sydney. The panel of antibodies used can be found in **Table 2** and **Supplementary Table 1**.

PBMCs were thawed in a 37°C water bath and washed twice with media (RPMI + 10% FBS) and once with CyFACS buffer

TABLE 2 | The antibody panel used for mass cytometry.

Metal tag	Target	Clone
141Pr	CD235ab	HIR2
142Nd	CD19	HIB19
143Nd	CD33	WM53
144Nd	CD11b	ICR544
145Nd	CD4	RPA-T4
146Nd	CD8	RPA-T8
147Sm	CD7	CD7-6B7
148Sm	CD16	3G8
149Sm	CD25	2A3
150Nd	pSTAT5 (Y694)	47
151Eu	CD123	6H6
152Sm	CD66b	80H3
153Eu	pSTAT1 (Y701)	58D6
154Sm	pAKT	J1-223.371
155Gd	CD27	L128
156Gd	pP38 (T180/Y182)	36/p38
158Gd	pSTAT3 (Y705)	4/p
159Tb	CD11c	Bu15
160Gd	CD14	M5E2
161Dy	CD69	FN50
162Dy	FoxP3	PCH101
163Dy	CD56 (NCAM)	HCD56
164Dy	CD45RO	UCHL1
166Er	pP65 (S529)	K10.895.12.50
167Er	CD197 (CCR7)	G043H7
168Er	pERK (T202/Y204)	D13.14.4E
169Tm	CD45RA	HI100
170Er	CD3	UCHT1
171Yb	CD66a/c/e	ASL-32
172Yb	CD130 (gp130)	2E1B02
173Yb	pMAPKAPK2 (Thr334)	27B7
174Yb	HLA-DR	L243
175Lu	Arginase 1	658922
176Yb	CD127 (IL-7Rα)	A019D5

(0.5% bovine serum albumin; BSA, 0.02% sodium azide, 2 mM ethylenediaminetetraacetic acid; EDTA, in phosphate-buffered saline; PBS) by centrifuging at 500 g for 5 min. A surface antibody master mix (surface marker antibodies diluted in CyFACS buffer) was applied to the samples and incubated for 30 min at 4°C. Samples were washed 3 times with CyFACS buffer by centrifuging at 500 g for 5 min at 4°C. The samples were stained for FoxP3 using the Foxp3/Transcription Factor staining Buffer Set (ebioscience™) according to the manufacturer's instructions. Briefly, the cells were fixed and permeabilisation using the provided fixation/permeabilisation buffer (30–60 min at 22°C). The cells were stained with FoxP3 antibody (diluted in the provided permeabilisation buffer) by incubating for 30 min at 22°C. The samples were washed with permeabilisation buffer and CyFACS buffer by centrifuging at 800 g for 8 min.

The samples were then permeabilised by adding 100% ice-cold methanol to each sample and incubating for 30 min on ice. The samples were washed once with CyFACS buffer and resuspended in a master phospho-antibody mixture (phospho-antibodies diluted in CyFACS buffer) and incubated for 45–60 min at 22°C. The cells were washed 3 times and resuspended in 4% paraformaldehyde and incubated overnight. The samples were washed with CyFACS buffer followed by resuspension in 0.125 μM of the Cell ID™ DNA intercalator-Ir (Fluidigm) and incubated for 20 min at 22°C. The cells were then washed three times with ultrapure water (18 MΩ-cm) and resuspended in normalisation beads (1X EQ™ four element calibration beads; Fluidigm) and filtered through a 35 μm nylon mesh and analysed on a CyTOF 2 Helios™ upgraded mass cytometer (Fluidigm). Normalisation procedure of the generated FCS files were carried out using the CyTOF acquisition software (Fluidigm) based on the concurrently run EQ beads.

Data Analysis

Analyses were performed using the Cytometry Analysis Pipeline for large and complex datasets (CAPX), a workflow for discovery of high-dimensional cytometry data providing a set of scripts using existing clustering and visualisation tools (18, 19). The pipeline uses the clustering algorithm, FlowSOM, an R package from Bioconductor, and visualisation using a t-Distributed Stochastic Neighbour Embedding (tSNE) plots. The data was pre-gated using FlowJo v10.4.1 (TreeStar, Inc.) on DNA$^+$, Single cells, CD235ab$^-$ CD66a/c/e$^-$ population and exported for further analysis (**Supplementary Figure 1**). The pre-processed samples were then clustered using the CAPX pipeline which was performed using RStudio. Cells were clustered on expression of lineage markers CD11b, CD11c, CD123, CD127, CD14, CD16, CD19, CD197 (CCR7), CD25, CD27, CD3, CD33, CD4, CD45RA, CD45RO, CD56, CD7, CD8, HLA-DR. An equal number of events were sampled without replacement from all files.

The mass cytometry results were also further analysed using a manual gating strategy on FlowJo. All samples underwent the same background gating strategy mentioned above (**Supplementary Figure 1**). Further gating strategies for NK cell subtypes are described in **Figure 2**. The frequency of cell populations was determined as a percentage of parent population. Absolute numbers of cell population was determined using the frequency as a percentage of PBMC population and the lymphocyte or monocyte counts. For instance, the absolute cell number of NK cells was measured using the formula:

$$\frac{\textit{frequency of cells (\% of total PBMCs)}}{\textit{frequncy of total lymphocytes (\% of total PBMCs)}} \; x \; \textit{lymphocyte count (cells/}\mu L)$$

Statistical Analysis

Statistical analysis was performed using GraphPad Prism 7.0. All data was statistically analysed using non-parametric tests. Mann-Whitney *U*-test was used for un-paired data including comparing healthy volunteers to patients. Wilcoxon test was used for paired data. In the cases of any missing data points (such as missing day 3 samples), only full pairs were used in the paired Wilcoxon test. *P* values <0.05 were considered significant. Multiple comparison testing was not performed as the analyses

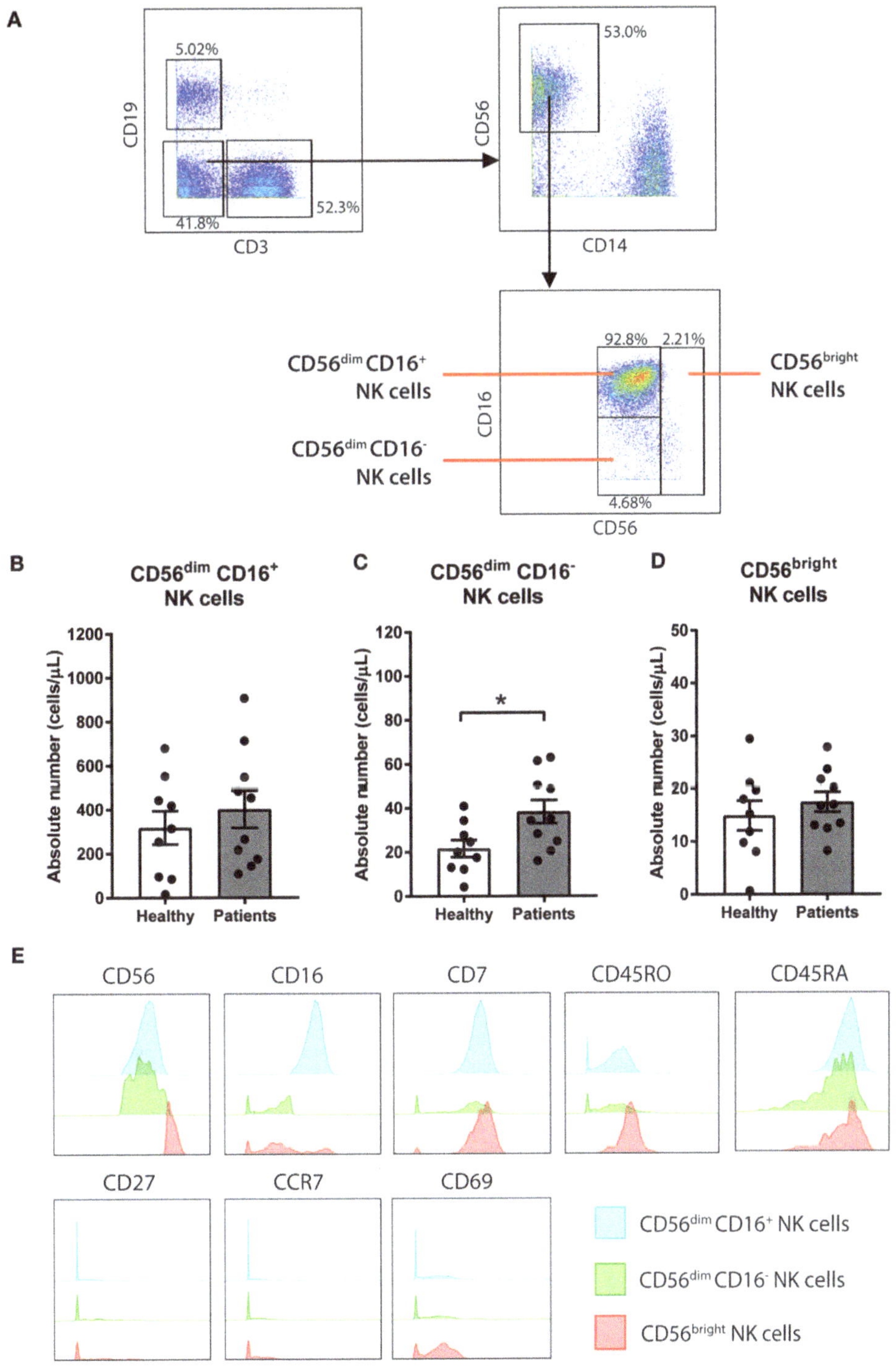

FIGURE 2 | CD56^{dim} CD16^{-} NK cells are increased in baseline of CRC patients compared to healthy volunteers. **(A)** The gating strategy used to identify the 3 sub-population of NK cells. CD3^{-} CD19^{-} population was gated out first followed by gating on the CD14^{-} CD56^{+} total NK cell population. The subtypes of NK cells were gated based on expression of CD56 and CD16 to characterise 3 sub-populations CD56^{dim} CD16^{+}, CD56^{dim} CD16^{-}, and CD56^{bright}. The differences in **(B)** CD56^{dim} CD16^{+}, **(C)** CD56^{dim} CD16^{-}, and **(D)** CD56^{bright} NK cells between the CRC patients pre-treatment compared to the healthy volunteers was statistically analysed using Mann-Whitney *U*-test. **(E)** The expression levels of various surface markers in each NK cell sub-population is visualised in a modal histogram. $^{*}p < 0.05$, $n = 19$.

were exploratory in nature and statistical results are to be viewed as hypothesis generating.

RESULTS

NK Cell Numbers Decline in CRC Patients Following Acute Chemotherapy

With the development of newer high dimensional analysis techniques, the data was analysed using an unsupervised, automated data clustering analysis; FlowSOM. FlowSOM is a clustering algorithm that analyses the data using self-organising maps based on the similarities of the marker expression between individual cells, followed by hierarchical consensus meta-cluster to merge cells into distinct clusters (20).

To determine the effect of an acute dose of cytotoxic chemotherapy on the immune cell populations, a clustering analysis was conducted using samples collected on days 1, 3, and 15 of the first cycle of chemotherapy (**Figure 1A**). We analysed the data into 20 clusters based on the expression of 19 surface markers, with the various clusters visualised using tSNE plots (**Figure 1B**). The FlowSOM clustering revealed a decrease in cluster 14 between days 1, 3, and 15, which can be seen in cluster size in the tSNE plots (**Figure 2B**). The expression of the median fluorescence intensity (MFI) of each surface marker for the clusters was visualised in a heatmap (**Figure 1C**). The heatmap showed that cluster 14 expressed CD56, CD16, and CD7 but lacked the expression of CD14, CD19, and CD3 thus we concluded that this population were NK cells (**Figure 1C**).

Statistical analysis of the absolute number of cells in cluster 14 showed a significant decrease in the population on day 3 compared to day 1 (358.4 $\pm$ 72.4 vs. 521.4 $\pm$ 101.4 cells/μL; $p = 0.0039$) and on day 15 compared to day 1 (287.2 $\pm$ 65.8 vs. 453.4 $\pm$ 126.3 cells/μL; $p = 0.0469$; **Figure 1D**). **Supplementary Figure 2** also shows the statistical difference between days 1, 3, and 15 across all clusters identified by the FlowSOM analysis. Of these populations, cluster 14 was the only population which demonstrated a sustained quantitative change following the first cycle or acute chemotherapy treatment therefore we chose to further investigate this population.

CD56^{dim} CD16$^-$ NK Cells Are Increased in CRC Patients

To further understand the impact of chemotherapy on sub-populations of NK cells, additional analysis of the NK cell population was conducted using a manual gating strategy. Total NK cell population was characterised as the CD3$^-$ CD19$^-$ CD14$^-$ CD56$^+$ using the gating strategy in **Figure 2A**. NK cell sub-populations were further gated based on the relative expression of CD56 and CD16 (**Figure 2A**). The 3 NK cell sub-populations characterised were CD56^{dim} CD16$^+$, CD56^{dim} CD16$^-$, and CD56^{bright}.

Statistical analysis was performed to determine the differences in the NK cells in the CRC patients at baseline compared to a healthy population. No differences in the absolute number of the total NK cell population were observed between the people with CRC and the healthy volunteers (**Supplementary Figure 3A**). Additionally, no difference in the absolute number of CD56^{dim} CD16$^+$ or CD56^{bright} population was seen between the people with CRC and the healthy volunteers (**Figures 2B,D**). However, there was an increase in the absolute numbers of CD56^{dim} CD16$^-$ population in people with CRC compared to the healthy volunteers (38.22 $\pm$ 5.29 vs. 21.6 $\pm$ 3.84 cells/μL; $p = 0.0279$; **Figure 2C**).

The phenotype of the NK cell sub-population was further assessed by examining the expression of various surface markers. As expected, the majority of the CD56^{bright} population expressed low or negative levels of CD16. In addition to CD56 and CD16, the NK cells sub-population expressed CD7, CD45RO, and CD45RA (**Figure 2E**). The NK cell subtypes also expressed low levels of CD69, particularly the CD56^{bright} population (**Figure 2E**).

Decrease in NK Cell Sub-populations Following Chemotherapy Treatment

Manual gating of the total NK cell population confirmed results obtained from the unsupervised clustering approach with a significant decrease in absolute numbers of the total NK cells on days 3 and 15 compared to day 1 (**Supplementary Figure 3B**). The effect of acute chemotherapy on each of the NK cell sub-population was further examined using manual gating. Results showed a significant decrease in the absolute numbers of CD56^{dim} CD16$^+$ population on day 3 compared to day 1 (286.5 $\pm$ 35.0 vs. 429.3 $\pm$ 88.63 cells/μL; $p = 0.0078$) and a decrease on day 15 compared to day 1, although this did not reach significance (227.9 $\pm$ 54.7 vs. 375.2 $\pm$ 109.2 cells/μL; $p = 0.0781$; **Figure 3A**). The CD56^{dim} CD16$^-$ population also decreased on day 3 (31.23 $\pm$ 4.5 vs. 40.19 $\pm$ 5.5 cells/μL; $p = 0.0547$) but no difference was seen on day 15 compared to day 1 (**Figure 3B**). Results also showed that the CD56^{bright} population significantly decreased on day 3 (10.7 $\pm$ 2.4 vs. 18.0 $\pm$ 2.0 cells/μL; $p = 0.0039$) compared to day 1. The CD56^{bright} population increased on day 15 but was still significantly lower than the baseline levels on day 1 (10.8 $\pm$ 2.6 vs. 16.1 $\pm$ 2.0 cells/μL; $p = 0.0469$; **Figure 3C**).

The effect of long-term chemotherapy treatment on the NK cell populations was also assessed. A decrease in the absolute number of cells in the total NK cell population was observed at cycles 2, 4, 6, and 8 (**Supplementary Figure 3C**). Results also showed a decrease in the absolute number of cells within the CD56^{dim} CD16$^+$ population throughout the chemotherapy treatment, with a significant decrease seen at cycle 4 (280.5 $\pm$ 94.2 vs. 368.3 $\pm$ 110.6 cells/μL; $p = 0.0313$), cycle 6 (196.2 $\pm$ vs. 384.6 $\pm$ 122.4 cells/μL; $p = 0.0313$), cycle 8 (233.7 $\pm$ 77.4 vs. 395.8 $\pm$ 117.7 cells/μL; $p = 0.0313$), and cycle 10 (203.3 $\pm$ 66.6 vs. 395.8 $\pm$ 117.7 cells/μL; $p = 0.0313$) compared to the baseline levels at cycle 1 (**Figure 3D**). No significant difference was seen in the absolute numbers of CD56^{dim} CD16$^-$ or CD56^{bright} populations through the later cycles of chemotherapy as seen in **Figures 3E,F**.

In addition to assessing the effect of long-term chemotherapy on the absolute numbers of NK cells, the effect on the frequency of NK cell sub-population was also assessed to investigate any shift in the NK cell sub-population frequency following chemotherapy. Results showed a decline in the CD56^{dim} CD16$^+$

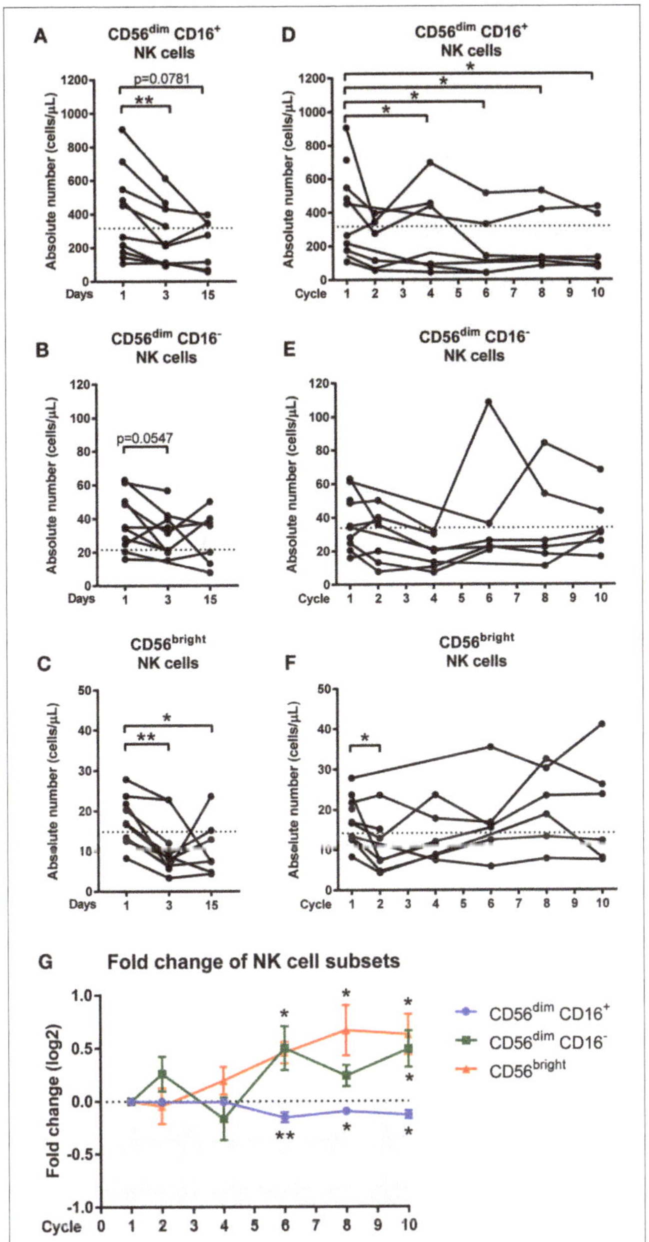

FIGURE 3 | Changes in NK cell sub-populations following chemotherapy treatment. Blood samples collected on day 1 (pre-treatment), day 3, and day 15 of the first cycle in CRC patients undergoing FOLFOX chemotherapy. Blood samples from later cycles were also collected to test the long term effect of chemotherapy. The absolute numbers of **(A)** CD56^{dim} CD16^{+}, **(B)** CD56^{dim} CD16^{-}, and **(C)** CD56^{bright} NK cells on days 1, 3, and 15 and the absolute numbers of **(D)** CD56^{dim} CD16^{+}, **(E)** CD56^{dim} CD16^{-}, and **(F)** CD56^{bright} NK cells throughout the later cycles of chemotherapy were statistically analysed using Wilcoxon test. **(G)** The fold change in the frequency of NK cell sub-populations as a percentage of total NK cells over the baseline levels were determined throughout the later cycles of chemotherapy and data presented as mean ± SEM. $^{*}p < 0.05$, $^{**}p < 0.01$. $n = 10$.

population during cycles 6 ($p = 0.0075$), 8, and 10 ($p = 0.0313$) and this is accompanied by increases in CD56^{dim} CD16^{-} at cycle 6 ($p = 0.0625$) and cycle 10 ($p = 0.0313$) and CD56^{bright} sub-population at cycles 6, 8, and 10 ($p = 0.0313$; **Figure 3G** and **Supplementary Figure 4**). This result indicated a shift in the NK cell sub-populations, particularly throughout the later cycles of chemotherapy.

Phosphorylation Signalling Responses in NK Cells of CRC Patients

Inflammatory cytokines and chemokines co-ordinate the recruitment, proliferation, activation, and survival of immune cells around the body to combat infections or inhibit tumour growth that can disrupt homeostasis. When bound to their cognate receptors on immune cells, these mediators will lead to the activation of the inflammatory signalling transcription factors and enable the immune cell to function appropriately in these situations (21, 22).

To assess the activation of the signalling pathways and function of the NK cells, we next investigated the phosphorylation status of 8 signalling proteins. Results showed significant changes in phosphorylation status between the CRC patients compared to healthy controls but chemotherapy did not significantly impact the signalling responses in any NK cell sub-population (**Supplementary Figure 5**).

No statistical difference in pP65, pAKT, pMAPKAPK2, or pSTAT1 was seen between people with CRC and the healthy volunteers (**Supplementary Figure 6**). However, results showed significant changes in pERK, pP38, pSTAT3, and pSTAT5 between the people with CRC at baseline and healthy volunteers (**Figure 4A**). The heatmap showed a global increase in pERK, and pSTAT5 but a decrease in pP38 and pSTAT3 in both the stage III and stage IV people with CRC compared to healthy.

Statistical analysis confirmed this observation as an increase was seen in pERK across all the NK cell sub-population, and this reached significance in the CD56^{bright} sub-population ($p = 0.0277$; **Figure 4B**). Similarly, results showed a significant decrease in pP38 in CD56^{dim} CD16^{+} ($p = 0.0028$), CD56^{dim} CD16^{-} ($p = 0.0172$), and CD56^{bright} sub-populations ($p = 0.0041$; **Figure 4C**).

Previous literature have demonstrated that NK cell development and survival is highly dependent on cytokines such as IL-2, IL-12, IL-15, IL-18, and IL-21, most of which signal through the JAK-STAT signalling pathway (23). A statistical analysis of the JAK/STAT signalling pathways found a significant decrease in pSTAT3 in CD56^{dim} CD16^{+} and CD56^{dim} CD16^{-} ($p = 0.0219$ and $p = 0.0030$, respectively, **Figure 4D**) and a significant increase in pSTAT5 across all 3 NK cell subtypes in CRC patients prior to undergoing chemotherapy ($p = 0.0044$, $p = 0.0330$, and $p = 0.0021$; **Figure 4E**).

DISCUSSION

We have used mass cytometry to enhance our understanding of the immune profile of advanced CRC patients undergoing standard cytotoxic chemotherapy. The unsupervised clustering analysis of our high-dimensional data following an acute dose of chemotherapy revealed a decrease in cluster 14, identified as NK cells. Further investigation of the NK cells using manual gating found a distinct and opposing shift in the NK cell subtypes with a

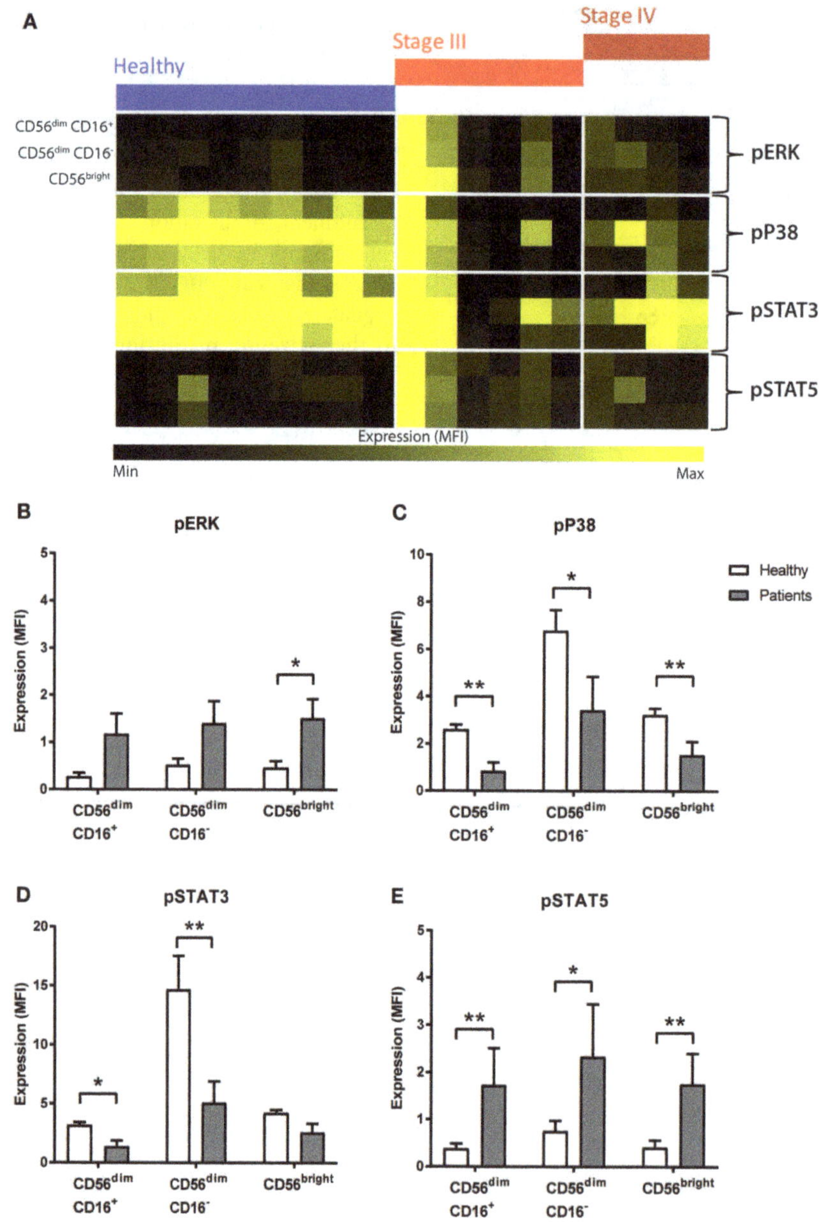

FIGURE 4 | Phosphorylation signalling responses in NK cells of CRC patients compared to healthy volunteers. **(A)** The median fluorescence intensity (MFI) of pERK, pP38, pSTAT3, and pSTAT5 in the NK cell sub-population between the healthy and the CRC patients were visually examined in a heatmap. The difference in the expression of **(B)** pERK, **(C)** pP38, **(D)** pSTAT3, and **(E)** pSTAT5 in the NK cell sub-populations between the CRC patients and healthy volunteers was statistically analysed using Mann-Whiteny *U*-test. Data presented as mean ± SEM. $^{*}p < 0.05$ $^{**}p < 0.01$. $n = 19$.

decrease in CD56^{dim} CD16^{+} population to CD56^{dim} CD16^{-} and CD56^{bright} population throughout the long-term chemotherapy, particularly at the later cycles of the treatment. Furthermore, we analysed the phosphorylation status of various signalling proteins and found an increase in pERK and pSTAT5 and a decrease in pP38 and pSTAT3 universally in all NK sub-populations of people with CRC compared to healthy volunteers.

The technological development in high dimensional data, including mass cytometry, has led to a surge in the development of unsupervised, automated clustering analysis. A study by Weber and Robinson (15) compared the clustering methods for high dimensional data and recommended FlowSOM, an R package from Bioconductor, as the first-choice clustering analysis as they found that it gave the best performance with a fast run-time. Therefore, we chose to analyse our data using FlowSOM. This clustering algorithm analyses data using self-organising maps (SOM), followed by hierarchical consensus meta-cluster to merge clusters (15, 20). The use of the clustering analysis of our high dimensional data allowed the rapid assessment of the effect of acute chemotherapy and identified a unique and under-appreciated finding that NK cells as the immune populations that were most affected by the cytotoxic treatment. Chemotherapy is known to induce cell death through apoptosis as well as other non-apoptotic death such as necrosis, autophagy, mitotic catastrophe, and senescence (24). Myeloid cells, granulocytes, and platelets are known to be reduced following cytotoxic chemotherapy and leucopoenia, neutropenia and thrombocytopenia are common toxicities in patients treated with FOLFOX therapy (25). However, the 14 day cycle is sufficient for repopulation of the hematopoietic stem cell population that both innate and adaptive cells, including NK cells, are derived (26). Therefore, it is interesting to note that the NK cells did not follow an equivalent cycle-dependent rebound.

NK cells are innate lymphoid cells that are involved in preventing tumours and controlling tumour growth (27). NK cells are able to directly and indirectly kill tumour cells without the requirement of prior sensitisation or antigen (28). In this study, we characterised 3 subtypes of NK cells; $CD56^{dim}$ $CD16^{+}$ and $CD56^{bright}$ $CD16^{-}$, and $CD56^{bright}$ cells. $CD56^{bright}$ NK cell sub-populations have low cytotoxic function but are highly proliferative and are specialised in cytokine production responsible for the activation and recruitment of macrophages and T cells into the tumour microenvironment (29, 30). In peripheral blood, $CD56^{bright}$ cells are classified as the stage 4 of NK cell maturation and development and are considered less mature (27, 31). The $CD56^{bright}$ population are known to transition and convert to the more mature sub-populations (stage 5) in a sequential manner, $CD56^{dim}$ $CD16^{-}$ cells followed by $CD56^{dim}$ $CD16^{+}$ NK cells which have lower proliferative ability but have high cytotoxic function (27, 31, 32). Although the $CD56^{dim}$ population are considered more mature as they are in a higher stage of maturation and development, both $CD56^{bright}$ and $CD56^{dim}$ population are both functionally active and are observed to perform different but equally important functions through either cytotoxicity or secretion of cytokines to induce an immunoregulatory environment (27, 31). In CRC, NK cells have long been shown to infiltrate the tumour microenvironment and are associated with an improved prognosis (33, 34). In addition, NK cells are also important in preventing recurrence by protecting against cancer-initiating cells (35).

The most abundant subtype of NK cells (~15% of all immune cells) identified in our study were the $CD56^{dim}$ $CD16^{+}$ sub-population, which was not found to be statistically different in the baseline peripheral blood samples of people with CRC compared to healthy people. Similarly, the $CD56^{bright}$ population was not statistically different in the peripheral blood of people with CRC compared to healthy people in baseline samples. In contrast, we found a statistical increase in the numbers of $CD56^{+}$ $CD16^{-}$ NK cells in CRC patients. CD16 is a low-affinity FcγRIII that binds antibody-coated targets and signals antibody dependent cellular cytotoxicity (ADCC) (36, 37). CD16 specifically binds to the Fc portion of the IgG antibodies on the surface of coated cells and triggers degranulation of intracellular granules, which kill the infected or tumour cells (30, 36). Previous studies have shown that in targeted therapies in CRC, such as cetuximab, NK cells contributes to ADCC and the higher frequency of NK cells predict patient response to therapy (38). The functional role of the NK cell subtypes in ADCC should be further investigated to understand the clinical relevance of the decrease in the NK cell population following cytotoxic chemotherapy.

Previous literature has shown contrasting results regarding the frequency of NK cells in the peripheral blood and tumours of CRC patients. A study by Rocca et al. (39) found no difference in the NK cell population, identified as $CD3^{-}$ $CD56^{+}$, in the peripheral blood of CRC patients compared to the healthy donors. Similar to our results, the study found no difference in the proportion of $CD56^{dim}$ and $CD56^{bright}$ in total NK cells. In contrast, the same group in 2016 found statistically higher levels of $CD3^{-}$ $CD56^{+}$ NK cell population in the peripheral blood of CRC patients (40). However, in both studies, the authors did not interrogate the expression of CD16 in the NK cell population.

To enhance our understanding of immune evasion during the lifetime of a cancer patient, we need to consider the impact of standard cytotoxic chemotherapy on the frequency and phenotype of immune populations that mediate these tumour promoting processes. Our results showed that an acute dose of chemotherapy (the first cycle) caused a decrease in the levels of the NK cell sub-populations, particularly the $CD56^{dim}$ $CD16^{+}$ and the $CD56^{bright}$ populations. Interestingly, long-term chemotherapy caused a phenotypic shift in the NK cell sub-populations, with a decrease in $CD56^{dim}$ $CD16^{+}$ population and an increase in the $CD56^{dim}$ $CD16^{-}$ and $CD56^{bright}$ populations. In contrast, a previous study in CRC showed that third-line treatment with the EGFR monoclonal antibody, cetuximab, was not shown to affect the frequency of $CD56^{+}$ or $CD56^{+}$ $CD16^{+}$ cells in advanced CRC patients (41).

As mentioned previously, $CD56^{dim}$ $CD16^{+}$ population has been shown to have high cytotoxic function but low cytokine production (27). In contrast, $CD56^{bright}$ population have low cytotoxic function but are specialised in cytokine production responsible for the activation and recruitment of macrophages and recruitment of T cells into the tumour microenvironment (29, 30). It remains unclear why the $CD56^{dim}$ $CD16^{+}$ population decreased throughout the chemotherapy treatment. As mentioned above chemotherapy may preferentially induce cellular cytotoxicity of the $CD56^{dim}$ $CD16^{+}$ population or cause inhibition of transition from $CD56^{bright}$ and $CD16^{dim}$ $CD16^{-}$ to a later maturation stage with an increase in cytotoxic function (27). Alternatively, migration of the $CD56^{dim}$ $CD16^{+}$ population to the tumour or other sites may also be a plausible explanation for the decreased frequency of this NK cell population. However, the role of chemotherapy impacting the migration of NK cells to other tissues, including tumours, is lacking evidence and will need to be explored in animal models due to the difficulties in obtaining clinically relevant tissues samples post-chemotherapy.

The increased frequency of $CD56^{dim}$ $CD16^{-}$ population may be due to increased loss of CD16 expression via shedding. Activation of NK cells through cytokines, such as IL-2, IL-15, and IL-18, TNF or target cells (such as tumour cells) can also lead to shedding of CD16 (42, 43). Many of these cytokines are increased in the circulation of colorectal cancer patients (44, 45). Activation of NK cells via signalling through CD16 or NKG2D leads to an increase in the metalloprotease ADAM17 which also cleaves CD16 on NK cells (30). Studies have shown that shedding or decrease of CD16 on NK cells via cytokine or direct tumour cell interactions are a common effect of several solid cancers including oral cancer (46), ovarian cancer (47), and melanoma (48). A decrease in the expression of CD16 on NK cells consequently led to a decrease in cytotoxic function of the NK cells, particularly decrease in ADCC, as well as production of IFNγ (46, 47, 49). The change in phenotype of NK cells from $CD16^{+}$ to $CD16^{-}$ as well as the decrease in cytotoxic activity following contact with target cells is known as "split anergy" (50–52). Split anergy can also be induced by stimulation with IL-2 and anti-CD16 antibodies or contact with monocytes (51). Further investigation using a larger cohort of stage IV CRC patients is needed to determine the effect of the decrease in frequency and anti-tumour function of NK cell sub-populations and response to therapy and survival outcome of the patients.

In addition to assessing the levels of NK cells sub-populations, this study was able to measure the phosphorylation status of numerous inflammatory signalling responses at a single-cell level in one small clinical sample using mass cytometry. In baseline samples, results in this study found a significantly lower expression of pSTAT3 and an increase in pSTAT5 across the NK cell subtypes in CRC patients. NK cell development in highly dependent on cytokines such as IL-2, IL-12, IL-15, IL-18, and IL-21, most of which signal through the JAK-STAT signalling pathway (23). Previous literature has shown that STAT3 is a negative regulator of NK cell function (53). *In vivo* studies by Gotthardt et al. (54) showed that a loss of STAT3 in NK cells enhanced the cytolytic activity resulting in enhanced tumour surveillance. In contrast, STAT5 has shown to be vital for NK cell development and survival through signalling from IL-2 and IL-15 (55). The decrease in pSTAT3 and increase in pSTAT5 suggest that the cytokines that target the pSTAT5 signalling pathway, such as IL-2 and IL-15, might play a more vital role in the activation and function of NK cells in this cohort of advanced CRC patients over cytokines that primarily signal through the STAT3 pathway, such as IL-12 and IL-21. Additionally supporting this finding is the increase in pERK and decrease in pP38 in the NK cell sub-populations, particularly in $CD56^{bright}$ population, in this study. Previous studies in NK cells found that IL-2 activated MAPK/ERK signalling but not the mitogen activated protein kinase (MAPK) P38 signalling pathway to regulate NK cell function (56). Interestingly, a study by Peruzzi et al. (57) also showed that IL-2 or IL-15 exposure led to the shedding of CD16 on the surface of NK cells which could also explain the decrease in CD16+ NK cells following chemotherapy.

There are important limitations to consider when using mass cytometry for discovery phase projects, such as this study. Statistical analysis of small datasets is challenging when obtaining the levels of high dimensional data obtained through a mass cytometry experiment. As this was a discovery project, we avoided using *post-hoc* corrections in our statistical analysis to reduce the risk of type II errors (false negatives) in this small cohort. However, this also increases the risk of type I error (false positives). As a recommendation following the mass cytometry discovery project, future studies need to utilise a larger cohort size and prospectively use *post-hoc* multiple comparison corrections (e.g., Bonferroni correction of pairwise comparisons or using a false discovery rate correction). Other sources of limitations were missing time points in some patients, particularly the end of infusion of day 3 sample, which could cause potential bias of results following a single acute dose of chemotherapy. Missing samples later during chemotherapy are due to unplanned discontinuation of chemotherapy for toxicity or progressive disease and would be difficult to predict when these random events occur. Finally, future experiments with mass cytometry should incorporate functional studies to validate the biological relevance of the changes in phenotype and how these are related to clinical outcomes. However, researchers do need to be mindful of the larger volumes of blood required to complete these more extensive functional assays in patients undergoing active chemotherapy and there may be challenges of acceptance by patients and ethics committees.

Despite only having access to a small number of patients, this study was nonetheless able to identify differences in the NK cell population in CRC patients undergoing standard chemotherapy treatment. Following the patients throughout their chemotherapy treatment (~5–6 months) in conjunction with use of mass cytometry proved to be a powerful combination that allowed us to profile the immune system of these patients as they underwent treatment and identify a novel phenotypic shift in the NK cell populations. Following standard cytotoxic chemotherapy, we have identified that there is an unrecognised deficiency in NK cell frequencies that needs to be considered in the therapeutic decisions and monitoring of treatment response and survival.

ETHICS STATEMENT

This study was approved by Northern Sydney Local Health District and North Shore Private Hospital Human Ethics Committees, and written, informed consent was obtained from all patients prior to participation in the study.

AUTHOR CONTRIBUTIONS

DS helped with enrolment of patients, performed experiments, analysed and interpreted data, and wrote the manuscript. HM helped with design of experiments, trained and helped DS run the samples on the mass cytometer, advised on analysis and interpreted obtained data, and critically revised the manuscript.

CD, NP, and SC helped with design of study, enrolment of patients, and reviewed the manuscript. SB interpreted obtained data and critically reviewed the manuscript. KC designed the study, enrolled patients, interpreted obtained data, participated in writing the manuscript, and critically reviewed the manuscript.

ACKNOWLEDGMENTS

We thank the patients and healthy donors for contributing to this study. We would also like to thank Thomas Ashhurst for his support in using CAPX pipeline for unsupervised clustering analysis. We thank Sydney Cytometry facility for access to the mass cytometer, Helios^{TM}, Caryn Van Vreden for technical assistance, and Ramaciotti Facility for Human Systems Biology for reagents used in the experiments.

REFERENCES

1. Favoriti P, Carbone G, Greco M, Pirozzi F, Pirozzi RE, Corcione F. Worldwide burden of colorectal cancer: a review. *Updates Surg.* (2016) 68:7–11. doi: 10.1007/s13304-016-0359-y
2. Andre T, Boni C, Mounedji-Boudiaf L, Navarro M, Tabernero J, Hickish T, et al. Oxaliplatin, fluorouracil, and leucovorin as adjuvant treatment for colon cancer. *N Engl J Med.* (2004) 350:2343–51. doi: 10.1056/NEJMoa032709
3. Brenner H, Kloor M, Pox CP. Colorectal cancer. *Lancet.* (2014) 383:1490–502. doi: 10.1016/S0140-6736(13)61649-9
4. Sclafani F, Cunningham D. Cetuximab or bevacizumab in metastatic colorectal cancer? *Lancet Oncol.* (2014) 15:1040–1. doi: 10.1016/S1470-2045(14)70360-2
5. Tol J, Koopman M, Cats A, Rodenburg CJ, Creemers GJM, Schrama JG, et al. Chemotherapy, bevacizumab, and cetuximab in metastatic colorectal cancer. *N Engl J Med.* (2009) 360:563–72. doi: 10.1056/NEJMoa0808268
6. Hanahan D, Weinberg RA. Hallmarks of cancer: the next generation. *Cell.* (2011) 144:646–74. doi: 10.1016/j.cell.2011.02.013
7. Wang K, Karin M. Tumor-elicited inflammation and colorectal cancer. *Adv Cancer Res.* (2015) 128:173–96. doi: 10.1016/bs.acr.2015.04.014
8. Albini A, Tosetti F, Benelli R, Noonan DM. Tumor inflammatory angiogenesis and its chemoprevention. *Cancer Res.* (2005) 65:10637–41. doi: 10.1158/0008-5472.CAN-05-3473
9. Hu T, Li LF, Shen J, Zhang L, Cho CH. Chronic inflammation and colorectal cancer: the role of vascular endothelial growth factor. *Curr Pharm Des.* (2015) 21:2960–7. doi: 10.2174/1381612821666150514104244
10. Overman MJ, Ernstoff MS, Morse MA. Where we stand with immunotherapy in colorectal cancer: deficient mismatch repair, proficient mismatch repair, and toxicity management. *Am Soc Clin Oncol Educ Book.* (2018) 38:239–47. doi: 10.1200/EDBK_200821
11. Le DT, Uram JN, Wang H, Bartlett BR, Kemberling H, Eyring AD, et al. PD-1 blockade in tumors with mismatch-repair deficiency. *N Engl J Med.* (2015) 372:2509–20. doi: 10.1056/NEJMoa1500596
12. Overman MJ, McDermott R, Leach JL, Lonardi S, Lenz HJ, Morse MA, et al. Nivolumab in patients with metastatic DNA mismatch repair-deficient or microsatellite instability-high colorectal cancer (CheckMate 142): an open-label, multicentre, phase 2 study. *Lancet Oncol.* (2017) 18:1182–91. doi: 10.1016/S1470-2045(17)30422-9
13. Tanner SD, Baranov VI, Ornatsky OI, Bandura DR, George TC. An introduction to mass cytometry: fundamentals and applications. *Cancer Immunol Immunother.* (2013) 62:955–65. doi: 10.1007/s00262-013-1416-8
14. Nair N, Mei HE, Chen SY, Hale M, Nolan GP, Maecker HT, et al. Mass cytometry as a platform for the discovery of cellular biomarkers to guide effective rheumatic disease therapy. *Arthritis Res Ther.* (2015) 17:127. doi: 10.1186/s13075-015-0644-z
15. Weber LM, Robinson MD. Comparison of clustering methods for high-dimensional single-cell flow and mass cytometry data. *Cytometry A.* (2016) 89:1084–96. doi: 10.1002/cyto.a.23030
16. eviQ. *Colorectal Adjuvant FOLFOX6 (Modified) (Fluorouracil Leucovorin Oxaliplatin).* eviQ Cancer Treatments Online, Cancer Institute NSW (2018). Available online at: https://www.eviq.org.au/medical-oncology/colorectal/adjuvant-and-neoadjuvant/637-colorectal-adjuvant-folfox6-modified-fluoro (accessed April 1, 2019).
17. Shinko D, Ashhurst TM, McGuire HM, and Charles KA. Staining of phosphorylated signalling markers protocol for mass cytometry. *Methods Mol Biol.* (2019) 1989:139–46. doi: 10.1007/978-1-4939-9454-0_10
18. Ashhurst TM. *Cytometry Analysis Pipeline for large and compleX Datasets v2.4.* GitHub repository (2018). Available online at: https://github.com/sydneycytometry/CAPX
19. Ashhurst TM, Cox DA, Smith AL, King NJC. Analysis of the murine bone marrow hematopoietic system using mass and flow cytometry. *Methods Mol Biol.* (2019) 1989:159–92. doi: 10.1007/978-1-4939-9454-0_12
20. Van Gassen S, Callebaut B, Van Helden MJ, Lambrecht BN, Demeester P, Dhaene T, et al. FlowSOM: using self-organizing maps for visualization and interpretation of cytometry data. *Cytometry A.* (2015) 87:636–45. doi: 10.1002/cyto.a.22625
21. Mantovani A, Allavena P, Sica A, Balkwill F. Cancer-related inflammation. *Nature.* (2008) 454:436–44. doi: 10.1038/nature07205
22. Shinko D, Diakos CI, Clarke SJ, Charles KA. Cancer-related systemic inflammation: the challenges and therapeutic opportunities for personalized medicine. *Clin Pharmacol Ther.* (2017) 102:599–610. doi: 10.1002/cpt.789
23. Di Santo JP. Natural killer cell developmental pathways: a question of balance. *Annu Rev Immunol.* (2006) 24:257–86. doi: 10.1146/annurev.immunol.24.021605.090700
24. Ricci MS, Zong W-X. Chemotherapeutic approaches for targeting cell death pathways. *Oncol.* (2006) 11:342–57. doi: 10.1634/theoncologist.11-4-342
25. Hochster HS, Hart LL, Ramanathan RK, Childs BH, Hainsworth JD, Cohn AL, et al. Safety and efficacy of oxaliplatin and fluoropyrimidine regimens with or without bevacizumab as first-line treatment of metastatic colorectal cancer: results of the TREE Study. *J Clin Oncol.* (2008) 26:3523–9. doi: 10.1200/JCO.2007.15.4138
26. Randall TD, Weissman IL. Phenotypic and functional changes induced at the clonal level in hematopoietic stem cells after 5-fluorouracil treatment. *Blood.* (1997) 89:3596–606. doi: 10.1182/blood.V89.10.3596.3596_3596_3606
27. Abel AM, Yang C, Thakar MS, Malarkannan S. Natural killer cells: development, maturation, and clinical utilization. *Front Immunol.* (2018) 9:1869. doi: 10.3389/fimmu.2018.01869
28. Nicholson SE, Keating N, Belz GT. Natural killer cells and anti-tumor immunity. *Mol Immunol.* (2017) 110:40–7. doi: 10.1016/j.molimm.2017.12.002
29. Freud AG, Mundy-Bosse BL, Yu J, Caligiuri MA. The broad spectrum of human natural killer cell diversity. *Immunity.* (2017) 47:820–33. doi: 10.1016/j.immuni.2017.10.008
30. Romee R, Foley B, Lenvik T, Wang Y, Zhang B, Ankarlo D, et al. NK cell CD16 surface expression and function is regulated by a

disintegrin and metalloprotease-17 (ADAM17). *Blood.* (2013) 121:3599–608. doi: 10.1182/blood-2012-04-425397

31. Poli A, Michel T, Theresine M, Andres E, Hentges F, Zimmer J. CD56bright natural killer (NK) cells: an important NK cell subset. *Immunology.* (2009) 126:458–65. doi: 10.1111/j.1365-2567.2008.03027.x
32. Jacobs R, Hintzen G, Kemper A, Beul K, Kempf S, Behrens G, et al. CD56bright cells differ in their KIR repertoire and cytotoxic features from CD56dim NK cells. *Eur J Immunol.* (2001) 31:3121–6. doi: 10.1002/1521-4141(2001010)31:10<;3121::AID-IMMU3121>;3.0.CO;2-4
33. Coca S, Perez-Piqueras J, Martinez D, Colmenarejo A, Saez MA, Vallejo C, et al. The prognostic significance of intratumoral natural killer cells in patients with colorectal carcinoma. *Cancer.* (1997) 79:2320–8. doi: 10.1002/(SICI)1097-0142(19970615)79:12<;2320::AID-CNCR5>;3.0.CO;2-P
34. Donadon M, Hudspeth K, Cimino M, Di Tommaso L, Preti M, Tentorio P, et al. Increased infiltration of natural killer and t cells in colorectal liver metastases improves patient overall survival. *J Gastrointest Surg.* (2017) 21:1226–36. doi: 10.1007/s11605-017-3446-6
35. Tallerico R, Todaro M, Di Franco S, Maccalli C, Garofalo C, Sottile R, et al. Human NK cells selective targeting of colon cancer-initiating cells: a role for natural cytotoxicity receptors and MHC class I molecules. *J Immunol.* (2013) 190:2381–90. doi: 10.4049/jimmunol.1201542
36. Cooper MA, Caligiuri MA. Isolation and characterization of human natural killer cell subsets. *Curr Protoc Immunol.* (2004) 60:7.34.1–12. doi: 10.1002/0471142735.im0734s60
37. Leibson PJ. Signal transduction during natural killer cell activation: inside the mind of a killer. *Immunity.* (1997) 6:655–61. doi: 10.1016/S1074-7613(00)80441-0
38. Trotta AM, Ottaiano A, Romano C, Nasti G, Nappi A, De Divitiis C, et al. Prospective evaluation of cetuximab-mediated antibody-dependent cell cytotoxicity in metastatic colorectal cancer patients predicts treatment efficacy. *Cancer Immunol Res.* (2016) 4:366–74. doi: 10.1158/2326-6066.CIR-15-0184
39. Rocca YS, Roberti MP, Arriaga JM, Amat M, Bruno L, Pampena MB, et al. Altered phenotype in peripheral blood and tumor-associated NK cells from colorectal cancer patients. *Innate Immun.* (2013) 19:76–85. doi: 10.1177/1753425912453187
40. Rocca YS, Roberti MP, Julia EP, Pampena MB, Bruno L, Rivero S, et al. Phenotypic and functional dysregulated blood NK cells in colorectal cancer patients can be activated by cetuximab plus IL-2 or IL-15. *Front Immunol.* (2016) 7:413. doi: 10.3389/fimmu.2016.00413
41. Matic IZ, Kolundzija B, Damjanovic A, Spasic J, Radosavljevic D, Dordic Crnogorac M, et al. Peripheral white blood cell subsets in metastatic colorectal cancer patients treated with cetuximab: the potential clinical relevance. *Front Immunol.* (2017) 8:1886. doi: 10.3389/fimmu.2017.01886
42. Felce JH, Dustin ML. Natural killers shed attachments to kill again. *J Cell Biol.* (2018) 217:2983. doi: 10.1083/jcb.201807105
43. Srpan K, Ambrose A, Karampatzakis A, Saeed M, Cartwright ANR, Guldevall K, et al. Shedding of CD16 disassembles the NK cell immune synapse and boosts serial engagement of target cells. *J Cell Biol.* (2018) 217:3267. doi: 10.1083/jcb.201712085
44. Mager LF, Wasmer M-H, Rau TT, Krebs P. Cytokine-induced modulation of colorectal cancer. *Front Oncol.* (2016) 6:96. doi: 10.3389/fonc.2016.00096
45. Yamaguchi M, Okamura S, Yamaji T, Iwasaki M, Tsugane S, Shetty V, et al. Plasma cytokine levels and the presence of colorectal cancer. *PLoS ONE.* (2019) 14:e0213602. doi: 10.1371/journal.pone.0213602
46. Jewett A, Cacalano NA, Head C, Teruel A. Coengagement of CD16 and CD94 receptors mediates secretion of chemokines and induces apoptotic death of naive natural killer cells. *Clin Cancer Res.* (2006) 12:1994–2003. doi: 10.1158/1078-0432.CCR-05-2306
47. Lai P, Rabinowich H, Crowley-Nowick PA, Bell MC, Mantovani G, Whiteside TL. Alterations in expression and function of signal-transducing proteins in tumor-associated T and natural killer cells in patients with ovarian carcinoma. *Clin Cancer Res.* (1996) 2:161–73.
48. Vujanovic L, Chuckran C, Lin Y, Ding F, Sander CA, Santos PM, et al. CD56dim CD16− natural killer cell profiling in melanoma patients receiving a cancer vaccine and interferon-α. *Front Immunol.* (2019) 10:14. doi: 10.3389/fimmu.2019.00014
49. Jewett A, Cavalcanti M, Bonavida B. Pivotal role of endogenous TNF-alpha in the induction of functional inactivation and apoptosis in NK cells. *J Immunol.* (1997) 159:4815–22.
50. Belyaev NN, Abramova VA. Transmission of "split anergy" from tumor infiltrating to peripheral NK cells in a manner similar to "infectious tolerance". *Med Hypotheses.* (2014) 82:129–33. doi: 10.1016/j.mehy.2013.11.019
51. Jewett A, Arasteh A, Tseng HC, Behel A, Arasteh H, Yang W, et al. Strategies to rescue mesenchymal stem cells (MSCs) and dental pulp stem cells (DPSCs) from NK cell mediated cytotoxicity. *PLoS ONE.* (2010) 5:e9874. doi: 10.1371/journal.pone.0009874
52. Jewett A, Tseng H-C. Potential rescue, survival and differentiation of cancer stem cells and primary non-transformed stem cells by monocyte-induced split anergy in natural killer cells. *Cancer Immunol Immunother.* (2012) 61:265–74. doi: 10.1007/s00262-011-1163-7
53. Cacalano NA. Regulation of natural killer cell function by STAT3. *Front Immunol.* (2016) 7:128. doi: 10.3389/fimmu.2016.00128
54. Gotthardt D, Putz EM, Straka E, Kudweis P, Biaggio M, Poli V, et al. Loss of STAT3 in murine NK cells enhances NK cell-dependent tumor surveillance. *Blood.* (2014) 124:2370–9. doi: 10.1182/blood-2014-03-564450
55. Gotthardt D, Putz EM, Grundschober E, Prchal-Murphy M, Straka E, Kudweis P, et al. STAT5 is a key regulator in NK cells and acts as a molecular switch from tumor surveillance to tumor promotion. *Cancer Discov.* (2016) 6:414–29. doi: 10.1158/2159-8290.CD-15-0732
56. Yu TK, Caudell EG, Smid C, Grimm EA. IL-2 activation of NK cells: involvement of MKK1/2/ERK but not p38 kinase pathway. *J Immunol.* (2000) 164:6244–51. doi: 10.4049/jimmunol.164.12.6244
57. Peruzzi G, Femnou L, Gil-Krzewska A, Borrego F, Weck J, Krzewski K, et al. Membrane-type 6 matrix metalloproteinase regulates the activation-induced downmodulation of CD16 in human primary NK cells. *J Immunol.* (2013) 191:1883–94. doi: 10.4049/jimmunol.1300313

5

Validation of CyTOF Against Flow Cytometry for Immunological Studies and Monitoring of Human Cancer Clinical Trials

Ramy Gadalla[1], Babak Noamani[1], Bethany L. MacLeod[1], Russell J. Dickson[1], Mengdi Guo[2], Wenxi Xu[1], Sabelo Lukhele[1], Heidi J. Elsaesser[1], Albiruni R. Abdul Razak[1], Naoto Hirano[1,2], Tracy L. McGaha[1,2], Ben Wang[1], Marcus Butler[1], Cynthia J. Guidos[2,3], Pam S. Ohashi[1,2], Lillian L. Siu[1] and David G. Brooks[1,2]*

[1] *Tumor Immunology Program, Princess Margaret Cancer Center, University Health Network, Toronto, ON, Canada,* [2] *Department of Immunology, University of Toronto, Toronto, ON, Canada,* [3] *Program in Developmental and Stem Cell Biology, Hospital for Sick Children Research Institute, Toronto, ON, Canada*

***Correspondence:**
David G. Brooks
dbrooks@uhnresearch.ca

Flow cytometry is a widely applied approach for exploratory immune profiling and biomarker discovery in cancer and other diseases. However, flow cytometry is limited by the number of parameters that can be simultaneously analyzed, severely restricting its utility. Recently, the advent of mass cytometry (CyTOF) has enabled high dimensional and unbiased examination of the immune system, allowing simultaneous interrogation of a large number of parameters. This is important for deep interrogation of immune responses and particularly when sample sizes are limited (such as in tumors). Our goal was to compare the accuracy and reproducibility of CyTOF against flow cytometry as a reliable analytic tool for human PBMC and tumor tissues for cancer clinical trials. We developed a 40+ parameter CyTOF panel and demonstrate that compared to flow cytometry, CyTOF yields analogous quantification of cell lineages in conjunction with markers of cell differentiation, function, activation, and exhaustion for use with fresh and viably frozen PBMC or tumor tissues. Further, we provide a protocol that enables reliable quantification by CyTOF down to low numbers of input human cells, an approach that is particularly important when cell numbers are limiting. Thus, we validate CyTOF as an accurate approach to perform high dimensional analysis in human tumor tissue and to utilize low cell numbers for subsequent immunologic studies and cancer clinical trials.

Keywords: CyTOF, flow cytometry, cancer clinical trials, immune studies, immunotherapy

INTRODUCTION

To discover immune correlates and biomarkers of disease requires global profiling of the immune system, the proteins differentially regulated by therapy and how these relate to disease outcome. Highly focused exploration may provide hypothesis-driven insight, but often the paradigm-altering discoveries come from unbiased global immune profiling. Flow cytometry (FC) has emerged as a key tool to profile multiple parameters of the immune system, including vital functional and exhaustion markers associated with the quality of the immune response (1). However, FC is limited by the number of parameters that can be analyzed at one time (generally 12 per staining panel).

This means that stains must be broken up into groups with redundancy of many of the cell lineage markers in different stains. As a result, FC requires large sample sizes for coverage of diverse immune subsets. This is particularly detrimental for tumor biopsies where sample sizes are often limiting and the broad array of FC staining panels often cannot be performed. Further, when only a few markers can be analyzed in a single sample, researchers must design panels using a priori knowledge of marker expression patterns to characterize cells of interest. If unusual marker expression patterns are encountered, as is often the case in disease states, follow-up studies that require time-consuming design and optimization of new panels must be performed, assuming more patient sample is available.

Recently, the use of high-dimensional time-of-flight mass cytometry (CyTOF) to identify 40+ parameters simultaneously has emerged as a technique for broad-scale immune profiling and biomarker discovery (1–7). Because CyTOF allows far more markers to be measured in a single tube, fewer cells are required per experiment than would be needed for traditional FC, which would require multiple tubes (with different antibody panels) to cover the same number of markers. By incorporating a large number of parameters into single stains, CyTOF enables acquisition of large amounts of immunologic data from limited sample sizes to better understand biologic systems, response to therapy (8) and signatures of disease(1, 5–7, 9–14). Examples include characterization of intra- and inter-tumor leukemia heterogeneity that correlates with clinical outcomes(15) as well as dissections of T and NK cell subtypes with high resolution (16–19), antiviral T cell responses (5, 7, 18, 20), and immune cell signatures linked to recovery from surgery (21). Thus, CyTOF has enormous potential to discover disease associated immunologic changes in cancer, identify functional changes to guide subsequent therapy and ultimately predict therapeutic outcomes.

Both FC and CyTOF utilize antibodies to label targets on cells. For FC these antibodies are labeled with fluorophores that are excited by lasers to emit light subsequently detected by the flow cytometer. Due to the range of wavelengths of these light emissions, there is overlap in their emission spectra that must be mathematically compensated, thus limiting the number of fluorophores that can be used simultaneously. CyTOF uses antibodies conjugated to rare heavy metal isotopes that are not normally present in biological specimens. As opposed to fluorescence, CyTOF uses an atomic mass cytometer to detect the time-of-flight (TOF) of each metal. Each atom's TOF is determined by its mass, allowing the composition of metal atoms on each cell to be ascertained. Detection overlap among heavy metal isotopes is generally limited to <2% (22) rather than the 5–100% spectral overlap seen in conventional FC, and backgrounds are very low because cells do not naturally contain heavy metals. Thus, the detection of low-expression markers is greatly enhanced even on cell populations such as myeloid cells with high auto-fluorescence.

The goal of this study is to validate CyTOF against FC for use in immune profiling for clinical trials. Panels were designed to include major (and most minor) immune lineage defining markers in combination with a wide array of functional, activation, exhaustion, differentiation, chemotaxis, immunomodulatory, and senescence markers (**Table 1**). Overall, our results demonstrate that CyTOF faithfully recapitulates FC data in PBMC and tumor tissues, providing reliable staining of >35 parameters for high dimensional analyses for analysis of cancer clinical trials.

MATERIALS AND METHODS

PBMC and Tumor Tissue Collection

All human tissues and blood were obtained through protocols approved by the institutional review board. Written informed consent was obtained from all donors. Peripheral blood samples were collected from 11 healthy donors into sterile anticoagulant-coated tubes from the Healthy Donor Blood Collection Study at the Princess Margret Cancer Center (IRB#11-0343). Five surgically resected tumor specimens; 2 ovarian (IRB#10-0335), 2 melanoma (IRB#05-0495), and 1 breast tumor (IRB#06-0801) were obtained from the UHN Biospecimen Program.

Sample Processing

Peripheral blood mononuclear cells (PBMCs) were isolated by Ficoll-paque density gradient centrifugation from the healthy donor's blood. After isolation, cells were directly stained for flow and mass cytometry. Excess cells were aliquoted in 10^7 cells per vial in freezing media (10% DMSO in heat-inactivated FBS) and cryopreserved in liquid nitrogen. Tissue samples were minced into 2–4 mm^3 fragments and digested enzymatically into single cell suspensions with the gentleMACS Dissociator (Miltenyi Biotech, catalog #130-093-235) and the human tumor dissociation kit (Miltenyi Biotech, catalog #130-095-929) to obtain single cell preparations. Cells were then aliquoted and cryopreserved in liquid nitrogen.

CyTOF and Flow Cytometry Antibodies

The same antibody clones were used for CyTOF and FC. The vendor from which each antibody was purchased is listed in **Tables 1**, **2**. For CyTOF, purified unconjugated antibodies used were Biolegend MaxPar Ready antibodies or custom-made with no additional protein carrier from Biolegend or Thermo Fisher. CyTOF antibodies were labeled with metal-tag at the SickKids-UHN Flow and Mass Cytometry Facility using the MaxPar Antibody Labeling kit from Fluidigm (catalog #201300).

Staining Procedure

After PBMCs isolation, cells were counted and viability measured by trypan blue exclusion. One million viable cells were aliquoted into 4 ml polystyrene V-bottom tubes for CyTOF staining. For FC staining, 1 million viable cells per well were added to 8 wells of into 96-well plate for the FC panels shown in **Table 2**. CyTOF and FC staining were performed simultaneously. Single cells suspensions from tumor tissues were handled analogously same way after thawing.

For FC staining, cells were incubated in Fc blocker (ThermoFisher, catalog #16-9161-73) for 10 min at room temperature, followed by incubation in the surface markers antibody cocktail for 30 min at 4°C. Cells were then fixed with

TABLE 1 | CyTOF Panel.

Mass and Tag	Specificity	Ab Clone	Replicates (PBMC)	Company
89Y	CD45	HI30	10	Fluidigm
141Pr	CD45RA	HI100	7	Biolegend
142Nd	HLA-DR	L243	8	Biolegend
143Nd	CD57	HCD57	8	Biolegend
144Nd	CD33	WM53	8	Biolegend
145Nd	CD183 (CXCR3)	G025H7	8	Biolegend
146Nd	CD8α	RPA-T8	11	Biolegend
147Sm	CD4	RPA-T4	11	Biolegend
149Sm	Perforin	B-D48	8	Biolegend
149Sm	FoxP3	236A-E7	8	ThermoFisher
150Nd	CD103	B-Ly7	9	ThermoFisher
150Nd	Tbet	4B10	7	Biolegend
151Eu	CD39	A1	10	Biolegend
152Sm	CD11c	Bu15	8	Biolegend
153Eu	CD3	UCHT1	11	Biolegend
154Sm	IgM	MHM-88	11	Biolegend
155Gd	CD45RO	UCHL1	7	Biolegend
156Gd	CD14	M5E2	8	Biolegend
158Gd	CD27	O323	11	Biolegend
159Tb	CD19	HIB19	11	Biolegend
160Gd	CD25	M-A251	9	Biolegend
161Sy	Ki67	Ki67	8	Biolegend
162Dy	CD28	CD28.2	11	Biolegend
163Dy	CD137 (41BB)	4B4-1	8	Biolegend
164Dy	CD34	581	8	Biolegend
165Ho	CD279 (PD1)	EH12.2H7	9	Biolegend
166Er	Tim3	F38-2E2	7	Biolegend
167Er	CD95 (Fas)	DX2	11	Biolegend
9168Er	CD185 (CXCR5)	MU5UBEE	8	ThermoFisher
169Tm	TCRγδ	5A6-E9	11	ThermoFisher
170Er	CD152 (CTLA4)	14D3	7	ThermoFisher
171Yb	GranzymeB	GB11	9	Biolegend
171Yb	Helios	22F6	6	Biolegend
172Yb	CD127 (IL-7Rα)	EBioRDR5	11	ThermoFisher
173Yb	CD56	HCD56		Biolegend
174Yb	TIGIT	MBSA43	11	ThermoFisher
175Lu	CD274 (PDL1)	29E.2A3	5	Biolegend
176Yb	CD223 (Lag3)	7H2C65	7	Biolegend
191Ir	DNA1 (Cell ID)			Fluidigm
193Ir	DNA2 (Cell ID)			Fluidigm
196Pt	Cisplatin (Viability)			BioVision
209Bi	CD16	3G8	6	Fluidigm

Antibodies used and their metal conjugation are shown in the table. Replicates indicates the number of different healthy PBMC donors that were used for the validation in ***Figures 1, 2****. Company indicates where each antibody was purchased.*

4% paraformaldehyde (PFA). For intracellular staining, cells were fixed and permeabilized by incubation with eBioscience Foxp3/Transcription Factor Staining Buffer Set (catalog #5523) for 30 min at 4°C, followed by incubation with intracellular antibody cocktail. Cells were washed by centrifugation at 480

TABLE 2 | Flow Cytometry Panels.

Fluorochrome	Specificity	Company
FLOW CYTOMETRY PANEL 1		
BUV395	CD3	BD Bioscience
BV605	CD4	BD Bioscience
FITC	TCRgd	ThermoFisher
PerCP	CD8	Biolegend
PE-Cy7	TIGIT	ThermoFisher
APC-Cy7	CD56	Biolegend
eFluor506	Viability	ThermoFisher
FLOW CYTOMETRY PANEL 2		
FITC	CD16	Biolegend
PE	CD14	Biolegend
PE-Cy7	CD11C	Biolegend
APC	PDL1	Biolegend
AlexaFluor 700	CD33	ThermoFisher
BV421	CD45RO	Biolegend
BV605	CD45	Biolegend
BV650	CD45RA	Biolegend
BV711	HLA-DR	Biolegend
eFluor506	Viability	ThermoFisher
FLOW CYTOMETRY PANEL 3		
BUV395	CD3	BD Bioscience
BV421	CD127	ThermoFisher
BV605	CD4	BD Bioscience
AlexaFluor700	CD8	ThermoFisher
PerCP-eF710	CD39	ThermoFisher
PE-CF594	CD95 (Fas)	BD Bioscience
eFluor506	Viability	ThermoFisher
FLOW CYTOMETRY PANEL 4		
BUV395	CD3	Biolegend
PE	CD103	ThermoFisher
PE-Cy7	CD28	ThermoFisher
APC	CXCR5	ThermoFisher
PerCP	CD8	Biolegend
AlexaFluor700	CD4	ThermoFisher
BV605	CXCR3	Biolegend
EFluor506	Viability	ThermoFisher
FLOW CYTOMETRY PANEL 5		
BUV395	CD3	BD Bioscience
BV605	CD4	BD Bioscience
PE	CD57	Biolegend
PerCP	CD8	Biolegend
APC-Cy7	CD27	Biolegend
BV421	IgM	Biolegend
AlexaFluor400	CD34	Biolegend
AlexaFluor700	CD19	ThermoFisher
eFluor506	Viability	ThermoFisher
FLOW CYTOMETRY PANEL 6		
BUV395	CD3	BD Bioscience
BV605	CD4	BD Bioscience
PE	FoxP3	ThermoFisher

(Continued)

TABLE 2 | Continued

Fluorochrome	Specificity	Company
PerCP	CD8	Biolegend
APC	CD25	Biolegend
APC-eF780	Helios	ThermoFisher
BV421	Tbet	Biolegend
eFluor506	Viability	ThermoFisher
FLOW CYTOMETRY PANEL 7		
BUV395	CD3	BD Bioscience
BV605	CD4	BD Bioscience
FITC	Perforin	Biolegend
PE	GranzymeB	ThermoFisher
PerCP	CD8	Biolegend
eFluor506	Viability	ThermoFisher
FLOW CYTOMETRY PANEL 8		
BUV395	CD3	BD Bioscience
BV421	Tim3	Biolegend
BV605	PD1	Biolegend
BV711	Ki67	Biolegend
PE	CD137	ThermoFisher
PerCP	CD8	Biolegend Biolegend
AlexaFluor700	CD4	ThermoFisher
PE-Cy7	Lag3	Biolegend
EFluor660	CTLA4	ThermoFisher
eFluor506	Viability	ThermoFisher

Eight different panels were used to span the antibodies needed for the single CyTOF panel. Each panel indicates the antibodies and their fluorescent conjugation.

× g for 3 min in phosphate buffer saline (PBS) to be ready for FC acquisition.

For CyTOF staining, cells were Fc blocked as for FC staining, followed by incubation with surface marker staining cocktail for 30 min at 4°C. For viability staining, cells were washed with PBS and incubated for 5 min in room temperature in 200 µl of 1 µM cisplatin solution (BioVision, catalog #1550-1000). Cisplatin was quenched by adding 2 ml of 5% serum-containing PBS. Cells were fixed and permeabilized immediately in eBioscience Foxp3/Transcription Factor Staining Buffer Set, followed by incubation in the intracellular markers antibody cocktail for 30 min at 4°C. EQ Four Element Calibration Beads (Fluidigm) were used to normalize signal intensity over time. For iridium labeling of cellular DNA, cells were suspended in 1 ml of 100 nM of iridium (Fluidigm, Catalog #201192B) in PBS containing 0.3% saponin and 1.6% formaldehyde for 1 h at 4 °C. Cells were then washed and kept in PBS with 1.6% formaldehyde in 4°C for 1 to 4 days before acquisition.

Data Acquisition and Analysis

Cells stained for FC were acquired on the day of or the day after staining using a 5-laser LSR Fortessa X-20 (BD) at the Flow Cytometry Core Facility at Princess Margaret Cancer Center. Single stain controls for each fluorochrome were prepared using UltraComp eBead Compensation Beads (ThermoFisher, catalog #01-2222-42). Data were analyzed using FlowJo V10.

For CyTOF data acquisition, cells were pelleted in Milli-Q water on the day of acquisition and transferred on ice to SickKids-UHN Flow and Mass cytometry Facility to be acquired on third-generation Helios mass cytometer (Fluidigm). Cells were then resuspended into 1 ml of EQ beads diluted 1:10 in Maxpar Cell Acquisition Solution and filtered through cell strainer cap tubes. Cells were acquired at rate of 100–250 events per second. Acquired raw FCS files were normalized with the preloaded normalizer algorithm on CyTOF software version 6.7. Normalized CyTOF FCS files were analyzed using Cytobank 6.2 (Cytobank, Inc) to manually gate different populations and create 2 dimensions and high dimensional plots. Parameters used for making the viSNE plots are CD3, CD4, CD8, CD25, Foxp3, CD19, CD56, CD16, HLA-DR, CD11c, CD33, CD14. Populations were then defined based on known lineage combinations of these proteins. viSNE analyses were performed using equal sampling per comparison, perplexity = 30, theta = 0.5, iterations = 1,000–5,000. **Figure 1** viSNE: event sampling = 49,998 cells per sample, 5,000 iterations, final KL divergence: 2.42. **Figure 4** viSNE: event sampling = 30,664 cells per sample, 2,000 iterations, final KL divergence: 2.53. **Figure 5** viSNE: event sampling = 6,910 cells per sample, 1,000 iterations, final KL divergence: 1.26.

For both FC and CyTOF, 1 million cells were stained and an average of 100,000 cells were acquired. Populations were gated based on their expression of linage defining markers (e.g., CD3 for T cells, CD19 for B cells) For manual gating on biaxial plots, the positive population of each marker (e.g., CD3+GzmB+) was defined as the events above the negative population (e.g., CD3-) on the same plot for both CyTOF and FC.

Raw flow cytometry and CyTOF data files from all experiments described herein are publicly available at www.flowrepository.org; http://flowrepository.org/id/RvFrkC3p2UldoMbc7kQpqboaZ6UYvg4alJi8JFKywZUnNbhULFhcOoSLOeDJVtwf.

Statistics

The equivalency between CyTOF and FC were compared using a paired TOST equivalence test. The paired TOST equivalence test reverses the null and alternative hypothesis to place the burden of proof on showing that two variables measured for the same subject are significantly equivalent (23). R package "equivalence" (version 0.7.2) was used to perform the equivalence test (24). We used an epsilon value of 5, indicating that a difference in proportion smaller than 5% is deemed equivalent. *P*-value $\leq$0.05 was considered statistically equivalent. GraphPad Prism 6 software (GraphPad Software, Inc.) was used to perform Pearson's correlation test.

RESULTS

Comparison of CyTOF vs. Flow Cytometry Staining in Freshly Isolated Peripheral Blood Mononuclear Cells

To appropriately compare staining patterns and expression of proteins of interest for cancer immunotherapy trials, we developed a 40+ parameter CyTOF panel that could identify

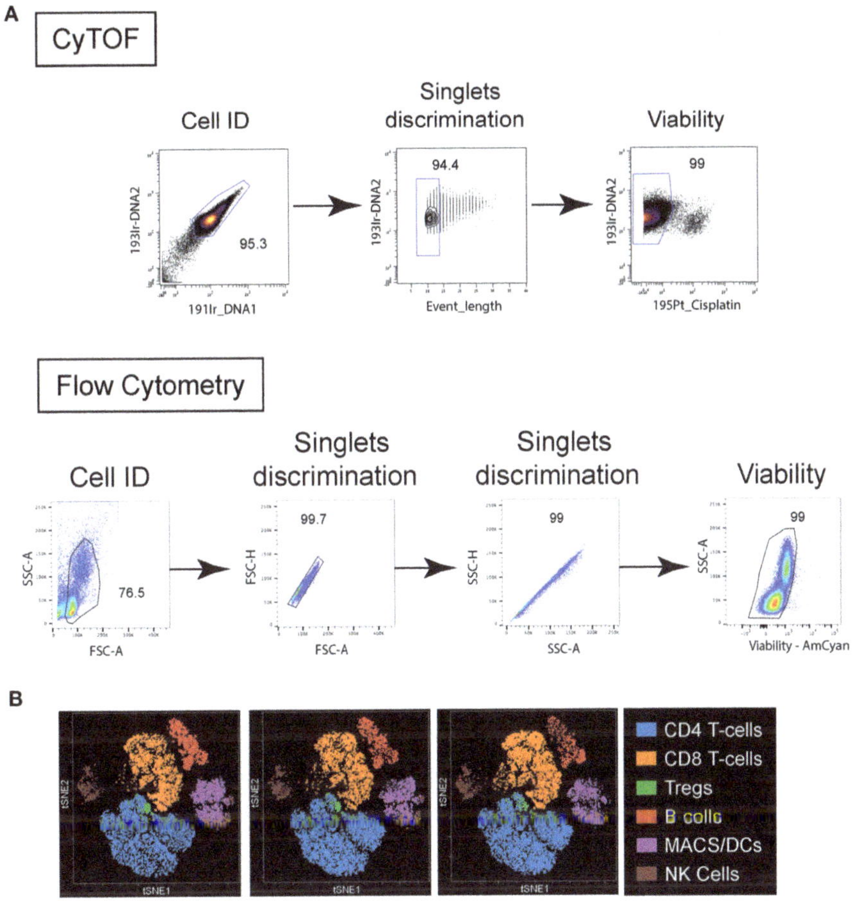

FIGURE 1 | Live/Dead cell gating and population clustering. **(A)** For CyTOF (top plots), cells were first identified based on DNA staining, singlet were selected based on event length and viability based on cisplatin exclusion. For FC (bottom plots) cells were identified based on forward scatter (FSC) vs. side scatter (SSC), singlets selected based on FSC-area vs. height and SSC-area vs. height, and viability based on dye exclusion. **(B)** Immune cell populations from 4 different PBMC donors stained by CyTOF were plotted on bivariate viSNE plots. Main cell populations were manually gated based on lineage marker expression and then the manual gates were used as the overlaid (colored) dimension. The main cell populations are shown by the indicated color profile.

all major (and most minor) cell lineage defining markers, in combination with transcription factors, activation/exhaustion, differentiation, and cytolytic factors (**Tables 1, 2**). These markers were chosen to broadly profile the differentiation and functional state of many cell types simultaneously instead of solely focusing on a single cell type (such as CD8 T cells or macrophages) as is often the case. For comparison of CyTOF to FC, the same antibody clones were used. Titrations were separately performed for CyTOF and flow cytometry antibodies to obtain the optimal concentration for use. In general, similar concentrations were optimal for both assays.

Comparisons were first performed using peripheral blood mononuclear cells (PBMC) isolated from healthy individuals. The PBMC were obtained, isolated and stained by flow cytometry or CyTOF on the same day. Standard FC utilizes the forward light scatter (cell size) and side light scatter (cells internal complexity/ granularity) to identify intact cells and from debris (**Figure 1A**). These same parameters are not feasible using mass cytometry, so a DNA-intercalator containing two iridium isotopes (191Ir and 193Ir) is used to detect cells by the CyTOF instrument (**Figure 1A**). These reagents additionally can be used for comparison with event length to distinguish single cells, doublets and other non-cellular particles (**Figure 1A**). Fluorescent reagents that are preferentially taken up by dead cells are used to distinguish live from dead cells by FC (**Figure 1A**). Similarly, short treatment of cells with the platinum-based reagent cisplatin is used in CyTOF to distinguish live from dead cells (25) (**Figure 1A**). For CyTOF, metal-containing beads (EQ Calibration beads from Fluidigm) are added to each sample to normalize signal variation (i.e., intensity of signal detected in each metal isotope "channel") resulting from instrument variability over time within each acquisition and between different samples acquired on the same day. In CyTOF, crosstalk between different mass channels can occur mainly due to potential isotopic impurities in the channels that detect other isotopes of the same element. Also, in cases of extremely high signal intensity, spillover, mainly in the mass (M) +1 and M-1 channels can occur as the instrument detectors becomes unable to separate ion peaks of adjacent channels. Another source of spillover in the M+16 channel occurs due to variable oxide formation (13). At the beginning of each analysis, any spillover was determined for each M+1, −1 and +16 channel and if observed, that channel was not used for subsequent analysis in the stain. Note, spillover was not observed in the experiments using this panel. Dimensionality reduction of the CyTOF data onto t-distributed stochastic neighbor embedding (t-SNE)-based visualization (viSNE) maps were used to simultaneously resolve the many distinct immune populations (**Figure 1B**) in combination with the numerous phenotypic/functional markers included in the panel, something less feasible by FC due to the restrictions in parameters that can be easily included in a given stain.

To compare the staining of individual proteins by FC and CyTOF, we directly measured their expression using bivariate dot plots. As shown in **Figure 2**, the frequency of cells expressing a given protein statistically equivalent between CyTOF and FC. We determined statistical equivalence by using the TOST equivalence test, which returns *p*- values below the significance threshold if the two proportions are deemed equivalent. This similarity was true whether the protein of interest was expressed on the cell surface or intracellularly (**Figure 2** and **Figure S1**). Further, a similar staining frequency of positive staining cells was observed whether the marker was expressed at high (e.g., CD28, CD127) or low (e.g., CD25, 4-1BB) levels (**Figure 2** and **Figure S1**). Visually, a few bivariate plots do not show the exact same staining pattern/intensity between CyTOF and FC, even though frequencies are equivalent (e.g., Helios, T-bet).

We next measured the change in staining intensity of each marker by flow cytometry and CyTOF comparing the mean fluorescence intensity (MFI) and the mean metal intensity (MMI), respectively, of each protein. This was done by gating on the negative and positive staining populations for each sample using the same logarithmic scale (same high and low end) for FC and CyTOF data, and then calculating the fold change. This approach was used instead of simply stating the MFI/MMI of the positive population to account for differences in the non-specific antibody binding, the background (autofluorescence or metal content) or due to inherent differences in the "brightness" of a given fluorochrome or metal tag. The fold change of a given protein was either the same between CyTOF and FC, or was higher by CyTOF (**Table 3**). It should be noted however that CyTOF background medians are often zero or close to zero, thereby increasing the fold change values for the CyTOF data. Thus, for the staining of human PBMC for cell lineage, activation, exhaustion, differentiation, and functional proteins of interest for immune monitoring and discovery in cancer immunotherapy trials, CyTOF data provides the same quality of staining as flow cytometry. Further, the ability to combine all the markers into one stain using CyTOF provides the opportunity to simultaneously measure changes across the immune system and to identify changes without preconceived bias of what proteins a cell "should" or "should not" express.

TABLE 3 | Comparison of MFI and MMI from healthy PBMC donors.

	Population	Fold change MFI+/− SE	Fold change MMI+/− SE
LAG3	CD3+ T-cells	54.3 ± 11.7	58.5 ± 12.5
CD27	CD3+ T-cells	72.3 ± 14.8	87.2 ± 12.2
CD28	CD3+ T-cells	63.7 ± 12.5	63.2 ± 8.3
CD25	CD3+ T-cells	26.76 ± 6.4	168 ± 73.4
4-1BB (CD137)	CD3+ T-cells	20.9 ± 3.8	167.8 ± 48.2
TCRγδ	CD3+ T-cells	38.8 ± 3.6	489.6 ± 97.6
CD57	CD3+ T-cells	167 ± 52.7	177.1 ± 36.5
CD103	CD3+ T-cells	186.8 ± 32.5	148.1 ± 43.4
Ki67	CD3+ T-cells	86.3 ± 70.2	38.9 ± 13.2
PD-1	CD3+ T-cells	9.3 ± 2.8	33.8 ± 6.1
CTLA4	CD3+ T-cells	10.9 ± 2.6	18.8 ± 5.6
CD127	CD3+ T-cells	7.7± 1.0	56.3 ± 12.3
TIGIT	CD3+ T-cells	55.0 ± 4.4	32.7 ± 5.4
TIM3	CD3+ T-cells	10.3 ± 1.5	167.9 ± 28.9
CD39	CD3+ T-cells	35.7± 11.9	29.6 ± 7.3
FOXP3	CD3+ T-cells	6.2 ± 0.7	41.0 ± 13.3
Granzyme B	CD3+ T-cells	52.9 ± 9.3	45.5 ± 6.2
Perforin	CD3+ T-cells	6.2 ± 0.9	21.6 ± 9.2
Fas	CD3+ T-cells	92.5 ± 33.4	72.2 ± 16.2
T-bet	CD3+ T-cells	4.8 ± 0.5	6.7 ± 1.4
Helios	CD3+ T-cells	12.3 ± 1.7	69.3 ± 42.7
CXCR5	CD3+ T-cells	37.2 ± 11.3	72.0 ± 19.1
CXCR3	CD3+ T-cells	11.7 ± 1.2	93.5 ± 25.1
PDL1	CD45+	83.5 ± 32.2	123.4 ± 24.7
CD45RA	CD45+	46.9 ± 17.2	80.0 ± 23.17
CD45RO	CD45+	56.6 ± 13.3	54.3 ± 11.6
IgM	B-cells	131.3 ± 14.9	199.8 ± 40.8

The Mean Fluorescence Intensity (MFI; flow cytometry) and the Mean Metal Intensity (MMI; CyTOF) were calculated for each stain. This was done by gating on the positive and negative populations for each stain and then calculating the fold change of positive staining over negative staining. The fold change shows the staining intensity of each antibody used, and that fluorescent and metal-tagged antibodies perform similarly in most cases, if not better by some CyTOF antibodies.

Comparison of CyTOF and Flow Cytometry in Frozen PBMC

Freezing of cells can lead to changes in protein detectability, however these are generally due to cleaving or loss of surface expression as opposed to changes in the technical aspects of the assay (26–28). As a result, we next compared whether CyTOF and FC were similarly effective using previously frozen PBMC. Note, the goal of this comparison is not to determine if freezing of cells disrupts certain markers, but instead to determine whether the two cytometric techniques perform equivalently on previously frozen cells. Viably frozen PBMC from healthy donors were thawed and stained for FC and CyTOF. For these analyses, PBMC had been frozen for at least 1 month prior to thawing and staining. Analogous to fresh PBMC, the percentage of positive cell staining for each marker was similar by CyTOF and FC, despite the inter-individual variability for each marker (**Figure 3**). Further, similar to fresh PBMC, the staining intensity

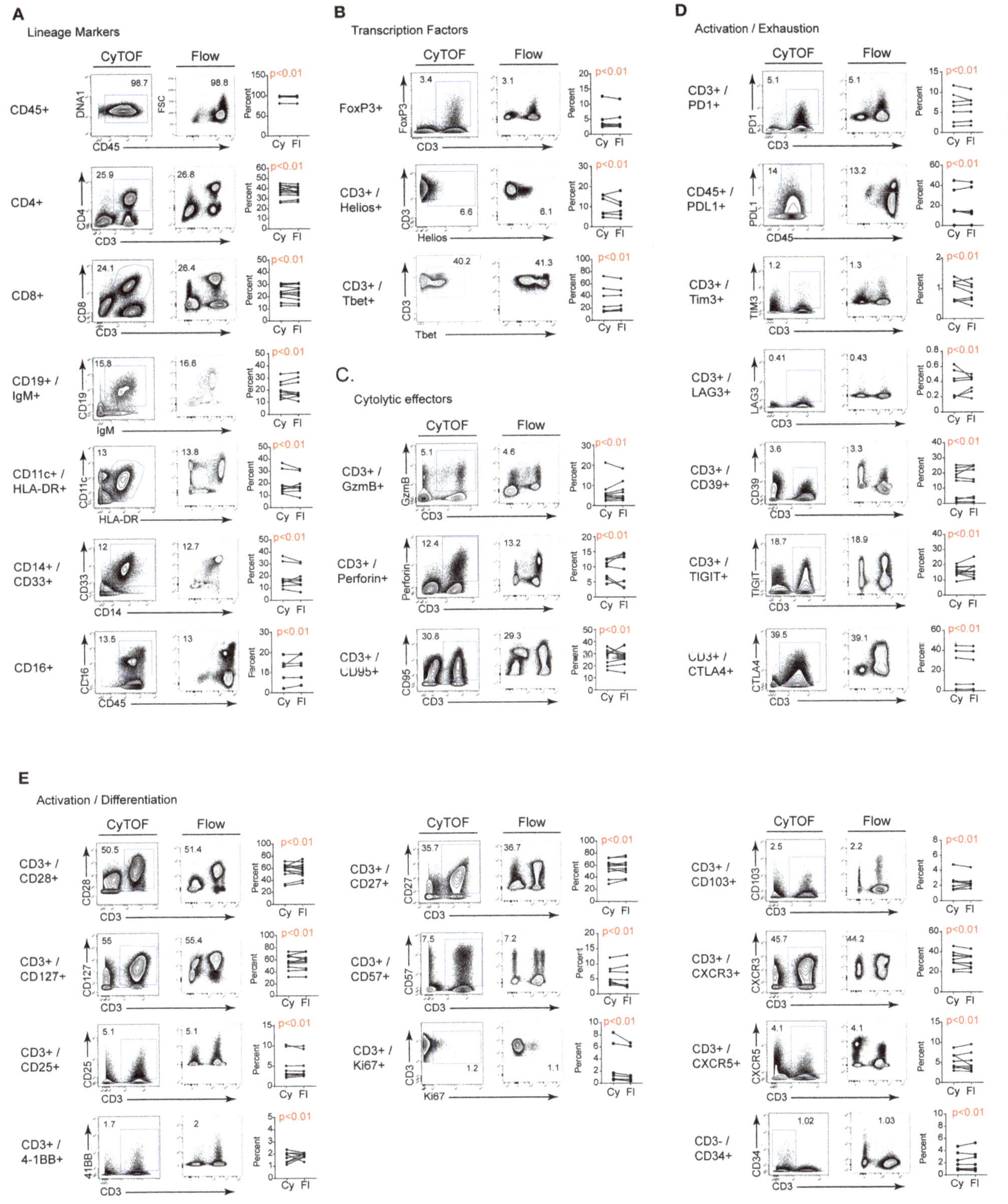

FIGURE 2 | Comparison of CyTOF and flow cytometry staining of freshly isolated human PBMC. Gates in each plot show the frequency of the indicated stained protein by CyTOF (left plots) or FC (right plots) for **(A)** cell lineage defining; **(B)** transcription; **(C)** cytolytic activity; **(D)** activation/exhaustion; and **(E)** activation/cellular differentiation. Graphs display donor sample paired expression of the frequency staining positive for the indicated protein by CyTOF (Cy) and FC (Fl). The number of donors for each stain is indicated in **Table 1**. Significance was determined by the TOST test for equivalence. $p \leq 0.05$ was considered statistically equivalent.

(i.e., the fold change in MFI and MMI) was similar or better using CyTOF (not shown). Thus, CyTOF is a robust approach to quantify cellular presence, phenotype and function in previously frozen PBMC.

Titration of PBMC Required for CyTOF Analysis

A critical issue limiting studies with small numbers of cells is the increased cell loss with staining procedures, the potential for increased "background" staining and for CyTOF in particular, the higher cell loss during acquisition. To overcome this issue, we developed a strategy in which serially diluted numbers of human PBMC were mixed with mouse splenocytes at a ratio such that the final number was always a million cells. Mouse splenocytes were used because they can be reliably distinguished from human hematopoietic cells based on expression of non-cross reactive clones of anti-mouse CD45 and anti-human CD45 antibodies (**Figure 4A**). We performed two-fold dilutions of human PBMC resulting in human cells comprising 100% (1 million PBMC), 50%, 25% or 12.5% (125,000 PBMC) of the total cells in the mix. These dilutions were subsequently stained for CyTOF analysis using the panel in **Table 1** and acquired. Comparison of the anti-mouse and anti-human CD45 antibody expression demonstrated the expected ratios of human PBMC based on the starting dilution and this was observed even at the lowest dilution containing only 125,000 human PBMC (**Figure 4A**). Further, titration down to 125,000 human PBMC did not alter their proportions or lead to loss of the smaller populations (**Figure 4B**). Of course, biologic restrictions still apply and at diminishing numbers of cells, small populations will increasingly fall below detection due to their loss in the population, similar to FC. Thus, by adjusting the cell numbers to maintain 1 million cells per stain, reliable CyTOF data can be obtained from as few as 125,000 human PBMC. This technique will be helpful in situations where cell numbers are limiting due to biologic restrictions (e.g., tumor biopsies) or multiple analyses are desired from a limited number of cells.

Validating CyTOF in Tumor Tissues

Many studies have used CyTOF to interrogate tumor tissues, yet a direct comparison of its validity compared to FC in human tumor samples is lacking. To validate CyTOF vs. FC in human tumor tissues, we used single cell suspensions of previously viably frozen tumors. For our analysis, we chose to compare five tumors made up of 3 types: 2 melanoma, 2 ovarian and 1 breast tumor. Initial viSNE analysis showed various amounts of inter-patient variability, but in all cases major immune cell populations were resolved, including T cells, Tregs, macrophages and MDSC (**Figure 5A**). Further, within these various populations, phenotypic, functional, and activation/exhaustion proteins with broad or restricted distribution could be identified, including high expression of PD1 in tumor infiltrating CD4 T cells and Tregs, with less PD1 expression observed in CD8 T cells, high level, and broad CD95 (Fas) and CD39 expression across many populations of tumor-infiltrating cells (although the latter was largely absent from CD8 T cells), and restricted expression of granzyme B, primarily by CD8 T cells (**Figure 5A**).

TABLE 4 | Statistical correlation between some CyTOF and Flow populations.

	Sample type	Pearson correlation	
		r	*p*
CD45RO+	Frozen PBMC	0.92	0.02
CD45+	Biopsy	0.99	0.000
CD3+ TIGIT+	Biopsy	0.97	0.006
CD3+ CTLA4+	Biopsy	0.97	0.005
CD3+ CD28+	Biopsy	0.98	0.002

Pearson correlation coefficient was calculated for populations that did not reach statistical significance using the TOST test for equivalence to indicate how closely their values are correlated.

Direct evaluation of CyTOF and FC staining in the different tumor types demonstrated similar proportions of immune cells in the tumor based on CD45 expression. Within the immune cell populations, staining for individual cell subsets was comparable between the two techniques (**Figure 5B** and **Figure S2**). Importantly, comparably to flow cytometry, CyTOF identified expression of numerous activation, differentiation, and functional proteins on tumor infiltrating cells (**Figure 5B** and **Figure S2**), and did so in a single stain as opposed to FC which required many separate panels with duplicate lineage markers to attain this same level of staining (**Tables 1**, **2**). Further, like PBMC, the fold change in MFI and MMI were similar or elevated with the CyTOF stain in the tumors (not shown).

Our results show that the two technologies provide highly equivalent values across markers and populations in fresh and frozen PBMC, and tumor biopsies. Values of few populations (CD45RO+ in Frozen PBMC, and CD45+, CD3+TIGIT+, CD3+CTLA4+, and CD3+CD28+ in tumor biopsies) did not give rise to statistically equivalent results using equivalence test. However, the values of these populations from CyTOF and FC showed highly significant correlation using Pearson correlation test as shown in **Table 4** (r ranges from 0.92 to 0.99, $p < 0.05$). We believe that the statistical inequivalence we observe in these populations is not due to differences in the two technologies. Instead, the sample size ($n = 5$) for both the frozen and biopsies specimens did not allow the values of these populations to reach the level of statistical significance using the TOST test for equivalence, although they correlated with high significance using the Pearson test and the fresh samples ($n = 11$) showed highly significant values for all populations.

DISCUSSION

The ability of CyTOF to combine many parameters into a single panel allows an unbiased and efficient approach for discovery of novel disease-associated cell populations or biomarkers from limited tumor samples (29). Yet, the comparability of CyTOF to the more standard use of FC of these tumor studies has not been stringently validated. Herein, we demonstrate that using our 40+ parameter panel on PBMC and tumor tissue samples, CyTOF is at least as effective, if not more so, than FC for the identification of diverse cell subsets and their subsequent

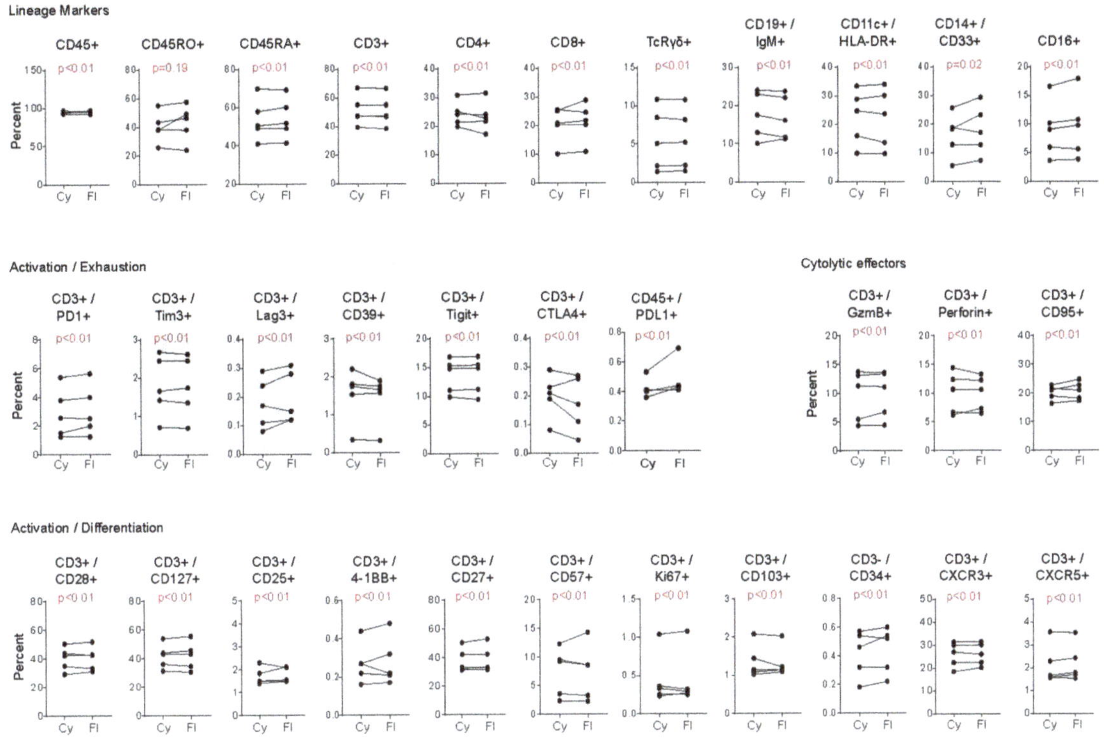

FIGURE 3 | Comparison of CyTOF and flow cytometry staining of viably frozen human PBMC. Analysis was performed as in **Figure 2**, except using PBMC that had been previously viably frozen. Each graph represents the donor paired frequency of cells staining positive for the indicated marked by CyTOF and FC. Data represent previously frozen PBMC samples from 5 healthy donors. Significance was determined by the TOST test for equivalence. $p \leq 0.05$ was considered statistically equivalent.

phenotyping. To validate the use of CyTOF we developed a 40+ parameter panel analyzing diverse cell lineages in combination with a comprehensive panel of differentiation, transcription, chemotactic, activation, exhaustion, senescence and functional factors, chosen for their observed and potential relevance for monitoring and discovery in cancer clinical trials. Both CyTOF and FC had comparable efficacy to identify proportions of cell subsets in human PBMC and tumors, including multiple subsets critical to cancer control and the immunotherapeutic response; e.g., T cells, Tregs, dendritic cells, macrophages, and MDSCs. These techniques were equally efficient whether the PBMC were fresh or previously viably frozen. On these subsets, proteins associated with cell function and differentiation state were stained with the same or better fidelity by CyTOF compared to flow cytometry. Since small numbers of cells are often obtained from tumor tissues, it is important to note that reliable data could be observed by CyTOF using as few as 125,000 PBMC when they were pre-mixed with carrier mouse splenocytes prior to staining to increase overall cell numbers and minimize the loss of human cells during staining procedures and washing steps. In addition, non-immune cells (including non-hematopoietic derived tumor cells) can also be identified based on the lack of CD45 expression or by addition of other tumor-antigen specific antibodies. Importantly, CyTOF was able to simultaneously measure all these parameters whereas FC required multiple panels with significant overlap to achieve this goal. This allowed detailed high-dimensional analyses to be performed and a large number of immune cell populations to be plotted on bivariate viSNE plots for subsequent interrogation. This approach is beneficial for immune monitoring, mechanistic understanding and biomarker discovery because it provides an unbiased and broad analysis of the immune system with combinations of markers that do not rely on a priori decisions of cell attributes.

Currently, most of the isotopic metals commercially available for conjugation with antibodies are from the lanthanides series. A panel of 40 antibodies can be used simultaneously without technical difficulties; alongside DNA parameters to identify cells, and viability dye to distinguish live from dead cells. Research is underway in the polymer chemistry field to develop use of metals from outside the lanthanides series, to increase the number of parameters researchers can use per panel. The cost of metal tagged-antibodies, antibodies conjugation kits, and the running reagents are quite high and may be impeding the widespread of CyTOF use. Hopefully, with increasing demands, and advancement in reagents and instruments manufacturing technology, prices will be more affordable to wide range of laboratories.

Designing an optimal CyTOF panel is as important as it is in flow cytometry. Although technically there is no signal

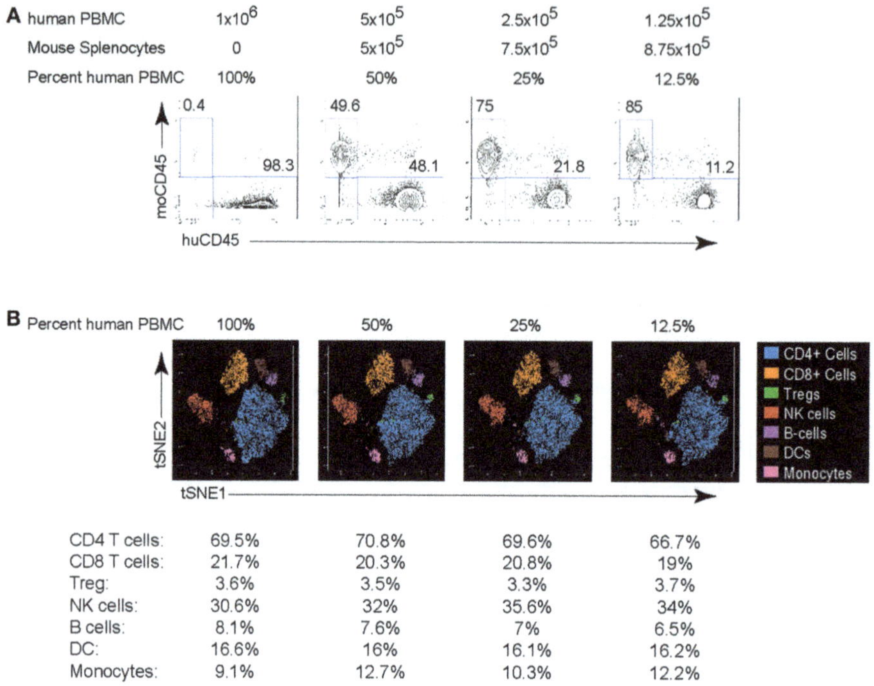

FIGURE 4 | Titration of PBMC for CyTOF staining. Human PBMC isolated from healthy donors were serially 2-fold diluted in mouse splenocytes at the indicated ration to maintain a total cell count of 1 million cells per stain. **(A)** Human and mouse cells were differentiated based on their expression of CD45. Numbers in the plots indicate the frequency of each population in the indicated dilution. **(B)** viSNE plots of major human PBMC populations from each dilution. The numbers under the viSNE plots indicate the frequency of each population in the dilution and the numbers in parenthesis indicate the number of cell events in the subset. Data are representative of 2 experiments using human PBMC from different donors.

interference between mass channels, isotopic impurities can cause a small amount of contamination between different channels. Therefore, the isotopic purity of the metal-tags used must be taken into consideration when assigning cellular biomarkers to each metal. Generally, less pure metals should be paired with low expression biomarkers, as this keeps the spillover at the background level in the channels where spillover is anticipated and reduces signal interference. Similar to flow cytometry, markers with low expression ideally are paired with high signal-intensity metals like 165Ho or 169Tm for better gating and resolution of the positive population. Again, like flow cytometry, to reduce signal "spillover" in CyTOF, it is good practice to try to use of markers exclusive to cell populations (e.g., CD3, CD19) on adjacent channels where "spillover" potential is highest. Antibody titration to find the optimal dilution is also equally important, as lower dilutions will result in lower resolution, while higher dilution will increase background and "spillover" on these susceptible channels.

The photobleaching process of fluorescent dyes in flow cytometry makes it paramount to acquire samples within a few hours after staining. On other hand, metal-tagged samples can be run up to 2 weeks after staining without notable loss of signal and can be cryopreserved up to 1 month without affecting the data quality or staining integrity of both surface and intracellular markers (30). This is very useful in clinical trials, wherein long-term preservation allows researchers to collect samples over a period of time and acquire them simultaneously.

The data analysis of CyTOF is perhaps the most challenging part of the workflow. With cytometry data in general, manual gating is the one of the main contributor to inter-laboratory variations (31). An optimally designed panel, with a well-matched biomarkers and metals-tags as mentioned above, will cause less trouble gating and resolving positive events. So, efforts must be made to design an optimal panel for good data quality. Some laboratories use mass minus one controls (similar to fluorescence-minus one in FC) to build a hierarchy of gates and set positivity threshold, but this does not take into account the inherent background staining of each antibody and the non-specific binding (even if isotype-matched control antibody is used) which leads to significant false positive signal. Further, it is impractical to prepare mass-minus one control for 40+ antibodies. However, mass-minus one controlling is ideal to investigate a potential spillover between channels. Fortunately, the unsupervised clustering and automated populations-detection algorithms, which accompanied the advent of CyTOF high-dimensional data, have decreased the need for manual gating (32). However, for the purpose of this article, we test the similarity between CyTOF and flow cytometry on a marker-by-marker basis and representative examples of the gating used for each marker

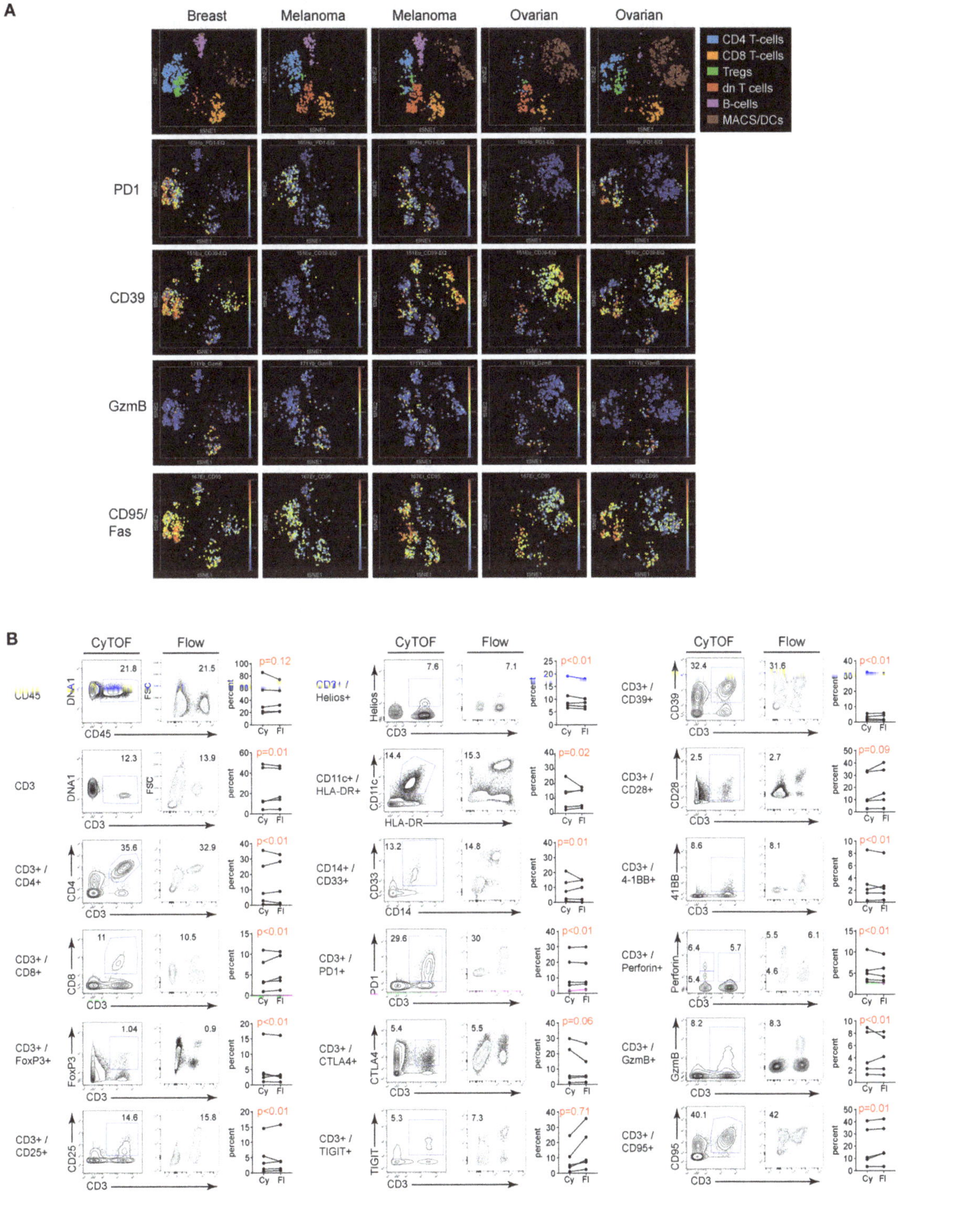

FIGURE 5 | Flow vs. CyTOF staining of tumor infiltrating leukocytes. Single cell suspensions of previously viably frozen tumors were stained for CyTOF and FC. Five tumors were chosen for analysis: 2 melanoma, 2 ovarian, and 1 breast. **(A)** CyTOF viSNE plots of major immune cell populations and expression of selected proteins from the tumor tissues gated on CD45 positive cells. dn T cells: CD3+, but CD4 and CD8 double negative T cells. **(B)** Gates in each plot show the frequency of the indicated stained protein by CyTOF (left plots) or FC (right plots). Graphs display donor sample paired expression of the frequency staining positive for the indicated protein by CyTOF (Cy) and FC (Fl). Significance was determined by the TOST test for equivalence. $p \leq 0.05$ was considered statistically equivalent.

are shown and scatter plots provided. Thus, manual gating on biaxial plots was employed with experience and knowledge of the brightness and purity of each of the metal tags used, their intrinsic background, and crosstalk, and also, familiarity with the staining pattern of each immune marker and the frequencies of cell populations.

A major drawback to CyTOF is acquisition flow rate. In comparison to flow cytometry (thousands of cells/second), CyTOF has a slower flow rate (~250–500 cells/second), resulting in longer acquisition time. Additionally, sample preparation for CyTOF requires extra caution to avoid contamination with heavy metals, which are common ingredient in laboratory detergents and other basic reagents. Further, because cells are ultimately vaporized in CyTOF, sorting out populations of interest for further analysis and downstream applications is not possible. This is something flow cytometers are able to do easily. Finally, the increase in number of parameters, made available by CyTOF technology, has intensified the complexity of data, which is a strong attribute of the technique, but also requires deeper analysis and in many cases new bioinformatics approaches to interpret and visualize the data. Importantly, neither FC nor CyTOF is the superior technique for all applications; rather, the choice must rest on the questions asked, the answers sought and the ability to analyze different data sets in meaningful ways. Thus, our data now validate CyTOF as an accurate approach to perform high dimensional analysis in human PBMC and tumor tissue for immunologic studies and cancer clinical trials.

ETHICS STATEMENT

All human tissues and blood were obtained through protocols approved by the Princess Margaret Cancer Center/University Health Network institutional review board. Written informed consent was obtained from all donors. All studies were performed using de-identified human data.

AUTHOR CONTRIBUTIONS

RG, BN, LS, and DB designed research. RG and HE performed experiments. RG, BN, and DB analyzed data. BM, RD, MG, WX, SL, HE, AR, NH, TM, BW, MB, CG, PO, LS, and DB provided intellectual input, critical discussion, and contributed technical expertise and discussion. RG and DB wrote the paper.

REFERENCES

1. Irish JM, Doxie DB. High-dimensional single-cell cancer biology. *Curr Top Microbiol Immunol.* (2014) 377:1–21. doi: 10.1007/82_2014_367
2. Bjornson ZB, Nolan GP, Fantl WJ. Single-cell mass cytometry for analysis of immune system functional states. *Curr Opin Immunol.* (2013) 25:484–94. doi: 10.1016/j.coi.2013.07.004
3. Nair N, Mei HE, Chen SY, Hale M, Nolan GP, Maecker HT, et al. Mass cytometry as a platform for the discovery of cellular biomarkers to guide effective rheumatic disease therapy. *Arthritis Res Ther.* (2015) 17:127. doi: 10.1186/s13075-015-0644-z
4. Ermann J, Rao DA, Teslovich NC, Brenner MB, Raychaudhuri S. Immune cell profiling to guide therapeutic decisions in rheumatic diseases. *Nat Rev Rheumatol.* (2015) 11:541–51. doi: 10.1038/nrrheum.2015.71
5. Huang AC, Postow MA, Orlowski RJ, Mick R, Bengsch B, Manne S, et al. T-cell invigoration to tumour burden ratio associated with anti-PD-1 response. *Nature.* (2017) 545:60–5. doi: 10.1038/nature22079
6. Lavin Y, Kobayashi S, Leader A, Amir ED, Elefant N, Bigenwald C, et al. Innate immune landscape in early lung adenocarcinoma by paired single-cell analyses. *Cell.* (2017) 169:750–65 e17. doi: 10.1016/j.cell.2017.04.014
7. Simoni Y, Becht E, Fehlings M, Loh CY, Koo SL, Teng KWW, et al. Bystander CD8(+) T cells are abundant and phenotypically distinct in human tumour infiltrates. *Nature.* (2018) 557:575–9. doi: 10.1038/s41586-018-0130-2
8. Bendall SC, Simonds EF, Qiu P, Amir el-AD, Krutzik PO, Finck R, et al. Single-cell mass cytometry of differential immune and drug responses across a human hematopoietic continuum. *Science.* (2011) 332:687–96. doi: 10.1126/science.1198704
9. Mair F, Hartmann FJ, Mrdjen D, Tosevski V, Krieg C, Becher B. The end of gating? An introduction to automated analysis of high dimensional cytometry data. *Eur J Immunol.* (2016) 46:34–43. doi: 10.1002/eji.201545774
10. Lowther DE, Goods BA, Lucca LE, Lerner BA, Raddassi K, van Dijk D, et al. PD-1 marks dysfunctional regulatory T cells in malignant gliomas. *JCI Insight.* (2016) 1:85935. doi: 10.1172/jci.insight.85935
11. van Unen V, Li N, Molendijk I, Temurhan M, Höllt T, van der Meulen-de Jong AE, et al. Mass cytometry of the human mucosal immune system identifies tissue- and disease-associated immune subsets. *Immunity.* (2016) 44:1227–39. doi: 10.1016/j.immuni.2016.04.014
12. Diggins KE, Ferrell PB Jr, Irish JM. Methods for discovery and characterization of cell subsets in high dimensional mass cytometry data. *Methods.* (2015) 82:55–63. doi: 10.1016/j.ymeth.2015.05.008
13. Leelatian N, Diggins KE, Irish JM. Characterizing phenotypes and signaling networks of single human cells by mass cytometry. *Methods Mol Biol.* (2015) 1346:99–113. doi: 10.1007/978-1-4939-2987-0_8
14. Nicholas KJ, Greenplate AR, Flaherty DK, Matlock BK, Juan JS, Smith RM, et al. Multiparameter analysis of stimulated human peripheral blood mononuclear cells: a comparison of mass and fluorescence cytometry. *Cytometry A.* (2016) 89:271–80. doi: 10.1002/cyto.a.22799
15. Levine JH, Simonds EF, Bendall SC, Davis KL, Amir el-AD, Tadmor MD, et al. Data-driven phenotypic dissection of AML reveals progenitor-like cells that correlate with prognosis. *Cell.* (2015) 162:184–97. doi: 10.1016/j.cell.2015.05.047
16. Horowitz A, Strauss-Albee DM, Leipold M, Kubo J, Nemat-Gorgani N, Dogan OC, et al. Genetic and environmental determinants of human NK cell diversity revealed by mass cytometry. *Sci Transl Med.* (2013) 5:208ra145. doi: 10.1126/scitranslmed.3006702
17. Wong MT, Chen J, Narayanan S, Lin W, Anicete R, Kiaang HT, et al. Mapping the diversity of follicular helper T cells in human blood and tonsils using high-dimensional mass cytometry analysis. *Cell Reports.* (2015) 11:1–12. doi: 10.1016/j.celrep.2015.05.022

18. Sen N, Mukherjee G, Arvin AM. Single cell mass cytometry reveals remodeling of human T cell phenotypes by varicella zoster virus. *Cell Reports.* (2014) 8:633–45. doi: 10.1016/j.celrep.2014.06.024
19. Mason GM, Lowe K, Melchiotti R, Ellis R, de Rinaldis E, Peakman M, et al. Phenotypic complexity of the human regulatory T cell compartment revealed by mass cytometry. *J Immunol.* (2015) 195:2030–7. doi: 10.4049/jimmunol.1500703
20. Snell LM, MacLeod BL, Law JC, Osokine I, Elsaesser HJ, Hezaveh K, et al. CD8+ T cell priming in established chronic viral infection preferentially directs differentiation of memory-like cells for sustained immunity. *Immunity.* (2018) 49:678–94 e5. doi: 10.1016/j.immuni.2018.08.002
21. Gaudillière B, Fragiadakis GK, Bruggner RV, Nicolau M, Finck R, Tingle M, et al. Clinical recovery from surgery correlates with single-cell immune signatures. *Sci Transl Med.* (2014) 6:255ra131. doi: 10.1126/scitranslmed.3009701
22. Leipold MD, Newell EW, Maecker HT. Multiparameter phenotyping of human PBMCs using mass cytometry. *Methods Mol Biol.* (2015) 1343:81–95. doi: 10.1007/978-1-4939-2963-4_7
23. Walker E, Nowacki AS. Understanding equivalence and noninferiority testing. *J Gen Intern Med.* (2011) 26:192–6. doi: 10.1007/s11606-010-1513-8
24. Anderson TR, Slotkin TA. *Equivalence R Package Version 0.7.2: Provides Tests And Graphics For Assessing Tests of Equivalence.* (2016). Available online at: https://cran.r-project.org/package=equivalence (accessed November 28, 2018).
25. Fienberg HG, Simonds EF, Fantl WJ, Nolan GP, Bodenmiller B. A platinum-based covalent viability reagent for single-cell mass cytometry. *Cytometry A.* (2012) 81:467–75. doi: 10.1002/cyto.a.22067
26. Costantini A, Mancini S, Giuliodoro S, Butini L, Regnery CM, Silvestri G, et al. Effects of cryopreservation on lymphocyte immunophenotype and function. *J Immunol Methods.* (2003) 278:145–55. doi: 10.1016/S0022-1759(03)00202-3
27. Zhang W, Nilles TL, Johnson JR, Margolick JB. The effect of cellular isolation and cryopreservation on the expression of markers identifying subsets of regulatory T cells. *J Immunol Methods.* (2016) 431:31–7. doi: 10.1016/j.jim.2016.02.004
28. Weinberg A, Song LY, Wilkening C, Sevin A, Blais B, Louzao R, et al. Optimization and limitations of use of cryopreserved peripheral blood mononuclear cells for functional and phenotypic T-cell characterization. *Clin Vaccine Immunol.* (2009) 16:1176–86. doi: 10.1128/CVI.00342-08
29. Yao Y, Liu R, Shin MS, Trentalange M, Allore H, Nassar A, et al. CyTOF supports efficient detection of immune cell subsets from small samples. *J Immunol Methods.* (2014) 415:1–5. doi: 10.1016/j.jim.2014.10.010
30. Sumatoh HR, Teng KW, Cheng Y, Newell EW. Optimization of mass cytometry sample cryopreservation after staining. *Cytometry A.* (2017) 91:48–61. doi: 10.1002/cyto.a.23014
31. Westera L, van Viegen T, Jeyarajah J, Azad A, Bilsborough J, van den Brink GR, et al. Centrally determined standardization of flow cytometry methods reduces interlaboratory variation in a prospective multicenter study. *Clin Transl Gastroenterol.* (2017) 8:e126. doi: 10.1038/ctg.2017.52
32. Li H, Shaham U, Stanton KP, Yao Y, Montgomery RR, Kluger Y. Gating mass cytometry data by deep learning. *Bioinformatics.* (2017) 33:3423–30. doi: 10.1093/bioinformatics/btx448

6

Mass Cytometry Imaging for the Study of Human Diseases—Applications and Data Analysis Strategies

Heeva Baharlou [1,2†], Nicolas P. Canete [1,2†], Anthony L. Cunningham [1,2], Andrew N. Harman [1,2] and Ellis Patrick [1,3]*

[1] The Westmead Institute for Medical Research, University of Sydney, Westmead, NSW, Australia, [2] Centre for Virus Research, The Westmead Institute for Medical Research, Westmead, NSW, Australia, [3] School of Mathematics and Statistics, University of Sydney, Sydney, NSW, Australia

***Correspondence:**
Ellis Patrick
ellis.patrick@sydney.edu.au

† These authors have contributed equally to this work

High parameter imaging is an important tool in the life sciences for both discovery and healthcare applications. Imaging Mass Cytometry (IMC) and Multiplexed Ion Beam Imaging (MIBI) are two relatively recent technologies which enable clinical samples to be simultaneously analyzed for up to 40 parameters at subcellular resolution. Importantly, these "Mass Cytometry Imaging" (MCI) modalities are being rapidly adopted for studies of the immune system in both health and disease. In this review we discuss, first, the various applications of MCI to date. Second, due to the inherent challenge of analyzing high parameter spatial data, we discuss the various approaches that have been employed for the processing and analysis of data from MCI experiments.

Keywords: imaging cytometry, analysis, multiplexed ion beam imaging, imaging mass cytometry (IMC), mass cytometry (CyTOF), cytometry, multiplexed imaging, single cell

INTRODUCTION

Multiplexed imaging methods are becoming an increasingly important tool for both basic science and clinical research (1–10). Recently, mass cytometry imaging (MCI) approaches, which enable imaging at subcellular resolution have been described (11, 12). MCI enables up to 40 parameters to be visualized in a single tissue section and is being rapidly adopted for various applications, including studies in cancer, diabetes and the definition of complex immune subsets during development and homeostasis (13–21).

Mass Cytometry Imaging Technologies

There are two approaches for MCI—Imaging Mass Cytometry (IMC) (11) and Multiplexed Ion Beam Imaging (MIBI) (12). In both methods, the first step is the labeling of tissue sections with up to 40 different antibodies conjugated to stable isotopes, mostly from the lanthanide series (**Figure 1A**). In IMC, the tissue is then ablated using a laser with a 1 μm spot size, which rasterizes over a selected region of interest. Plumes of tissue matter are then aerosolized, atomized, and ionized, and then fed into a time-of-flight mass spectrometer for analysis of isotope abundance (**Figure 1B**). In MIBI, an oxygen duoplasmatron primary ion beam rasterizes over the tissue, ablating a thin layer of the tissue surface, which then liberates antibody-bound metal isotopes as ions. Similar to IMC, these secondary ions are then fed into a time-of-flight mass spectrometer for the estimation of isotope abundance [**Figure 1C**; (13)]. In both methods, the isotope abundance of each "spot" can then be mapped back to the original co-ordinates, producing a high dimensional image qualitatively similar to a fluorescence microscopy image (**Figure 1D**).

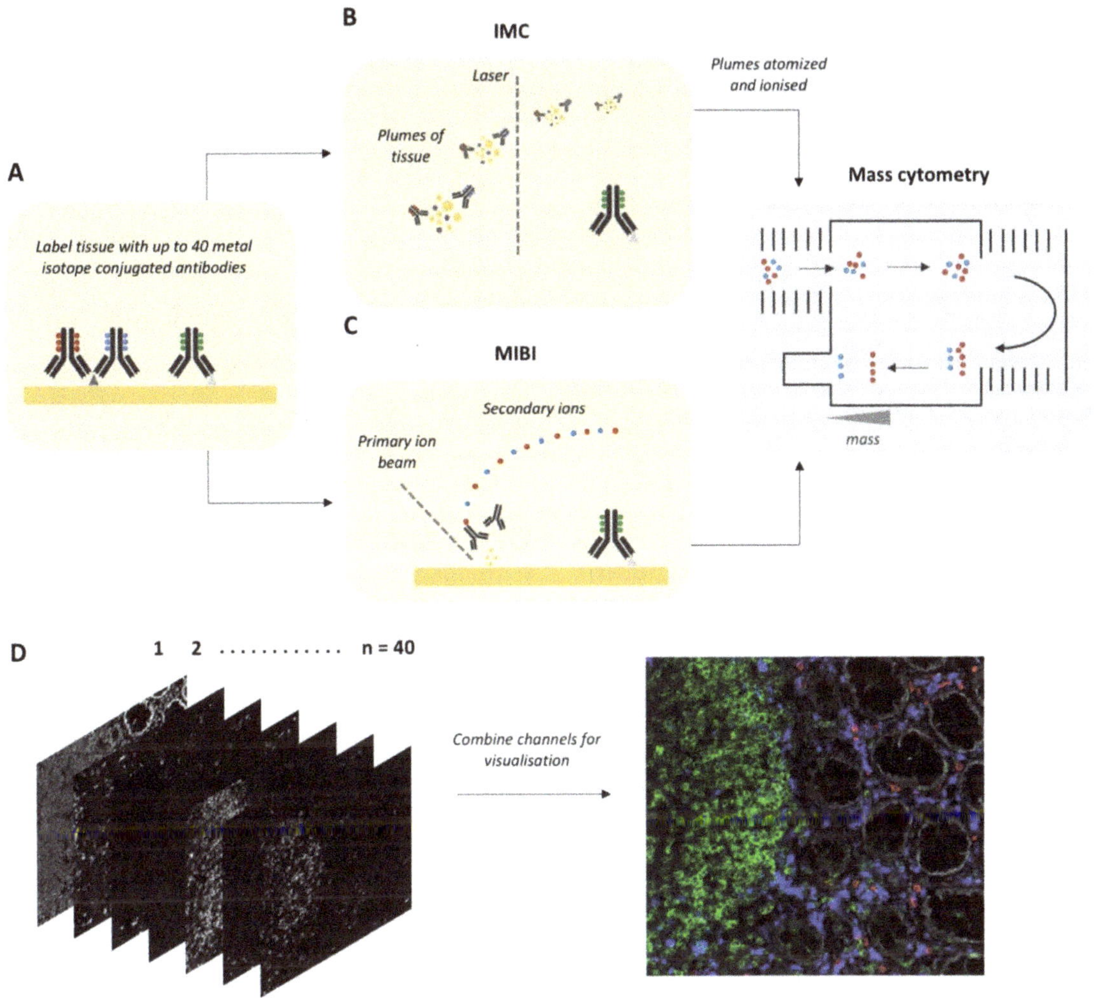

FIGURE 1 | Workflow for Mass Cytometry Imaging. **(A)** Tissue sections are first labeled with a cocktail of metal-isotope-tagged antibodies. **(B)** In Imaging Mass Cytometry the tissue is ablated using a laser with 1 μm spot size. Plumes of tissue matter are then aerosolized, atomized and ionized, and then fed into a time-of-flight mass spectrometer, where metal ions are separated based on mass. **(C)** In Multiplexed Ion Beam Imaging a thin layer of the sample surface is ablated using an oxygen-based primary ion beam. Metal isotypes are liberated from antibodies as secondary ions which are then delivered to a time-of-flight mass spectrometer. **(D)** A high dimensional image is generated, which when combined and visualized, resembles a traditional fluorescence microscopy image. Parts of this figure were made Biorender.

The differences between IMC and MIBI have previously been reviewed (2). However, MIBI has undergone extensive improvements since its initial description, overcoming many of the limitations relating to speed of acquisition and multiplexing capacity (13). Accordingly, there are no up-to-date published comparisons of these two technologies. Both have recently been used to successfully analyse 30–40 parameters *in situ* in patient tissue samples (13, 17, 18). Two important differences we will mention relate to sample ablation and image resolution. IMC uses a laser for sample acquisition and is designed to ablate the entire sample with a fixed lateral resolution of 1,000 nm. However, MIBI utilizes a tuneable ion beam which can be adjusted for varying depth of sample acquisition and also ion spot size (image resolution). This means that the same area can be scanned at a lower resolution to gain an overview and then potential areas of interest rescanned at a higher resolution, reportedly as low as 260 nm, though with a trade-off of longer acquisition times. A comparison of features between IMC and MIBI is summarized in **Table 1**.

Significance of Mass Cytometry Imaging

MCI is a landmark development because it allows for upward of 40 markers to be simultaneously stained, acquired and visualized, enabling a variety of distinct cell types to be analyzed concurrently in their native microenvironment. The microenvironment consists of a complex matrix of fluids, proteins and cells which provide signals that shape a given cells phenotype and function within an organ in both health and disease (22–26). Indeed, there is increasing evidence that cellular functions are programmed not just by cell ontogeny but also

TABLE 1 | Highly multiplexed imaging technologies.

	Serial staining immunofluorescence	Metal tagged antibodies	
Examples	CycIF, GEMultiOmyx, 4i, CODEX	IMC	MIBI
Resolution	~200 nm	~1,000 nm	~260 nm*
Simultaneous detection limit	1–5	40	40
Max number of epitopes imaged per section**	~60	40	40
Throughput***	Hours or 1 day per cycle per tissue section	1 mm^2/2 h	1 mm^2/5 h (500 nm resolution)
References	(3, 4, 6–8)	(11)	(12, 13)

**A smaller spot size (resolution) results in longer acquisition times. A lower limit of 260 nm is referenced in a recent publication, but the actual data acquired in the study was at a resolution of 500 nm (13).*

***There is no hard upper limit for serial staining protocols, but published data has shown approximately 60 markers per section (4, 7, 8). A limit of 40 markers for IMC and MIBI is derived from interpretation, based on both the indicated references and current reagent availability.*

****The rate-limiting step for serial staining protocols is the antibody incubation period which can take hours and is often performed overnight. Throughput for IMC is listed in the Fluidigm product specification sheet for acquisition at 200 Hz. Throughput for MIBI is based on correspondence with IONpath and is expected to be published later this year in a paper describing the current specifications of MIBI.*

by signals from the surrounding microenvironment. Examples include Monocytes and Dendritic Cells and T cells which exist in several functionally diverse subsets, which vary across tissues so as to meet the requirements of their local environment (27–31). Specific subsets of Dendritic Cells, Innate Lymphoid Cells and T cells can carry out distinct functions at a given point in time, inducing either tolerance or inflammation depending on a host of signals derived from both cytokines and direct cell contact (32–35). In the context of disease pathogenesis, the tumor microenvironment is now appreciated as a complex signaling network between transformed and non-transformed cells, with the latter being corrupted to promote tumor function (36, 37). The importance of the microenvironment for cell function is clear. The major contribution of MCI is that it provides spatial data for a large number of parameters at subcellular resolution. As such, we are now positioned to discover interdependencies between complex cell subsets in health and disease. These interactions can be further investigated *ex vivo* to determine their functional outcome and contribution to disease progression.

MCI is also an important development for practical reasons as it enables complete studies to be performed on archival samples. This is particularly useful as research questions evolve with time and it is invaluable to be able to repeatedly interrogate the same sample for different parameters. This feature will be particularly helpful for investigations of inflammatory disorders where significant heterogeneity can exist, making it difficult to accurately characterize the cell types involved and thus the immune motifs underlying the disease; such is the case for dendritic cell subsets which are partly defined by surface markers that are labile during inflammation (38). Furthermore, many studies can only be performed using small biopsies or precious post-mortem samples, as in brain and pancreatic tissues, with samples typically curated through biobank networks (39, 40). As such large gaps remain in our understanding of disease pathogenesis in these tissues; a gap which MCI is poised to fill.

Other Approaches for Highly Multiplexed Imaging

Serial Staining Immunofluorescence

Other approaches exist which are fluorescence-based and involve iterative rounds of staining, imaging, and removal of fluorescent signals (3, 4, 6–9). In these serial staining approaches, typically 2–3 parameters are acquired per round, thus requiring 13–20 rounds to acquire 40 parameters which is the current limit for MCI. Advantages of this approach relate to broad compatibility with many fluorescence-based imaging systems and the capacity to acquire large areas across multiple tissue sections in a short period of time, which allows parallel processing of many slides. However, there are several disadvantages including lengthy acquisition times which can span weeks, extensive tissue manipulation and perturbance of antigens between staining cycles, autofluorescence, and the lower dynamic range of fluorescence compared to MCI (3, 8, 41, 42). Further, considerable expertise and computing power is required to process the resultant large images, which if acquired at a high resolution in multiple Z planes, can form gigabytes and even terabytes of raw data, which must be deconvolved, projected and registered prior to analysis. For basic science research, our evaluation is that these methods could complement each other; where MCI captures a global overview and serial staining immunofluorescence could be used to quickly answer targeted questions with fewer parameters, using a large cohort of samples. However, in the clinical setting, a serial staining method that relies on chemically induced signal removal is unlikely to be adopted, as there will always be questions relating to incomplete signal removal and also antigenic stability over time. A comparison of features between serial staining and MCI methods is provided in **Table 1**.

Mass Spectrometry Imaging

It is worth noting that MCI differs significantly from other Mass Spectrometry Imaging (MSI) approaches such as Matrix Assisted Laser Desorption/Ionization (MALDI) MSI. In MALDI-

MSI, a laser and mass spectrometer are used to ablate and ionize molecules on the surface of a sample and the mass spectrum of each pixel on the section is collected. This is performed in a label-free manner, whereby the identity of molecules, such as proteins and metabolites, is determined either by fragmentation of ionized species at each pixel, or by comparing the intact mass to a database of known molecules (43–45). In this way, MALDI-MSI has much greater coverage compared to MCI techniques. However, MALDI-MSI has several limitations compared to MCI, such as lower resolution, lower sensitivity (often limiting analysis to larger proteins) and compatibility issues with common sample preservation methods such as formalin fixation or embedding in optimal cutting temperature compound (OCT) (46–49). The MSI community is currently at work to address these limitations and this has recently been reviewed (46). In particular, once limitations in resolution and sample preparation requirements are bridged, this could offer exciting opportunities for multi-modal imaging protocols which combine the breadth of MSI with the sensitivity of MCI, allowing for in-depth molecular profiling of targeted cell subsets.

The purpose of this review is two-fold. First, we provide an overview of the published applications of MCI. Second, as analysis is a significant challenge in MCI projects, we provide an overview and evaluation of the data processing and analysis strategies that have been successfully employed. The reader will take away an understanding of the applications and questions that can be answered with MCI, as well as the various possible approaches for analysis to address these.

APPLICATIONS OF MASS CYTOMETRY IMAGING

In this section we will discuss all applications of MCI to date which are summarized in **Table 2** with associated references and also graphically represented in **Figure 2**. MCI has been primarily used in the fields of cancer research and more recently in studies of autoimmune disorders such as type 1 diabetes mellitus and multiple sclerosis. MCI has also been used for immunophenotyping studies to define complex cell types, their interactions and also location *in situ*. Additionally, there have been many recent expansions, which include a counterstaining method, RNA detection, drug discovery, and also 3D imaging. For each study we will refer to the specific technology applied—IMC or MIBI—and also to the application of these technologies generally, as MCI.

Cancer

The first published examples using primary cancer tissues were the original papers describing IMC and MIBI (11, 12). These were more proof of principle studies largely confirming pathologist observations and findings from the literature. Subsequent studies in cancer research adapted IMC for the analysis of very small clinical samples (14, 15) (**Figure 2A**). Gerdtsson et al. showed that IMC can be effectively integrated into the established high definition single cell analysis (HD-SCA) assay for liquid biopsies. HD-SCA involves coating glass slides with millions of cells from a blood draw and using immunofluorescence to identify and characterize very rare tumor cells among millions of leukocytes (60). The major advantages of performing microscopy in this context, is that it allows small samples to be analyzed and is an almost lossless strategy capturing cells that might otherwise be missed using suspension cytometry (60). The HD-SCA assay has been shown to generate useful data for clinical decision making (61). Gerdtsson et al. used a combination approach where immunofluorescence identified regions with tumor cells, which were then acquired by IMC for in-depth phenotyping. This approach was later used by the same group on touch preparations of bone marrow and prostate tissue from a patient with polymetastatic prostate cancer (14). A key finding from their IMC analysis was the lower expression of EpCAM on tumor cells in the bone marrow compared to the prostate. This would suggest that for the patient under study, anti-EpCAM therapies may have limited effect on metastatic tumor cells in the bone marrow. Therefore, these studies highlight the utility of MCI to examine multiple clinically relevant markers in small samples, which can be used to guide therapeutic interventions. The identification of biomarkers of metastases is an active field of research and combined genomics and MCI data would be a powerful approach for discovery analysis in limited patient samples (62, 63).

IMC has also been used to investigate the spatial distribution, and effect on relevant cell populations, of platinum-based drugs *in situ*, which are used to treat solid tumors (50). In this study the drug cisplatin was detected by its atomic mass of 195, in a patient-derived pancreatic ductal adenocarcinoma xenograft model (**Figure 2A**). Traditionally, cisplatin distribution has been measured using inductively coupled plasma mass spectrometry which does not allow cellular resolution (64, 65). However, the use of IMC has overcome this limitation, successfully showing differential cisplatin entry into tissue compartments as well as cell-type dependent effects on DNA damage and proliferation (50). Furthermore, a recent pre-print from the Nolan lab has described an expansion of MIBI capable of super-resolution 3D imaging (discussed further below) (51). This technology was used to map the intracellular distribution of cisplatin in an ovarian cancer cell line. Together, these MCI modalities offer complementary approaches to studying the effects of cisplatin on both tumor and normal host cells. This will be particularly useful for the development of therapeutic interventions targeting the kidney and cochlea tissues where cisplatin accumulation often leads to loss of kidney function (66) and hearing, respectively (67, 68).

Recent studies have used MCI to analyse the tumor microenvironment for patterns of prognostic value. The first such study was performed by Keren et al., who published a landmark paper using MIBI to profile the tumor immune landscape in archival samples from 41 triple-negative breast cancer patients (13). Importantly, this study was the first to use MCI as a standalone technique for the comprehensive profiling of immune cells and their spatial orientation *in situ*. As such, this study provides a framework for the analysis of MCI data which is discussed throughout the section below on "Image Processing and Analysis." Through the innovative use of spatial analysis techniques, the authors found that patients could be stratified

TABLE 2 | Summary of MCI applications and associated publications.

Application	Description of applications	References
Original papers	Landmark papers describing IMC and MIBI	(11, 12)
Cancer	Phenotyping cancer cells in Liquid Biopsies & tissue touch preparations	(14, 15)
	Distribution and cellular effects of platinum-based drug Cisplatin	(50, 51)
	Analyzing tumor-microenvironment to predict patient outcomes	(13, 52, 53)
Autoimmune disorders	Immune system involvement in type 1 diabetes progression	(17, 18)
	Profiling immune cells in lesions at different stages of lesion progression	(54)
	Landscape of microglia and astrocytes in MS lesions	(55)
Immunophenotyping	Resolving phenotype, location and function of murine kidney myeloid subsets	(19)
	Demonstration of interactions between antigen presenting cells and memory T cells in the fetal small intestine	(20)
	Mapping location myeloid subsets in human tonsil tissue	(56)
	Mapping location of memory and marginal zone B cells in human appendiceal tissue	(21)
Other applications and expansions	Counterstaining method for IMC, generating H&E like image.	(57)
	Simultaneous detection of RNA transcripts and protein by IMC.	(16)
	3D super-resolution MIBI	(51, 58)
	High content drug screening	(59)

into two groups defined as either "mixed," with extensive tumor and immune cell mixing, or "compartmentalized," in which regions comprised mostly of either tumor or immune cells (**Figure 2A**). This stratification turned out to be meaningful and was predictive of many differences between patients, including immune cell composition, immunoregulatory protein expression and even patient survival, where "compartmentalized" patients were significantly more likely to survive compared to their "mixed" counterparts (**Figure 2A**). Importantly, this example demonstrates how sophisticated computational tools can be used to model high dimensional spatial data, revealing immune network patterns which are predictive of disease outcome.

Another recent study by Carvajal-Hausdorf et al. used an IMC panel to investigate the tissue microenvironment in breast cancer patients and risk of relapse following trastuzumab (HER2 extracellular domain-targeted) treatment (52). They showed that the ratio of the HER2 extracellular/intracellular domain expression correlated with benefit from trastuzumab treatment, and were able to relate this to CD8 T cell proximity to tumor cells. Worth noting, the authors mention that they were previously unable to generate a reliable predictive ratio using fluorescence microscopy due to difficulty normalizing for variable quantum yield between fluorophores, an issue overcome through the use of IMC, again highlighting its potential for clinical applications.

In all, MCI is an emerging and powerful tool for applications in clinical management, and also preclinical studies examining drug effects and the tumor microenvironment.

Autoimmune Disorders

Diabetes

Two papers recently published back-to-back in Cell Metabolism, have set the scene for the use of IMC to investigate the immune correlates of type 1 diabetes mellitus (T1DM) progression (17, 18). These studies compared the pancreas of healthy organ donors to that of T1DM patients at various times since diagnosis (**Figure 2B**). To date human T1DM studies have been limited by both sample availability and the availability of highly multiplexed imaging methods to comprehensively analyse these archival tissue samples. Here we highlight a few key results from these studies which used IMC as a standalone tool for their investigations.

A hallmark of T1DM is the progressive loss of beta cells in the islets of the pancreas and we are only beginning to understand the role the immune system plays in this loss which includes the generation of islet-reactive CD8 T cells (69, 70) and how their function is promoted by (71, 72) or inhibited (73) by other resident immune cell subsets. In their study, Damond et al. developed a 35 parameter panel to investigate the correlates of beta cell loss. They showed that at the time of T1DM onset, beta cell levels are similar to that of healthy pancreata, but that the expression of beta-cell markers varies widely across islets of the same donor, with only some resembling that of late stage disease (>8 years) (**Figure 2B**). In essence, this revealed that at the time of initial diagnosis beta cells, which normally produce insulin, are present but look different; thus, highlighting the possibility of therapeutic interventions to rescue beta cells during early stage disease.

Both studies found a temporal correlation between beta cell destruction and CD4/CD8 T cell infiltration into the islets (**Figure 2B**). Considering the coincident downregulation of beta cell markers, it has been hypothesized that this may be a form of "immunological camouflage" in an attempt to escape immune attack (74). Furthermore, alpha cells, which are also resident within islets, were shown to upregulate the beta-cell transcription factor NKX6, which supports the idea of alpha cell trans-differentiation into beta cells in the case of beta cell loss. Together these studies illustrate the enormous utility of MCI for understanding the causes of T1DM and for developing new strategies for prevention and cure.

Multiple Sclerosis

Multiple sclerosis is a progressive disease characterized by the appearance of demyelinating lesions in the central nervous

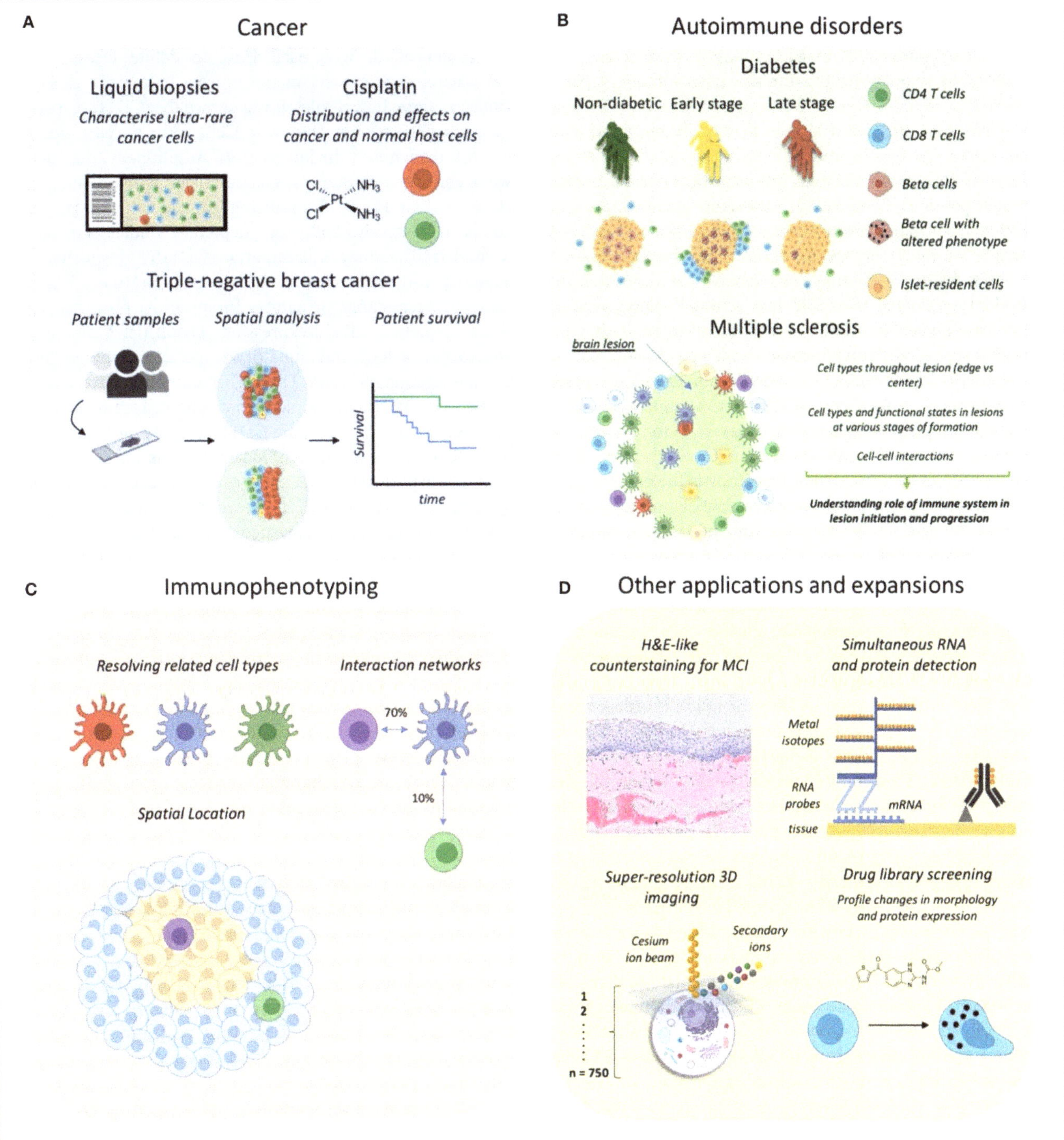

FIGURE 2 | Applications of Mass Cytometry Imaging. **(A)** MCI has been utilized for cancer studies examining rare circulating tumor cells in liquid biopsies, the distribution and effects of anti-cancer drugs such as cisplatin, and for profiling the tumor-immune landscape in tripe-negative breast cancer. **(B)** IMC has been used to investigate the immune correlates of autoimmune disorder progression, including type 1 diabetes mellitus and multiple sclerosis lesion formation in the central nervous system. **(C)** Some studies have begun to use MCI for immunophenotyping so as to discriminate cell subsets, their interactions and anatomical distribution. **(D)** Several recent expansions of MCI, including the development of a counterstaining method, simultaneous RNA and protein detection, 3D super-resolution imaging of single cells, and applications for drug screening. Parts of this figure were made Biorender.

system (75). The formation of these lesions occurs in stages which have been formally characterized (76). Importantly, lesion formation is considered an immune-mediated pathology. However, similar to T1DM, dissecting the role of the immune system has been challenging, due to both difficulty obtaining samples and the lack of technologies to simultaneously characterize the repertoire, functional state and spatial location of lesion-associated immune cell populations (77–79). Accordingly, two recent pre-prints by Ramaglia et al. and Park et al. have utilized IMC to characterize the immune environment of post-mortem MS brain tissue which we discuss in this section (54, 55).

The study by Ramaglia et al. was specifically purposed as a proof of principle as to the utility of IMC to profile the immune landscape of MS lesions (54). Accordingly, their results largely recapitulate previous literature, but importantly demonstrate that a wealth of information from previous studies can be captured in a single section. One specific example is the finding that the majority of demyelinating macrophages are derived from the resident microglial pool and not activated blood-derived macrophages. Such information may be useful to guide therapy design, as it suggests existing therapies, which block the influx of inflammatory cells, may need to be complemented with therapies targeting the factors that drive microglia activation (80–82).

Park et al. used a panel of 13 markers to perform a targeted examination of myeloid and astrocyte phenotypes in MS lesions (55). A key strength of this study is the employment of sophisticated computational tools which demonstrate both diversity and specific ordering of immune networks within MS lesions. They were able to identify five subtypes of astrocytes and six subtypes of myeloid cells within MS lesions, the latter of which were shown to localize to different areas of the lesion, suggesting distinct functional states. Further they were able to show there were significant cell-cell interactions between specific immune subsets in hypercellular regions of lesions indicating that cell to cell communication within the lesion is ordered and not random. However, the limited parameters in this study did not allow for the assessment of the functional consequence of these interactions. Furthermore, they were able to quantify the influence of cell intrinsic and extrinsic factors on cellular marker expression. This showed that microglia on the edge of the lesion are more responsive to cues from the extracellular environment, whilst microglia within the lesion are more driven by cell intrinsic programs potentially instigated by myelin phagocytosis.

Together, these studies provide a strong rationale for follow-up MCI studies with increased parameters and patient samples to further characterize the immune networks that are active in various stages of lesion development. The use of complementary technologies such as laser-capture microdissection and RNA-sequencing may aid in this characterization through the selective capture and in-depth profiling of selected areas of interest (83).

Immunophenotyping of Cell Subsets

The definition of distinct immune cell subsets is an important area of research for the study of human diseases. For example, cells that are ontogenically and therefore phenotypically closely related, can have distinct immunological functions and consequently play very different roles in disease pathogenesis (38, 84). Furthermore, these many and varied subsets will have their own specific interaction networks, which adds another layer of complexity. Accordingly, some studies have begun to use MCI for the definition of complex cell subsets, their anatomical location and potential interacting neighbors (**Figure 2C**).

The deep phenotyping enabled by MCI enables phenotypically similar cell types to be distinguished. This was demonstrated by Brahler et al. who used IMC to define Dendritic Cell and Macrophage subsets in the murine kidney. In this work, contrary to previous studies, it was shown that CD11c-expressing Macrophages and not Dendritic Cells form a dense dendritic network throughout the kidney (19). Additionally, they defined two Dendritic Cell subsets, characterized as expressing either CD103 or CD11b and localizing to large and small blood vessels, respectively. Follow-up depletion studies showed that in models of kidney inflammation CD11b+ Dendritic Cells played a pro-inflammatory role, whilst CD103+ Dendritic Cells were regulatory in nature. Importantly, previous studies which depleted CD11c-expressing Dendritic Cells showed attenuation of local inflammatory responses in mouse models of inflammation (85, 86). The high parameter characterization enabled by IMC demonstrated that among Dendritic Cells, it was likely the depletion of the CD11b-expressing Dendritic Cell subset that led to mitigation of local inflammation.

In its early adoption IMC has proven a useful tool for making qualitative observations of the location of multiple cell subsets and their interactions. In particular it has been used to show clustering of activated memory CD4+ T cells with specific antigen presenting cells in the fetal small intestine, potentially indicative of immune priming by antigen presenting cells (20). This helped cement the results from their *ex vivo* data which demonstrated a diverse and active memory T cell compartment within the fetal small intestine, a site previously considered to be protected from foreign antigens (87). Another study by Durand et al. investigated the role of myeloid cell subsets in CD4+ T follicular helper (Tfh) cell priming, which is critical for the generation of effective humoral responses (56). IMC analysis was used to map the anatomical location of myeloid cell subsets in human tonsil tissue. Critically, Macrophages were shown to cluster with Tfh cells which supported *ex vivo* data showing that Macrophages are potent inducers of Tfh cells. Finally, a study by Zhao et al. investigated the relationship between memory B cells and their marginal zone counterparts which are related but reported to play distinct roles in memory responses and the generation of innate responses independent of T cell antigens, respectively (21, 88, 89). In their study, IMC revealed that class switched memory B cells (CD27+IgM-) are located toward the periphery of appendiceal lymphoid tissue, closer to the follicle associated epithelium, and surround their marginal zone B cell (CD27+IgM+IgD+) counterparts. The differential location supports the notion of differing functional roles of these subsets, however the significance of the differential localization observed here remains to be elucidated (19, 20).

With increased adoption, MCI will likely become an indispensable tool for atlas studies of immune cell composition, interactions, and anatomical location in health and disease.

Other Applications and Expansions

The first adaptation of IMC was its aforementioned use for phenotyping liquid biopsies from cancer patients (14, 15). Beyond this, several techniques have been developed which either add to, or extend on, IMC and MIBI (**Figure 2D**).

In histology, counterstaining, most commonly using haematoxylin, is useful as it provides an overview of tissue architecture and can assist in the assessment of tissue pathology. Accordingly, Catena et al. developed a counterstaining method for IMC using ruthenium tetraoxide, which achieves good uniformity, paralleling that of a haemotoxylin stain (57). In combination with the DNA intercalator, iridium, the output images, when pseudo-colored appropriately, are similar to that of a traditional H&E stain (**Figure 2D**). Importantly, this method was shown to not interfere with detection of signals due to metal-tagged antibodies. Furthermore, H&E images have been shown to provide sufficient information for Dermatologist-level classification of skin cancer using deep neural networks (90). Accordingly, the counterstaining method described here could provide useful textual information for automated classification of anatomically distinct structures.

IMC has been used for the detection of proteins and compounds with appropriate atomic mass. However, Schulz et al. have described an extension of IMC which includes the detection of RNA transcripts *in situ* (16). This entailed a modification of the popular RNAscope technique where the final amplification steps use lanthanide-tagged, rather than enzyme-tagged, oligonucleotides [**Figure 2D**; (91)]. The authors show a good correlation of both protein and RNA signals between the modified and usual fluorescence-based version of the RNAscope assay. However, they note a lower limit of detection of 6–14 transcripts per cell, which is significantly lower than the single transcript sensitivity of the original assay. This lower sensitivity is likely due to the loss of enzyme-substrate amplification present in the original assay. This could potentially be improved through the use of lanthanide-tagged substrates, or using lanthanide-tagged antibodies targeting the deposited substrate.

The capacity to detect RNA transcripts by IMC represents a significant extension of this technique. For example, many pathogens, such as HIV, cannot reliably be detected *in situ* using antibodies and require RNA-based detection (92). This opens the door to the investigation of host-pathogen interactions in a high parameter setting. In addition, difficult to target or lowly expressed proteins, such as cytokines, can now be detected *in situ,* and mapped to the cell types producing these functional molecules (93–95). Indeed, this was demonstrated by Schulz et al., where they assessed CXCL10 expression in breast cancer tissues. They found that CXCL10-expressing cells clustered together and that their frequency correlated with T cell presence. CXCL10 expression has been associated with poor survival in various cancers (96–98). As such, further profiling of the specific T cell subsets recruited, their phenotype and localization in the tumor microenvironment, could help explain the oncogenic effects of CXCL10 in driving metastasis and poor clinical outcome.

Two recent pre-prints from the Nolan lab have described an extension of MIBI which allows three-dimensional imaging at sub 100 nm resolution (51, 58). This technique involves taking multiple axial scans of single cells using a cesium ion beam, which can then be reconstructed to form a 3D image with lateral (XY) and axial (Z) resolutions of approximately 30 and 5 nm, respectively (**Figure 2D**). One drawback of this approach is that the cesium beam cannot efficiently ionize lanthanide-tagged antibodies. Accordingly, the authors developed a novel antibody tagging method, where stable isotopes (for example ^{19}F, ^{81}Br, ^{127}I) are embedded into single-stranded DNA oligonucleotide-tagged antibodies, which can be efficiently ionized by the cesium ion beam. The inutility of lanthanides suggests a trade-off of resolution for multiplexing capacity. This form of "super-resolution" MIBI is designed for the analysis of single cells rather than large fields of view containing thousands of cells, as in IMC and MIBI. Accordingly, the types of questions which can be asked and answered differ vastly. As such, we will not further discuss the use of "super resolution" MIBI for remainder of this review.

Finally, a recent preprint by Bouzekri et al. has described a workflow for the use of IMC for high content drug screening [**Figure 2D**; (59)]. A key challenge of these screens is the labor and cost of testing thousands of compounds across many cell lines. However, it has been shown that high-dimensional profiling of drug responses in a single cell line can help select a subset of compounds with diverse biological performance, which by definition is a good library for screening drug effects (99). Accordingly, as the speed and resolution of IMC improves, it could become a useful tool for the improved screening of preclinical drug candidates (100).

Summary of MCI Applications

Despite its recency, MCI has already proven a useful tool for various applications, particularly in the domain of clinical and translational research (**Figure 1**, top panel). As outlined here, several recent studies have begun to use MCI as a primary research tool for the systems level interrogation of patient samples (13, 16–18). Accordingly, a variety of techniques for image processing and analysis were employed to identify changes in cell composition, phenotype and spatial organization, which we have comprehensively reviewed here. A common feature of these studies was the use of panels to define canonical cell types (Macrophages, T cells, B cells etc.) along with a selection of disease-relevant markers such beta cell markers in the diabetes studies (17, 18) and immunoregulatory protein markers in the breast-cancer cohort study (13). This provided a valuable overview of the distinct lineages that may play a role in disease pathogenesis and is therefore a good approach for pilot studies seeking to understanding the role of the immune system in disease etiology. Going forward, however, we anticipate studies that will become more tailored, examining specific lineages and functional markers which are known players in a specific disease context. Indeed, as discussed here, data from the few comprehensive MCI studies to date have provided a rationale for the detailed examination of specific subsets of T cells (16–18) in the patient samples studied. In the context of translational research, these targeted investigations are necessary as interventions that enhance or inhibit the activity of specific cell types require their precise definition (53, 101–106).

Finally, it is important to discuss the potential of MCI in deciphering the nature of unknown targets. This relates to the definition of "novel cell subsets" and "novel phenotypes," respectively. In terms of cell subsets, with the large number of parameters offered by MCI, it may be tempting to characterize potential "novel" cell subsets. However, caution should be exercised as cell segmentation will always be imperfect, potentially leading to the erroneous classification of new cell types. In saying that, information gleaned from MCI may provide a useful hint at phenotypes which could be validated using more robust single-cell techniques such as flow or mass cytometry (15). MCI will likely be more useful in defining the relative spatial distribution of cell subsets classified using unbiased approaches such as single-cell RNA-seq (107). Regarding novel phenotypes, disease often accompanies phenotypic changes in known target cells, which has been demonstrated in several MCI papers discussed in this review (13, 16–18). Markers of known relevance to each disease were studied, however it is possible for MCI to be combined with other multi-omics tools in donor matched samples to screen for differentially expressed molecules in health and disease (101, 108, 109). This form of guided panel design would potentiate novel discoveries through the mapping of functionally relevant markers to specific target cells or spatial niches.

IMAGE PROCESSING AND ANALYSIS

Due to its ease of use, MCI is poised to be a useful tool in clinical research. However, a key bottleneck in MCI is related to both image processing and the inherent difficulty of analyzing up to 40 parameters with added spatial dimensions. In this section, we first cover all techniques that have been used for processing MCI data. Broadly, this includes image denoising, single-cell segmentation and finally tissue and cell-type annotation. Next, we discuss approaches for the analysis of MCI images that have been implemented in MCI studies at present for studying disease models. The analysis section is formatted as a series of general biological questions which can be answered using image analysis. For each question we discuss both its clinical significance and the specific techniques used in MCI studies to answer each question.

Processing

In this section, we outline the steps taken to process MCI images, allowing downstream analysis with a single-cell approach.

Denoising

An important issue common to all image analysis is the presence of noise and artifacts which must be removed prior to analysis (**Figure 3A**, left). Robust and stable methods for denoising will become increasingly important if MCI is to be applied within the clinical setting, allowing for accurate patient sample characterization. There are noise profiles that are specific to MCI, in contrast to other imaging technologies, and may be specific to tissue types (13, 17, 18, 102). To comprehensively analyse the images obtained, various computational methods for denoising to preserve real signal and remove technical artifacts have been proposed (13, 17, 18, 102). At present there is no consensus on the most appropriate way to denoise images with research to date employing homebrew approaches based on the level and composition of noise observed by the investigators. Such approaches include correcting for channel cross-talk (18, 102), removing objects that differ from real signals in terms of size and pixel distributions (13, 18), and by using image filters to identify artifacts (13, 18). Here, we describe methods proposed to eliminate noise and artifacts in MCI images.

Crosstalk is the phenomenon in which signals from one channel are introduced into adjacent channels. This has been observed when comparing channels within $\pm$ 3 atomic masses from each other, occurring due to the presence of contaminating isotopes of similar masses (103–105). Crosstalk can even occur within 16 atomic masses due to oxidation (105). This confounding phenomenon needs to be corrected as it can lead to the misidentification of real signal within a single channel, particularly if adjacent channels correspond to markers that may be co-expressed. To correct for crosstalk, two methods have been proposed. Wang et al. observed a linearly correlated increase in pixel intensities at high pixel values for adjacent channels when plotting the intensities for two channels (18). They classified these pixels as crosstalk, and compensation was performed by resampling their intensity values in the given channel, providing a post-acquisition method for correcting for crosstalk. Chevrier et al. presents a bead-based compensation workflow to account for crosstalk, made available as the CATALYST R/Bioconductor package (102). Damond et al. implements this solution, measuring channel crosstalk using a slide with the metal isotopes used. There are trade-offs between using a fully post-acquisition approach, as opposed to a bead-guided approach. The post-acquisition method by Wang et al. is advantageous as it minimizes IMC acquisition time and resources required. However, it is unclear if their approach is valid for other images, and it is difficult to assess if real signals are removed. Additionally, correction may not be necessary if the marker panel employed is well-designed and titrated. If certain markers are expressed at vastly different levels across samples, panel design alone may not eliminate crosstalk. Hence, users should make a judgement as to whether crosstalk correction is necessary for their study.

Background noise and the corrections required can be specific to certain tissue types and experimental setups. As such, several "homebrew" computational methods have been developed to identify and remove noise in MCI images. Wang et al. observed horizontal streak artifacts within their image (18). The authors accounted for this by using a 5 $\times$ 5 μm^2 median filter which excludes the middle row. For each pixel, the median pixel value within this filter is measured, and the central pixel is removed if it is brighter than this median and is in the top 2% of pixel intensity values, characteristic of these streaks. Keren et al. observed a background artifact in areas of the slide outside of tissue in all channels (13). To correct for this, a background channel, not containing antibody derived signals, was obtained. The area corresponding to background was identified with a threshold, and the pixel intensities were reduced in all other channels within this area. The authors also observed that low density pixel signals (those with few neighboring pixel signals) were associated with noise, while real signals tended to aggregate together, corresponding to cellular staining. To remove the interfering low density pixels, each pixel in the image was assigned a score by calculating the average distance to the 25 nearest positive counts. A bimodal distribution was obtained, and pixels above the crossing point of the distributions were removed, corresponding to the low-density noise. This background removal method complements wet-lab based optimizations of blocking methods and antibody concentrations. Indeed, it can be very challenging to address all signal-to-noise issues for large antibody panels. As such, computational methods, as described here, are an important preprocessing step to ensure reliable downstream analysis.

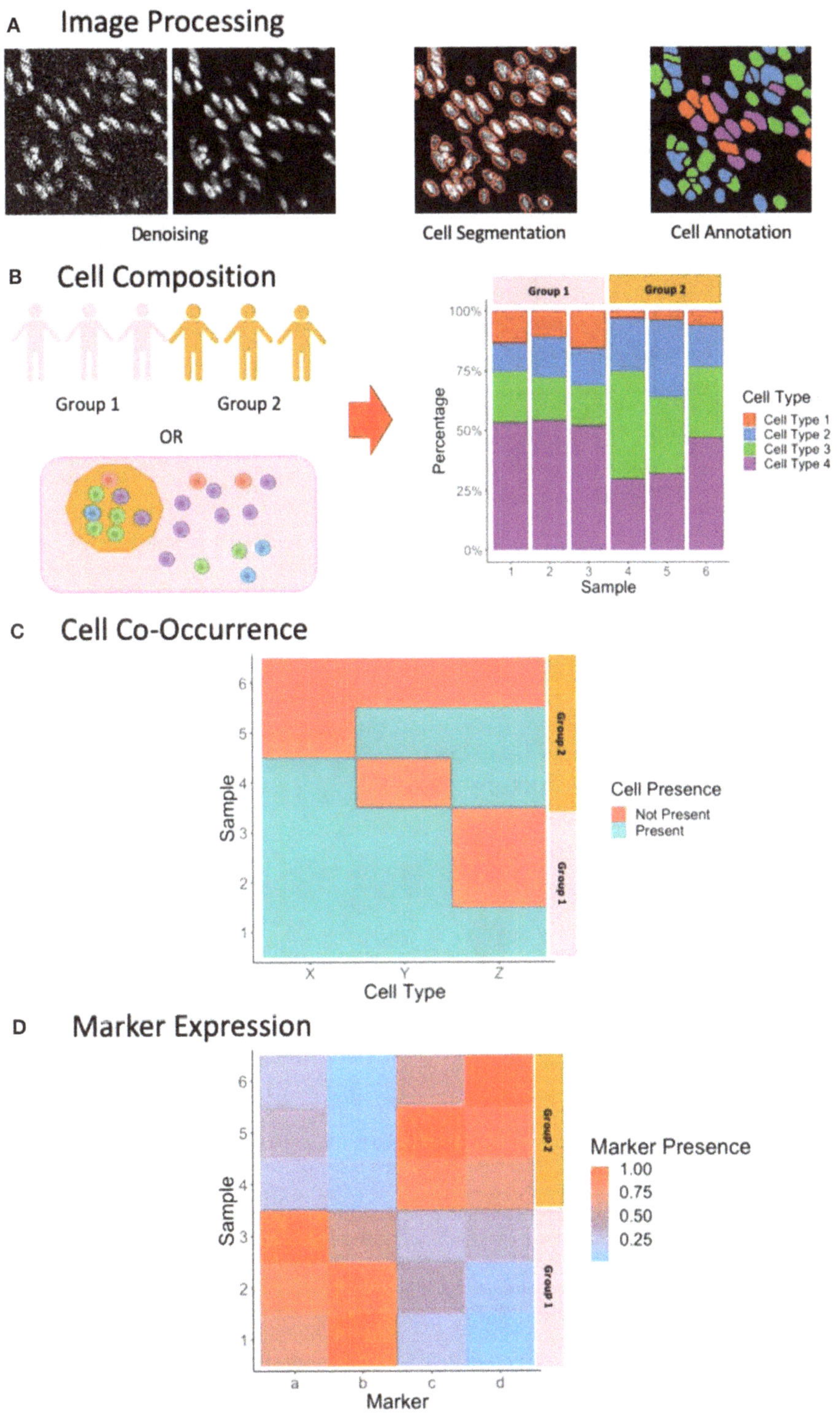

FIGURE 3 | Continued

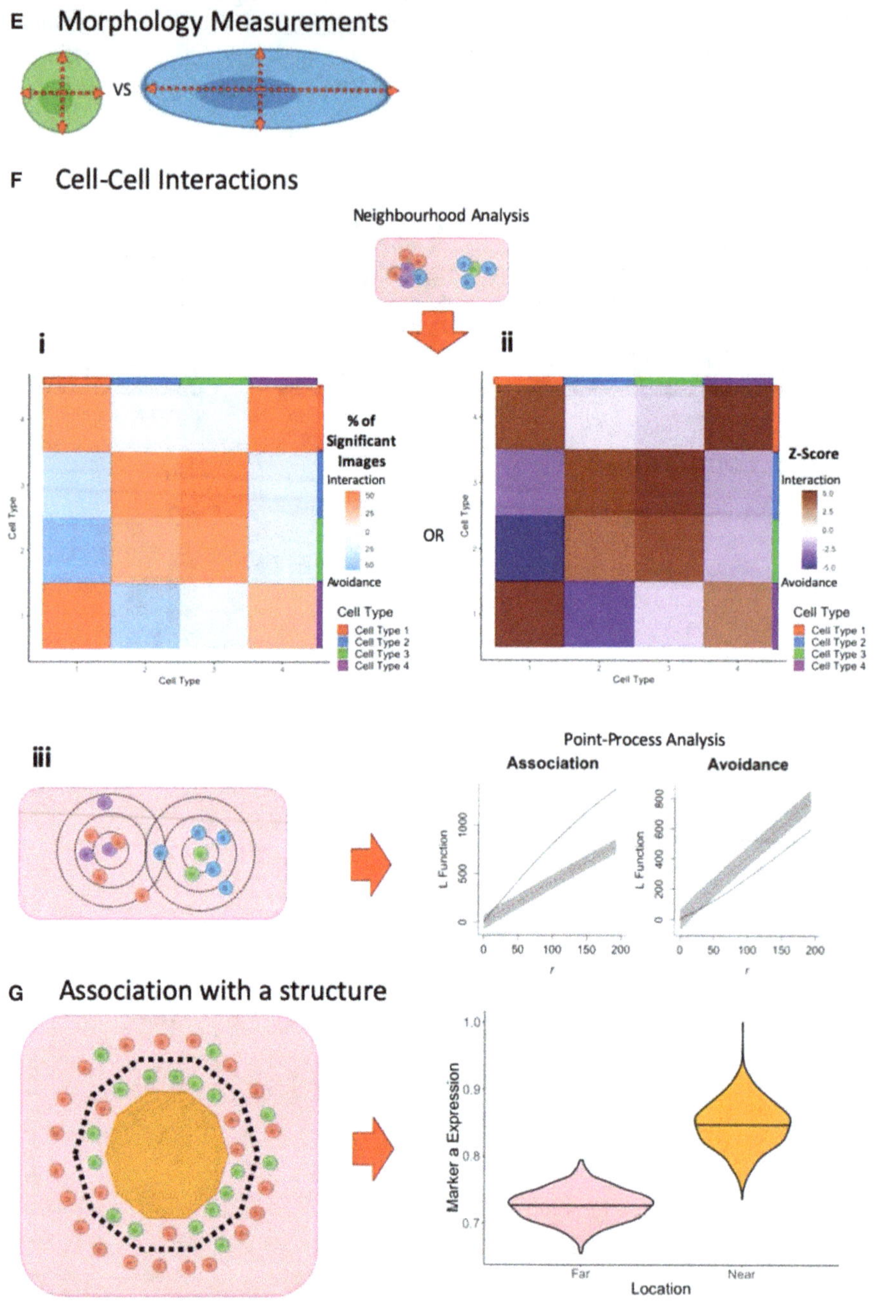

FIGURE 3 | Summary of Image Processing and Analysis Techniques in MCI. **(A)** Following the acquisition of MCI, image processing is performed to denoise the images, perform single-cell segmentation to identify cell outlines, and to classify these cells based on marker expression. **(B)** One way of exploring cell composition between groups is to compare the change in the cell fractions. **(C)** Another way to explore cell composition is to classify patients as being positive and negative for a particular cell population. The co-occurrence of cells can be presented similar to what is presented here, and significance of co-occurrence can be identified using a chi-square test. **(D)** Differences in marker expression between patients can be visualized using a heatmap. **(E)** Cell morphology measurements can be used to explore cell phenotypes. **(F)** Cell-cell interactions can be measured using neighborhood analysis or point-process analysis. With a neighborhood analysis, percentage of significant images (i) or Z-scores (ii) of the cell-cell interactions can be represented as a heatmap, with significant associations associated with a more positive Z-score and significant avoidance is associated with a more negative Z-score. With a point-process analysis, an L function can be used to assess the significance of cell-cell interactions. The L function being above or below the gray envelope generated by bootstrapping corresponds to association and avoidance, respectively (iii). **(G)** One way of measuring cell or marker association with a marker is to classify cells as being near or far away from the border. A cell composition analysis can be used to explore differences, or differences in marker expression can be explored, as shown here. Parts of this figure were made Biorender.

While various custom algorithms have been successful for denoising in previous studies, the application of MCI within a clinical setting will require an improved understanding of the sources of noise for specific samples. The standardization of "best practice" procedures for sample processing, staining, and acquisition in addition to image post-processing methods will be necessary going forward.

Cell Segmentation

Fundamental to the study of tissues in health and disease is the identification and characterization of individual cells. In microscopy this is achieved through single-cell segmentation, which involves identifying the boundary of individual cells (**Figure 3A,** middle). While single-cell segmentation has been applied to higher resolution fluorescence images, MCI images present a unique challenge because of its lower resolution, making the identification of cell boundaries more difficult both visually and computationally. Accordingly, this section discusses several approaches which have been applied for segmenting MCI data (summarized in **Table 3**).

Pipelines for single-cell segmentation established for other imaging modalities are also popular for MCI. These pipelines typically apply a threshold to a nuclear image and implement watershed segmentation to identify nuclear boundaries. Dilation of the cells, or the use of a cell-membrane marker, identifies the remaining cell body. The popular CellProfiler software (53) is often used for single-cell segmentation, with the user being able to provide inputs on the size filters, smoothing, and thresholding applied among other parameters to achieve segmentation. This is implemented by Wang et al., taking advantage of the many parameters used in IMC by using a range of non-immune and immune cell membrane markers for cell segmentation (18). This approach has the advantage of not requiring user training, requiring few user inputs for implementation. However, CellProfiler may not be able to segment cells that are packed tightly, as in tumors and lymphoid tissues, especially when the resolution is low as in the case of MCI. Schüffler et al. proposes a method in which multiple membrane proteins are weighted together to define the cell membrane (106). The proposed method performs an exhaustive search for an appropriate weighting and smoothing of all cell membrane channels, and provides a score based on how successful segmentation is performed. This self-reflective scoring may be useful for assessing the success of segmentation, but it is unknown whether it is successful for difficult, high-density images. Finally, Durand et al. employs an in-house-developed segmentation pipeline to achieve single-cell segmentation of tonsil tissue (56). First, a Laplacian-of-Gaussian filter is applied, which resolves nuclei as spots with a local minimum. A h-minima transform is then applied to identify these local minima (115). Finally, a single-cell segmentation mask is obtained by applying a watershed transformation to the linear combination distance map obtained from the h-minima transform and the average image of all membrane-bound marker proteins. The cellular regions are restricted by a defined radius of 8 pixels around each local minimum to avoid oversized cells. Ultimately, these pipelines allow cell boundaries to be identified without user training.

For more precise single-cell segmentation in MCI, supervised classifiers have been successful. These approaches require humans outlining single-cells to produce a set of well-annotated cells that can be used to train machine learning algorithms, with the advantage that humans may be better at identifying the subtle details that separate cells. Schulz et al. (16) and Damond et al. (17) implement the popular Ilastik toolkit (112, 113), employing a random forest classifier for cell segmentation, while Keren et al. (13) implements DeepCell (116), which employs deep-learning for cell segmentation. With both tools, training sets are developed using nuclear, cytoplasmic, and membrane markers, and a probability map is produced describing whether a pixel is nuclear, cytoplasmic, or background. CellProfiler, or conventional thresholding and watershed segmentation is then used to identify cells and their bodies based on the probability maps. This workflow of performing segmentation on probability maps was first demonstrated by Schapiro et al. (53). These supervised methods have been successful at separating cells that are clustered together, and can be advantageous to using CellProfiler in a standalone manner. However, these techniques require users to generate substantial training data with a new classifier needing to be generated for each experimental panel and tissue type which can be time consuming.

In general, if the outline of cells is obvious, using CellProfiler may be sufficient for performing single-cell segmentation. However, if cell shapes are more complex, as in the case of neural tissue, or if dense cell structures are present within tissue structures, then the use of classifiers will be more suitable. In fluorescence images, these classifiers have been shown to outperform classical methods for segmentation (117), but an extensive comparison using MCI has not yet been performed. As the use of MCI becomes more universal and applied within a clinical setting, there will be an increased need for more precise segmentation. It is likely that the most appropriate method will be to use a well-trained classifier. For generally applicable classifiers, users may have to contribute to an existing online classifier, creating a diverse training set to perform cell segmentation. Much investigation will hence be necessary in the future for improved and more generalized segmentation.

Tissue and Cell Annotation

Immune cells exist in great diversity within both healthy and diseased contexts. Along with canonical cell types such as Dendritic Cells, Macrophages, T cells, and B cells, each cell type is comprised of diverse subsets which differ throughout the body. Importantly, specific subsets can play a crucial role in disease manifestation, even when their prevalence is extremely low. As such, accurate and high throughput methods for the annotation of cell types (**Figure 3A,** right) and the tissue compartments in which they reside, are essential. Here we discuss several approaches that have been employed for the annotation of MCI data (summarized in **Table 2**).

The simplest approach for identifying cells is by selecting manual gates based on scatter plots of marker expression, similar to other single-cell technologies such as flow cytometry. Marker expression is typically quantified by summing the ion counts within a single cell as outlined by segmentation and dividing by

TABLE 3 | Software for cell segmentation and cell classification.

	Technique	Description	References
Cell Segmentation	CellProfiler	Identify primary object with nuclear marker, secondary object with membrane marker	(110)
	Weighted sum of membrane markers	Segments using a weighted sum of membrane markers	(111)
	Ilastik	Uses a random forest classifier, defining pixels as nuclear, cytoplasm, and background based on user training data. Probability maps can be used as an input for segmentation in CellProfiler	(112, 113)
	DeepCell	Identifies cell nuclei based on training data, using deep-learning	(114)
Cell Classification	Manual gating	Users manually identify their cells based on marker expression	
	Hierarchical Clustering	Identifies clusters in a hierarchical cluster by grouping together cells or clusters that are most similar to each other	
	Phenograph	Models cells as a nearest-neigh graph in high-dimensional space	(115)
	FlowSOM	Self-organizing maps used to identify cell populations. Meta-clustering is then performed to find a given number of populations	(116)
	Ilastik	Uses a trained random forest classifier to classify identified single cells	(112, 113)

the area of the cell. The histoCAT package (53) provides a tool which allows users to gate on cells and visualize the presence of these cells within their image. Furthermore, the single cell data can be exported from histoCAT for downstream analysis using commercial platforms such as FlowJo or Cytobank, and also open source platforms such as Flowing Software. However, a key advantage of histoCAT is that cell selections can be visualized on the image in real-time, which facilitates greater accuracy when selecting gates. However, while manual gating provides a user with full control over the cells being classified, this can be time consuming, especially when many markers are considered. Nevertheless, manual gating may be useful for exploratory analysis of image data.

One approach for semi-automated gating is by using a mixture model, such as the implementation by the *mclust* R package (106). This package is used to classify cells as being positive or negative for a marker, based on the mean pixel intensity in that specific marker channel. Another approach is by Boolean rules based on whether cells are positive or negative for these markers to classify cell types. Wang et al. implement this method, but set additional manual cutoffs as informed by the mixture models to identify positive and negative populations (18). This approach will only be applicable for markers with which cells can be discretely positive and negative for, but not when cell-type definition relies on a continuum of marker expression (e.g., low, mid, and high).

Automated gating strategies employing clustering techniques to group cells by similarities in marker intensity have become popular in all high-parameter imaging assays. This provides a quick and unbiased approach for classifying cells in tissue. Schulz et al. (16) employs PhenoGraph (115) to cluster cells, employing a nearest-neighbor graph to identify phenotypically coherent subpopulations. Here, they use both marker expression as well as RNA expression to cluster cells. Durand et al. use a hierarchical clustering approach on all markers, obtaining 60 clusters which was arbitrarily chosen to overclassify cells (56). This allowed the authors to identify smaller yet distinct clusters with some similar clusters manually merged when the clusters were annotated based on known cellular phenotypes. Keren et al. (13) clusters cells into immune and non-immune cells using FlowSOM (116), which employs a self-organizing map to identify cell populations. Lineage marker expression was used to cluster cells. This was applied iteratively, first to distinguish between immune and non-immune cells, then to classify non-immune cells into epithelial, mesenchymal, endothelial, and unidentified cells, and finally to classify immune cells into specific subsets. The approach taken by Keren et al. employs only canonical cell markers, leading to the identification of canonical cell subsets. Expression of functionally significant markers was then assessed on the defined cell subsets in different tissue compartments. In contrast, Schulz et al. clusters using all markers, leading to canonical cells being divided by marker expression. For example, two CD3 high T cell clusters were obtained, one of which expressed CD3 only, and the other being a potential memory T cell subset. Importantly, this clustering revealed the identification of rare cells that express CXCL10 RNA. Durand et al., however, merges clusters with a similar phenotype. Hence, a choice needs to be made as to whether to include all markers or only lineage markers when investigating cell phenotypes.

Finally, users can employ supervised classifiers, providing training data to predict cell types based on both marker expression and the visual texture of the signals. For example, membrane markers will be localized only to the membrane of the cell. This can be achieved using an interactive classifier such as Ilastik, where users can annotate cells as the cell subsets they are interested in Ilastik uses both marker expression level and morphology to classify cells based on the provided training data. Damond et al. implements this classification iteratively, first to classify cells as islet, immune, exocrine, and "other" cells. A second round of training and classification was then performed to classify the different immune, islet, and exocrine cells, and "other" cells were classified as endothelial, stromal or unknown cells. The classifier is advantageous as classification is informed by both marker expression and texture as defined based on more reliable human judgement. However, the training of a classifier can be time consuming, and this approach will only be able to identify user-defined cells. Hence, supervised classifiers will not identify other cell marker phenotypes that automated gating may identify.

Following cell classification, tissue compartment identification can be performed. This is useful for exploring the role of tissue structures in the context of disease. Keren et al. (13) and Wang et al. (18) use classified tumor cells and islet cells to identify the tumor and islet areas, respectively. Damond et al. uses Ilastik to identify islets and blood vessels by constructing training data using a range of structural markers, while Durand et al. uses E-Cadherin, CD19, and CD3 to identify the crypt, B cell zone, and T cell zone of tonsil tissue. The identification of these tissue structures is important because of their role in disease pathology. For example, the tumor-immune boundary has been used as a prognostic indicator for tumor progression, and islet cell composition and morphology have been observed to change with disease progression (118–120). Identifying these key compartments and their borders hence allow their role to be observed with MCI.

Similar to the segmentation of individual cells, cell-type annotation in the clinical setting would require automated and standardized methods for cell-type classification. At present, classifiers used for annotation are trained on a study-by-study basis. Although accurate, it has not been established that these approaches are generalizable or time efficient for use in the clinical setting. Ultimately, classifiers will need to be constructed and trained to account for patient and experimental variation.

Analysis

In this section, the key biological questions that are answered through image analysis is discussed (summarized in **Table 4**).

How to Stratify Data for Analysis?

To understand the biological processes underlying disease, the appropriate stratification of patient data for analysis is important. The simplest method is to group data based on clinically defined categories such as "time since diagnosis" or "patient survival." This approach is implemented by both Wang et al. (18) and Damond et al. (17) in their study of T1DM. Here, they stratified their patient groups based on time since diagnosis, with an additional control group. Although this method is often appropriate, stratification based on a biologically meaningful model of disease can offer a powerful and complementary approach for revealing disease specific relationships that simple clinical groupings could miss. For example, as diabetes is a progressive disease, Damond et al. performed pseudotime analysis (discussed below) to group islets into three "pseudostages" of disease. This followed from their observation that islet profiles followed a spectrum during the early-stages of disease, resembling both healthy islets and late-stage islets as well-intermediate stages in between. Additionally, as tumor-immune organization is known to predict survival for certain cancers, Keren et al. performed a spatial enrichment analysis (discussed below), generating a metric for tumor-immune cell mixing and allowing the investigators to stratify patients based on tumor organization (13). The decision on how to best group data for analysis is crucial for the discovery of disease specific immunological motifs. In reality, this part of the analysis stretches back to experimental design. To effectively use MCI as a primary research tool, it is important to carefully consider beforehand, choice of patient samples, availability of clinical data and also MCI panel design. These three aspects will inform the types of data stratification that are possible and therefore the scope of questions that can be asked and answered using MCI.

How Does Cell Composition Change With the Disease Context?

The prevalence of specific cell subsets is associated with disease outcomes, both in the clinical setting and in models of disease. As such, the basic analysis of cell composition is an important first step which can also inform downstream analyses. In present MCI studies, this has taken two approaches. The first is to quantify cell compositions and then compare these between different patient groups. This is done as either absolute counts of a specific cell subset, a measure of its proportion among a larger group of cells, or as a cell density per mm^2 of tissue. The second is to examine the co-occurrence or anti-occurrence of cell types, providing an insight on any causal pathways that may underlie disease. In this section we summarize how MCI studies have explored cell composition within tissue.

In MCI studies, the cell subset composition can be presented as the proportion of the total cells (or all immune, tumor, islet cells, etc.) (**Figure 3B**), the total number of cells, or the cell density. There are many advantages and disadvantages to these different approaches for quantification. Total counts can allow for patient-patient comparisons, allowing interpatient variations to be observed. When comparing between groups of patients, the cell proportion may be more appropriate for comparison, normalizing the data to account for interpatient variation. Cell density per mm^2 of tissue may be appropriate when comparing cells within compartments, with the data being normalized by the area of the compartment. The density measurement is also useful for comparing small changes that are overwhelmed by the abundance of another cell type. Ultimately, the choice of measurements used is dependent on the question being asked.

This cell composition analysis is implemented by both Damond et al. (17) and Wang et al. (18) in studying how the islet cell composition changes with T1DM progression. Both studies observed a decrease in beta cell fraction, and an increase in gamma cell fraction with disease progression, relative to all other islet cells. Damond et al. further observed a small decrease between pseudostage 1 and 2 islets, followed by a significant decrease between pseudostage 2 and 3 islets. Additionally, Damond et al. and Keren et al. present the proportion of immune cell subsets within their images, assessing the composition of immune infiltration within tissue. Data obtained from cell composition analysis can also reveal meaningful biological relationships. For example, Keren et al. ordered patients by number of infiltrating immune cells and found that patients with more immune cells were more likely to have a "compartmentalized" phenotype. Additionally, Damond et al. found that when ordering patients by the number of islet cells, stratified by patient diabetes status, mid-sized islets had a higher

TABLE 4 | Summary of analytical questions with clinical examples and the techniques used to answer these questions.

Analytical question	Clinical example	Analytical techniques
How does cell composition change with disease context?	How does cell composition change with type-1 diabetes progression? (17, 18)	Measurements such as cell counts, cell proportions, or cell densities can be used to compare between different disease contexts Pearson's correlation of the above measurements can be used to identify the co-occurrence or anti-occurrence of cell types Cell types can be considered present or not present within an image if the cell count is greater than a given cut-off (e.g., 10 cells). A chi-square test can then be used to identify cell type co-occurrence
Does marker expression or co-expression change with diseased context?	How does islet marker expression change with type 1 disease progression? (17)	Heatmaps can be utilized for visualizing marker changes across images Markers can be considered present or not present within an image. A chi-square test can then be used to identify marker co-occurrence Pseudotime analysis such as SCORPIUS (121, 122) allow marker changes associated with cell dynamic processes to be investigated
Does cell or structural morphology change with diseased context?	Does islet morphology change with disease progression? (17)	Morphology measurements can be identified using image analysis software such as histoCAT (53), CellProfiler (110), and ImageJ (123)
Are there any interactions between specific cell types, and does this change with disease context?	Are tumor-immune interactions present and significant within tissue compared to immune-immune interactions? (13, 53)	Neighborhood analysis using histoCAT (53), or by setting a distance cut-off to define neighbors (13), can be used to identify cell interaction or avoidance, visualized with a heatmap Marked point process models using the R package "*spatstat*" can be used to determine cell co-localization or anti-co-localization (124, 125)
Do cells localize to histological structures and does this vary with disease context?	In breast cancer sections that exhibit compartmentalized structures, are there differences in marker expression with distance from the tumor-immune boundary? (13)	Within binned distances away from a histological boundary, differences in cell composition (17, 18) or marker expression (13) can be identified Marked point process models using the R package "*spatstat*" can be used to explore the distribution of cells as a function of distance from a histological boundary (124, 125)
What is the role of the cell microenvironment in a diseased setting?	In multiple sclerosis brain lesions, how does the environment influence variations in cell marker expression? (55)	Spatial variance component analysis (126) can be used to decompose the sources of variation of a marker into intrinsic effects, environmental effects, and cell-cell interactions

proportion of beta cells. Presentation of data in this manner can aid in the interpretation of single-cell MCI data.

To assess cell subset co-occurrence or anti-occurrences, two approaches have been used in present MCI studies. The first approach is to observe whether the count or proportion of one cell subset is correlated with that of another cell subset, assessed using Pearson's Correlation. This measurement is useful when investigators want to show that an increased presence of one cell type is accompanied by an increase or decrease of another cell type, and is appropriate when both cell types are often or always present within that tissue type. The second approach is to convert cell counts into categorical data by classifying images as being positive or negative for a given cell subset if the count exceeds a user-defined cutoff (**Figure 3C**). A chi-square test is then used to quantify the significance of co-occurrence. This measurement is not very useful when both cell types are often or always present within that tissue type. Hence, this measurement is suitable only when the cell types being investigated are not consistently present within that tissue type.

The co-occurrence approaches mentioned above have been applied by Keren et al. and Damond et al. In studying immune infiltration into tumors, Keren et al. observed that there was a correlated increase in CD4+ T cell proportion and a correlated decrease in macrophage proportion. Similarly, when studying immune cell infiltration into the islets, Damond et al. observed a correlated increase in CD4+ helper, and CD8+ cytotoxic T cells in pseudostage 2 islets. This revealed that both CD4+ and CD8+ T cells are recruited simultaneously into the islets during the onset of diabetes, potentially co-operating to mediate beta cell destruction. Furthermore, to assess co-occurrence of cells in tumor infiltration, Keren et al. classified each patient as being positive for a given immune cell if the cell count is >10, and negative otherwise. A chi-square test subsequently revealed relationships such as patients with B cell infiltration into their tumors also had CD4+ and CD8+ T cell infiltration. The relationships observed by these analyses reveal a potential coordination in the immune response in both tumors and islets, with the recruitment of several cell types occurring.

Does the Expression or Co-expression of Cell Markers Change With Disease Context?

In addition to changes in cell composition, understanding variations in functionally relevant markers is essential for understanding disease pathology. Indeed, many interventions targeting cancer, infectious diseases and autoimmune diseases use antibodies and small molecule inhibitors targeting cytokines or cell-associated ligands/receptors (127–129). Through the many markers afforded by MCI, these diverse markers can be studied within the disease pathology setting. This section will explore how marker expression is examined in IMC images.

In MCI studies so far, the exploration of cell marker expression has taken many pathways. One approach is to compare marker expression among canonical cell subsets, with fold-changes being expressed as a heatmap (**Figure 3D**). Marker expression can also be measured at the tissue compartment or patient level, with expression level visualized as a heatmap for each sample (**Figure 3D**). By stratifying samples into groups, direct comparisons can be made. To assist with the analysis of the many markers used by MCI imaging, dimensionality reduction techniques have been used. These include principal components analysis, t-Distributed Stochastic Neighbor Embedding (t-SNE), and pseudotime analysis. Finally, the investigation of preferential co-expression of markers can be assessed by classifying images as being positive or negative for a given marker and using a chi-square test to quantify the significance of co-occurrence. Each of these approaches can be used to investigate differences in marker expression within different samples, with each analysis telling different aspects of the overall pathophysiological story. Investigators should use the appropriate investigation required depending on the question being asked, and the cellular pathway being explored.

In their investigation of T1DM progression, Damond et al. studied the change of islet marker expression within islets (17). While the investigators observed a decrease in beta cell fraction as described previously (120), they wanted to further investigate whether this was a result of beta cell loss, a downregulation of beta cell marker expression, or both. To investigate this, the authors performed a pseudotime analysis using the trajectory inference algorithm SCORPIUS (121, 122). This was performed by measuring the islet marker expression profiles of each individual islet. The algorithm finally assigns a value between 0 and 1 to each islet, relating the marker expression profile of islets to the T1DM development timeline, and allowing the investigators to stratify the islets into three pseudostages. Specifically, they observed a strong downregulation of beta cell markers between pseudostages 1 and 2, and stability between pseudostages 2 and 3. The authors concluded that progression from pseudostages 1 and 2 may be driven by the down regulation of beta cell markers, while the transition between pseudostages 2 and 3 is reflective of cell death. The assessment of changes in marker expression, combined with cell composition analysis, can reveal the mechanisms behind a disease timeline.

Keren et al. investigated the expression of the immunoregulatory proteins PD-1, PD-L1, IDO, and LAG3 in their study of breast cancer (13). Through a chi-square test, they found that patients expressing one of these proteins expressed another, implying that multiple immunosuppressive pathways are present within the tumor environment. Additionally, it was found that the presence of regulatory T cells accompanied the presence of at least one of these markers, reflecting the potential for these proteins to induce the differentiation of naïve T cells toward a regulatory T cell phenotype. Such results provide insight as to the signaling pathways that are present within the disease setting, and relate molecular expression profiles to the histological structure of the tissue.

Ultimately, it is important to understand the distribution and expression level of functional markers relevant to disease. These maybe chosen based on the literature as in the MCI studies discussed here, or alternatively using other omics technologies, such as genomics and proteomics platforms (130, 131), to pre-screen samples for suitable candidates. Importantly, the inclusion of such markers allows one to infer biologically processes from static 2D images.

Does Cell or Structural Morphology Vary With Disease Context?

Another important aspect of cellular phenotype is its morphology (**Figure 3E**). Just as with marker expression, cell morphology can also be associated with disease context or with drug treatment. Morphology measurements such as area, perimeter, solidity, eccentricity, and circularity can be made with analysis software such as histoCAT (53), as well as most image analysis packages (110, 123). These measurements allow structural changes to cell or tissue to be identified with changing disease context, or with drug treatment. However, the reliability of the measurements is dependent on how accurately segmentation of objects are obtained. This can be difficult with the lower resolution of MCI images, but may be reliable when classifiers are used, as mentioned previously.

Morphological measurements can be used to assess the integrity of histological structures. Damond et al. applies these measurements to their islets to assess changes with diabetes progression (17). The authors measured the islet extent (islet area divided by islet bounding box) and solidity (portion of pixels in the islet convex hull that are also in the islet), indicative of shape regularity. These two measurements were found to decrease between pseudostages 2 and 3, indicative of a more irregular islet shape, associated with beta cell loss and diabetes progression. Thus, morphology measurements can provide an unbiased quantification of tissue structure, identifying degradation as described here, but may also be used to highlight swelling or growth.

Cell morphology can be affected by drugs and has utility in drug-discovery (132). Bouzekri et al. uses morphology measurements to assess drug effects on breast cancer cell lines as visualized by IMC. The authors found that certain drugs led to an increase in size, with morphological measurements such as area, perimeter, and major- and minor-axes increasing following drug application. In combination with protein measurements, these observations may allow researchers to propose transduction pathways affected in response to drug treatment (133, 134).

Are There Any Interactions Between Specific Cell Types Within Tissue, and Does This Change With Disease Context?

Within previous MCI studies, two methods have been used to investigate cell-cell interactions. The first is through the neighborhood analysis algorithm described by Schapiro et al. (53). This method identifies whether a cell of type X is within a user-defined neighborhood of cell type Y, and vice-versa. This is performed by dilating each cell in a single-cell mask by a user-defined number of pixels (usually 4–6) and counting the cell types that it overlaps with. To assess significance, a bootstrapping approach was implemented, in which the annotated cell labels are randomly reassigned. The mean number of cells of type X within the neighborhood of cells of type Y are calculated for each simulation and for the real distribution. The statistic obtained for the real distribution is then ranked against the simulated statistics with two one-tailed permutation tests to obtain a p-value. The upper-tailed test corresponds to interaction, while the lower-tailed test corresponds to avoidance. When applied to a large number of donors, this can be represented on a heatmap as the percentage of significant avoidance or interactions for each cell pair (**Figure 3Fi**). The second method was to count the number of cells of type X within a user-set distance away from cells of type Y. A similar bootstrapping approach was implemented, and the number of cells was remeasured to generate a distribution from which Z-scores are obtained. This relabeling can be performed with all cells, providing context of global organizational patterns of the cells, or by constraining within a specific group of cells (e.g., immune cells, tumor cells, T cells, etc.), providing a more context dependent answer. A negative Z-score corresponds to avoidance, while a positive Z-score corresponds to association, and these values can be visualized on a heatmap (**Figure 3Fii**). These two approaches are effective for identifying cell-cell interactions. However, they do not provide any context of the cell-cell interactions over a wider distance, and does not reveal whether cells traffick toward a particular target. Additionally, an arbitrary distance needs to be chosen, and the sign of the Z-score and hence the interpretation of cell-cell interactions, can vary with scale.

This neighborhood analysis technique has been applied by Damond et al., who observed reduced beta cell associations in the third pseudostage, representative of beta cell destruction, while immune cell associations with other immune cells was increased in the second and third pseudostages, indicative of an immune response (17). They also found that the number of interactions of beta cells with CD4+ helper and CD8+ cytotoxic T cells was much higher during pseudostage 2, in line with their previous results.

Additionally, Keren et al. counted the number of cells positive for marker X located within 39 μm from marker Y. This resulted in the identification of three distinct levels of tumor and immune cell mixing: "cold," with low immune infiltration, "mixed," with high immune infiltration, and "compartmentalized," with tumor and immune cells forming distinct clusters separated from each other. The authors developed a mixing score to quantify this, defined as the number of immune-tumor interactions divided by the number of immune-immune interactions. Furthermore, when plotting Kaplan-Meier curves, which showed survival as a function of time for patients, they observed higher survivability in patients with "compartmentalized" tumors compared to patients with "mixed" tumors. Here, the spatial organization of tumor was related to patient survivability.

To explore avoidance or association at a range of distances, cells can be modeled as a marked point process model (135), in which cells are represented as labeled points on a plane. One approach is to use Ripley's K and L functions to model cell-cell interactions, with the variance stabilized L function being a useful transformation to the K function (plotted in **Figure 3Fiii**). Simply, Ripley's K function is a function which models the number of cells of type X a certain distance away from cells of type Y, as a function of distance. Bootstrapping is once again used to generate significance. This was used by Setiadi et al. in fluorescence imaging to show that B cells cluster in tumor-draining lymph nodes compared to healthy lymph nodes (136). While applied to the same cell type in this example, this can be applied to pairs of cells of different types, or with cells of a specific type to a pathogen. This can provide context of the significance of these interactions along a wider range, and to observe how interactions can change with scale, and may give insight to any cellular trafficking from a steady-state image. These functions, along with other functions and methods for comparison between samples, are readily available in the R package *spatstat* (124). However, a disadvantage of these models is that no single Z-score is given, making visualization and interpretation difficult. Baddeley et al. (125) proposes envelope-based tests to measure the statistical power of the interaction or avoidance, while another strategy may be to determine the percentage of images with which interaction or avoidance was significant, similar to Schapiro et al. (53). An investigation on the appropriate spatial statistic will be necessary to make robust conclusions about any cell-cell interactions, especially in the context of MCI images where many cell subsets are being investigated simultaneously.

With MCI, spatial analysis can be applied to a wider range of cell subsets compared to conventional microscopy over a range of distances. This allows a diverse range of cell-cell interactions to be performed, with the possibility of cell-pathogen interactions to be investigated in the future. Although these images only provide a snapshot of the tissue environment, the identification of significant interactions may bypass the need for more complicated techniques using live imaging. As well, interactions observed in the native microenvironment provide a sound rationale for *ex vivo* co-culture experiments, to investigate the functional outcome of certain cell-cell interactions. Given that specific cell-cell interactions have already been associated with patient outcomes (13, 17), such interactions metrics could prove a useful prognostic indicator in a variety of disease settings.

Do Cells Localize to Histological Structures and Does This Vary With Disease Context?

In addition to cell-cell or cell-pathogen interactions, it is useful to understand whether cells or pathogens localize to a specific histological structure, such as epithelium, tumors, and islets, which have been implicated to have an involvement in disease pathology.

In previous MCI studies so far, the number of cells or the amount of cell expression was measured within user-selected binned distances from the structure to investigate cell localization. This can be visualized as a heatmap, if 2 bins are used to represent "near" or "far" from a border. Dividing distance from a structure into user-selected bins essentially turns the problem into a comparison of cell composition or marker expression between bins. While simple, this approach discretizes continuous data, and results can vary depending on the bins used. In particular, it is hard to ascertain whether there truly is a continuous trend in the change in cell composition or marker expression toward a border. The use of a point process model as described in the previous section may prove to be suitable for analyzing the spatial dependence of cells or markers from a structure, but further investigation is required to assess the robustness of such measurements.

Keren et al. hypothesized that there are differences in the cell phenotype near or far from the tumor-immune border in "compartmentalized" patients (13). To investigate this, the authors applied a cut-off of 39 um to stratify cells as being close to or far from the border. In addition to counting cells, they observed whether marker expression was higher or lower away from the border (**Figure 3G**). The authors observed that the ratio of H3K27me3 (methylated DNA) to H3K9ac (acetylated DNA) increased for tumor cells that are far from the border in two patients, indicating that cells closer to the border may be more transcriptionally active. However, this strategy fails to provide any insight as to how this marker ratio varied continuously as a function of distance from the border. It would be interesting to see whether or not the marker ratio increased with distance, coinciding with the binned approach, or whether it alternates between increasing and decreasing. Furthermore, to simplify the spatial relationships observed, a principal component analysis was performed, revealing a subset of patients that had increased immunoregulatory protein expression in CD11c+CD11b+ immune cells. This is suggestive of myeloid derived suppressor cells, which may inhibit the immune response (137). Hence, the examination of a spatial binning to analyse the spatial dependence of marker expression from a structure was able to reveal subgroups of patients with unique phenotypes. An interesting progression may be to compare how the survival varies between these subgroups.

What Is the Role of the Cell Microenvironment in a Diseased Setting?

Multiparameter imaging provides the opportunity for cellular microenvironments to be examined within a diseased setting. Spatial variance component analysis (SVCA) (126) is a technique that has been applied to MCI data which allows the sources of variation of gene or protein markers in an image to be identified, without the need for cell classification. The sources of variation of cell markers are decomposed into intrinsic effects, environmental effects, and cell-cell interactions. SVCA was applied by Park et al. to investigate how multiple sclerosis (MS) brain lesion environments influence variations in cell marker expression (55). They found that toward the center of a lesion, the relative influence of intrinsic and environmental effects increased, while the relative influence of cell-cell interactions had decreased. The authors suggest that cells in the lesion rim are more responsive to cues from the microenvironment, such as cytokines or receptor-ligand interactions, while cells respond to cell-intrinsic programs in the lesion center. There have been additional methods proposed for measuring associations between cell microenvironment and marker expression, however these methods have not been applied to MCI data (7, 138). Ultimately such analysis approaches can provide insight on the role of the microenvironment within a diseased state.

Summary of Image Processing and Analysis

Through image processing and analysis, researchers are in a position to interrogate high parameter MCI data in a single-cell manner. This approach allows key clinical and biological questions to be explored and answered, providing insight on the cellular dynamics that are present in the diseased context. In addition, these results can inform further experimentation within or outside the cytometry setting.

There is potential for the development of statistical tests to identify associations between disease outcomes and the spatial relationships between cells, implementing spatial information with multiple markers. Current methods are able to classify cells, but still perform simple spatial analysis that is implemented in other imaging cytometry assays (135). Complex machine learning algorithms will eventually benefit from including both spatial and marker information provided by MCI, constructing predictive models in a higher dimensional space.

Deep learning has become a well-established tool for image analysis. Its consistent use in a variety of applications has been driven by its ability to deconstruct and model highly complex images (112, 113, 115, 116). However, deep learning methods require many observations to train effective models. In MCI, deep learning is ideal for cell type prediction, where thousands of cells can be trained from a single image. Though, it is unclear whether it will be effective for classifying heterogeneous global spatial interactions in datasets with relatively small sample sizes, as observed in many exploratory clinical studies. Such approaches may become useful in large cohorts generated after MCI has been implemented in routine clinical use, allowing for improved accuracy.

There is still an exciting opportunity to develop analytic algorithms for summarizing spatial cell-cell interaction relationships into simple, easy to interpret summary statistics. Such algorithms are characterized by the discussed methods for tumor-immune mixing quantification and pseudotime analysis, which stratify patients into risk groups or assigns groups to a disease progression gradient. It is important to simplify such complex relationships as it will allow scores or statistics to be developed for interpretable decision making. This may also facilitate the ability for MCI data to be included in disease risk scores, incorporating the data with other clinical and pathological and genetic information (13, 117–119).

Finally, to establish confidence in the use of MCI in the clinical setting, it will be important to identify methods that are both accurate and robust in a variety of applications. This focus applies to both methods for quantifying differences in cell-type compositions and spatial interactions, as well as strategies for image processing and quality control. Within the MCI analysis community, there has been an established culture of making code available on repositories such as github, as well as supplemental information when research is published, with image data also being openly accessible. It is important that this culture continues, supporting methods that are well-annotated, easily implemented, and actively maintained for reliable integration with multiple pipelines. This will ensure that robust and novel analytical development strengthens the potential for MCI, pushing the technology closer toward clinical application.

CONCLUSIONS

In this review we have outlined the various applications of Mass Cytometry Imaging for studying the immune system in health and disease *in situ*. MCI is a more recent addition to the repertoire of tools for high parameter imaging. However, despite its recency it has already been adopted in diverse contexts ranging from oncology to autoimmunity where it has shown promise for predicting clinical outcome and understanding the role of the immune system in disease progression. Underlying these studies are common questions relating to the composition, phenotype and location of cell subsets and how they interact. Given the fundamental similarities, these studies also share similar computational strategies which we have linked to the general biological questions they answer. MCI is currently limited by its speed of acquisition, which often restricts analysis to smaller areas, and also the availability of commercially available pure isotopes. The speed has improved substantially since the initial papers describing IMC and MIBI, and will likely continue to improve as new advancements are made. At present, this limitation can be mitigated by using MCI with complementary assays such as immunofluorescence microscopy which can guide the selection of regions to be acquired by MCI. As advancements are made in instrumentation and reagent availability, computational tools, which are still in their infancy, must also develop to realize the full potential of high parameter image data. We anticipate MCI in combination with other high dimensional assays will play an important role in furthering our understanding of the etiology of disease and in clinical decision making.

AUTHOR CONTRIBUTIONS

HB, NC, AC, AH, and EP conceived and planned the manuscript. HB and NC performed the literature search. HB, NC, and EP drafted the manuscript. AC and AH provided critical revisions.

REFERENCES

1. Zrazhevskiy P, Gao X. Quantum dot imaging platform for single-cell molecular profiling. *Nat Commun.* (2013) 4:1619. doi: 10.1038/ncomms2635
2. Bodenmiller B. Multiplexed epitope-based tissue imaging for discovery and healthcare applications. *Cell Syst.* (2016) 2:225–38. doi: 10.1016/j.cels.2016.03.008
3. Lin J-R, Fallahi-Sichani M, Sorger PK. Highly multiplexed imaging of single cells using a high-throughput cyclic immunofluorescence method. *Nat Commun.* (2015) 6:8390. doi: 10.1038/ncomms9390
4. Lin J-R, Izar B, Wang S, Yapp C, Mei S, Shah PM, et al. Highly multiplexed immunofluorescence imaging of human tissues and tumors using t-CyCIF and conventional optical microscopes. *eLife.* (2018) 7:e31657. doi: 10.7554/eLife.31657
5. Tsujikawa T, Kumar S, Borkar RN, Azimi V, Thibault G, Chang Y, et al. Quantitative multiplex immunohistochemistry reveals myeloid-inflamed tumor-immune complexity associated with poor prognosis. *Cell Rep.* (2017) 19:203–17. doi: 10.1016/j.celrep.2017.03.037
6. Gut G, Herrmann MD, Pelkmans L. Multiplexed protein maps link subcellular organization to cellular states. *Science.* (2018) 361:eaar7042. doi: 10.1126/science.aar7042
7. Goltsev Y, Samusik N, Kennedy-Darling J, Bhate S, Hale M, Vazquez G, et al. Deep profiling of mouse splenic architecture with CODEX multiplexed imaging. *Cell.* (2018) 174:968–81.e15. doi: 10.1016/j.cell.2018.07.010
8. Gerdes MJ, Sevinsky CJ, Sood A, Adak S, Bello MO, Bordwell A, et al. Highly multiplexed single-cell analysis of formalin-fixed, paraffin-embedded cancer tissue. *Proc Natl Acad Sci USA.* (2013) 110:11982–7. doi: 10.1073/pnas.1300136110
9. McKinley ET, Sui Y, Al-Kofahi Y, Millis BA, Tyska MJ, Roland JT, et al. Optimized multiplex immunofluorescence single-cell analysis reveals tuft cell heterogeneity. *JCI Insight.* (2017) 2:93487. doi: 10.1172/jci.insight.93487
10. Gerner MY, Kastenmuller W, Ifrim I, Kabat J, Germain RN. Histo-Cytometry: A method for highly multiplex quantitative tissue imaging analysis applied to dendritic cell subset microanatomy in lymph nodes. *Immunity.* (2012) 37:364–76. doi: 10.1016/j.immuni.2012.07.011
11. Giesen C, Wang HA, Schapiro D, Zivanovic N, Jacobs A, Hattendorf B, et al. Highly multiplexed imaging of tumor tissues with subcellular resolution by mass cytometry. *Nat Methods.* (2014) 11:417–22. doi: 10.1038/nmeth.2869
12. Angelo M, Bendall SC, Finck R, Hale MB, Hitzman C, Borowsky AD, et al. Multiplexed ion beam imaging of human breast tumors. *Nature Medicine.* (2014) 20:nm.3488. doi: 10.1038/nm.3488
13. Keren L, Bosse M, Marquez D, Angoshtari R, Jain S, Varma S, et al. A structured tumor-immune microenvironment in triple negative breast cancer revealed by multiplexed ion beam imaging. *Cell.* (2018) 174:1373–87.e19. doi: 10.1016/j.cell.2018.08.039
14. Malihi PD, Morikado M, Welter L, Liu ST, Miller ET, Cadaneanu RM, et al. Clonal diversity revealed by morphoproteomic and copy number profiles of single prostate cancer cells at diagnosis. *Conv Sci Phys Oncol.* (2018) 4:015003. doi: 10.1088/2057-1739/aaa00b
15. Gerdtsson E, Pore M, Thiele JA, Gerdtsson A, Malihi PD, Nevarez R, et al. Multiplex protein detection on circulating tumor cells from liquid biopsies using imaging mass cytometry. *Conver Sci Phys Oncol.* (2018) 4:015002. doi: 10.1088/2057-1739/aaa013
16. Schulz D, Zanotelli V, Fischer J, Schapiro D, Engler S, Lun XK, et al. Simultaneous multiplexed imaging of mRNA and proteins with subcellular resolution in breast cancer tissue samples by mass cytometry. *Cell Syst.* (2018) 6:25–36.e5. doi: 10.1016/j.cels.2017.12.001
17. Damond N, Engler S, Zanotelli V, Schapiro D, Wasserfall CH, Kusmartseva I, et al. A map of human type 1 diabetes progression by imaging mass cytometry. *Cell Metab.* (2019) 29:755–68.e5. doi: 10.1016/j.cmet.2018.11.014
18. Wang YJ, Traum D, Schug J, Gao L, Liu C, Consortium H, et al. Multiplexed *in situ* imaging mass cytometry analysis of the human endocrine pancreas and immune system in type 1 diabetes. *Cell Metab.* (2019) 29:769–83.e4. doi: 10.1016/j.cmet.2019.01.003
19. Brähler S, Zinselmeyer BH, Raju S, Nitschke M, Suleiman H, Saunders BT, et al. Opposing roles of dendritic cell subsets in experimental GN. *J Am Soc Nephrol.* (2017) 29:138–54. doi: 10.1681/ASN.2017030270
20. Li N, van Unen V, Abdelaal T, Guo N, Kasatskaya SA, Ladell K, et al. Memory CD4+ T cells are generated in the human fetal intestine. *Nat Immunol.* (2019) 20:301–12. doi: 10.1038/s41590-018-0294-9

21. Zhao Y, Uduman M, Siu JH, Tull TJ, Sanderson JD, Wu YC, et al. Spatiotemporal segregation of human marginal zone and memory B cell populations in lymphoid tissue. *Nat Commun.* (2018) 9:3857. doi: 10.1038/s41467-018-06089-1
22. Sachs PC, Mollica PA, Bruno RD. Tissue specific microenvironments: a key tool for tissue engineering and regenerative medicine. *J Biol Eng.* (2017) 11:34. doi: 10.1186/s13036-017-0077-0
23. Snijder B, Pelkmans L. Origins of regulated cell-to-cell variability. *Nat Rev Mol Cell Biol.* (2011) 12:119. doi: 10.1038/nrm3044
24. Rani B, Cao Y, Malfettone A, Tomuleasa C, Fabregat I, Giannelli G. Role of the tissue microenvironment as a therapeutic target in hepatocellular carcinoma. *World J Gastroenterol.* (2014) 20:4128–40. doi: 10.3748/wjg.v20.i15.4128
25. Brábek J, Mierke CT, Rösel D, Veselý P, Fabry B. The role of the tissue microenvironment in the regulation of cancer cell motility and invasion. *Cell Commun Signal.* (2010) 8:22. doi: 10.1186/1478-811X-8-22
26. Oliver AJ, Lau PK, Unsworth AS, Loi S, Darcy PK, Kershaw MH, et al. Tissue-dependent tumor microenvironments and their impact on immunotherapy responses. *Front Immunol.* (2018) 9:70. doi: 10.3389/fimmu.2018.00070
27. Geissmann F, Manz MG, Jung S, Sieweke MH, Merad M, Ley K. Development of monocytes, macrophages, and dendritic cells. *Science.* (2010) 327:656–61. doi: 10.1126/science.1178331
28. Guilliams M, Dutertre CA, Scott CL, McGovern N, Sichien D, Chakarov S, et al. Unsupervised high-dimensional analysis aligns dendritic cells across tissues and species. *Immunity.* (2016) 45:669–84. doi: 10.1016/j.immuni.2016.08.015
29. Granot T, Senda T, Carpenter DJ, Matsuoka N, Weiner J, Gordon CL, et al. Dendritic cells display subset and tissue-specific maturation dynamics over human life. *Immunity.* (2017) 46:504–15. doi: 10.1016/j.immuni.2017.02.019
30. Wong M, Ong D, Lim F, Teng K, McGovern N, Narayanan S, et al. A high-dimensional atlas of human T cell diversity reveals tissue-specific trafficking and cytokine signatures. *Immunity.* (2016) 45:442–56. doi: 10.1016/j.immuni.2016.07.007
31. Sathaliyawala T, Kubota M, Yudanin N, Turner D, Camp P, Thome J, et al. Distribution and compartmentalization of human circulating and tissue-resident memory T cell subsets. *Immunity.* (2013) 38:187–97. doi: 10.1016/j.immuni.2012.09.020
32. Geginat J, Paroni M, Maglie S, Alfen J, Kastirr I, Gruarin P, et al. Plasticity of human CD4 T cell subsets. *Front Immunol.* (2014) 5:630. doi: 10.3389/fimmu.2014.00630
33. Bauché D, Joyce-Shaikh B, Jain R, Grein J, Ku KS, Blumenschein WM, et al. LAG3+ regulatory T cells restrain interleukin-23-producing CX3CR1+ gut-resident macrophages during group 3 innate lymphoid cell-driven colitis. *Immunity.* (2018) 49:342–52.e5. doi: 10.1016/j.immuni.2018.07.007
34. Guilliams M, Mildner A, Yona S. Developmental and functional heterogeneity of monocytes. *Immunity.* (2018) 49:595–613. doi: 10.1016/j.immuni.2018.10.005
35. Bluestone JA, Mackay CR, O'Shea JJ, Stockinger B. The functional plasticity of T cell subsets. *Nat Rev Immunol.* (2009) 9:811–6. doi: 10.1038/nri2654
36. Balkwill FR, Capasso M, Hagemann T. The tumor microenvironment at a glance. *J Cell Sci.* (2012) 125:5591–6. doi: 10.1242/jcs.116392
37. Palma M, Biziato D, Petrova TV. Microenvironmental regulation of tumour angiogenesis. *Nat Rev Cancer.* (2017) 17:nrc.2017.51. doi: 10.1038/nrc.2017.51
38. Collin M, Bigley V. Human dendritic cell subsets: an update. *Immunology.* (2018) 154:3–20. doi: 10.1111/imm.12888
39. Bycroft C, Freeman C, Petkova D, Band G, Elliott LT, Sharp K, et al. The UK Biobank resource with deep phenotyping and genomic data. *Nature.* (2018) 562:203–9. doi: 10.1038/s41586-018-0579-z
40. Campbell-Thompson M, Wasserfall C, Kaddis J, Albanese-O'Neill A, Staeva T, Nierras C, et al. Network for pancreatic organ donors with diabetes (nPOD): developing a tissue biobank for type 1 diabetes. *Diabetes Metab Res Rev.* (2012) 28:608–17. doi: 10.1002/dmrr.2316
41. Croce AC, Bottiroli G. Autofluorescence spectroscopy and imaging: a tool for biomedical research and diagnosis. *Eur J Histochem.* (2014) 58:2461. doi: 10.4081/ejh.2014.2461
42. Levenson RM, Borowsky AD, Angelo M. Immunohistochemistry and mass spectrometry for highly multiplexed cellular molecular imaging. *Lab Investig.* (2015) 95:397–405. doi: 10.1038/labinvest.2015.2
43. Zhang Y, Buchberger A, Muthuvel G, Li L. Expression and distribution of neuropeptides in the nervous system of the crab *Carcinus maenas* and their roles in environmental stress. *Proteomics.* (2015) 15:3969–79. doi: 10.1002/pmic.201500256
44. Bergman H-M, Lundin E, Andersson M, Lanekoff I. Quantitative mass spectrometry imaging of small-molecule neurotransmitters in rat brain tissue sections using nanospray desorption electrospray ionization. *Analyst.* (2016) 141:3686–95. doi: 10.1039/c5an02620b
45. El-Aneed A, Cohen A, Banoub J. Mass spectrometry, review of the basics: electrospray, MALDI, and commonly used mass analyzers. *Appl Spectrosc Rev.* (2009) 44:210–30. doi: 10.1080/05704920902717872
46. Buchberger A, DeLaney K, Johnson J, Li L. Mass spectrometry imaging: a review of emerging advancements and future insights. *Analyt Chem.* (2017) 90:240–65. doi: 10.1021/acs.analchem.7b04733
47. Chen B, Lietz CB, Li L. *In situ* characterization of proteins using laserspray ionization on a high-performance MALDI-LTQ-orbitrap mass spectrometer. *J Am Soc Mass Spectr.* (2014) 25:2177–80. doi: 10.1007/s13361-014-0986-9
48. Oetjen J, Lachmund D, Palmer A, Alexandrov T, Becker M, Boskamp T, et al. An approach to optimize sample preparation for MALDI imaging MS of FFPE sections using fractional factorial design of experiments. *Anal Bioanal Chem.* (2016) 408:6729–40. doi: 10.1007/s00216-016-9793-4
49. O'Rourke MB, Raymond BB, Djordjevic SP, Padula MP. A versatile cost-effective method for the analysis of fresh frozen tissue sections via matrix-assisted laser desorption/ionisation imaging mass spectrometry. *Rapid Commun Mass Sp.* (2015) 29:637–44. doi: 10.1002/rcm.7138
50. Chang Q, Ornatsky OI, Siddiqui I, Straus R, Baranov VI, Hedley DW. Biodistribution of cisplatin revealed by imaging mass cytometry identifies extensive collagen binding in tumor and normal tissues. *Sci Rep.* (2016) 6:36641. doi: 10.1038/srep36641
51. Rovira-Clave X, Jiang S, Bai Y, Barlow G, Bhate S, Coskun A, et al. Subcellular localization of drug distribution by super-resolution ion beam imaging. *bioRxiv.* (2019) 557603. doi: 10.1101/557603
52. Carvajal-Hausdorf DE, Patsenker J, Stanton KP, Villarroel-Espindola F, Esch A, Montgomery RR, et al. Multiplexed measurement of signaling targets and cytotoxic T cells in Trastuzumab-treated patients using imaging mass cytometry. *Clin Cancer Res.* (2019) 25:3054–62. doi: 10.1158/1078-0432.ccr-18-2599
53. Schapiro D, Jackson HW, Raghuraman S, Fischer JR, Zanotelli VR, Schulz D, et al. histoCAT: analysis of cell phenotypes and interactions in multiplex image cytometry data. *Nat Methods.* (2017) 14:873–6. doi: 10.1038/nmeth.4391
54. Ramaglia V, Sheikh-Mohamed S, Legg K, Park C, Rojas OL, Zandee S, et al. Multiplexed imaging of immune cells in staged multiple sclerosis lesions by mass cytometry. *eLife.* (2019) 8:e48051. doi: 10.7554/eLife.48051
55. Park C, Ponath G, Levine-Ritterman M, Bull E, Swanson EC, Jager PL, et al. The landscape of myeloid and astrocyte phenotypes in acute multiple sclerosis lesions. *bioRxiv.* (2019) 632554. doi: 10.1101/632554
56. Durand M, Walter T, Pirnay T, Naessens T, Gueguen P, Goudot C, et al. Human lymphoid organ cDC2 and macrophages play complementary roles in T follicular helper responses. *J Exp Med.* (2019) 216:1561–81. doi: 10.1084/jem.20181994
57. Catena R, Montuenga LM, Bodenmiller B. Ruthenium counterstaining for imaging mass cytometry. *J Pathol.* (2018) 244:479–84. doi: 10.1002/path.5049
58. Coskun AF, Han G, Chen S-Y, Rovira-Clave X, Jiang S, Huerch C, et al. Ion beam subcellular tomography. *bioRxiv.* (2019)557728. doi: 10.1101/557728
59. Bouzekri A, Esch A, Ornatsky O. Multidimensional profiling of drug-treated cells by Imaging Mass Cytometry. *FEBS Open Biol.* (2019) 9:1652–69. doi: 10.1002/2211-5463.12692
60. Marrinucci D, Bethel K, Kolatkar A, Luttgen MS, Malchiodi M, Baehring F, et al. Fluid biopsy in patients with metastatic prostate, pancreatic and breast cancers. *Phys Biol.* (2012) 9:016003. doi: 10.1088/1478-3975/9/1/016003
61. Scher HI, Lu D, Schreiber NA, Louw J, Graf RP, Vargas HA, et al. Association of AR-V7 on circulating tumor cells as a treatment-specific biomarker with outcomes and survival in castration-resistant prostate cancer. *JAMA Oncol.* (2016) 2:1441–9. doi: 10.1001/jamaoncol.2016.1828
62. Gupta GP, Massagué J. Cancer metastasis: building a framework. *Cell.* (2006) 127:679–95. doi: 10.1016/j.cell.2006.11.001
63. Lambert AW, Pattabiraman DR, Weinberg RA. Emerging biological principles of metastasis. *Cell.* (2017) 168:670–91. doi: 10.1016/j.cell.2016.11.037

64. Brouwers E, Tibben M, Rosing H, Schellens J, Beijnen JH. The application of inductively coupled plasma mass spectrometry in clinical pharmacological oncology research. *Mass Spectrom Rev.* (2008) 27:67–100. doi: 10.1002/mas.20159
65. Tothill P, Matheson LM, Smyth JF, McKay K. Inductively coupled plasma mass spectrometry for the determination of platinum in animal tissues and a comparison with atomic absorption spectrometry. *J Analyt Atomic Spectr.* (1990) 5:619–22. doi: 10.1039/JA9900500619
66. Dentino M, Luft FC, Yum M, Williams SD, Einhorn LH. Long term effect of Cis-diamminedichloride platinum (CDDP) on renal function and structure in man. *Cancer.* (1978) 41:1274–81. doi: 10.1002/1097-0142(197804)41:4<1274::aid-cncr2820410410>3.0.co;2-f
67. Breglio AM, Rusheen AE, Shide ED, Fernandez KA, Spielbauer KK, McLachlin KM, et al. Cisplatin is retained in the cochlea indefinitely following chemotherapy. *Nat Commun.* (2017) 8:1654. doi: 10.1038/s41467-017-01837-1
68. van Zeijl L, Conijn E, Rodenburg M, Tange R, Brocaar M. Analysis of hearing loss due to cis-diamminedichloroplatinum-II. *Arch Otorhinolaryngol.* (1984) 239:255–62. doi: 10.1007/bf00464252
69. Gonzalez-Duque S, Azoury M, Colli ML, Afonso G, Turatsinze J-V, Nigi L, et al. Conventional and neo-antigenic peptides presented by β cells are targeted by circulating naïve CD8+ T cells in type 1 diabetic and healthy donors. *Cell Metab.* (2018) 28:946–60.e6. doi: 10.1016/j.cmet.2018.07.007
70. Culina S, Lalanne A, Afonso G, Cerosaletti K, Pinto S, Sebastiani G, et al. Islet-reactive CD8+ T cell frequencies in the pancreas, but not in blood, distinguish type 1 diabetic patients from healthy donors. *Sci Immunol.* (2018) 3:eaao4013. doi: 10.1126/sciimmunol.aao4013
71. Marro BS, Legrain S, Ware BC, Oldstone M. Macrophage IFN-I signaling promotes autoreactive T cell infiltration into islets in type 1 diabetes model. *JCI Insight.* (2019) 4:e125067. doi: 10.1172/jci.insight.125067
72. Espinosa-Carrasco G, Saout C, Fontanaud P, Stratmann T, Mollard P, Schaeffer M, et al. CD4+ T helper cells play a key role in maintaining diabetogenic CD8+ T cell function in the pancreas. *Front Immunol.* (2018) 8:2001. doi: 10.3389/fimmu.2017.02001
73. Haque M, Lei F, Xiong X, Das J, Ren X, Fang D, et al. Stem cell-derived tissue-associated regulatory T cells suppress the activity of pathogenic cells in autoimmune diabetes. *JCI Insight.* (2019) 4:126471. doi: 10.1172/jci.insight.126471
74. Pozzilli P, Signore A. The reconstructed natural history of type 1 diabetes mellitus. *Nat Rev Endocrinol.* (2019) 15:256–57. doi: 10.1038/s41574-019-0192-8
75. Lucchinetti C, Brück W, Parisi J, Scheithauer B, Rodriguez M, Lassmann H. Heterogeneity of multiple sclerosis lesions: Implications for the pathogenesis of demyelination. *Ann Neurol.* (2000) 47:707–17. doi: 10.1002/1531-8249(200006)47:6<707::AID-ANA3>3.0.CO;2-Q
76. Kuhlmann T, Ludwin S, Prat A, Antel J, Brück W, Lassmann H. An updated histological classification system for multiple sclerosis lesions. *Acta Neuropathol.* (2017) 133:13–24. doi: 10.1007/s00401-016-1653-y
77. Machado-Santos J, Saji E, Tröscher AR, Paunovic M, Liblau R, et al. The compartmentalized inflammatory response in the multiple sclerosis brain is composed of tissue-resident CD8+ T lymphocytes and B cells. *Brain.* (2018) 141:2066–82. doi: 10.1093/brain/awy151
78. Podjaski C, Alvarez JI, Bourbonniere L, Larouche S, Terouz S, Bin JM, et al. Netrin 1 regulates blood–brain barrier function and neuroinflammation. *Brain.* (2015) 138:1598–612. doi: 10.1093/brain/awv092
79. Frischer JM, Bramow S, Dal-Bianco A, Lucchinetti CF, Rauschka H, Schmidbauer M, et al. The relation between inflammation and neurodegeneration in multiple sclerosis brains. *Brain.* (2009) 132:1175–89. doi: 10.1093/brain/awp070
80. Torkildsen Ø, Myhr K-M, Bø L. Disease-modifying treatments for multiple sclerosis – a review of approved medications. *Eur J Neurol.* (2016) 23:18–27. doi: 10.1111/ene.12883
81. Sun D, Whitaker JN, Huang Z, Liu D, Coleclough C, Wekerle H, et al. Myelin antigen-specific CD8+ T cells are encephalitogenic and produce severe disease in C57BL/6 mice. *J Immunol.* (2001) 166:7579–87. doi: 10.4049/jimmunol.166.12.7579
82. Storch MK, Piddlesden S, Haltia M, Iivanainen M, Morgan P, Lassmann H. Multiple sclerosis: *in situ* evidence for antibody- and complement-mediated demyelination. *Ann Neurol.* (1998) 43:465–71. doi: 10.1002/ana.410430409
83. Nichterwitz S, Chen G, Benitez J, Yilmaz M, Storvall H, Cao M, et al. Laser capture microscopy coupled with Smart-seq2 for precise spatial transcriptomic profiling. *Nat Commun.* (2016) 7:12139. doi: 10.1038/ncomms12139
84. Simoni Y, Newell EW. Dissecting human ILC heterogeneity: more than just three subsets. *Immunology.* (2018) 153:297–303. doi: 10.1111/imm.12862
85. Riedel J-H, Paust H-J, Turner J-E, Tittel AP, Krebs C, Disteldorf E, et al. Immature renal dendritic cells recruit regulatory CXCR6+ invariant natural killer T cells to attenuate crescentic GN. *J Am Soc Nephrol.* (2012) 23:1987–2000. doi: 10.1681/ASN.2012040394
86. Scholz J, Lukacs-Kornek V, Engel DR, Specht S, Kiss E, Eitner F, et al. Renal dendritic cells stimulate IL-10 production and attenuate nephrotoxic nephritis. *J Am Soc Nephrol.* (2008) 19:527–37. doi: 10.1681/ASN.2007060684
87. Thome JJ, Bickham KL, Ohmura Y, Kubota M, Matsuoka N, Gordon C, et al. Early-life compartmentalization of human T cell differentiation and regulatory function in mucosal and lymphoid tissues. *Nat Med.* (2015) 22:72–7. doi: 10.1038/nm.4008
88. Mebius RE, Nolte MA, Kraal G. Development and function of the splenic marginal zone. *Crit Rev Immunol.* (2004) 24:449–64. doi: 10.1615/CritRevImmunol.v24.i6.40
89. Seifert M, Küppers R. Molecular footprints of a germinal center derivation of human IgM+(IgD+)CD27+ B cells and the dynamics of memory B cell generation. *J Exp Med.* (2009) 206:2659–69. doi: 10.1084/jem.20091087
90. Esteva A, Kuprel B, Novoa RA, Ko J, Swetter SM, Blau HM, et al. Dermatologist-level classification of skin cancer with deep neural networks. *Nature.* (2017) 542:115. doi: 10.1038/nature21056
91. Wang F, Flanagan J, Su N, Wang L-C, Bui S, Nielson A, et al. RNAscope a novel *in situ* RNA analysis platform for formalin-fixed, paraffin-embedded tissues. *J Mol Diagn.* (2012) 14:22–9. doi: 10.1016/j.jmoldx.2011.08.002
92. Deleage C, Wietgrefe SW, Prete G, Morcock DR, Hao X-P, Piatak J, et al. Defining HIV and SIV reservoirs in lymphoid tissues. *Pathog Immun.* (2016) 1:68–106. doi: 10.20411/pai.v1i1.100
93. Silver JS, Kearley J, Copenhaver AM, Sanden C, Mori M, Yu L, et al. Inflammatory triggers associated with exacerbations of COPD orchestrate plasticity of group 2 innate lymphoid cells in the lungs. *Nat Immunol.* (2016) 17:ni.3443. doi: 10.1038/ni.3443
94. Gupta M, Babic A, Beck AH, Terry K. TNF-α expression, risk factors, and inflammatory exposures in ovarian cancer: evidence for an inflammatory pathway of ovarian carcinogenesis? *Hum Pathol.* (2016) 54:82–91. doi: 10.1016/j.humpath.2016.03.006
95. Yu S-H, Zheng Q, Esopi D, Macgregor-Das A, Luo J, Antonarakis ES, et al. A paracrine role for IL6 in prostate cancer patients: lack of production by primary or metastatic tumor cells. *Cancer Immunol Res.* (2015) 3:1175–84. doi: 10.1158/2326-6066.CIR-15-0013
96. Mulligan A, Raitman I, Feeley L, Pinnaduwage D, Nguyen LT, O'Malley FP, et al. Tumoral lymphocytic infiltration and expression of the chemokine CXCL10 in breast cancers from the ontario familial breast cancer registry. *Am Assoc Cancer Res.* (2013) 19:336–46. doi: 10.1158/1078-0432.CCR-11-3314
97. Ming I, Chen X, Ba YI. CXCL10/CXCR3 overexpression as a biomarker of poor prognosis in patients with stage II colorectal cancer. *Mol Clin Oncol.* (2016) 4:23–30. doi: 10.3892/mco.2015.665
98. Bronger H, Singer J, Windmüller C, Reuning U, Zech D, Delbridge C, et al. CXCL9 and CXCL10 predict survival and are regulated by cyclooxygenase inhibition in advanced serous ovarian cancer. *Br J Cancer.* (2016) 115:553. doi: 10.1038/bjc.2016.172
99. Wawer MJ, Li K, Gustafsdottir SM, Ljosa V, Bodycombe NE, Marton MA, et al. Toward performance-diverse small-molecule libraries for cell-based phenotypic screening using multiplexed high-dimensional profiling. *Proc Natl Acad Sci USA.* (2014) 111:10911–16. doi: 10.1073/pnas.1410933111
100. Moffat JG, Vincent F, Lee JA, Eder J, Prunotto M. Opportunities and challenges in phenotypic drug discovery: an industry perspective. *Nat Rev Drug Discov.* (2017) 16:531–43. doi: 10.1038/nrd.2017.111
101. Aebersold R, Mann M. Mass spectrometry-based proteomics. *Nature.* (2003) 422:198–207. doi: 10.1038/nature01511

102. Chevrier S, Crowell HL, Zanotelli V, Engler S, Robinson MD, Bodenmiller B. Compensation of signal spillover in suspension and imaging mass cytometry. *Cell Syst.* (2018) 6:612–20.e5. doi: 10.1016/j.cels.2018.02.010
103. Bendall SC, Nolan GP, Roederer M, Chattopadhyay PK. A deep profiler's guide to cytometry. *Trends Immunol.* (2012) 33:323–32. doi: 10.1016/j.it.2012.02.010
104. Bandura DR, Baranov VI, Ornatsky OI, Antonov A, Kinach R, Lou X, et al. Mass cytometry: technique for real time single cell multitarget immunoassay based on inductively coupled plasma time-of-flight mass spectrometry. *Anal Chem.* (2009) 81:6813–22. doi: 10.1021/ac901049w
105. Ornatsky OI, Kinach R, Bandura DR, Lou X, Tanner SD, Baranov VI, et al. Development of analytical methods for multiplex bio-assay with inductively coupled plasma mass spectrometry. *J Anal Atomic Spectrom.* (2008) 23:463–9. doi: 10.1039/B710510J
106. Scrucca L, Fop M, Brendan T, Adrian RE. mclust 5: clustering, classification and density estimation using gaussian finite mixture models. *R J.* (2016) 8:289. doi: 10.32614/RJ-2016-021
107. Hwang B, Lee J, Bang D. Single-cell RNA sequencing technologies and bioinformatics pipelines. *Exp Mol Med.* (2018) 50:96. doi: 10.1038/s12276-018-0071-8
108. Uhlén M, Fagerberg L, Hallström BM, Lindskog C, Oksvold P, Mardinoglu A, et al. Tissue-based map of the human proteome. *Science.* (2015) 347:1260419. doi: 10.1126/science.1260419
109. Fagerberg L, Hallström BM, Oksvold P, Kampf C, Djureinovic D, Odeberg J, et al. Analysis of the human tissue-specific expression by genome-wide integration of transcriptomics and antibody-based proteomics. *Mol Cell Proteomics.* (2014) 13:397–406. doi: 10.1074/mcp.M113.035600
110. Carpenter AE, Jones TR, Lamprecht MR, Clarke C, Kang I, Friman O, et al. CellProfiler: image analysis software for identifying and quantifying cell phenotypes. *Genome Biol.* (2006) 7:R100. doi: 10.1186/gb-2006-7-10-r100
111. Schüffler PJ, Schapiro D, Giesen C, Wang HA, Bodenmiller B, Buhmann JM. Automatic single cell segmentation on highly multiplexed tissue images. *Cytometry.* (2015) 87:936–42. doi: 10.1002/cyto.a.22702
112. Sommer C, Straehle C, Kothe U, Hamprecht FA. Ilastik: Interactive learning and segmentation toolkit. 2011 IEEE International Symposium on Biomedical Imaging: from nano to macro. *IEEE.* (2011) 1:230–3. doi: 10.1109/ISBI.2011.5872394
113. Berg S, Kutra D, Kroeger T, Straehle CN, Kausler BX, Haubold C, et al. ilastik: Interactive machine learning for (bio)image analysis. *Nat Methods.* (2019) 16:1–7. doi: 10.1038/s41592-019-0582-9
114. Van Valen DA, Kudo T, Lane KM, Macklin DN, Quach NT, DeFelice MM, et al. Deep learning automates the quantitative analysis of individual cells in live-cell imaging experiments. PLoS Comput Biol. (2016) 12:e1005177. doi: 10.1371/journal.pcbi.1005177
115. Levine JH, Simonds EF, Bendall SC, Davis KL, Amir ED, Tadmor MD, et al. Data-driven phenotypic dissection of AML reveals progenitor-like cells that correlate with prognosis. *Cell.* (2015) 162:184–97. doi: 10.1016/j.cell.2015.05.047
116. Van Gassen S, Callebaut B, Van Helden MJ, Lambrecht BN, Demeester P, Dhaene T, et al. FlowSOM: using self-organizing maps for visualization and interpretation of cytometry data. *Cytometry Part A.* (2015) 87:636–45. doi: 10.1002/cyto.a.22625
117. Caicedo JC, Roth J, Goodman A, Becker T, Karhohs KW, Broisin M, et al. Evaluation of deep learning strategies for nucleus segmentation in fluorescence images. *bioRxiv.* (2019) 335216. doi: 10.1101/335216
118. Fortis SP, Sofopoulos M, Sotiriadou NN, Haritos C, Vaxevanis CK, Anastasopoulou EA, et al. Differential intratumoral distributions of CD8 and CD163 immune cells as prognostic biomarkers in breast cancer. *J Immunother Cancer.* (2017) 5:39. doi: 10.1186/s40425-017-0240-7
119. Atkinson MA, Eisenbarth GS. Type 1 diabetes: new perspectives on disease pathogenesis and treatment. *Lancet.* (2001) 358:221–9. doi: 10.1016/S0140-6736(01)05415-0
120. Atkinson MA, Eisenbarth GS, Michels AW. Type 1 diabetes. *Lancet.* (2014) 383:69–82. doi: 10.1016/S0140-6736(13)60591-7
121. Cannoodt R, Saelens W, Saeys Y. Computational methods for trajectory inference from single-cell transcriptomics. *Eur J Immunol.* (2016) 46:2496–506. doi: 10.1002/eji.201646347
122. Saelens W, Cannoodt R, Todorov H, Saeys Y. A comparison of single-cell trajectory inference methods: towards more accurate and robust tools. *bioRxiv.* (2018) 276907. doi: 10.1101/276907
123. Schneider CA, Rasband WS, Eliceiri KW. NIH Image to ImageJ: 25 years of image analysis. *Nat Methods.* (2012) 9:671–5. doi: 10.1038/nmeth.2089
124. Baddeley A, Turner R. spatstat: An R Package for analyzing spatial point patterns. *J Stat Softw.* (2005) 12:1–42. doi: 10.18637/jss.v012.i06
125. Baddeley A, Diggle PJ, Hardegen A, Lawrence T, Milne RK, Nair G. On tests of spatial pattern based on simulation envelopes. *Ecol Monogr.* (2014) 84:477–89. doi: 10.1890/13-2042.1
126. Arnol D, Schapiro D, Bodenmiller B, Saez-Rodriguez J, Stegle O. Modeling cell-cell interactions from spatial molecular data with spatial variance component analysis. *Cell Rep.* (2019) 29:202–11.e6. doi: 10.1016/j.celrep.2019.08.077
127. Mahoney KM, Freeman GJ, Rmott DF. The next immune-checkpoint inhibitors: PD-1/PD-L1 blockade in melanoma. *Clin Ther.* (2015) 37:764–82. doi: 10.1016/j.clinthera.2015.02.018
128. Kanmogne G, Woollard S. Maraviroc: a review of its use in HIV infection and beyond. *Drug Design Dev Ther.* (2015) 9:5447–68. doi: 10.2147/DDDT.S90580
129. Chan AC, Carter PJ. Therapeutic antibodies for autoimmunity and inflammation. *Nat Rev Immunol.* (2010) 10:301–16. doi: 10.1038/nri2761
130. Navin N, Kendall J, Troge J, Andrews P, Rodgers L, McIndoo J, et al. Tumour evolution inferred by single-cell sequencing. *Nature.* (2011) 472:90–4. doi: 10.1038/nature09807
131. Cho WC. Proteomics in translational cancer research: biomarker discovery for clinical applications. *Expert Rev Proteomics.* (2014) 11:131–3. doi: 10.1586/14789450.2014.899908
132. Ljosa V, Caie PD, ter Horst R, Sokolnicki KL, Jenkins EL, Daya S, et al. Comparison of methods for image-based profiling of cellular morphological responses to small molecule treatment. *J Biomol Screen.* (2013) 18:1321–9. doi: 10.1177/1087057113503553
133. Boutros M, Heigwer F, Laufer C. Microscopy-based high-content screening. *Cell.* (2015) 163:1314–25. doi: 10.1016/j.cell.2015.11.007
134. Tanaka M, Bateman R, Rauh D, Vaisberg E, Ramachandani S, Zhang C, et al. An unbiased cell morphology–based screen for new, biologically active small molecules. *PLoS Biol.* (2005) 3:e128. doi: 10.1371/journal.pbio.0030128
135. Lagache T, Sauvonnet N, Danglot L, Olivo-Marin J. Statistical analysis of molecule colocalization in bioimaging. *Cytometry Part A.* (2015) 87:568–79. doi: 10.1002/cyto.a.22629
136. Setiadi FA, Ray NC, Kohrt HE, Kapelner A, Carcamo-Cavazos V, Levic EB, et al. Quantitative, architectural analysis of immune cell subsets in tumor-draining lymph nodes from breast cancer patients and healthy lymph nodes. *PLoS ONE.* (2010) 5:e12420. doi: 10.1371/journal.pone.0012420
137. Gabrilovich DI, Nagaraj S. Myeloid derived suppressor cells as regulators of the immune system. *Nat Rev Immunol.* (2009) 9:162–74. doi: 10.1038/nri2506
138. Battich N, Stoeger T, Pelkmans L. Control of transcript variability in single mammalian cells. *Cell.* (2015) 163:1596–610. doi: 10.1016/j.cell.2015.11.018

7

Mass Cytometry Analysis Reveals Complex Cell-State Modifications of Blood Myeloid Cells During HIV Infection

Sixtine Coindre[1], Nicolas Tchitchek[1], Lamine Alaoui[1], Bruno Vaslin[1], Christine Bourgeois[1], Cecile Goujard[2,3], Camille Lecuroux[1], Pierre Bruhns[4], Roger Le Grand[1], Anne-Sophie Beignon[1], Olivier Lambotte[1,2] and Benoit Favier[1]*

[1] CEA-Université Paris Sud-INSERM U1184, IDMIT Department, IBFJ, DRF, Fontenay-aux-Roses, France, [2] Service de médecine interne et d'immunologie clinique, Hôpital Bicêtre, APHP, Le Kremlin Bicêtre, France, [3] INSERM U1018-Université Paris Sud, CESP (Centre for Research in Epidemiology and Population Health), Le Kremlin Bicêtre, France, [4] Unit of Antibodies in Therapy and Pathology, Institut Pasteur, UMR1222 INSERM, Paris, France

***Correspondence:**
Benoit Favier
benoit.favier@cea.fr

Dendritic cells (DC), which are involved in orchestrating early immune responses against pathogens, are dysregulated in their function by HIV infection. This dysregulation likely contributes to tip the balance toward viral persistence. Different DC subpopulations, including classical (cDCs) and plasmacytoid (pDCs) dendritic cells, are subjected to concomitant inflammatory and immunoregulatory events during HIV infection, which hampers the precise characterization of their regulation through classical approaches. Here, we carried out mass cytometry analysis of blood samples from early HIV-infected patients that were longitudinally collected before and after 1 year of effective combination antiretroviral therapy (cART). Blood samples from HIV controller patients who naturally control the infection were also included. Our data revealed that plasma HIV RNA level was positively associated with a loss of cDC and pDC subpopulations that display high expression of LILR immunomodulatory receptors. Conversely, specific monocyte populations co-expressing high levels of HLA-I, 3 immunomodulatory receptors, CD64, LILRA2, and LILRB4, and the restriction factor CD317 (also known as BST2/Tetherin), were more abundant in early HIV-infection. Finally, our analysis revealed that the blood of HIV controller patients contained in a higher abundance a particular subtype of CD1c$^+$ cDCs, characterized by elevated co-expression of CD32b inhibitory receptor and HLA-DR antigen-presentation molecules. Overall, this study unravels the modifications induced in DC and monocyte subpopulations in different HIV$^+$ conditions, and provides a better comprehension of the immune regulation/dysregulation mechanisms induced during this viral infection.

Keywords: LILRB1 (ILT2), LILRB2 (ILT4), LILRA4 (ILT7), CD32 (FcgRII), CD38, immune checkpoints, primary HIV infection, elite controllers

INTRODUCTION

HIV infection is characterized by the dysregulation of immune responses leading to viral persistence and disease progression (1–3). During the last few decades, most studies of HIV pathogenesis have focused on T-cell immune responses. Nevertheless, dendritic cells (DCs) including, classical (cDCs) and plasmacytoid (pDCs) cells, play a pivotal role in the early defenses against viruses by bridging innate and adaptive immune responses (4, 5). After viral sensing, cDCs rapidly mature and migrate toward secondary lymphoid organs to stimulate T-cell responses. Several studies indicate that in HIV or SIV infections, cDCs are prone to apoptosis and demonstrate attenuated capacities of antigen presentation and cytokine production leading to inefficient T-cell proliferation (1, 6–8). *Ex vivo* analysis of cDCs from HIV-infected patients illustrates phenotypic changes induced early during infection and that are associated with cDC dysregulation (9, 10). Further studies in rhesus macaques identify dysregulation of cDCs induced in early SIV infection as a predictive marker of disease progression (11). These studies suggest a critical role for cDCs in the regulation of early immune responses, where deficiencies in functions tip the balance of disease outcomes toward viral persistence.

Because pDCs show unique capacities to regulate immune responses and viral replication through massive production of type I interferon (IFN), their role in HIV and SIV infection has also been investigated. pDCs from chronically HIV-infected patients show dysregulated immunophenotypic attributes (12). *In vitro* experiments indicate that HIV attenuates the production of type I-IFNs mediated by pDCs (13). Moreover, during early SIV infection, pDCs rapidly move toward lymph nodes, are subjected to apoptosis and renewal, and only a small fraction of these cells produce type-I-IFNs (14, 15). These data suggest that SIV infection induces heterogeneous functional capacities among pDCs.

Massive monocyte turnover is induced during SIV and HIV infection and has been directly linked to disease progression (3, 14). In addition, microbial translocation induces overactivation of monocytes, which in turn participate in the inflammatory events associated with viral persistence (3, 15). Finally, the production of soluble CD14 and CD163, which reflects monocyte/macrophage activation, has been associated with HIV mortality in primary and chronic infection (3, 15–17).

Even though these studies indicate that DC and monocyte subpopulations are dysregulated in HIV infection, a precise view of their dysregulation mechanisms at the molecular level is difficult to decipher through classical approaches. In this respect, HIV infection induces concomitant inflammatory and immunoregulatory events, which can differentially influence cell maturation/activation phenotype within the same populations due to proximity and/or exposure to different stimuli (virus and host mediators). Phenotypic heterogeneity among subpopulations may be further enhanced by perturbation of hematopoiesis and egress of less differentiated DCs from bone marrow to replenish dying cells as has been explored in SIV infection (18, 19).

In this study, we carried out a mass cytometry analysis to unravel the heterogeneity and dynamics of myeloid cell subsets occurring from the acute phase of HIV infection to the control of viral replication through successful combination antiretroviral therapy (cART). For this purpose, we collected samples from primary HIV-infected patients longitudinally, prior to and after 1 year of effective cART. Samples from elite controllers, who naturally control HIV replication in the absence of treatment, were also included as well as control samples from healthy donors. Interestingly, myeloid cells from elite controllers were previously shown to display enhanced functions and a specific expression profile of Leukocyte Immunoglobulin-Like Receptors (LILRs), a family of receptors that play important roles in the regulation of myeloid cell maturation and functions (20–22). In this regard, LILRs could represent key markers that account for DC-associated regulation/dysregulation mechanisms (23). Therefore, markers for the most well-characterized LILRs were included in our mass cytometry panel.

Our data reveal an association between a high level of HIV RNA and a loss in the blood of cDC and pDC clusters that highly expressed specific members of LILR family. In contrast, early HIV infection was positively associated with clusters of monocytes displaying high expression of HLA-I ligands, CD64, LILRA2, LILRB4 immunoregulatory receptors and restriction factor CD317 (also known as BST2 or tetherin), a ligand of LILRA4. Finally, a subtype of cDCs defined by high expression of CD32b and HLA-DR was more abundant in elite controllers than in other conditions. Altogether, our results provide a unique view of the diversity and various phenotypic changes induced in DCs and monocytes during early HIV infection, before and after effective cART, but also in patients that naturally control HIV infection. Overall, this study reveals new insights on the mechanisms driving the dysregulation of early myeloid immune responses, which may account for inefficient adaptive immune responses and viral persistence.

RESULTS

Phenotypical Characterization of Dendritic Cell and Monocyte Populations Among Patient Samples

To characterize the phenotypic diversity of DC and monocyte subsets in HIV primary and controlled infections, we developed a mass-cytometry panel of 29 markers mainly dedicated to myeloid cells (**Table S1**). We applied this panel to PBMCs from three groups of individuals. The first group included six patients who were longitudinally sampled during the primary phase of HIV infection, as previously described (24), before (primary HIV) and after 1 year of combination antiretroviral therapy (HIV cART). The second group was composed of six HIV-infected elite controller patients (HIV controllers) that naturally control viral replication. Finally, the third group encompassed six healthy subjects (Healthy). Clinical characteristics of these groups are shown in **Table 1**. These groups allow us to question the changes in the dynamics, diversification, and regulatory events among DCs and monocytes during both primary infection and potential normalization on cART, and in HIV controllers.

The mass cytometry panel was designed to detect lineage, migration and adhesion markers, as well as activation and inhibitory immunoreceptors known to play an important role in myeloid cell functions and maturation (**Figure 1**). After the acquisition of all samples by mass-cytometry, we applied a first step of manual gating strategy to exclude lymphocyte subsets, followed by the positive selection of cell populations expressing HLA-DR (**Figure S1**) to select DCs and other myeloid

TABLE 1 | Summary of patient and subject clinical parameters.

	Primary HIV ($n = 6$)	HIV cART ($n = 6$)	HIV controllers ($n = 6$)	Healthy ($n = 6$)
Age median (min-max), in years	34 (24–47)	35 (25–48)	39 (25–49)	35 (25–45)
Gender	M	M	M	M
Days since HIV-1 diagnosis median (min-max), in days	28 (18–29)	361 (290–372)	1,825 (1,825–7,300)	N/A
Treatment	Naive	cART	Naive	Naive
RNA HIV load at diagnosis median (min-max), in $\log_{10}$ copies/ml of plasma	6.67 (5.47–7.26)	1 (1–1.63)	1.54 (1.43–1.69)	N/A
CD4 T-cell count median (min-max), in 10^3 cells/μl of blood	470 (258–669)	843 (570–1,247)	827 (652–1,180)	856 (634–1,412)

Eighteen Caucasian men were involved in this study to constitute four groups of conditions. These groups are composed of six primary HIV-infected patients before treatment (primary HIV) and after 1 year of combination antiretroviral therapy (HIV cART), six elite controllers (HIV controllers), and six healthy subjects (Healthy). The gender and median patient age, days since HIV-1 diagnosis, RNA viral load, and CD4$^+$ T-cell count are indicated for each group. cART, combination antiretroviral therapy; N/A, not applicable; M, male.

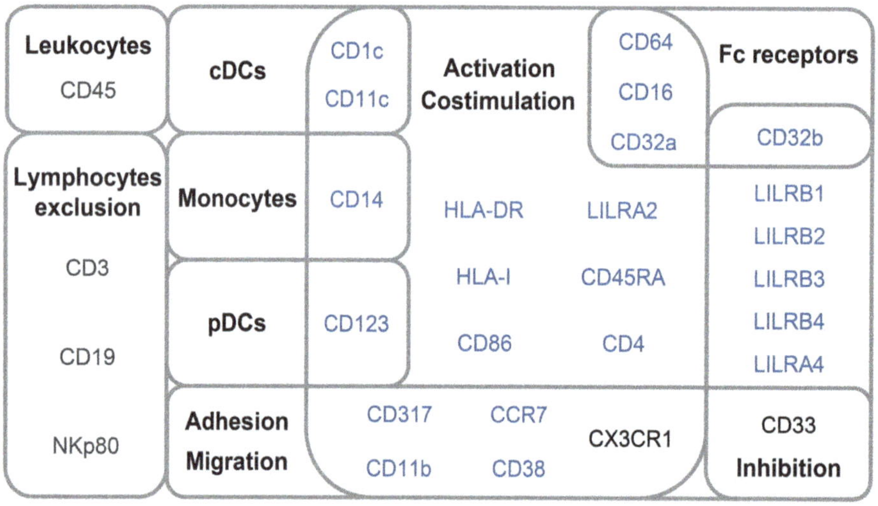

FIGURE 1 | Mass-cytometry panel. Mass-cytometry panel of 29 cell parameters used to characterize myeloid cell population diversity in PBMC samples. Markers used to select leukocytes and exclude lymphocytes from the analysis are indicated in gray. Markers used for SPADE clustering of myeloid cells are indicated in blue. Markers used for the phenotypic characterization of myeloid cells are indicated in blue or black.

cells. We next characterized the simultaneous expression of markers from our panel on these myeloid cells. For this purpose, we used the Spanning-tree Progression Analysis of Density-normalized Events (SPADE) clustering algorithm to identify myeloid cell clusters having similar expressions for selected markers regardless of their sample cell origin (25, 26). A categorical heatmap was generated using hierarchical clustering to visualize more easily the respective relative marker expression of each myeloid cell cluster identified (**Figure 2A**). The overall phenotype distribution of all clusters was visualized in **Figure S2**. For each cluster, the correlation with plasma RNA viral load and its variation in abundance across patient groups was also analyzed (**Figures 2B,C**).

Based on the cell cluster dendrogram, 12 families of cell clusters were defined (**Figure 2A**). A tSNE representation generated to represent the similarities between cell cluster phenotypes confirmed the segregation of cell cluster families defined by the heatmap dendrogram (**Figure S3**). Seven cluster families exhibited a monocyte phenotype (HLA-DR$^+$, CD14$^+$) and 4 cluster families exhibited a cDC phenotype (CD14$^-$, CD11c$^+$, HLADR$^+$). Among the 4 cluster families with a cDC phenotype, one family highly expressed CD123, CD86, and CD16. Finally, a family of cell clusters corresponding to the phenotype of pDC (CD14$^-$, CD11c^{low}, CD123$^+$, CD4$^+$, HLADR$^+$) was defined. A total of 76 cell clusters were associated with the monocyte families, whereas cDC and pDC families

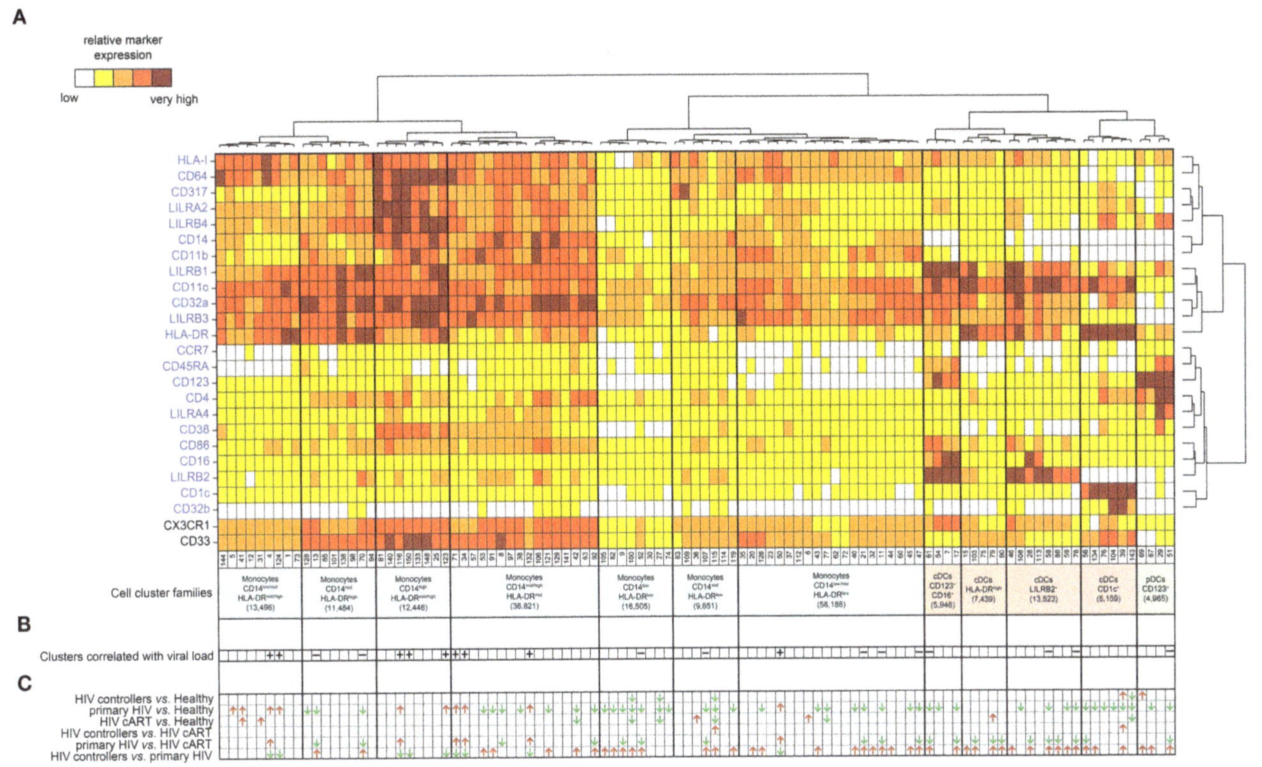

FIGURE 2 | Phenotypic landscape, variation in cell abundance and association with HIV-infection of myeloid cell clusters from HIV-infected and healthy donor samples. **(A)** Heatmap showing relative marker expression for myeloid cell clusters. The mean of the median expression of each marker was determined and classified using a five-tiered color scale ranging from white (not expressed) to dark red (highly expressed), according to their relative ranges of expression (5th–95th percentile) throughout the dataset. Clustering markers are shown in blue. Hierarchical clustering of both the cell clusters and clustering markers were performed and represented using dendrograms. Based on the cluster dendrogram, several cluster families were identified and represented in blue for monocyte families, red for cDC families and green for pDC family. **(B)** Chart summarizing clusters having cell abundance correlated with HIV RNA load (Correlated Clusters). Clusters positively correlated are indicated with a "+," whereas clusters negatively correlated are indicated with a "−." **(C)** Chart summarizing the clusters showing significantly differences of cell abundances between the biological conditions (Differentially Abundant Clusters). For each identified DACs, red arrows indicate an increase of the cell cluster abundance, whereas green arrows indicate a decrease of the cell cluster abundance.

consisted of 23 and 4 cell clusters, respectively. Cell abundance of each cluster was represented in **Figure S4**.

These results indicate that monocytes and DCs in the dataset include heterogeneous and discrete cell subpopulations carrying a specific combination of markers that may reflect a divergence in functions or differentiation that could be associated with HIV infection.

Primary HIV-Infection Induces a Significant Loss of Peripheral cDC2 and pDCs

Previous reports show the loss of DC subpopulations during early HIV and SIV infection (10, 11). To assess this process in our dataset, we first analyzed the variations of cell cluster abundances for the cDC2 (CD1c$^+$ cDC) and pDC families among the different conditions. The percentage of cells in each condition relative to the number of cells in the CD45$^+$ parent population were compared (**Figure 3**). We observed significant decreases of the percentages of cDC2 (80% of decline, $p = 0.0142$) and pDC (69% of decline, $p = 0.00263$) in the blood of primary HIV-infected patients compared to the same patients 1 year after effective cART. These significant decreases were also observed for primary HIV-infected patients in comparison to HIV controllers (85% of cDC2 decline, $p = 0.0003$ and 66% of pDC decline, $p = 0.0022$) and to healthy donors (92% of cDC2 decline, $p = 0.0065$ and 74% of pDC decline, $p = 0.0059$). Interestingly, our results also demonstrated significantly higher percentages of cDC2 ($p = 0.0302$) in the healthy group than in the HIV cART-treated group (**Figure 3A**). No significant difference was observed between these two groups for pDCs (**Figure 3B**). Concordantly with previous studies, our dataset demonstrates that primary HIV-infection induces a profound decline of peripheral cDC2s and pDCs abundance that seems to be partially recovered under cART, but to a lesser extent for cDC2s.

Elevated Plasma HIV Load Is Associated With Modifications in the Abundance of Specific Dendritic Cell and Monocyte Subpopulations

We next investigated if the abundance of specific myeloid cell subsets was associated with HIV RNA levels across HIV$^+$ and healthy samples.

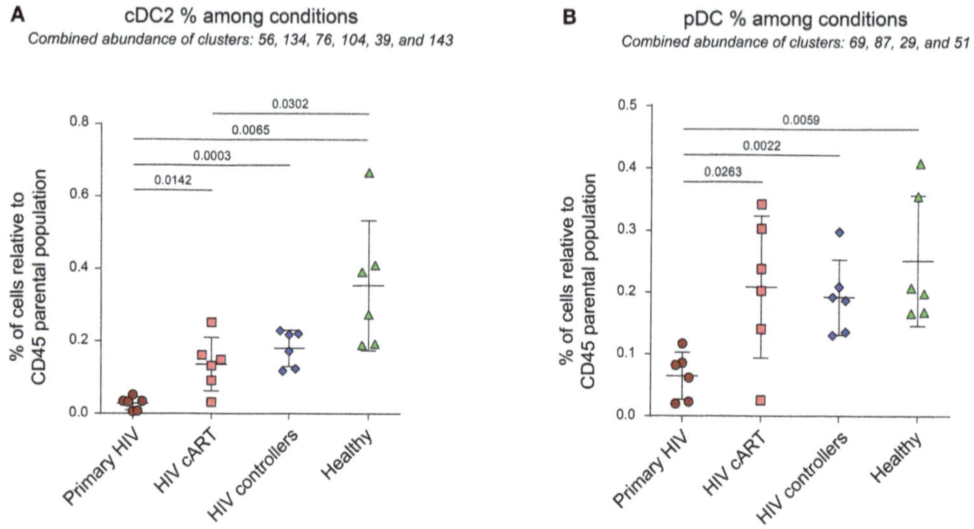

FIGURE 3 | Percentages of cDC2 and pDC among CD45^{+} cells from HIV-infected patients and healthy donors. **(A,B)** Percentage analyses of cDC2 (left panel) and pDC (right panel) relative to CD45^{+} cells among conditions. Percentages were compared among primary HIV-infected patients before (Primary HIV, red circles) and after 1 year of cART (HIV cART, pink squares), HIV-infected elite controller patients (HIV controllers, blue rhombus), and healthy donors (Healthy, green triangles). Statistical differences between conditions were calculated using a two-tailed unpaired Welch's t-test with a p-value threshold of 0.05.

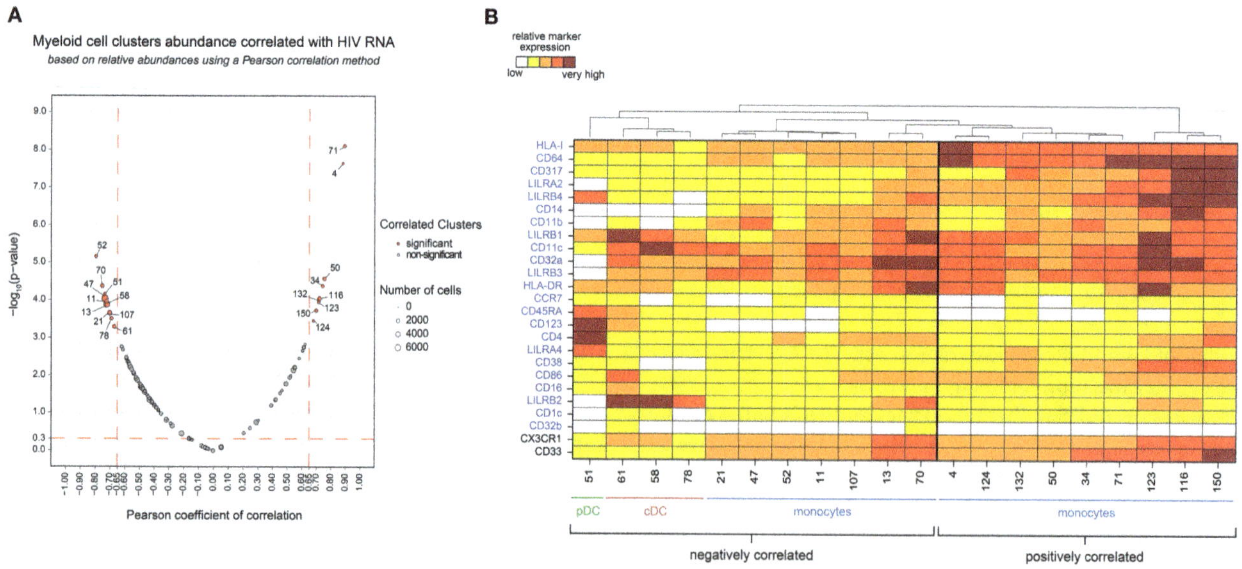

FIGURE 4 | Association analysis of myeloid cell cluster abundances with HIV RNA levels and phenotypic characterization. **(A)** Two-dimensional chart representing the correlation between myeloid cell clusters abundances and the total HIV RNA. Correlations were identified based on the number of cells associated with each cluster relative to the number of cells in the CD45^{+} parent population. Each dot in the representation corresponds to a cell cluster. The size of the dot is proportional to the number of cells of the whole dataset associated with the cluster. Significantly positively (right) or negatively (left) correlated clusters are indicated in red with a Pearson correlation coefficient >0.65 and a $p < 0.05$. The Pearson correlation coefficient is represented on the X-axis and the associated p-value, shown as $-\log_{10}$, on the Y-axis. **(B)** Heatmap representation showing the phenotype of the clusters positively and negatively correlated with HIV RNA levels. The relative marker expression for each cluster was indicated by a five-tiered color scale ranging from white (not expressed) to dark red (highly expressed). Clustering markers are indicated in blue. Using cluster dendrogram and CD14, CD11c, and CD123 expression level, clusters were annotated as monocyte, cDC or pDC.

We found 20 clusters significantly correlated (CCs) with plasma viral load (**Figure 4A**). These clusters were split into two groups based on the positive or negative correlation of their cell abundance with HIV RNA load (**Figure 4B**). On the one hand, nine clusters that were positively correlated with viral load were exclusively monocyte populations. On the other hand, eleven clusters that negatively correlated with viral load included monocyte and DC populations. The monocyte clusters that positively correlated with viral load were mainly characterized by strong expression of CD64 and HLA-I. These

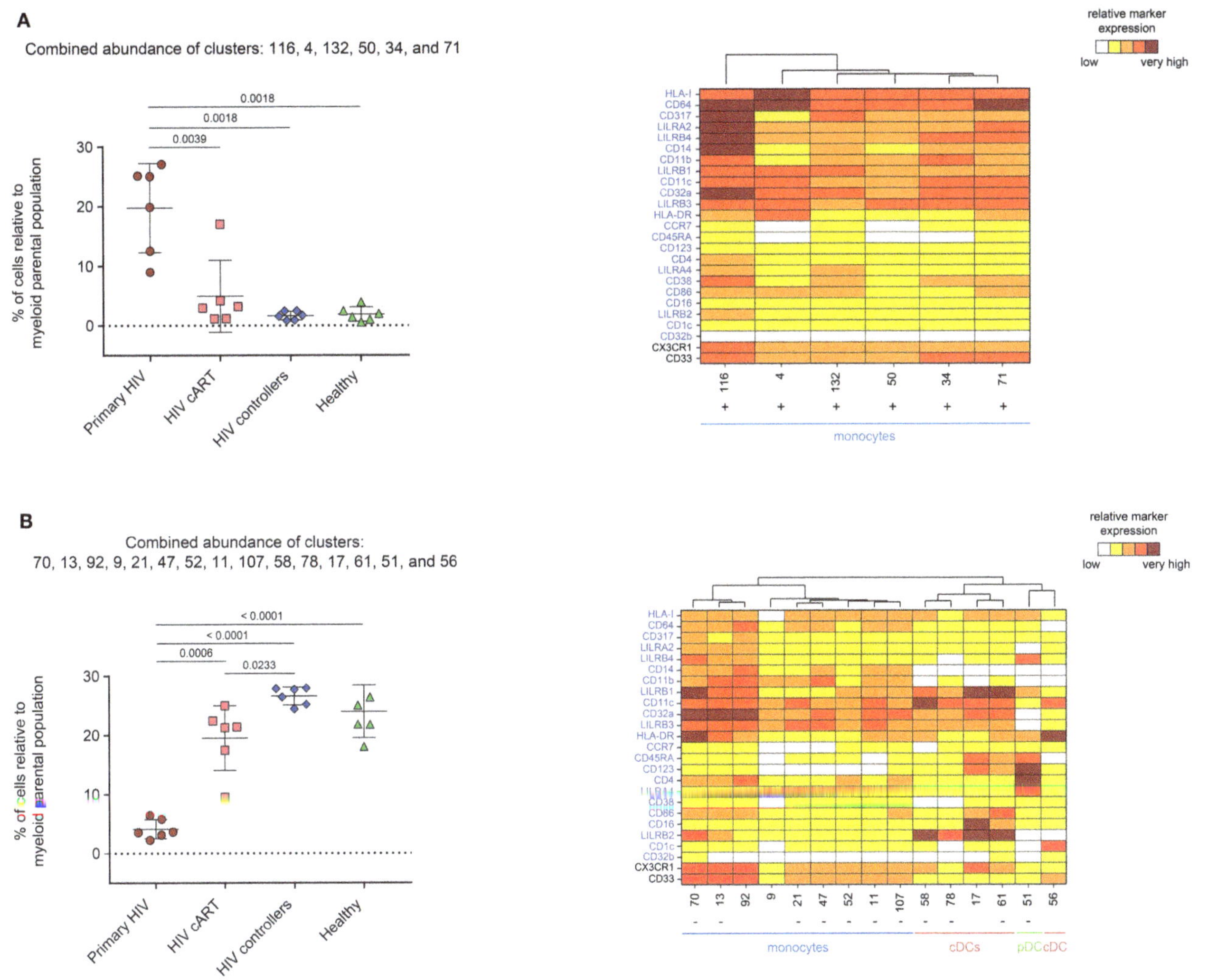

FIGURE 5 | Characterization of myeloid cell clusters showing significant differences in cell abundance for primary HIV condition. **(A)** Graph showing the cell abundance of the clusters #116, #4, #132, #50, #34, and #71 relative to myeloid cells for all samples, and heatmap representation illustrating the phenotype of these clusters. These six clusters were significantly more abundant under primary HIV (red circles) compared to HIV cART (pink squares), HIV controllers (blue rhombus), and Healthy (green triangles) conditions. **(B)** Graph showing the cell abundance of the clusters #70, #13, #92, #9, #21, #47, #52, #11, #107, #58, #78, #17, #61, #51, and #56 relative to myeloid cells for all samples, and heatmap representation illustrating the phenotype of these clusters. These 15 clusters were significantly less abundant under primary HIV (red circles) compared to HIV cART (pink squares), HIV controllers (blue rhombus), and Healthy (green triangles) conditions. These clusters were also significantly less abundant under HIV cART condition compared to HIV controllers condition. In the abundance graph representations, for each condition, the mean cell abundance is indicated (black lines). Statistical differences between conditions were calculated using a two-tailed unpaired Welch's t-test with a p-value threshold of 0.05. For heatmap representations, the relative marker expression for each cluster was indicated by a five-tiered color scale ranging from white (not expressed) to dark red (highly expressed). Clustering markers are indicated in blue. Using cluster dendrogram and CD14, CD11c, and CD123 expression level, clusters were annotated as monocyte, cDC or pDC. Clusters positively correlated with HIV RNA levels are indicated with a "+" while clusters negatively correlated are indicated with a "–".

clusters also displayed high expression of HIV restriction factor CD317, and the immunomodulatory receptors LILRA2 and LILRB4. It is important to note that among them, only some clusters, displayed a medium or high-level expression of CD38 (a transmembrane glycoprotein involved in myeloid cell adhesion, activation, and metabolism). Among the dendritic cell clusters that negatively correlated with the viral load, pDC cluster #51 ($R = -0.65$) demonstrated a strong expression of LILRA4 and LILRB4. Furthermore, cDC clusters #61 ($R = -0.59$), #58 ($R = -0.66$), and #78 ($R = -0.60$) expressed high levels of LILRB2 inhibitory receptor. Meanwhile, the seven monocyte clusters that negatively correlated with viral load expressed moderated levels of HLA-I, CD64, CD317, LILRA2, LILRB4, and CD38, in contrast to the other monocyte clusters that were positively correlated with HIV RNA. Interestingly, the negatively correlated monocyte clusters #13 and #70 displayed a medium and high expression of LILRB2, respectively, with high coexpression of CX3CR1 and CD33.

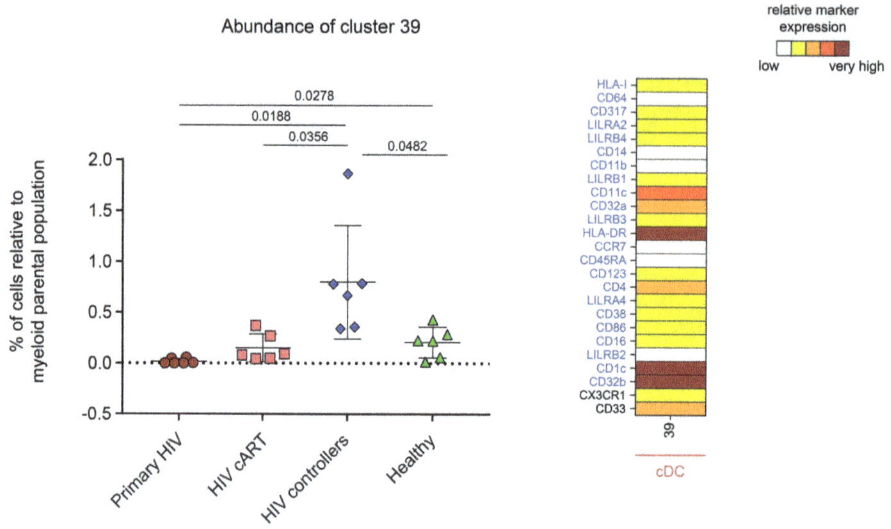

FIGURE 6 | Characterization of a myeloid cell cluster specifically and significantly more abundant in HIV controller patients. Graph showing the cell abundance of the cluster #39 relative to myeloid cells for all samples, and heatmap representation illustrating the phenotype of this cluster. Cluster #39 was significantly more abundant in HIV controllers (blue rhombus) compared to primary HIV (red circles), HIV cART (pink squares), and Healthy (green triangles) conditions. This cluster was also significantly more abundant in Healthy donors compared to primary HIV infected patients. In the abundance graph representations, for each condition, the mean cell abundance is indicated (black lines). Statistical differences between conditions were calculated using a two-tailed unpaired Welch's *t*-test with a *p*-value threshold of 0.05. For heatmap representation, the relative marker expression for cluster #39 was indicated by a five-tiered color scale ranging from white (not expressed) to dark red (highly expressed). Clustering markers are indicated in blue. Using cluster CD14, CD11c, and CD123 expression level, cluster #39 was annotated as cDC.

Our data show that an increase in HIV viral load was associated with the specific loss of discrete DC populations in blood. These populations included pDC clusters that were characterized by high expression of LILRA4 and LILRB4, but also cDCs highly expressing LILRB2. Conversely, specific subsets of monocytes strongly expressing HLA-I, CD64, CD317, LILRA2, LILRB4, and for some of them, CD38, seemed to be enriched when viral load increased.

Primary HIV-Infected Patients and HIV Controllers Display Differentially Abundant Clusters

We then aimed to identify myeloid cell clusters undergoing contraction or expansion within the different patient groups. These clusters were named Differentially Abundant Clusters (DACs) and were summarized in **Figure 2C**. We first identified clusters having different cell abundances between healthy and each HIV$^+$ conditions (**Figures S5A–C**). We found that DACs were mainly enriched in healthy condition. This may indicate expression level modification of surface markers or a loss in the blood of specific myeloid cell subsets in HIV-infected patients even under cART or natural control, compared to healthy donors. We then identified clusters with differences in cell abundances for the comparisons between all HIV$^+$ groups (**Figures S5D–F**). The comparison between HIV controllers and primary HIV samples displayed the greatest number of DACs, with 43 out of 52 being more abundant in samples from HIV controllers (**Figure S5F**). Conversely, the comparison between samples from HIV controllers and HIV-infected patients once under cART displayed the lowest number of DACs, with only 2 DACs more abundant in HIV controllers (**Figure S5D**). These changes may indicate important differences in myeloid cell dynamics between primary HIV$^+$ and HIV-controller patients, whereas the myeloid cell dynamics between cART treated HIV$^+$ and HIV-controller patients is more similar.

We next analyzed the phenotype and abundance of all DACs that were significantly more abundant in primary HIV$^+$ patients when compared to the other conditions (HIV cART, HIV controllers, and Healthy; **Figure 5A**). We found that six DACs, clusters #116, #4, #132, #50, #34, and #71, were more abundant in primary HIV$^+$ samples and displayed monocyte phenotypes. Interestingly, these six clusters were positively correlated with plasma viral load (**Figure 4**). These results confirmed that individuals in the primary HIV infection state had a higher abundance of monocytes that strongly expressed HLA-I, CD64, CD317, LILRA2, and LILRB4, with some subpopulations also expressing mid- to high- levels of CD38.

We then focused on DACs that were less abundant in primary HIV$^+$ patients than in all other conditions (**Figure 5B**). These clusters included: monocyte clusters #70, #13, #21, #47, #52, #11, and #107; cDC clusters #58, #78, and #61; and pDC cluster #51. These 11 clusters were previously identified as negatively correlated with viral load. The four remaining DACs less abundant in primary HIV$^+$ samples displayed monocyte phenotypes (clusters #92 and #9), and cDC phenotypes (clusters #17, and #56). Furthermore, cDC clusters #58, #78, #17, and #61 strongly expressed LILRB2 immunoreceptor, with clusters #17 and #61 also expressing CD123, CD86, and CD16. Cluster #56 did not express LILRB2, but strongly expressed CD1c. The pDC cluster #51, which was also found correlated with HIV RNA in **Figure 4**, strongly expressed LILRA4 and LILRB4. It is interesting to note that all the DACs that were less abundant in primary HIV condition had a weaker expression of HLA-I, CD64, CD317, LILRA2, and LILRB4 compared to clusters more abundant in the same condition (**Figure 5A**). In addition, none of these DACs expressed a medium or high-level of CD38.

One DAC was shown to be more abundant in HIV controllers compared to other HIV$^+$ and healthy conditions (**Figure 6**). This DAC, cluster #39, displayed a CD1c$^+$ cDC phenotype strongly expressing inhibitory receptor CD32b (low-affinity receptor for IgG also known as FcγRIIB) and HLA-DR. Furthermore, this cluster expressed moderate levels of CD32a (activatory counterpart of CD32b), CD4 and CD33. Using a Kolmogorov–Smirnov distance (KS) test to quantify the differences in marker expression between this cluster and all CD1c$^+$ cDC subsets (**Figure S6**), we identified CD32b as the marker with the highest difference (KS = 0.7672). In addition, when we quantified the differences in marker expression between this cluster and the other CD32b$^+$ CD1c$^+$ cDC clusters (**Figure S7**), CD32b was the second most distant marker (KS = 0.5021). Thus, high CD32b expression was specific to this CD1c$^+$ cDC subset found enriched in the blood of HIV controllers.

Altogether, we found that a modification in the balance of monocyte and DC subpopulations is induced from the early stages of HIV infection. Monocytes with a strong expression of HLA-I, CD64, CD317, LILRA2, LILRB4, and CD38 were most prominent in primary HIV$^+$ patients when compared to cART, HIV controllers and healthy donors. In addition, primary HIV$^+$ patients had significantly fewer pDCs that expressed high levels of LILRA4 and LILRB4. Moreover, they had considerably less LILRB2^{hi} cDCs. Finally, we discovered a unique CD1c$^+$ CD32b^{hi} HLA-DR^{hi} cDC cluster that was specifically enriched in HIV elite controllers.

DISCUSSION

DCs and monocytes play an important role in the initiation of immune responses against HIV. However, the study of their regulation and dynamics during early HIV infection is hindered by late disease diagnosis. Moreover, early immune responses against HIV induce complex concomitant inflammatory and immunoregulatory events that can be difficult to decipher through classical approaches. In this regard, we carried out a mass cytometry analysis to characterize phenotypic heterogeneity among myeloid cell subpopulations under various conditions of HIV infection.

Our high dimensional analysis illustrates that specific DC and monocyte subpopulations found in peripheral blood are differentially affected by HIV infection. After mapping the different phenotypes of DC and monocyte subsets from PBMC samples, we highlighted a global loss of cDC2s and pDCs under primary HIV-infection in the blood. No DC clusters were enriched during primary infection, suggesting that this decrease could result from cell death rather than phenotypic changes (7, 10, 11). However, it is also well-established that cDCs and pDCs rapidly migrate toward peripheral lymph nodes after HIV or SIV infection to elicit adaptive immune response (27, 28). Therefore, the loss of DC subsets observed in primary HIV infection might result from various physiological mechanisms.

We also investigated the abundance variation of myeloid cell clusters among the different conditions and determined their association with HIV RNA level. We found that specific monocyte clusters were enriched in primary HIV-infected patients and/or positively correlated with the plasma viral load. These subpopulations of monocytes expressed high levels of HLA-I and CD64. In the context of viral infection, HLA-I molecules present peptides derived from intracellular viral proteins to CD8$^+$ T lymphocytes to activate their cytolytic activity (29). CD64 is a high-affinity Fc receptor for IgG, which allows for immune complex internalization driving cross-presentation of viral epitopes on HLA-I (30). Thus, it seems consistent that monocytes positively correlated with the viral load exhibit strong co-expression of HLA-I and CD64. Increased HLA-I and CD64 expressions by monocytes were previously reported in acute and chronic HIV-infection, respectively (8, 31). However, our data demonstrate further the strong expression of CD317, LILRA2, and LILRB4 for these subsets, and for some subclusters, a medium or high-level expression of CD38. In agreement with our data, the HIV-restriction factor CD317 was previously shown to be up-regulated at the surface of monocytes and CD4$^+$ T-cells during acute HIV/SIV infection (32, 33). The activating immune-receptor LILRA2 is expressed by monocytes and neutrophils and recognizes bacterially cleaved immunoglobulin, leading to the activation of signaling pathways and subsequent immune responses (34). However, LILRA2 can selectively modulate LPS-mediated cytokine production by monocytes, and could inhibit CD64-dependent phagocytosis (35). Finally, increased expression of LILRB4 was shown to induce tolerogenic monocytes and cDCs (8, 36–38). Previous studies have also demonstrated that LILRB4 interaction with CD64 is a potent inhibitor of monocyte activation, and CD64-mediated clathrin-dependent endocytosis and phagocytosis (39, 40). Thus, expression of these molecules could explain the dysregulated ability of phagocytosis and cytokine production observed in monocytes from HIV$^+$ patients (41). The up-regulation of inhibitory receptors on immune cells could also constitute a retro control mechanism to dampen chronic inflammation.

Conversely, monocyte clusters that were negatively correlated with viral load, and/or less abundant in primary HIV-infected patients, did not exhibit high level expression of HLA-I, CD64, CD317, LILRA2, LILRB4, and CD38. Therefore, these monocyte subpopulations seemed to be specifically differentiated and/or contracted under primary HIV infection. Our mass cytometry panel included CD16 marker to detect inflammatory monocytes. However, we only detected few clusters of CD16^{hi} cDCs and no CD16^{hi} monocyte clusters. The attenuation of CD16 staining on monocytes could result from the freezing procedure of PBMCs that was shown to modify staining of some FcRs on specific cell subsets (42).

Among the DC populations characterized in our study, the clusters of cDCs that highly expressed LILRB2, and a cluster of pDCs that highly expressed LILRA4 and LILRB4, were also less abundant in primary HIV-infected patients. The majority of these clusters were also negatively correlated with plasma viral load. Functional studies indicate that cDCs and pDCs show dysregulated functions in early and chronic HIV/SIV infections. cDCs have an impaired maturation with reduced capacity for antigen presentation and cytokine production, whereas pDCs have reduced capacities to produce type-I IFNs (1, 9, 13, 43–45). In this respect, HIV infection enhances LILRB2/HLA-I and LILRA4/CD317 axes leading to the dysregulation of cDC and pDC functions, respectively (8, 9, 13, 46–49). Moreover, it has been reported that the strength of the LILRB2/HLA-I interaction is enhanced by HLA-I presentation of HIV-derived peptides, or genetic variation of HLA-I haplotypes, and correlates with the level of cDC dysregulation in HIV-infected patients (46, 47). Previous studies showed that LILRB2 was up-regulated on cDCs from blood in the acute phase of HIV and SIV infection (9, 10). LILRB2 expression was even higher in cDCs from peripheral lymph nodes than those from peripheral blood during early SIV infection (10). Therefore, in our study, the loss of LILRB2^{hi} cDC and LILRA4^{hi} pDC clusters observed in the blood from primary HIV infected patients could correspond in part to the migration of these subpopulations toward secondary lymphoid organs. Consequently, inhibitory impulses induced by the LILRB2/HLA-I and LILRA4/CD317 axes on cDCs and pDCs that have migrated into secondary lymphoid organs during primary HIV infection may enhance their dysfunctions and impaired the establishment of an effective adaptive immune response.

We also found that HIV controllers had an enrichment of a CD1c^{+} CD32b^{hi} HLA-DR^{hi} cDC cluster. These data are concordant with the recent discovery of a new CD1c^{hi}, CD32b^{hi} cDC subset, using a single-cell RNA sequencing approach (50). This cDC subset was a potent stimulator of naive T-cell proliferation, and was more likely to secrete high levels of CCL19, IL-8, IL-10, and IL-12b (50). However, further studies will be necessary to better characterize the function of this DC subset in the context of HIV infection, in particular its implication in the mechanisms leading to the natural control of viral replication in elite controller patients. Since natural control of HIV infection can occur through various mechanisms, it will be important to also characterize the abundance of CD1c^{+} CD32b^{hi} HLA-DR^{hi} cDCs in additional elite controller patients, to assess whether this feature is shared by all elite controllers.

New populations of cDCs, called pre-DCs, were recently identified in the peripheral blood from healthy donors (51). These populations can differentiate into cDC1 or cDC2 subsets *in vitro* and were proposed to be cDC precursors. However, the relationship between pre-DCs and HIV infection is still unknown. Therefore, future mass cytometry studies including additional dendritic cell markers such as CD141, CD2, Siglec-6, and Axl will be helpful to better understand the dynamics and regulation of cDC1 and pre-DC subsets during HIV infection.

In conclusion, our results unravel the diversity and various phenotypic changes induced in cDCs, pDCs, and monocytes during early stage, anti-retroviral treatment control, and naturally controlled HIV infections. These results should be helpful when trying to better understand the cellular and molecular basis of the events driving the regulation/dysregulation of myeloid immune responses involved in the progression or control of HIV infection.

MATERIALS AND METHODS

Study Subjects and Ethics Statements

This study involved six patients with primary HIV-1 infection estimated, as previously described (17), to have been infected <30 days before inclusion. These patients were enrolled from the French ANRS CO6 PRIMO cohort and has approval by the Ethics Committee of Cochin Hospital. Blood samples were collected from patients at enrolment, who were antiretroviral naïve and negative for hepatitis B and C viruses. The six primary HIV-infected patients were then placed under cART, and blood samples were collected after 1 year. As previously described for these individuals (24), after 1 year of cART viral load was undetectable and CD4^{+} T cell count was restored (CD4^{+} T cells > 500/μl of blood). This study also involved blood samples of six HIV controller patients from the French ANRS CO21 CODEX. This cohort was approved by the ethics review committee of Ile de France VII. HIV controllers were defined as patients infected by HIV-1 for at least 5 years, who never received cART and whose last five consecutive plasma HIV RNA values were <400 copies/ml. Finally, blood samples of six healthy subjects were obtained from the Etablissement Français du Sang (EFS). All subjects gave written informed consent to participate in the study.

Sample Processing and Storage

As previously described (24), peripheral blood mononuclear cells (PBMCs) were isolated by Ficoll density gradient centrifugation, and $\sim 1 \times 10^7$ PBMCs per sample were cryopreserved at −150°C.

Antibody Labeling and Cell Staining

To avoid batch variation effects, all samples were stained with the same batch of antibodies and on the same day. All samples were acquired in 1 day to avoid instrument signal fluctuation. Antibodies (listed in **Table S1**) were either pre-conjugated from the manufacturer (Fluidigm, San Francisco, CA) or conjugated in-house with the appropriate metal isotopes as previously described (24). Cells were thawed and 5.10^6 PBMCs were transferred per well. As previously described (24), PBMCs were incubated with Rhodium DNA-intercalator (Fluidigm), first stained with the primary surface antibody mix for 1 h, and then stained with the secondary surface antibody mix for 15 min. Next, samples were resuspended in 1.6% PFA and incubated 20 min. Cells were finally incubated 30 min in permeabilization buffer with 1 μM Iridium DNA-intercalator before a 4°C overnight incubation in 1.6% PFA with 0.1 μM Iridium DNA intercalator. For acquisition, cells were washed and filtered through a cell strainer cap of a 5-ml polystyrene round-bottom tube (BD Biosciences). Normalization beads (Fluidigm) were added to each sample. Then, samples were acquired using a mass cytometer (CyTOF-I; Fluidigm) and following the standard procedure recommended by the manufacturer. An average of 200,264 ± 13,472 events was acquired per sample.

Data Normalization

Raw cytometry profiles generated by CyTOF-I were normalized using normalization beads and MatLab Compiler normalizer software (52).

Manual Gating of CD45$^+$ Myeloid Cells

Normalized events were gated using the Cytobank analysis platform. First, cells with only one Iridium level were selected to exclude cell doublets from the analysis. Second, normalization beads and dead cells were removed by selecting cells negative for Cerium (Ce140) and Rhodium, respectively. Thirdly, leukocytes were selected based on the positive expression of CD45. Myeloid cells were then selected based on the absence of CD3, CD19, and NKp80, and expression of HLA-DR (**Figure S1**).

Automatic Identification of Cell Clusters

SPADE algorithm was used to perform automatic identification of cell clusters (25). We observed large differences in the number of manually gated myeloid cells in each sample, ranging from 2,255 to 35,658 cells. Consequently, we first down-sampled 2,255 cells from each sample to avoid over-representation of samples with high number of cells. These uniformly down-sampled events were up-sampled at the end of the SPADE analysis. The SPADE clusters were generated using the entire and singular dataset (24 samples from 18 individuals, including 6 during primary infection and 1 year later after effective cART). Cells having similar expression of the 23 selected clustering markers (shown in blue in **Figure 1**) were grouped into clusters, regardless of donor origin. Moreover, SPADE was configured to identify 150 cell clusters (down-sampling of 40%). These parameters were defined to obtain the highest number of clusters with uniform phenotypes (26). The SPADE heatmap was generated with the SPADE clusters using the 23 clustering markers. CD45, CD3, CD19, and NKp80 were discarded from the SPADE analysis as we used them to pre-select cells of interest. Both CX3CR1 and CD33 markers were not included in the set of clustering markers due to their high heterogeneity of expression among samples. However, CX3CR1 and CD33 were added to the 23 clustering markers on heatmaps for the phenotypic characterization of myeloid cells.

Phenotypic Characterization of Identified Cell Clusters

We used the SPADEVizR R-package to perform the phenotypic categorization of the 150 cell clusters (26). Expression level of each marker was classified into five categories, which were defined based on the range of expression (5th–95th percentile) relative to the myeloid population gate across all samples. The five uniform categories represent negative, low, medium, high, and very high levels of marker expression. The categories of expression were displayed using a color scale, which ranged from white to dark red. The dendrogram, represented in the heatmap, was constructed using Euclidian distance and the complete linkage method.

There were 36 clusters that displayed a lymphoid phenotype (based on the negative expression of CD33, CD123, CD14, and LILRB3), which were identified among the total 150 cell clusters and were removed from the SPADE analysis to leave only myeloid cell clusters. Additionally, 11 myeloid cell clusters with <350 cells associated were removed from the analysis, as their phenotypes cannot be assessed accurately. Thus, 103 myeloid cell clusters were remaining from the 150 SPADE clusters.

Families of cell clusters were determined using hierarchical clustering, represented by a dendrogram on the top of the marker categorical heatmap. Thanks to this clustering method, cell clusters with similar marker expression profiles were grouped together in the heatmap. The dendrogram was cut so that the different cluster families with homogeneous expression profiles were separated. This resulted in 12 different cluster families. These cluster families were also represented in a tSNE representation. The tSNE representation was generated using the original 23 clustering markers and Barnes-Hut t-Distributed Stochastic Neighbor Embedding (53), based on a perplexity parameter of 3. Distances between cell cluster phenotypes were calculated based on the Manhattan distance.

Identification of Differentially Abundant Clusters and Correlating Clusters

We used the SPADEVizR R-package to identify differentially abundant clusters (DACs), and correlated clusters (CCs) (26). DACs identification was based on the percentage of cells in the clusters, relative to total myeloid cells by unpaired Student t tests (absolute fold-change > 2 and $p < 0.05$). CCs identification was based on the percentage of cells in clusters relative to the total myeloid cells that correlated with HIV RNA levels (absolute Pearson correlation coefficient > 0.65 and $p < 0.05$).

Quantification of Cluster #39 Phenotypic Specificity

Detailed phenotypic characterization of cluster #39 relative to CD1c$^+$ cDC and CD32b$^+$ CD1c$^+$ cDC clusters was performed using CytoCompare R-package (54), based on the Kolmogorov-Smirnov distance, using a threshold of 0.30.

Statistical Analysis of Cluster Abundances Among Conditions

A two-tailed unpaired Welch's t-test, with a p-value threshold of 0.05, was used to compare the percentages of cDC2 and pDC among CD45$^+$ cells and the differences in cluster cell abundance between each biological condition. All statistical analyses were performed using GraphPad Prism 7.0 (GraphPad Software).

ETHICS STATEMENT

This study and the associated protocol were approved by the Ethics Committee of Cochin Hospital and ethics review committee of Ile de France VII. All subjects gave written informed consent in accordance with the Declaration of Helsinki.

AUTHOR CONTRIBUTIONS

SC, A-SB, OL, RL, and BF: conceptualization. SC, NT, LA, A-SB, OL, and BF: methodology. SC, NT, LA, BV, CB, CG, CL, PB, RL, A-SB, OL, and BF: validation. SC, NT, BV, A-SB, OL, and BF: formal analysis and writing—review and editing. SC, NT, and BF: investigation. CG, CL, PB, and A-SB: resources. SC, NT, and BF: writing—original draft. BF: supervision.

ACKNOWLEDGMENTS

We thank the ANRS (French National Agency for AIDS research) CO6 PRIMO and CO21 CODEX cohort for helpful collaboration and all the medical professionals involved in blood sampling at the Hôpital Kremlin-Bicêtre. We also thank Bruno Iannascoli (Institut Pasteur) for the *in vitro* production of anti-CD32b antibodies and Oscar Haigh and Jean-Louis Palgen for critical reading of the manuscript.

SUPPLEMENTARY MATERIAL

Figure S1 | Myeloid gating strategy. "Singlets" were identified using cell length vs. Ir191-DNA intercalator and calibration beads signal was excluded (cells no beads). Living leukocytes were identified by selecting Rhodium (Rh103)Di-negative cells, and then $CD45^+$ cells. Finally, myeloid cells were identified by gating on $CD3^-$, $CD19^-$, and then $NKp80^-$ $HLA\text{-}DR^+$ cells.

Figure S2 | Categorization of marker expressions. Marker expression ranges were used to characterize the phenotypes of identified SPADE clusters. Ranges of marker expression were obtained after manual gating of myeloid cells and are presented as arcsine transformed Mean Signal Intensity (MSI) signals. The range of expression for each marker was defined based on the 5th–95th percentiles of expression throughout the dataset, and were divided into five categories represented using a five-tiered color scale ranging from white (not expressed) to dark red (highly expressed). For each expressed marker of a particular cluster, the average of the median marker expression level was used to determine the expression category of that marker. Combined marker ranges define the phenotype of each cluster. Clustering markers are shown in blue.

Figure S3 | tSNE representation showing the phenotypical similarities between cell clusters identified by SPADE. Each dot corresponds to a cell cluster and the dots are positioned in a 2-dimensional space that best represents the phenotypical proximity between cell clusters. Cell clusters have been colored based on their associated cell cluster family, blue for monocyte families, red for cDC families and green for pDC family.

Figure S4 | Cell number in each myeloid SPADE cluster. This representation shows the number of cells associated with each myeloid cell cluster, regardless of sample cell origin. Cluster names are indicated on the X-axis and the corresponding number of cells on the Y-axis. The size of the dots is proportional to the number of cells in the cluster. Cell clusters are ordered based on the dendrogram represented in **Figure 2**.

Figure S5 | Identification of differentially abundant clusters for each biological condition comparison. **(A–C)** Volcano plot representations showing Differentially Abundant Clusters (DACs) in HIV controllers, primary HIV and HIV cART samples compared to Healthy samples. **(D–F)** Volcano plot representations showing DACs in HIV controllers and primary HIV samples compared to HIV cART samples and HIV controllers compared to primary HIV samples. Each dot in the representation corresponds to a cell cluster and is proportional in size to the number of cell associated. Log_2 fold-changes are indicated in the X-axis, and the associated p-values, shown as $-log_{10}$, are indicated in the Y-axis. DACs were identified using a paired Student t-test with a p-value threshold of 0.05 and a fold-change cutoff of 2. Red dots correspond to significantly abundant clusters.

Figure S6 | Marker expression densities showing the phenotypic specificity of cluster #39 relative to $CD1c^+$ cDC clusters. The expression densities of all clustering markers, as well as CD33 and CX3CR1 are shown for cluster #39 and $CD1c^+$ cDC clusters. The marker expression densities for cluster #39 are shown in blue whereas the marker expression densities for all $CD1c^+$ cDC clusters are shown in gray. The differences between marker expression densities were quantified using the Kolmogorov–Smirnov distances (KS) using the entire and singular dataset.

Figure S7 | Marker expression densities showing the phenotypic specificity of cluster #39 relative to $CD32b^+$ $CD1c^+$ cDC clusters. The expression densities of all clustering markers, CD33 and CX3CR1 are shown for cluster #39 and $CD32b^+$ $CD1c^+$ cDC clusters. The marker expression densities for cluster #39 are shown in blue whereas the marker expression densities for all $CD32b^+$ $CD1c^+$ cDC clusters are shown in gray. The differences between marker expression densities were quantified using the Kolmogorov–Smirnov distances (KS) using the entire and singular dataset.

Table S1 | Overview of the mass cytometry panel. The metal, antigen, clone, isotype, and supplier are indicated for each antibody. *Not used for cell clustering.

REFERENCES

1. Miller E, Bhardwaj N. Dendritic cell dysregulation during HIV-1 infection. *Immunol Rev.* (2013) 254:170–89. doi: 10.1111/imr.12082
2. Boasso A, Shearer GM, Chougnet C. Immune dysregulation in human immunodeficiency virus infection: know it, fix it, prevent it? *J Intern Med.* (2009) 265:78. doi: 10.1111/j.1365-2796.2008.02043.x
3. Deeks SG, Tracy R, Douek DC. Systemic effects of inflammation on health during chronic HIV infection. *Immunity.* (2013) 39:633–45. doi: 10.1016/j.immuni.2013.10.001
4. Steinman RM. Decisions about dendritic cells: past, present, and future. *Annu Rev Immunol.* (2012) 30:1–22. doi: 10.1146/annurev-immunol-100311-102839
5. Reizis B. Plasmacytoid dendritic cells: development, regulation, and function. *Immunity.* (2019) 50:37–50. doi: 10.1016/j.immuni.2018.12.027
6. Wonderlich ER, Wu WC, Normolle DP, Barratt-Boyes SM. Macrophages and myeloid dendritic cells lose T cell-stimulating function in simian immunodeficiency virus infection associated with diminished IL-12 and IFN-α production. *J Immunol.* (2015) 195:3284–92. doi: 10.4049/jimmunol.1500683
7. Laforge M, Campillo-Gimenez L, Monceaux V, Cumont MC, Hurtrel B, Corbeil J, et al. HIV/SIV infection primes monocytes and dendritic cells for apoptosis. *PLoS Pathog.* (2011) 7:e1002087. doi: 10.1371/journal.ppat.1002087
8. Huang J, Al-Mozaini M, Rogich J, Carrington MF, Seiss K, Pereyra F, et al. Systemic inhibition of myeloid dendritic cells by circulating

HLA class I molecules in HIV-1 infection. *Retrovirology*. (2012) 9:11. doi: 10.1186/1742-4690-9-11

9. Huang J, Yang Y, Al-Mozaini M, Burke PS, Beamon J, Carrington MF, et al. Dendritic cell dysfunction during primary HIV-1 infection. *J Infect Dis*. (2011) 204:1557–62. doi: 10.1093/infdis/jir616
10. Alaoui L, Palomino G, Zurawski S, Zurawski G, Coindre S, Dereuddre-Bosquet N, et al. Early SIV and HIV infection promotes the LILRB2/MHC-I inhibitory axis in cDCs. *Cell Mol Life Sci*. (2018) 75:1871–87. doi: 10.1007/s00018-017-2712-9
11. Wijewardana V, Soloff AC, Liu X, Brown KN, Barratt-Boyes SM. Early myeloid dendritic cell dysregulation is predictive of disease progression in simian immunodeficiency virus infection. *PLoS Pathog*. (2010) 6:e1001235. doi: 10.1371/journal.ppat.1001235
12. Benlahrech A, Yasmin A, Westrop SJ, Coleman A, Herasimtschuk A, Page E, et al. Dysregulated immunophenotypic attributes of plasmacytoid but not myeloid dendritic cells in HIV-1 infected individuals in the absence of highly active anti-retroviral therapy. *Clin Exp Immunol*. (2012) 170:212–21. doi: 10.1111/j.1365-2249.2012.04647.x
13. Bego MG, Côté É, Aschman N, Mercier J, Weissenhorn W, Cohen ÉA. Vpu exploits the cross-talk between BST2 and the ILT7 receptor to suppress anti-HIV-1 responses by plasmacytoid dendritic cells. *PLoS Pathog*. (2015) 11:e1005024. doi: 10.1371/journal.ppat.1005024
14. Hasegawa A, Liu H, Ling B, Borda JT, Alvarez X, Sugimoto C, et al. The level of monocyte turnover predicts disease progression in the macaque model of AIDS. *Blood*. (2009) 114:2917–25. doi: 10.1182/blood-2009-02-204263
15. Sandler NG, Douek DC. Microbial translocation in HIV infection: causes, consequences and treatment opportunities. *Nat Rev Microbiol*. (2012) 10:655–66. doi: 10.1038/nrmicro2848
16. Sandler NG, Wand H, Roque A, Law M, Nason MC, Nixon DE, et al. Plasma levels of soluble CD14 independently predict mortality in HIV infection. *J Infect Dis*. (2011) 203:780–90. doi: 10.1093/infdis/jiq118
17. Krastinova E, Lecuroux C, Leroy C, Seng R, Cabie A, Rami A, et al. High soluble CD14 levels at primary HIV-1 infection predict more rapid disease progression. *J Infect Dis*. (2015) 212:909–13. doi: 10.1093/infdis/jiv145
18. Prost S, Le Dantec M, Augé S, Le Grand R, Derdouch S, Auregan G, et al. Human and simian immunodeficiency viruses deregulate early hematopoiesis through a Nef/PPARgamma/STAT5 signaling pathway in macaques. *J Clin Invest*. (2008) 118:1765–75. doi: 10.1172/JCI33037
19. Bruel T, Dupuy S, Démoulins T, Rogez-Kreuz C, Dutrieux J, Corneau A, et al. Plasmacytoid Dendritic cell dynamics tune interferon-alfa production in SIV-infected cynomolgus macaques. *PLoS Pathog*. (2014) 10:e1003915. doi: 10.1371/journal.ppat.1003915
20. Favier B. Regulation of neutrophil functions through inhibitory receptors: an emerging paradigm in health and disease. *Immunol Rev*. (2016) 273:140–55. doi: 10.1111/imr.12457
21. Baudhuin J, Migraine J, Faivre V, Loumagne L, Lukaszewicz AC, Payen D, et al. Exocytosis acts as a modulator of the ILT4-mediated inhibition of neutrophil functions. *Proc Natl Acad Sci USA*. (2013) 110:17957–62. doi: 10.1073/pnas.1221535110
22. Lichterfeld M, Yu XG. The emerging role of leukocyte immunoglobulin-like receptors (LILRs) in HIV-1 infection. *J Leukoc Biol*. (2012) 91:27–33. doi: 10.1189/jlb.0811442
23. Huang J, Burke PS, Cung TD, Pereyra F, Toth I, Walker BD, et al. Leukocyte immunoglobulin-like receptors maintain unique antigen-presenting properties of circulating myeloid dendritic cells in HIV-1-infected elite controllers. *J Virol*. (2010) 84:9463–71. doi: 10.1128/JVI.01009-10
24. Coindre S, Tchitchek N, Alaoui L, Vaslin B, Bourgeois C, Goujard C, et al. Mass cytometry analysis reveals the landscape and dynamics of CD32a+ CD4+ T cells from early HIV infection to effective cART. *Front Immunol*. (2018) 9:1217. doi: 10.3389/fimmu.2018.01217
25. Qiu P, Simonds EF, Bendall SC, Gibbs KD, Bruggner RV, Linderman MD, et al. Extracting a cellular hierarchy from high-dimensional cytometry data with SPADE. *Nat Biotechnol*. (2011) 29:886–91. doi: 10.1038/nbt.1991
26. Gautreau G, Pejoski D, Le Grand R, Cosma A, Beignon AS, Tchitchek N. SPADEVizR: an R package for visualization, analysis and integration of SPADE results. *Bioinformatics*. (2016) 33:btw708. doi: 10.1093/bioinformatics/btw708
27. Smed-Sörensen A, Loré K. Dendritic cells at the interface of innate and adaptive immunity to HIV-1. *Curr Opin HIV AIDS*. (2011) 6:405–10. doi: 10.1097/COH.0b013e328349b06b
28. Malleret B, Manéglier B, Karlsson I, Lebon P, Nascimbeni M, Perié L, et al. Primary infection with simian immunodeficiency virus: plasmacytoid dendritic cell homing to lymph nodes, type I interferon, and immune suppression. *Blood*. (2008) 112:4598–608. doi: 10.1182/blood-2008-06-162651
29. Krensky AM. The HLA system, antigen processing and presentation. *Kidney Int Suppl*. (1997) 58:S2–7.
30. Guilliams M, Bruhns P, Saeys Y, Hammad H, Lambrecht BN. The function of Fcγ receptors in dendritic cells and macrophages. *Nat Rev Immunol*. (2014) 14:94–108. doi: 10.1038/nri3582
31. Dugast AS, Tonelli A, Berger CT, Ackerman ME, Sciaranghella G, Liu Q, et al. Decreased Fc-receptor expression on innate immune cells is associated with impaired antibody mediated cellular phagocytic activity in chronically HIV 1 infected individuals. *Virology*. (2012) 415:160–7. doi: 10.1016/j.virol.2011.03.012
32. Homann S, Smith D, Little S, Richman D, Guatelli J. Upregulation of BST-2/Tetherin by HIV infection *in vivo*. *J Virol*. (2011) 85:10659–68. doi: 10.1128/JVI.05524-11
33. Mussil B, Javed A, Töpfer K, Sauermann U, Sopper S. Increased BST2 expression during simian immunodeficiency virus infection is not a determinant of disease progression in rhesus monkeys. *Retrovirology*. (2015) 12:92. doi: 10.1186/s12977-015-0219-8
34. Hirayasu K, Saito F, Suenaga T, Shida K, Arase N, Oikawa K, et al. Microbially cleaved immunoglobulins are sensed by the innate immune receptor LILRA2. *Nat Microbiol*. (2016) 1:16054. doi: 10.1038/nmicrobiol.2016.54
35. Lu HK, Mitchell A, Endoh Y, Hampartzoumian T, Huynh O, Borges L, et al. LILRA2 selectively modulates LPS-mediated cytokine production and inhibits phagocytosis by monocytes. *PLoS ONE*. (2012) 7:e33478. doi: 10.1371/journal.pone.0033478
36. Anderson KJ, Allen RL. Regulation of T-cell immunity by leucocyte immunoglobulin-like receptors: innate immune receptors for self on antigen-presenting cells. *Immunology*. (2009) 127:8–17. doi: 10.1111/j.1365-2567.2009.03097.x
37. Chang CC, Ciubotariu R, Manavalan JS, Yuan J, Colovai AI, Piazza F, et al. Tolerization of dendritic cells by T(S) cells: the crucial role of inhibitory receptors ILT3 and ILT4. *Nat Immunol*. (2002) 3:237–43. doi: 10.1038/ni760
38. Brenk M, Scheler M, Koch S, Neumann J, Takikawa O, Häcker G, et al. Tryptophan deprivation induces inhibitory receptors ILT3 and ILT4 on dendritic cells favoring the induction of human CD4+CD25+ Foxp3+ T regulatory cells. *J Immunol*. (2009) 183:145–54. doi: 10.4049/jimmunol.0803277
39. Lu HK, Rentero C, Raftery MJ, Borges L, Bryant K, Tedla N. Leukocyte Ig-like receptor B4 (LILRB4) is a potent inhibitor of FcgammaRI-mediated monocyte activation via dephosphorylation of multiple kinases. *J Biol Chem*. (2009) 284:34839–48. doi: 10.1074/jbc.M109.035683
40. Park M, Raftery MJ, Thomas PS, Geczy CL, Bryant K, Tedla N. Leukocyte immunoglobulin-like receptor B4 regulates key signalling molecules involved in FcγRI-mediated clathrin-dependent endocytosis and phagocytosis. *Sci Rep*. (2016) 6:35085. doi: 10.1038/srep35085
41. Espíndola MS, Soares LS, Galvão-Lima LJ, Zambuzi FA, Cacemiro MC, Brauer VS, et al. Epigenetic alterations are associated with monocyte immune dysfunctions in HIV-1 infection. *Sci Rep*. (2018) 8:5505. doi: 10.1038/s41598-018-23841-1
42. Wittner M, Dunay GA, Kummer S, Bockhorn M, Hüfner A, Schmiedel S, et al. Cd32 expression of different memory T cell subpopulations in the blood and lymph nodal tissue of HIV patients and healthy controls correlates with immune activation. *JAIDS J Acquir Immune Defic Syndr*. (2017) 77:345–9. doi: 10.1097/QAI.0000000000001622
43. Martin-Gayo E, Buzon MJ, Ouyang Z, Hickman T, Cronin J, Pimenova D, et al. Potent cell-intrinsic immune responses in dendritic cells facilitate HIV-1-specific T cell immunity in HIV-1 elite controllers. *PLoS Pathog*. (2015) 11:e1004930. doi: 10.1371/journal.ppat.1004930
44. Wijewardana V, Bouwer AL, Brown KN, Liu X, Barratt-Boyes SM. Accumulation of functionally immature myeloid dendritic cells in lymph nodes of rhesus macaques with acute pathogenic simian immunodeficiency virus infection. *Immunology*. (2014) 143:146–54. doi: 10.1111/imm.12295

45. Sabado RL, O'Brien M, Subedi A, Qin L, Hu N, Taylor E, et al. Evidence of dysregulation of dendritic cells in primary HIV infection. *Blood.* (2010) 116:3839–52. doi: 10.1182/blood-2010-03-273763
46. Bashirova AA, Martin-Gayo E, Jones DC, Qi Y, Apps R, Gao X, et al. LILRB2 interaction with HLA class I correlates with control of HIV-1 infection. *PLoS Genet.* (2014) 10:e1004196. doi: 10.1371/journal.pgen.1004196
47. Huang J, Goedert JJ, Sundberg EJ, Cung TD, Burke PS, Martin MP, et al. HLA-B*35-Px–mediated acceleration of HIV-1 infection by increased inhibitory immunoregulatory impulses. *J Exp Med.* (2009) 206:2959–66. doi: 10.1084/jem.20091386
48. Lichterfeld M, Kavanagh DG, Williams KL, Moza B, Mui SK, Miura T, et al. A viral CTL escape mutation leading to immunoglobulin-like transcript 4-mediated functional inhibition of myelomonocytic cells. *J Exp Med.* (2007) 204:2813–24. doi: 10.1084/jem.20061865
49. Cao W, Bover L, Cho M, Wen X, Hanabuchi S, Bao M, et al. Regulation of TLR7/9 responses in plasmacytoid dendritic cells by BST2 and ILT7 receptor interaction. *J Exp Med.* (2009) 206:1603–14. doi: 10.1084/jem.20090547
50. Villani AC, Satija R, Reynolds G, Sarkizova S, Shekhar K, Fletcher J, et al. Single-cell RNA-seq reveals new types of human blood dendritic cells, monocytes, and progenitors. *Science.* (2017) 356:eaah4573. doi: 10.1126/science.aah4573
51. See P, Dutertre CA, Chen J, Günther P, McGovern N, Irac SE, et al. Mapping the human DC lineage through the integration of high-dimensional techniques. *Science.* (2017) 356:eaag3009. doi: 10.1126/science.aag3009
52. Finck R, Simonds EF, Jager A, Krishnaswamy S, Sachs K, Fantl W, et al. Normalization of mass cytometry data with bead standards. *Cytom Part A.* (2013) 83A:483–94. doi: 10.1002/cyto.a.22271
53. van der Maaten L, Hinton G. Visualizing data using t-SNE. *J Mach Learn Res.* (2008) 9:2579–605.
54. Platon L, Pejoski D, Gautreau G, Targat B, Le Grand R, Beignon AS, et al. A computational approach for phenotypic comparisons of cell populations in high-dimensional cytometry data. *Methods.* (2018) 132:66–75. doi: 10.1016/j.ymeth.2017.09.005

8

Deep Phenotyping of Urinary Leukocytes by Mass Cytometry Reveals a Leukocyte Signature for Early and Non-Invasive Prediction of Response to Treatment in Active Lupus Nephritis

Martina Bertolo[1†], *Sabine Baumgart*[2†], *Pawel Durek*[2], *Anette Peddinghaus*[2], *Henrik Mei*[2], *Thomas Rose*[3], *Philipp Enghard*[1] and *Andreas Grützkau*[2*]

[1] *Department of Nephrology, Charité Universitätsmedizin Berlin, Berlin, Germany,* [2] *Deutsches Rheuma-Forschungszentrum Berlin (DRFZ), a Leibniz-Institute, Berlin, Germany,* [3] *Department of Rheumatology and Clinical Immunology, Charité Universitätsmedizin Berlin, Berlin, Germany*

***Correspondence:**
Andreas Grützkau
gruetzkau@drfz.de

† *These authors have contributed equally to this work*

Non-invasive biomarkers are necessary for diagnosis and monitoring disease activity in lupus nephritis (LN) to circumvent risks and limitations of renal biopsies. To identify new non-invasive cellular biomarkers in the urine sediment of LN patients, which may reflect kidney inflammation and can be used to predict treatment outcome, we performed in-depth urinary immune cell profiling by mass cytometry. We established a mass cytometric workflow to comparatively analyze the cellular composition of urine and peripheral blood (PB) in 13 patients with systemic lupus erythematosus (SLE) with active, biopsy-proven proliferative LN. Clinical and laboratory data were collected at the time of sampling and 6 months after induction of therapy in order to evaluate the clinical response of each patient. Six patients with different acute inflammatory renal diseases were included as comparison group. Leukocyte phenotypes and composition differed significantly between urine and paired PB samples. In urine, neutrophils and monocytes/macrophages were identified as the most prominent cell populations comprising together about 30%–83% of nucleated cells, while T and B lymphocytes, eosinophils, and natural killer (NK) cells were detectable at frequencies of <10% each. The majority of urinary T cells showed phenotypical characteristics of activated effector memory T cells (EM) as indicated by the co-expression of CD38 and CD69 – a phenotype that was not detectable in PB. Kidney inflammation was also reflected by tissue-imprinted macrophages, which phenotypically differed from PB monocytes by an increased expression of HLA-DR and CD11c. The presence of activated urinary T cells and macrophages could be used for differential diagnosis of proliferative LN forms and other renal pathologies. Most interestingly, the amount of EM in the urine sediment could be used as a biomarker to stratify LN patients in terms of response to induction therapy. Deep immunophenotypic profiling of urinary cells in LN allowed us to identify a signature of activated T cells and macrophages, which appear to reflect leukocytic infiltrates in the kidney. This explorative study has not only confirmed but also extended the knowledge about urinary cells as a future non-invasive biomarker platform for diagnosis and precision medicine in inflammatory renal diseases.

Keywords: systemic lupus – erythematosus, lupus nephritis, lupus nephritis biomarker, mass cytometry, urinary leukocytes

INTRODUCTION

Systemic lupus erythematosus (SLE) is a rare potentially life-threatening autoimmune disease with a complex and not fully understood immune pathophysiology (1).

Almost half of SLE patients develop lupus nephritis (LN) (2), which is responsible for a significant increase in mortality (18% over 5 years) and morbidity (end-stage renal disease, cardiovascular events) (3). There are several types of renal diseases in SLE, which are mainly immune complex-mediated glomerulonephritis. These can be differentiated by histopathological examination of renal biopsies. Morphological changes are divided into six different classes according to the International Society of Nephrology/Renal Pathology Society (ISN/RPS) 2003 classification of LN and are critical to the issue of patient care (4, 5). While class I and class II are characterized by pure mesangial involvement and do not need specific therapy, class III and class IV LN present with focal (III) or diffuse (IV) endocapillary proliferation and are often treated with potent immunosuppression. Finally, class V membranous glomerulonephritis and class VI, presenting with advanced sclerotic lesions, may be managed conservatively with antiproteinuric, renoprotective measures (6). Combinations of proliferative (III or IV) and membranous (V) lesions can be observed. In addition, renal diseases as pauci-immune glomerulonephritis may be rarely seen in SLE patients.

When LN is suspected by an increased serum creatinine level, new onset proteinuria, erythrocyturia with the occurrence of urinary acanthocytes or casts, a kidney biopsy is indispensable to confirm the diagnosis and define the nature of renal involvement (2). However, several clinical situations might occur in which kidney biopsy is contraindicated, due to severe hypertension, bleeding diathesis, or solitary kidney, or is not performed, such as in mild proteinuria and silent LN (7). In these cases, the diagnosis is uncertain and initiation of induction therapy might be delayed, potentially resulting in ongoing inflammation and subsequent chronic organ damage, while early diagnosed and treated LN patients have a better outcome (8, 9). Moreover, when response to induction therapy has not been achieved after 6 months and a change in the histopathologic classification of the kidney or chronic renal damage is suspected, additional biopsies are required to aid therapeutic decision-making and predicting outcomes (2). In fact, laboratory parameters on which current remission criteria are based (10), especially serum creatinine and proteinuria, cannot distinguish between active disease and established organ damage, and several studies showed their poor sensitivity for predicting disease outcomes (11, 12).

To overcome the limitations of kidney biopsy and to improve LN prognosis, reliable non-invasive biomarkers for early diagnosis and outcome prediction are required. For this purpose, the urine sediment of LN patients was already investigated by conventional flow cytometry before, and the presence of mononuclear cells in urine of patients with active renal disease was described (13–15). Remarkably, these studies showed that the phenotype of urinary immune cells differs from that of peripheral blood (PB) leukocytes while it resembles that of kidney-infiltrating inflammatory cells, suggesting that urinary leukocytes most likely originate from the leukocytic kidney infiltrate intrarenal resident cells and not from blood leaking into urine (12–15). In particular, urinary T cells were revealed as promising biosensors to identify an active proliferative LN. While their frequencies correlated with the extent of renal inflammation, the disappearance of urinary T cells under induction therapy was associated with better outcome. SLE patients with inactive LN or non-proliferative LN forms showed an "immunologically inactive" urine sediment (13, 14). These results support the initial hypothesis that urinary cells yield reliable biomarkers for clinical use.

Conventional flow cytometry has been employed in a hypothesis-based manner to analyze urine with respect to particular cell types. There, not only the limited number of cytometric readouts but also autofluorescence of urinary cells and problems to compensate for spectral spillover artifacts restricted the power of fluorescence-based analyses. Therefore, we have used for the first time fluorescence-free mass cytometry (cytometry by time-of-flight, CyTOF) to systematically map all major and many minor leukocyte subsets typically detectable in PB at unprecedented detail in human urine. This technology uses metal isotope-conjugated monoclonal antibodies to detect for today up to 50 parameters simultaneously at the single-cell level and circumvents the technical limitations of conventional flow cytometry mentioned before (16). This technology allowed us an in-depth analysis of leukocytes of urine with respect to their particular phenotypes associated to cellular differentiation and activation. The identification of a robust cell signature in urine is of potential interest as a non-invasive biomarker for the diagnosis of LN.

MATERIALS AND METHODS

Study Population

Urine and PB samples were collected from patients fulfilling at least 4 of the 2010 American College of Rheumatology revised criteria for SLE (17) and suspected active renal involvement. Active renal involvement was suspected clinically by worsening kidney function, abnormal proteinuria, and/or erythrocyturia of unknown origin. All SLE patients (n = 16) underwent renal biopsy and were diagnosed with active LN. Histological findings were evaluated according to the ISN/RPS 2003 classification of LN (4). One patient (P12) was diagnosed with a focal LN (class III), nine patients were diagnosed with a diffuse LN (class IV), three patients (P01, P10, and P15) were diagnosed with mixed proliferative and membranous LN (class IV + V), one patient (P05) was diagnosed with pure membranous LN (class V), and two patients (P07 and P08) showed a pauci-immune, crescentic glomerulonephritis (**Table 1**).

In a subgroup of 13 patients with proliferative LN (LN class III, IV, and mixed forms), paired urine and blood samples were analyzed to identify proliferative LN-specific urinary biomarkers. For P01 und P16, no blood samples were available, so urine samples were analyzed only. Samples from SLE patients with pauci-immune LN forms (P07 and P08), with biopsy-proven anti-neutrophil cytoplasmic antibodies (ANCA)-associated glomerulonephritis (P17 and P19) and with acute granulomatous interstitial tubulonephritis (gITN; P18) were used as non-proliferative control group (**Table 1**). P05 (class V) was not used for further analysis, because relatively low numbers of urine cells were detectable and most of them were granulocytes.

For each SLE patient, SLE Disease Activity Index (SLEDAI) (18) was assessed; SLEDAI elements accounting for kidney disease (proteinuria, leukocyturia, erythrocyturia, and casts) are presented as renal SLEDAI, whereby each positive element is weighted with four points. Routine laboratory values as well as urine sediment findings were retrieved from the medical records.

All patients with proliferative LN received induction therapy with combinations of high-dose corticosteroids (>1 mg/kg body weight) and either cyclophosphamide (CYC) or mycophenolate mofetil (MMF) for 6 months (in case of patient 03 only 3 months) (**Table 2**). Patients were clinically monitored for 6 months. At this time, the response to induction therapy was assessed by adopting a simplified version of the ACR renal response criteria and verifying clinician's judgment (**Table 2**). We defined patients as responders when creatinine remained stable (if estimated glomerular filtration rate (eGFR) was >60 ml/min at baseline) or improved of at least 50% (if eGFR was <60 ml/min at baseline), and/or proteinuria showed an improvement of at least 50% without worsening of other findings (creatinine, proteinuria, and urine sediment/hematuria) over time. Patients who did not fulfill these criteria were considered as non-responders. According to this assessment, nine patients were responders and four were non-responders (**Table 2**).

All patients were recruited in a time period of 4 years (between 2014 and 2017) from the ward of the Department of Rheumatology and Clinical Immunology, Charité University Hospital, Berlin, Germany. Informed consent was obtained from all patients. The study was approved by the ethics committee of the Charité University Hospital (EA1/356/14) and was conducted in accordance with the Declaration of Helsinki.

TABLE 1 | Baseline characteristics and medication of all included patients.

Patient ID	Sex Age	ISN/RPS class LN/Other GN	SLEDAI	renal SLEDAI	Active urine sediment	Proteinuria (mg/24h)	Creatinine (mg/dl)	Immunosuppressive therapies
01	F, 34	IV - G(A/C) + V	12	8	no	907	0.72	AZA, HCQ
02	F, 31	IV - S (C)	10	8	yes	500	3.49	AZA, HCQ
03	F, 20	IV - G(A)	14	8	yes	393	1.69	
04	F, 29	IV	11	12	no	4327	0.91	
05	F, 46	V	8	4	no	1254	0.74	MMF, HCQ
06	F, 38	IV - G(A)	10	8	no	4812	0.74	HCQ
07	F, 51	pauci-immune*	13	8	yes	1424	1.17	CS
08	F, 33	pauci-immune** + V	12	8	yes	1019	1.69	
09	F, 25	IV	18	12	yes	1584	0.62	
10	F, 30	IV - G(A) + V	16	12	yes	2994	2.45	
11	F, 19	IV - G(A/C)	22	16	yes	1264	0.79	HCQ
12	F, 33	III - S(A)	26	16	yes	637	0.79	CS
13	F, 24	IV - G(A/C)	12	8	no	654	0.80	AZA, HCQ
14	F, 40	IV - G(A)	13	8	no	1097	0.67	AZA, Belimumab
15	F, 56	IV - G(A/C) + V	18	12	yes	3384	2.79	AZA
16	F, 20	IV - S(A)	14	8	yes	393	1.89	
17	M,40	AAV	n.a.	n.a.	yes	568	4.63	
18	F, 29	gITN	n.a.	n.a.	no	128	4.44	
19	F, 64	AAV	n.a.	n.a.	yes	76	0.92	

*Proliferative LN cohort in white; control cohort in gray. *Focal necrotizing, crescentic glomerulonephritis by SLE. **Focal crescentic and sclerotic glomerulonephritis by SLE, later by antineutrophil cytoplasmic antibody positivity als LN overlap AAV diagnosed. LN, lupus nephritis; GN, glomerulonephritis; G, global; S, segmental; A, active, C, chronic lesions; AAV, ANCA-associated glomerulonephritis; gITN; granulomatous interstitial tubulonephritis; SLEDAI, Systemic Lupus Erythematosus Disease Activity Index; AZA, azathioprine; HCQ, hydroxycloroquine; MMF, mycophenolate mofetil; CS, corticosteroids.*

TABLE 2 | Clinical and laboratory response to induction therapy.

Patient ID	Induction Therapy*	Creatinine [mg/dl]; eGFR		Proteinuria#		Clinical valuation	Response to Treatment
		Before	After	Before	After		
01	CS+ CYC	0.72; >90	0.55; >90	907	204	good response to CYC, switch to maintenance therapy	R
02	CS+ CYC	3.55; 16	3.13; 19	505	220	proteinuria improved, stabile GFR by chronic renal failure	R
03	CS+ CYC (3 months)	1.69; 43	0.64; >90	393	42	good response so far (after 3 months)	R
04	CS+ CYC	0.91; 73	0.76; >90	4327	231	good response, switch to maintenance therapy	R
06	CS+MMF	0.74; >90	n.d.	4812	>3000	active disease, induction therapy has to be continued	NR
09	CS+ CYC	0.62; >90	0.68; >90	1584	228	no more disease activity, switch to maintenance therapy	R
10	CS+MMF	2.45; 26	0.85; >90	3151#	610#	good response to induction therapy	R
11	CS+ CYC	0.79; 89	0.55; >90	1264	1074	active disease, switch to MMF	NR
12	CS+MMF	0.56; >90	0.71; >90	668	189#	good response to MMF, switch to maintenance therapy	R
13	CS+ CYC	0.80; >90	0.93; 86	654	1527	worsening of proteinuria, switch to MMF	NR
14	CS+MMF	0.67; >90	0.86; 87	535#	272#	good response to induction	R
15	CS+ CYC	2.79; 18	1.40; 48	3384	1651	incomplete response to CYC, switch to MMF	NR
16	CS+ CYC	1.89; 38	0.62; >90	617#	108#	good response, switch to maintenance therapy	R

Induction therapy was given for 6 months (except for Patient P 03) Proteinuria is expressed as mg/24h or as uPCR. uPCR values are labeled with #. eGFR, estimated Glomerular Filtration Rate (ml/min); uPCR, urinary Protein Creatinin Ratio (mg Protein/mg Creatinine); n.d., not determined; R, response; NR, non-response; CS, corticosteroids; CYC, cyclophosphamide; MMF, mycophenolate mofetil.

Sample Preparation

Buffers, Chemicals, and Materials

The following buffers and chemicals were used: erythrocyte lysis buffer (Qiagen, Hilden, Germany), 1 × PBS, made from 10 × PBS (Rockland, Gilbertsville, PA, United States; pH 7.2) using Millipore water, 0.1% cell permeabilization buffer, made from 10 × saponin-based permeabilization buffer (eBioscience), 4% formaldehyde solution in PBS made from 16% paraformaldehyde (EMS, Hatfield, PA, United States), PBS supplemented with 0.5% BSA (PAN Biotech, Aidenbach, Germany), and 0.02% sodium azide (Sigma-Aldrich, St. Louis, MO, United States) (PBS/BSA). Buffers were sterile-filtered through 0.22-μm membranes and stored in Stericup disposable bottles (Merck, Darmstadt, Germany). Blood, urine, and cells were processed in 50-ml, 15-ml, and 5-ml round-bottom polystyrene/polypropylene tubes (Corning, Corning, NY, United States and Sarstedt, Nümbrecht, Germany).

MAXPAR antibody labeling kits, EQ Four element calibration beads, washing and tuning solution, and DNA intercalators were purchased from Fluidigm Corporation (South San Francisco, CA, United States). Pre-conjugated and unlabeled antibodies are summarized in the **Supplementary Table S1**.

Cis-Platinum (II)-diamine dichloride (cisplatin) was purchased from Enzo Life Sciences GmbH (Lörrach, Germany). A 25 mM stock solution was prepared in DMSO (Sigma-Aldrich) and aliquots were stored at -20°C.

Sample Collection and Preservation of Urinary Cells

EDTA anti-coagulated blood and fresh voided urine samples (50 to 150 ml) were collected from each patient. Patients with active urinary infections or menstruation at the time of urine collection were excluded. Fresh urine was diluted with 30% v/v PBS supplemented with 1% BSA and promptly centrifuged (300 × *g*, 10 min, 4°C) within 60 min after collection in order to minimize artifacts resulting from delayed sample processing. Urinary cells were washed twice with PBS/BSA. Blood was subjected to erythrocyte lysis within 1 h after collection. One volume of whole blood was mixed with 4 volumes of EL buffer, incubated for 10 min on ice, and centrifuged (300 × *g*, 10 min, 4°C), and cells were washed once with EL buffer and twice with PBS/BSA.

The number of leukocytes and their viability were checked by conventional flow cytometry staining successively with CD45 (Miltenyi Biotec; Vio770 conjugate diluted 1:50) and 4,6-diamidino-2-phenylindole dihydrochloride (DAPI) (Sigma-Aldrich; final concentration 1 μg/ml) just before measuring on a MACSQuant flow cytometer (Miltenyi Biotec, Bergisch-Gladbach, Germany). Urine samples with at least 1 × 10^5 viable CD45-positive cells were used for mass cytometric analysis. While the viability of blood cells was always >95%, a large variability was seen for urine cells, which ranged from 5% to 55% (mean 33%; SD ± 29%).

Sample Processing for Mass Cytometric Analysis

Up to 3 × 10^6 cells were incubated with cisplatin as described before to stain dead cells. A cocktail including 26 anti-human monoclonal antibodies (**Supplementary Table S1**) was used to stain blood and urinary cells for 30 min at room temperature as described before (19). All in-house-conjugated antibodies were titrated before using blood cells. Commercial antibodies were used as recommended by the manufacturer.

After washing, cells were fixed overnight using 4% PFA. On the next day, samples were washed and nucleated cells were stained with iridium intercalator in permeabilization buffer for 30 min at RT. After washing twice with PBS/BSA and subsequently twice with Millipore water, cells were adjusted to 0.5 × 10^6 cells/ml using Millipore water supplemented with 1/10 v/v EQ Four element beads.

Mass Cytometric Measurement

Cell suspensions were acquired on a CyTOF v1 instrument controlled by CyTOF software v5.1.6.4.8 and v6.0.626) (Fluidigm). The instrument was set up and tuned daily according to the manufacturer's recommendations. Cells were injected into a 450-μl loop at a flow rate of 45 μl/min. Data were acquired in dual calibration mode, with noise reduction turned on and lower and upper cell length parameter thresholds set to 10 and 75. Absolute cell numbers of each particular sample are summarized in **Supplementary Figure S1**. For blood samples, about 2.5×10^6 total events were acquired.

Data Analysis and Statistics

Data were normalized based on signals of the internal standard beads. Zero values were randomized to values between -1 and 0. Data were then analyzed by manual gating using FlowJo 10.6 software (Treestar, Ashland, OR, United States). Blood and urinary leukocytes were identified by the expression of CD45. The gating strategy applied to urine and blood samples is shown in **Supplementary Figure S2**. viSNE analyses of paired urine and blood samples were performed by Cytobank premium (Santa Clara, CA, United States)[1] using the following parameters: perplexity = 100, theta = 0.5, iterations = 1000.

Statistical analyses were conducted using GraphPad Prism 8.0 (GraphPad Software, San Diego, United States). Non-parametric Wilcoxon test was used for paired analyses of blood and urine. Correlation analyses with disease activity were assessed using Spearman's rank correlation. Non-parametric Mann–Whitney *U* test was adopted to analyze differences between responder and non-responder groups. Two-tailed *p*-values of less than 0.05 were considered statistically significant. The hierarchical cluster analysis was generated based on *z*-score standardized frequencies of cell subpopulations obtained from urine samples of patients with active LN and other acute renal diseases. Cell frequencies were obtained by manual gating of mass cytometric data. Hierarchical clustering was performed based on Spearman distance and the Ward linkage criterion.

RESULTS

Identification of Viable, Nucleated Cells in PB and Urine

At first, the presence of live, single nucleated cells was evaluated according to the manual gating strategy exemplarily shown for PB and urine cells in **Supplementary Figure S2**. While stable amounts of live single $CD45^+$ cells were recovered from PB samples, corresponding urine samples of LN patients showed large variations with respect to cell density in the urine and in cell viability ranging from 5% to 55%. In **Supplementary Figure S1** absolute numbers of nucleated cells acquired by mass cytometry are summarized.

[1] www.cytobank.org

Which Immune Cells Can Be Found in Urine of LN Patients?

The application of a comprehensive mass cytometry antibody panel allowed an in-depth analysis of the urinary leukocyte composition in comparison to autologous blood samples. Neutrophils, monocytes/macrophages, and T lymphocytes were identified as predominating leukocyte populations in the urine, adding to 32–84% of all nucleated cells (**Figure 1A**). In addition, minor frequencies (<4% of nucleated cells) of B lymphocytes, eosinophils, and natural killer (NK) cells were detectable (**Figure 1A**).

In contrast to the paired PB samples, no reasonable numbers of dendritic cells, basophils, or plasma cells/plasmablasts were ascertainable in urine samples. If compared to PB samples, a large variability was seen in the cellular composition of the urine cell sediment regarding neutrophils (17–53% of nucleated cells), monocytes/macrophages (12–78% of nucleated cells), and T cells (0.2–16% of nucleated cells) (**Figure 1A**). In the **Supplementary Table S2** all phenotypes identified by the manual gating are summarized.

The results obtained by manual gating could be confirmed by t-SNE analysis, which revealed similar cell clusters (**Figure 3B**). The most obvious difference between PB and urine was seen within the myeloid compartments. Here clusters of granulocytes and monocytes/macrophages showed clear changes in their spatial classification. The changed phenotype of granulocytes seen in urine samples most probably reflects their sensitive behavior in response to the chemical nature of urine.

Can Urine-Specific Immune Cell Phenotypes Be Identified?

Beyond the abundance of major leukocyte subsets, we further analyzed the immunophenotypic characteristics of urinary T cells and monocytes in more detail. Urinary T cells showed a significant lower CD4/CD8 ratio as compared to the paired PB samples (0.8 ± 0.8 vs. 1.6 ± 0.7, p = 0.02) and only a poor correlation between blood and urine was observed (r = 0.2760, p = n.s.).

T cells lacking CD4 and CD8 (DN) were significantly increased in urine as compared to blood (28% ± 13% vs. 8% ± 5% of $CD3^+$ cells; p = 0.002).

Naïve ($CD45RA^+CCR7^+$), central memory (CM, $CD45RA^-CCR7^+$), effector memory (EM, $CD45RA^-CCR7^-$), and terminally differentiated effector memory (TEMRA, $CD45RA^+CCR7^-$) T cell subsets showed a significantly different distribution in urine and blood (**Figures 1B,C**). In urine, both $CD4^+$ and $CD8^+$ effector memory T cells represented by far the largest T cell subset ($CD4^+$ EM, 68% ± 24%; $CD8^+$ EM, 84% ± 19% of $CD4^+$ and $CD8^+$ cells, respectively), while in PB, naïve T cells were dominating ($CD4^+$ naïve: 46% ± 16%; $CD8^+$ naïve: 55% ± 28% in relation to all $CD4^+$ and $CD8^+$ cells, respectively).

We further investigated the expression of activation markers on particular T cell subsets, i.e., HLA-DR, CD69, and CD38. The majority of urinary T cells showed a $CD69^+CD38^+$ double-positive phenotype (52% ± 23% of $CD3^+$ cells), while this

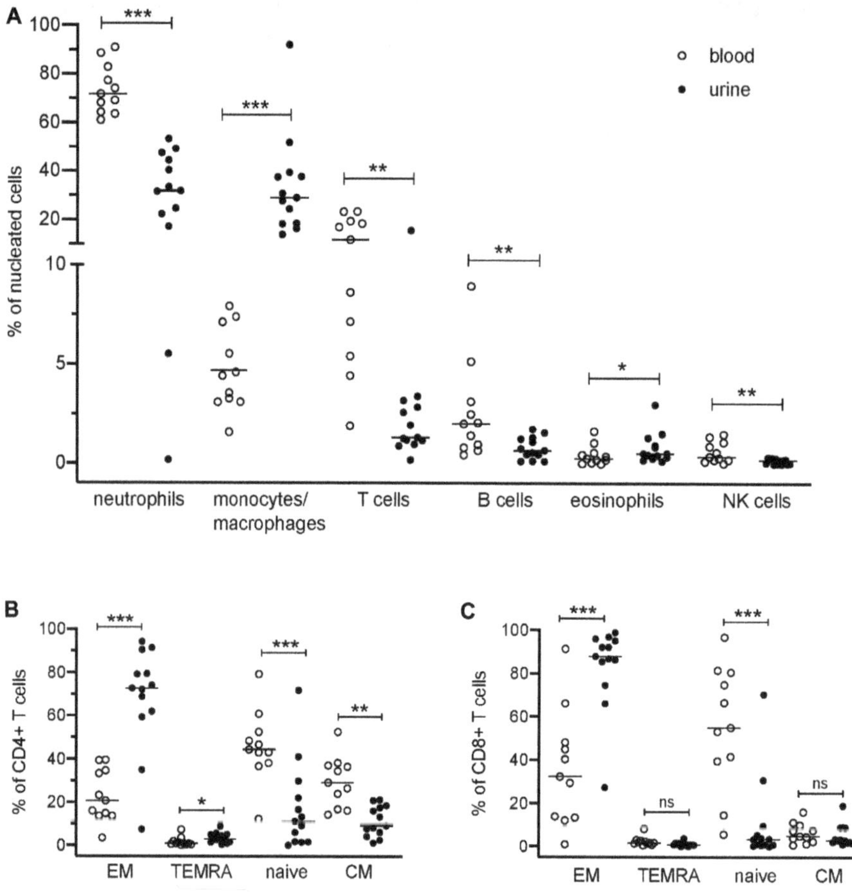

FIGURE 1 | Distribution of blood and urinary immune cells. **(A)** Frequencies of urinary leukocytes (% of nucleated cells) in comparison to blood. **(B)** Frequencies of $CD4^+$ naïve and effector cell subsets in urine and blood (% of $CD4^+$ T cells). **(C)** Frequencies of $CD8^+$ naïve and effector cell subsets in urine and blood (% of $CD8^+$ cells). EM, effector memory T cells; TEMRA, terminally differentiated effector memory T cells; CM, central memory T cells. Wilcoxon test for paired samples, *p*-values: $^*p < 0.05$, $^{**}p < 0.01$, $^{***}p < 0.001$, n.s.: not significant.

phenotype was almost absent in blood (3% ± 3%) (**Figure 2A**). The percentage of $CD69^+CD38^+$ T cells was highest among $CD8^+$ EM cells (66% ± 21%) followed by $CD4^+$ EM cells (45% ± 13%) (**Figure 2A**).

The activated phenotype of urinary T cells was also reflected by a higher expression of HLA-DR (**Figure 2B**). Here, $CD4^+$ EM cells showed twofold higher mean intensity values than $CD8^+$ EM cells.

The results obtained by manual gating could be confirmed by t-SNE analysis, which revealed similar cell clusters (**Figure 3A**). The most obvious difference between PB and urine was seen within the myeloid compartments. Here, clusters of granulocytes and monocytes/macrophages showed clear changes in their spatial classification. The changed phenotype of granulocytes seen in urine samples most probably reflects their sensitive behavior in response to the chemical nature of urine. t-SNE analyses allowed an in-depth phenotypic characterization of the monocyte/macrophage clusters exemplarily shown in **Figure 3B**. While monocytes were detectable by the co-expression of CD14, CD36, CD16, and HLA-DR in PB, obviously tissue-imprinted macrophages were characterized by high expression values for HLA-DR and CD11c in urine (**Figures 3A,B**). CD36, CD14, and CD38 were significantly lower expressed on urine macrophages as compared to PB monocytes (**Figure 3C** and **Supplementary Figure S3**).

Can a Urinary Leukocyte Signature Be Used to Identify Proliferative LN Patients?

Next, we analyzed whether the cellular phenotypes identified in the urine of LN patients can be used to distinguish proliferative from non-proliferative LN forms and other acute inflammatory renal diseases. For this analysis, cell populations were considered when at least 25 cell counts were detectable; i.e., CM, TEMRA cells, Treg's, and DC's were excluded. This was the reason why P05 (membranous LN) was omitted from analysis because, here, urinary neutrophils were almost exclusively detected. As shown in the hierarchical cluster analysis of **Figure 4**, the frequencies of 23 urinary leukocyte subsets as summarized in the **Supplementary Table S2** allowed a separation of patients into two main clusters. This classification is largely in agreement

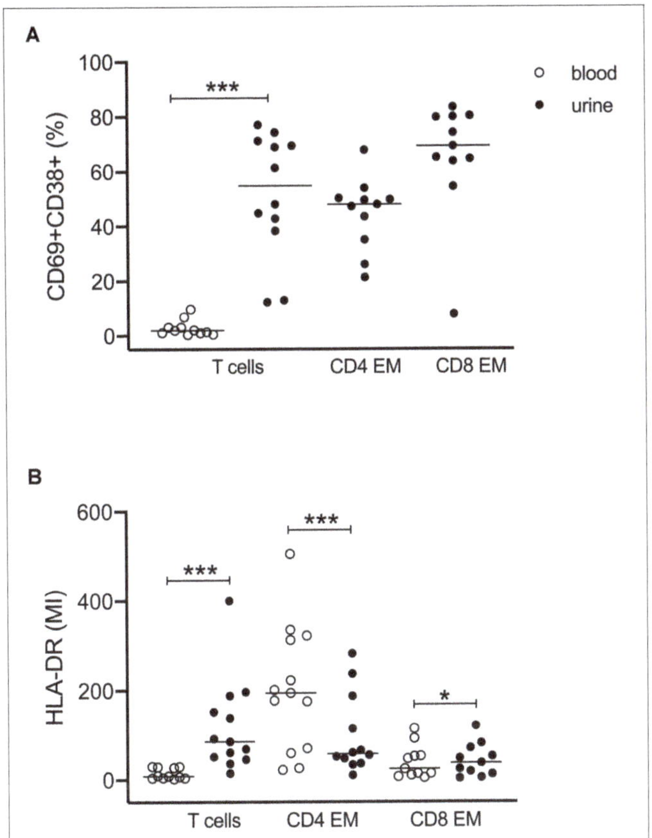

FIGURE 2 | Activated T cells in urine and blood. (A) Frequencies of $CD69^{+}CD38^{+}$ double-positive T cell subsets related to all $CD3^{+}$ and to $CD4^{+}$ EM and $CD8^{+}$ EM cell subsets. Since almost no activated T cells were found in blood, CD4- and CD8-related analyses were shown for urinary cells only (closed symbols). **(B)** Mean intensity of HLA-DR expression on all $CD3^{+}$, $CD4^{+}$ EM, and $CD8^{+}$ EM cells in urine (closed symbols) and blood (open symbols). Wilcoxon test for paired samples, *p*-values: $^{*}p < 0.05$, $^{***}p < 0.001$.

with histopathological evaluation of kidney biopsies. In fact, 11 out of 13 proliferative LN samples clustered together and clearly separated from the other ones (**Figure 4**). Interestingly, P02 and P16, which clustered separately together with non-lupus samples, were the only class IV patients showing segmental lesions in the glomeruli instead of global lesions observed in all the other class IV patients. Two of five controls (P17 and P18) clustered together with proliferative LN samples.

Do Urinary T Cell Subsets Correlate With Clinical Parameters?

Next, we investigated which urinary cell subsets correlate with clinical parameters. The only significant correlation observed was between $CD4^{+}$ T cells and proteinuria. Here, a negative correlation could be ascertained, which reflects the low CD4/CD8 ratio detected in PB and urine of LN patients (**Supplementary Figure S4**). Other clinical parameters such as renal SLEDAI, active urinary sediment, and creatinine did not show significant correlations with any of the cell subsets identified.

Can Urinary Cell Signatures Be Used as Therapy Response Predictors?

Finally, it was interesting to know whether urinary cell subsets can be used to predict response to induction therapy. LN patients were classified 6 months after starting induction therapy as responders or non-responders (**Table 2**). In 9 out of 13 LN patients, clinical improvement was observed in response to standard immunosuppressive therapies. High frequencies of $CD4^{+}$ EM cells (>90% of total $CD4^{+}$) were identified at baseline as the most promising predictor to indicate insufficient response to therapy (**Figure 5**). All other urinary cell subsets did not allow prediction of therapy response or non-response.

With regard to PB, we could not identify any leukocyte subset predictive for therapy response.

DISCUSSION

The availability of non-invasive biomarkers in LN, which could be diagnostically used to clarify renal injury and which would help in individualized therapeutic decision-making, is hitherto unmet clinical needs. Therefore, this study used state-of-the-art mass cytometry to enable an in-depth profiling of urinary leukocytes in comparison to PB with respect to identifying new cell-associated biomarkers that can be used along with humoral markers of serum and urine for an innovative, non-invasive management of LN.

Although the cellular composition of the urine sediment has already been analyzed in several studies (13–15, 20–23), these commonly fluorescence-based flow cytometric analyses were restricted by methodological limitations, such as limited number of parameters necessary for deep and comprehensive profiling of leukocyte subsets, issues emerging from autofluorescence of cells present in the urine, and how these can be appropriately compensated for when spilled over in the fluorescence channels of interest. As mass cytometry eliminates these technical limitations, we have used it for a deep comparative profiling of blood and urinary leukocytes. So, we were able to identify significant differences in the distribution of leukocyte subsets and phenotypic features, which are exclusively expressed by urinary cells, supporting the assumption that urinary leukocytes may reflect the inflammatory infiltrate in LN. This assumption is supported by data of a recent study analyzing urine and kidney-related cell clusters in LN by single-cell transcriptomics (24). Here, different macrophage subsets, NK cells, and lymphocyte subsets were identified in urine, which were also assignable to tissue-located leukocytes in the inflamed kidney. Contrary to the study of Arazi et al. (24), our mass cytometry approach allowed the detection of neutrophils, which, along with monocytes/macrophages, are the dominant leukocyte subsets detectable in the urine sediment and, consequently, have a strong influence on the relative quantitative composition of urinary cells.

With the present data, we could not only confirm the occurrence of main inflammatory cell types in the urine from affected kidneys but also detect rare cell types such as B cells, NK cells, or eosinophils at the single-cell level. With the exception of Brito's investigation of urinary eosinophils

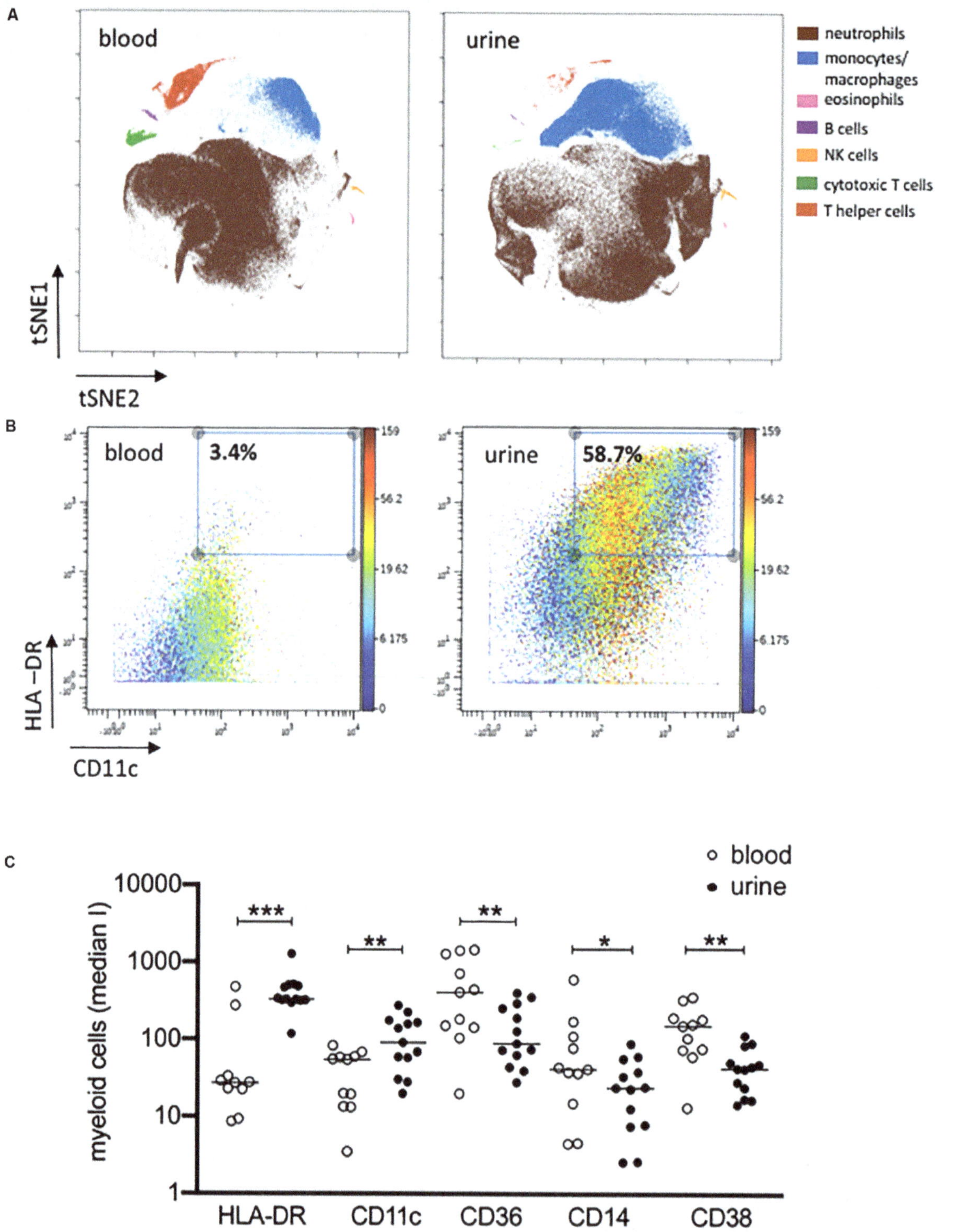

FIGURE 3 | Activated monocytes/macrophages in urine and blood. **(A)** viSNE analysis of all pre-gated viable nucleated cells from urine and blood (plot 5, **Supplementary Figure S1**) with cell populations defined based on basic phenotypic markers exemplarily shown for patient 04 (equal sampling per comparison, event sampling = 200,000 cells per sample; 1,000 iterations, final KL divergence: 5.11). **(B)** HLA-DR and CD11c expression on pre-gated monocyte/macrophages cell population shown in a two-dimensional plot; color corresponds to CD14 expression exemplarily shown for patient 04 in urine and blood. **(C)** Myeloid cells gated before for HLA-DR and CD11c were further analyzed for the expression of HLA-DR, CD11c, CD36, CD14 and CD38 as median intensities (median I). Wilcoxon test for paired samples, *p*-values: **p* < 0.05; ***p* < 0.01; ****p* < 0.001.

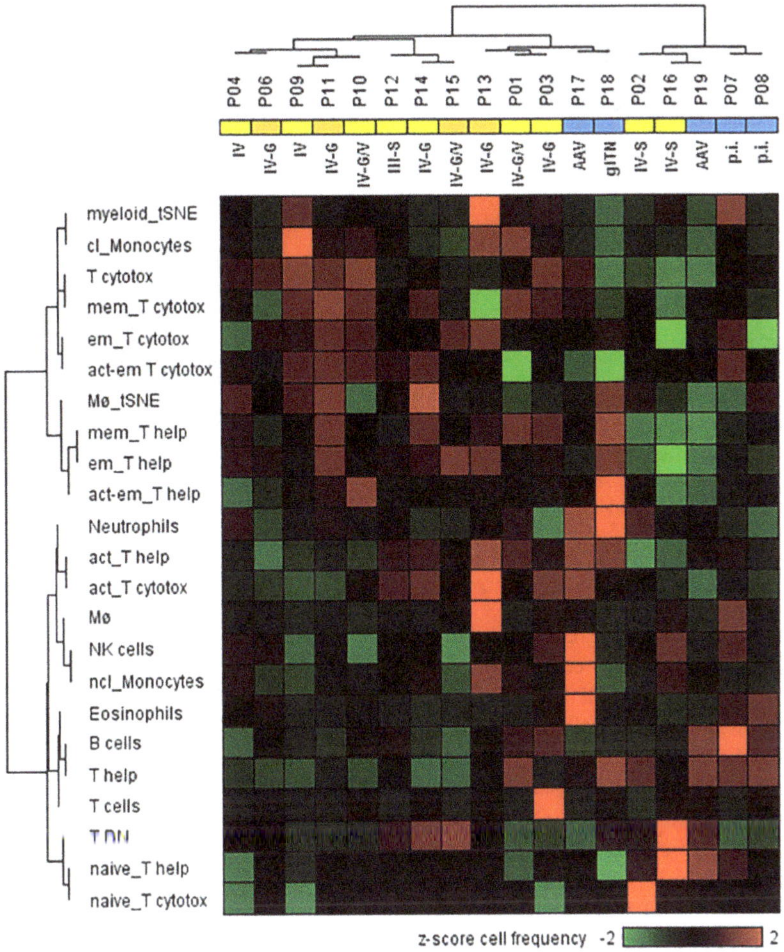

FIGURE 4 | Two-dimensional hierarchical cluster analysis using 23 urinary cellular phenotypes for the classification of active proliferative LN (n = 13) and other renal diseases (n = 5). The heat map was generated based on z-score standardized frequencies of cell subpopulations obtained from urine samples of patients with active LN and other acute renal diseases that were obtained by manual gating of mass cytometric data. Hierarchical clustering was performed based on Spearman distance and Ward linkage criterion. Values above 2 and below -2 standard deviations are highlighted by light red and green, respectively. Proliferative LN patients who did not respond to induction therapy were marked in dark yellow. Analysis revealed two main clusters of patients consistent with histological results for proliferative LN patients (yellow) and kidney disorders with different diagnoses (blue). However, two proliferative LN patients clustered within the control group and two controls clustered in the proliferative LN group. Abbreviations according to **Table 1** and **Supplementary Table S2** respectively, p.i.: pauci-immune.

(20), most studies conducted so far focused on mononuclear cell subsets, although they account for only 20% of total cells detectable in urine of LN patients (21). Several recent publications indicate that granulocytes (neutrophils, basophils, and eosinophils) play an important role in SLE pathogenesis by promoting innate and adaptive aberrant autoimmune responses and enhancing tissue damage (25). Therefore, our antibody panel was conceived to investigate both granulocytic and mononuclear cell populations. According to our data, neutrophilic granulocytes and mononuclear cells account for roughly 50% of nucleated cells in the urine. Comparing neutrophils from urine and blood, phenotypic differences were detectable according to the t-SNE analyses. It was not possible to assign clearly defined phenotypes since the granulocytic compartment showed high inter-individual differences, which may be induced by the chemical nature of the urine. Obviously, granulocytes are particularly very sensitive to this kind of cell stress and apoptotic programs will be initiated.

The second largest urinary cell population consisted of monocytes/macrophages. When compared to blood monocytes, urinary cells showed a more differentiated macrophage-like phenotype as indicated by an increased expression of HLA-DR and CD11c (26).

T cells are most frequently investigated in LN urine (21–23). The predominant appearance of urinary T cells and monocytes besides granulocytes confirms histopathologic findings of the inflamed tissue in LN (22, 27–29), again supporting the view that leukocytes attracted into the inflamed kidney may escape from damaged glomerular capillaries and tubules into the urine. Our data allowed an in-depth phenotyping of urinary T cells, which have been already described as reliable biomarkers in proliferative LN (14). In line with the findings of Dolff et al. (15),

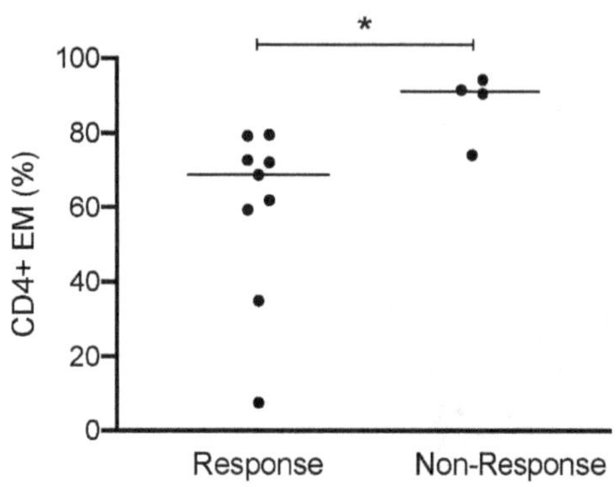

FIGURE 5 | CD4$^+$ EM cells as predictors of responsiveness at baseline of induction therapy in active proliferative LN patients (n = 13). Frequencies of effector memory CD4$^+$ cells at baseline in patient responder and non-responder groups. Responsiveness was calculated 6 months after starting induction therapy as described in **Table 2**. Mann–Whitney test for unpaired samples, p-value: $^*p < 0.05$.

we could confirm that urinary T cells have predominantly an effector memory phenotype, but additionally could show that they co-expressed the activation markers CD38 and CD69. Comparable results were obtained by single-cell transcriptome analyses of LN kidneys, in which CD69-positive central memory and effector memory T helper cells were identified as one of the main lymphocyte clusters (24). Most strikingly, the amount of effector memory T cells was predictive for the response to immunosuppressive induction therapy. Furthermore, most of the CD4$^+$ EM cells could be identified as CCR5-expressing Th1 cells in a subgroup of patients analyzed by a second antibody panel (**Supplementary Figure S5**), which are known to be primarily responsible for disease progression in LN (30–32).

Besides CD4$^+$ and CD8$^+$ T cell subsets, double-negative (DN) CD3$^+$ T cells were identified in both blood and urine. These cells were discussed to be producers of IL-17 and were found to be increased in glomerulonephritis (33).

Although promising, the expression of this T cell-related activation signature (CD69, CD38, and HLA-DR) did not show any prognostic relevance in our cohort. Instead, it was a striking finding that those patients having high percentages of urinary EM T cells at baseline (especially CD4$^+$ EM) were not appropriately responding to therapy.

According to current data, urinary immune cells are not only detectable in active proliferative LN but also present in other inflammatory renal diseases. However, the distribution of leukocyte populations and their respective phenotypes varies among patient groups (22, 23, 34), probably disclosing the differences in the respective renal infiltrates. To show that urinary leukocyte signatures can possibly be used for differential diagnosis of different renal pathologies, we performed a supervised hierarchical cluster analysis including proliferative LN samples as well as non-proliferative LN forms and other acute inflammatory diseases, and could demonstrate that 11 out of 13 proliferative LN samples clustered together and clearly separated from the others. Interestingly, one of both misclassified proliferative LN samples (P16) showed a cellular composition that was very similar to that of LN blood samples and may be caused by a superimposed bleeding derived from an infection of the genitourinary tract. Two of the controls clustered together with proliferative LN samples and therefore the disease specificity of urinary cell signature has to be validated in a larger cohort.

In summary, we could show that the multiplexing power of mass cytometry did allow a more detailed description of urinary T cell and monocyte signatures, disclosing promising biomarker tools for clinical purposes and also revealing some new knowledge about those phenotypes, which drive the inflammation in proliferative LN. Due to the limited number of patients included in this study, we are aware of its explorative nature. Therefore, the conclusions drawn from our results have to be proven by independent and larger cohorts to reliably evaluate the diagnostic and prognostic value of urinary cell signatures for precision medicine in LN patients.

Somehow unclear is the observation that a wide array of dead cells can be found in the urine sediment. On the one hand, the viability is certainly influenced by pH and hyper- or hypo-osmotic nature of the urine, but on the other hand, urinary dead and apoptotic cells may reflect the defective clearance of apoptotic cells in the inflamed kidney, which is unequivocally implicated in the etiopathogenesis of SLE (35, 36). Besides leukocytes, epithelial cells from damaged parenchymal structures, such as glomerula, tubules, and collecting ducts, might also be found in the urine sediment. Accordingly, a more detailed analysis of dead cells with respect to apoptosis-related molecules and epithelial markers might provide additional information about the pathophysiological state of the injured kidney. Nevertheless, we propagate to dilute urine with PBS/BSA buffer immediately after voiding as a simple pre-diagnostic processing procedure to achieve a more standardized collection of urine samples.

In conclusion, urinary cells, being accessible in a non-burdensome manner, would perfectly allow a real-time longitudinal monitoring of cellular changes in the inflamed kidney. It seems to be undisputed that singular markers alone are not likely to have sufficient sensitivity and specificity as required in patients' clinical management. Hence, urinary multi-parametrical panels including humoral factors, micro RNAs, and cellular markers should be tested in appropriately designed clinical studies. The deeper the knowledge about robustly assessed urinary signatures is, the more likely is the successful establishment of a non-invasive tool for differential diagnosis and prognostic stratification of LN patients.

ETHICS STATEMENT

The studies involving human participants were reviewed and approved by the Ethics Committee of the Charité University

Hospital (EA1/356/14). The patients/participants provided their written informed consent to participate in this study.

AUTHOR CONTRIBUTIONS

MB, SB, and AG wrote the manuscript. MB, SB, PE, HM, and AG have designed the study and the experimental strategy. MB, SB, and PD were responsible for data analysis. MB, TR, and PE were responsible for patient selection and their clinical characterization. SB and AP performed the sample preparations and measurements.

agreement # 777357 and e:Med research and funding concept sysINFLAME, grant # 01ZX1606_B, the Leibniz ScienceCampus Chronic Inflammation (www.chronischeentzuendung.org), and Berlin Institute of Health - Clinical Innovator Program.

ACKNOWLEDGMENTS

We especially thank Marianna – without her, manuscript preparation would have literally taken years.

REFERENCES

1. Rose T, Dörner T. Drivers of the immunopathogenesis in systemic lupus erythematosus. *Best Pract Res Clin Rheumatol.* (2017) 31:321–33. doi: 10.1016/j.berh.2017.09.007
2. Bertsias GK, Tektonidou M, Amoura Z, Aringer M, Bajema I, Berden JHM, et al. Joint European League against Rheumatism and European renal association–European dialysis and transplant association (EULAR/ERA-EDTA) recommendations for the management of adult and paediatric lupus nephritis. *Ann Rheum Dis.* (2012) 71:1771–82. doi: 10.1136/annrheumdis-2012-201940
3. Hermansen M-L, Lindhardsen J, Torp-Pedersen C, Faurschou M, Jacobsen S. The risk of cardiovascular morbidity and cardiovascular mortality in systemic lupus erythematosus and lupus nephritis: a Danish nationwide population-based cohort study. *Rheumatology.* (2017) 56:709–15. doi: 10.1093/rheumatology/kew475
4. Weening JJ, D'agati VD, Schwartz MM, Seshan SV, Alpers CE, Appel GB, et al. The classification of glomerulonephritis in systemic lupus erythematosus revisited. *Kidney Int.* (2004) 65:521–30. doi: 10.1111/j.1523-1755.2004.00443.x
5. Austin HA, Boumpas DT, Vaughan EM, Balow JE. Predicting renal outcomes in severe lupus nephritis: contributions of clinical and histologic data. *Kidney Int.* (1994) 45:544–50.
6. Almaani S, Meara A, Rovin BH. Update on lupus nephritis. *Clin J Am Soc Nephrol.* (2017) 12:825–35. doi: 10.2215/CJN.05780616
7. Zabaleta-Lanz M, Vargas-Arenas RE, Tápanes F, Daboin I, Atahualpa Pinto J, Bianco NE. Silent nephritis in systemic lupus erythematosus. *Lupus.* (2003) 12:26–30. doi: 10.1191/0961203303lu259oa
8. Fiehn C, Hajjar Y, Mueller K, Waldherr R, Ho AD, Andrassy K. Improved clinical outcome of lupus nephritis during the past decade: importance of early diagnosis and treatment. *Ann Rheum Dis.* (2003) 62:435–9.
9. Faurschou M, Starklint H, Halberg P, Jacobsen S. Prognostic factors in lupus nephritis: diagnostic and therapeutic delay increases the risk of terminal renal failure. *J Rheumatol.* (2006) 33:1563–9.
10. Gordon C, Jayne D, Pusey C, Adu D, Amoura Z, Aringer M, et al. European consensus statement on the terminology used in the management of lupus glomerulonephritis. *Lupus.* (2009) 18:257–63. doi: 10.1177/0961203308100481
11. Wofsy D, Hillson JL, Diamond B. Abatacept for lupus nephritis: alternative definitions of complete response support conflicting conclusions. *Arthritis Rheum.* (2012) 64:3660–5. doi: 10.1002/art.34624
12. Zickert A, Sundelin B, Svenungsson E, Gunnarsson I. Role of early repeated renal biopsies in lupus nephritis. *Lupus Sci Med.* (2014) 1:e000018. doi: 10.1136/lupus-2014-000018
13. Enghard P, Humrich JY, Rudolph B, Rosenberger S, Biesen R, Kuhn A, et al. CXCR3+CD4+ T cells are enriched in inflamed kidneys and urine and provide a new biomarker for acute nephritis flares in systemic lupus erythematosus patients. *Arthritis Rheum.* (2009) 60:199–206. doi: 10.1002/art.24136
14. Enghard P, Rieder C, Kopetschke K, Klocke JR, Undeutsch R, Biesen R, et al. Urinary CD4 T cells identify SLE patients with proliferative lupus nephritis and can be used to monitor treatment response. *Ann Rheum Dis.* (2014) 73:277–83. doi: 10.1136/annrheumdis-2012-202784
15. Dolff S, Abdulahad WH, van Dijk MCRF, Limburg PC, Kallenberg CGM, Bijl M. Urinary T cells in active lupus nephritis show an effector memory phenotype. *Ann Rheum Dis.* (2010) 69:2034–41. doi: 10.1136/ard.2009.124636
16. Bandura DR, Baranov VI, Ornatsky OI, Antonov A, Kinach R, Lou X, et al. Mass cytometry: technique for real time single cell multitarget immunoassay based on inductively coupled plasma time-of-flight mass spectrometry. *Anal Chem.* (2009) 81:6813–22. doi: 10.1021/ac901049w
17. Petri M. Review of classification criteria for systemic lupus erythematosus. *Rheum Dis Clin North Am.* (2005) 31:245–54. doi: 10.1016/j.rdc.2005.01.009
18. Gladman DD, Ibañez D, Urowitz MB. Systemic lupus erythematosus disease activity index 2000. *J Rheumatol.* (2002) 29:288–91.
19. Baumgart S, Peddinghaus A, Schulte-Wrede U, Mei HE, Grützkau A. OMIP-034: comprehensive immune phenotyping of human peripheral leukocytes by mass cytometry for monitoring immunomodulatory therapies. *Cytometry A.* (2017) 91:34–8. doi: 10.1002/cyto.a.22894
20. Brito TNS, Vilar MJ, Almeida JB, Faria ALSB, Medeiros SDV, Medeiros MCC, et al. Measuring eosinophiluria, urinary eosinophil cationic protein and urinary interleukin-5 in patients with Lupus Nephritis. *Allergy Asthma Clin Immunol.* (2014) 10:61. doi: 10.1186/s13223-014-0061-x
21. Chan RW-Y, Lai FM-M, Li EK-M, Tam L-S, Chung K-Y, Chow K-M, et al. Urinary mononuclear cell and disease activity of systemic lupus erythematosus. *Lupus.* (2006) 15:262–7. doi: 10.1191/0961203306lu2287oa
22. Scott E, Dooley MA, Vilen BJ, Clarke SH. Immune cells and type 1 IFN in urine of SLE patients correlate with immunopathology in the kidney. *Clin Immunol.* (2016) 168:16–24. doi: 10.1016/j.clim.2016.04.005
23. Kopetschke K, Klocke J, Grießbach A-S, Humrich JY, Biesen R, Dragun D, et al. The cellular signature of urinary immune cells in Lupus nephritis: new insights into potential biomarkers. *Arthritis Res Ther.* (2015) 17:94. doi: 10.1186/s13075-015-0600-y
24. Arazi A, Rao DA, Berthier CC, Davidson A, Liu Y, Hoover PJ, et al. The immune cell landscape in kidneys of patients with lupus nephritis. *Nat Immunol.* (2019) 20:902–14. doi: 10.1038/s41590-019-0398-x
25. Kaplan MJ. Neutrophils in the pathogenesis and manifestations of SLE. *Nat Rev Rheumatol.* (2011) 7:691–9. doi: 10.1038/nrrheum.2011.132
26. Tang PM, Nikolic-Paterson DJ, Lan H. Macrophages: versatile players in renal inflammation and fibrosis. *Nat Rev Nephrol.* (2019) 15:144–58. doi: 10.1038/s41581-019-0110-2

27. D'Agati VD, Appel GB, Estes D, Knowles IIDM, Pirani CL. Monoclonal antibody identification of infiltrating mononuclear leukocytes in lupus nephritis. *Kidney Int.* (1986) 30:573–81. doi: 10.1038/ki.1986.223
28. Alexopoulos E, Seron D, Barrie Hartley R, Stewart Cameron J. Lupus nephritis: correlation of interstitial cells with glomerular function. *Kidney Int.* (1990) 37:100–9. doi: 10.1038/ki.1990.14
29. Fiore N, Castellano G, Blasi A, Capobianco C, Loverre A, Montinaro V, et al. Immature myeloid and plasmacytoid dendritic cells infiltrate renal tubulointerstitium in patients with lupus nephritis. *Mol Immunol.* (2008) 45:259–65. doi: 10.1016/j.molimm.2007.04.029
30. Segerer S, Mack M, Regele H, Kerjaschki D, Schlöndorff D. Expression of the C-C chemokine receptor 5 in human kidney diseases. *Kidney Int.* (1999) 56:52–64. doi: 10.1046/j.1523-1755.1999.00544.x
31. Masutani K, Akahoshi M, Tsuruya K, Tokumoto M, Ninomiya T, Kohsaka T, et al. Predominance of Th1 immune response in diffuse proliferative lupus nephritis. *Arthritis Rheum.* (2001) 44:2097–106. doi: 10.1002/1529-0131(200109)44:93.0.CO;2-6
32. Caligaris-Cappio F, Bergui L, Tesio L, Ziano R, Camussi GHLA-DR. + T cells of the Leu 3 (helper) type infiltrate the kidneys of patients with systemic lupus erythematosus. *Clin Exp Immunol.* (1985) 59:185–9.
33. Apostolidis SA, Crispín JC, Tsokos GC. IL-17-producing T cells in lupus nephritis. *Lupus.* (2011) 20:120–4. doi: 10.1177/0961203310389100
34. Hotta O, Yusa N, Ooyama M, Unno K, Furuta T, Taguma Y. Detection of urinary macrophages expressing the CD16 (Fc gamma RIII) molecule: a novel marker of acute inflammatory glomerular injury. *Kidney Int.* (1999) 55:1927–34. doi: 10.1046/j.1523-1755.1999.00431.x
35. Makino H, Sugiyama H, Yamasaki Y, Maeshima Y, Wada J, Kashihara N. Glomerular cell apoptosis in human lupus nephritis. *Virchows Arch.* (2003) 443:67–77. doi: 10.1007/s00428-003-0827-x
36. Mahajan A, Herrmann M, Muñoz LE. Clearance deficiency and cell death pathways: a model for the pathogenesis of SLE. *Front Immunol.* (2016) 7:35. doi: 10.3389/fimmu.2016.00035

9

Use of Mass Cytometry to Profile Human T Cell Exhaustion

Frances Winkler[1,2] *and Bertram Bengsch*[1,3*]

[1] Department of Medicine II, Gastroenterology, Hepatology, Endocrinology, and Infectious Diseases, Faculty of Medicine, University Medical Center Freiburg, Freiburg, Germany, [2] Faculty of Biology, University of Freiburg, Freiburg, Germany, [3] Signalling Research Centres BIOSS and CIBSS, University of Freiburg, Freiburg, Germany

***Correspondence:**
Bertram Bengsch
bertram.bengsch@uniklinik-freiburg.de

Mass cytometry has become an important technique for the deep analysis of single cell protein expression required for precision systems immunology. The ability to profile more than 40 markers per cell is particularly relevant for the differentiation of cell types for which low parametric characterization has proven difficult, such as exhausted $CD8^+$ T cells (T_{EX}). T_{EX} with limited effector function accumulate in many chronic infections and cancers and are subject to inhibitory signaling mediated by several immune checkpoints (e.g., PD-1). Of note, T_{EX} represent considerable targets for immune-stimulatory therapies and are beginning to be recognized as a major correlate of successful checkpoint blockade approaches targeting the PD-1 pathway. T_{EX} exhibit substantial functional, transcriptomic and epigenomic differences compared to canonical functional T cell subsets [such as naïve (T_N), effector (T_{EFF}) and memory T cells (T_{MEM})]. However, phenotypic distinction of T_{EX} from T_{EFF} and T_{MEM} can often be challenging since many molecules expressed by T_{EX} can also be expressed by effector and memory T cell populations. Moreover, significant heterogeneity of T_{EX} has been described, such as subpopulations of exhausted T cells with progenitor-progeny relationships or populations with different degrees of exhaustion or homeostatic potential that may directly inform about disease progression. In addition, T_{EX} subsets have essential clinical implications as they differentially respond to antiviral and checkpoint therapies. The precise assessment of T_{EX} thus requires a high-parametric analysis that accounts for differences to canonical T cell populations as well as for T_{EX} subset heterogeneity. In this review, we discuss how mass cytometry can be used to reveal the role of T_{EX} subsets in humans by combining exhaustion-directed phenotyping with functional profiling. Mass cytometry analysis of human T_{EX} populations is instrumental to gain a better understanding of T_{EX} in chronic infections and cancer. It has important implications for immune monitoring in therapeutic settings aiming to boost T cell immunity, such as during cancer immunotherapy.

Keywords: T cell differentiation, systems immunology, mass cytometry (CyTOF), T cell exhaustion, chronic infections, cancer, immune checkpoint blockade, immunotherapy

INTRODUCTION

Mass cytometry has become a transformative technology for human immune cell profiling. The use of purified metal isotopes as labels for specific antibodies to stain individual cells and detection of these label isotopes on ionized cells by time-of-flight mass spectroscopy allows the analysis of the protein expression of >40 insightful markers on single cells. The lack of relevant spectral overlap of metal isotopes is a major advantage over traditional fluorescence-based flow cytometry, in which multiplexing of reagents is frequently limited by the need to compensate for overlapping emission spectra of different fluorophores. The ability to integrate the information from more than 40 detection channels for single-cell profiling has been particularly valuable for comprehensive immune monitoring (i.e., analysis of many immune cell lineages) in the setting of translational studies that involve patient cohorts with limited sample access. However, in addition to this "horizontal" profiling approach, mass cytometry also represents a key tool suitable for deep "vertical" profiling of a given immune cell population and may reveal previously unknown heterogeneity within this population, such as complexity within $CD8^+$ T cells (1). In this review, we will discuss how deep immune profiling of exhausted $CD8^+$ T cells by mass cytometry has led to significant insights into their heterogeneity and role in pathophysiology across chronic infections and disease. Characterization of exhausted T cells using mass cytometry is of particular relevance in many immuno-oncologic trials that aim to enhance T cell function.

T CELL EXHAUSTION: BACKGROUND AND MAIN CONCEPTS

Exhausted T cells (T_{EX}) are increasingly recognized as a distinct T cell population with a key role in many chronic infections and cancer. T_{EX} were initially described in chronic viral infection, and many subsequent reports have highlighted the accumulation of T_{EX} in the context of ongoing bacterial and parasitic infection, as well as cancer and autoimmunity (2). T_{EX} are characterized by the co-expression of inhibitory receptors and reduced effector function preventing optimal control of viral infection or tumor progression. Targeting inhibitory signaling, such as by interference with inhibitory receptor PD-1 signaling or other immune checkpoints, can reinvigorate T_{EX} function and contribute to disease control or elimination. Consequently, T_{EX} have recently been identified as a major correlate of the clinical response of patients undergoing checkpoint therapy (3, 4), highlighting the need for better immune profiling of T_{EX} as a relevant biomarker for immune therapy trials.

Based on the reduced effector function due to inhibitory signaling in T_{EX} compared to canonical effector T cells (T_{EFF}), T_{EX} have been perceived long-term as a population of suppressed effector T cells according to a "loss-of-function" model (5–7). However, in recent years, it has become clear that the signals inducing T cell exhaustion following T cell activation can drive these cells dynamically into a distinct differentiation fate compared to T_{EFF} and memory T cells (T_{MEM}) that is characterized by massive changes in their metabolism, transcriptome, and epigenome (8–16) (**Figure 1**).

Exhausted T cells as well as functional effector and memory T cell differentiation are most thoroughly characterized in the Lymphocytic choriomeningitis virus (LCMV) models of acute and chronic viral infection. In these models, genetic differences between acute and chronic LCMV strains are minimal and immunodominant T cell epitopes are identical, facilitating cross-comparison of T cell phenotypes at the level of endogenous responses or by analysis of transferred virus-specific T cells sharing the same T cell receptor. During acute resolving viral infection, viral clearance after induction of functional effector T cells is followed by the establishment of a pool of memory T cells (17, 18) (**Figure 1**). In sharp contrast, antigen-specific T cells during chronic infection progressively develop major features of exhaustion, including the up-regulation of inhibitory receptor expression and functional impairment (e.g., consecutive loss of IL-2, TNF and IFN-γ production) (6, 7, 19, 20). While in the first week of chronic infection, the exhaustion program appears to remain flexible and can be altered, as evidenced after transfer of T cells into non-chronically infected hosts, exhaustion appears to become more fixed following the second week of infection (21, 22). Notably, at later time points, the global differentiation program of T_{EX} assessed on the transcriptional and epigenetic level remains stable even after checkpoint blockade intervention and functional reinvigoration (12).

CHALLENGES FOR THE ASSESSMENT OF EXHAUSTED T CELLS IN HUMANS

Many insights into T_{EX} have been obtained by the study of antigen-specific T cells in chronic infection and cancer, and multiplexed tetramer analysis together with surface and intracellular markers by mass cytometry has allowed important insights into antigen-specific T cells (1, 23). Identification of T_{EX} without prior knowledge of antigen specificity has remained challenging and is a major obstacle for immune phenotyping in human disease—in particular in cancer—where many tumor antigens especially neoantigens are unknown and tools for assessment of antigen-specific T cell populations are limited. Moreover, established models for T cell differentiation in humans based on markers such as CCR7/CD62L, CD45RA/CD45RO, or CD27/CD28 that allow assessment of naïve T cells (T_N), T_{EFF}, and T_{MEM} and additional subpopulations (e.g., central and effector memory T cells) cannot reliably distinguish T_{EX} from the effector or effector memory T cell phenotype (24). A likely explanation is that T_{EX}, similar to T_{EFF}, initially undergo T cell activation programs that include the downregulation of markers of naïvety (such as lymph node homing markers CCR7 and CD62L or preferential CD45RA to CD45RO alternative splicing linked to activation and memory programs), while activation markers, such as CD38 are also induced.

Many investigators have therefore turned to the profiling of inhibitory receptors with a relevant role in T_{EX} biology, such as PD-1 (alone or in combination with other inhibitory receptors such as CTLA-4, Tim-3, Lag-3, 2B4, CD160, TIGIT, and others) for the assessment of exhausted T cells in chronic infections and cancer (20, 25–35). However, it has become clear that those inhibitory receptors can also be expressed by functional effector T cells and may also be present on memory T cell populations and therefore lack specificity (36–39). Moreover, heterogeneous subpopulations of T_{EX} exist for which progenitor-progeny relationships or partial expression of memory-related programs has been described that present further challenges

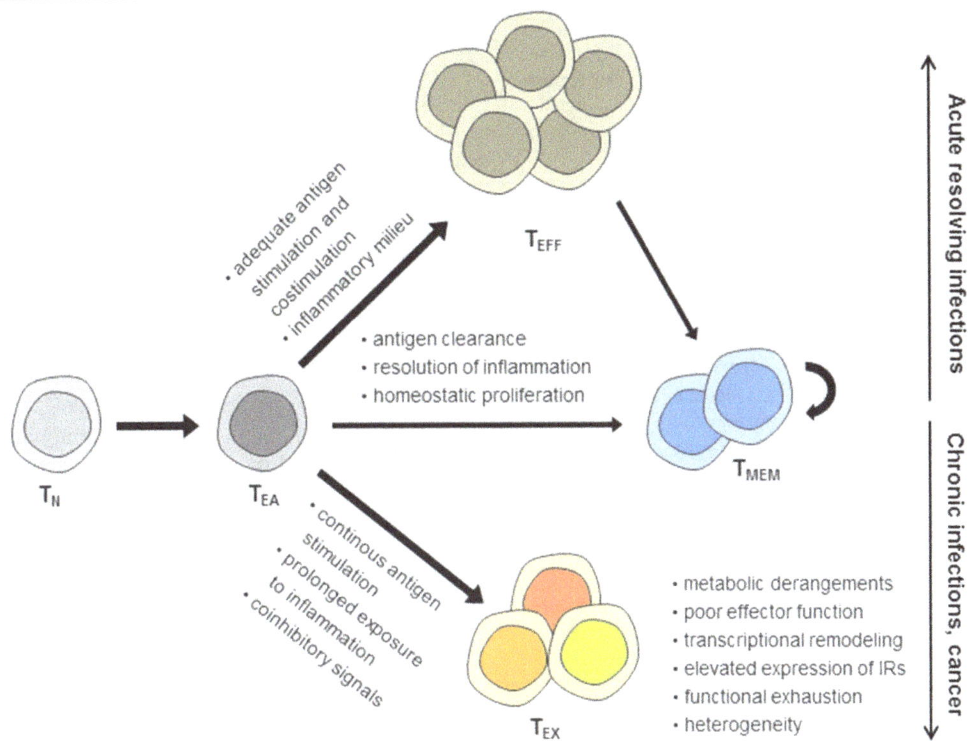

FIGURE 1 | Model of post-thymic CD8$^+$ T cell differentiation. According to this model, after activation of naïve T cells (T_N) during priming, early activated effector T cells (T_{EA}) receive signals driving functional differentiation to effector T cells (T_{EFF}) and memory T cells (T_{MEM}) depending on the recognition of antigen, costimulation, and the inflammatory milieu. In contrast, persistent antigen stimulation, reduced costimulation in the presence of coinhibitory signals and prolonged exposure to inflammatory cues are main drivers of the differentiation toward the exhausted T cell (T_{EX}) fate, including an up-regulation of inhibitory receptors (IRs).

for phenotypic characterization (40–44). Nevertheless, while no single phenotypic marker can reliably assess T_{EX} in humans, the utility of combining several inhibitory receptors for the analysis of differences in antigen-specific exhausted T cells suggests that a combinatorial strategy integrating several exhaustion markers might overcome the limitations for immune profiling.

SELECTION STRATEGY FOR SUITABLE MARKERS TO IDENTIFY T_{EX} USING MASS CYTOMETRY

Markers convenient for the identification of T_{EX} and discrimination from T_N, T_{EFF}, and T_{MEM} cells display different levels of expression on T_{EX} compared to these canonical functional T cell populations and across several disease models. To identify such appropriate exhaustion-specific markers, differences in the transcriptional and epigenomic programs between canonical T cell populations and exhausted T cells from the well-controlled LCMV model can be harnessed as specific candidate genes.

Following such an approach, sets of epigenomically regulated exhaustion-specific genes have been recently identified, including 313 genes specifically up-regulated in T_{EX} compared to T_N, T_{EFF}, and T_{MEM} that displayed higher gene expression by transcriptome analysis and concomitant changes in enhancer accessibility (45). Moreover, 182 genes down-regulated in T_{EX} were identified that were specifically suppressed on a transcriptional level and lacked accessibility of adjacent enhancers. These exhaustion-specific genes identified in the LCMV infection model were thus predicted as sufficient markers of T_{EX}. The authors then validated individual genes by comparing them for their enrichment in other murine and human settings of infection and cancer, for which T cell exhaustion has been described. Specific genes for exhaustion-directed immune profiling with strong enrichment of gene expression in multiple settings of exhaustion for which suitable reagents were available for cytometry were then selected for further analysis (**Table 1**).

This approach confirmed several markers of exhausted T cells frequently used for the profiling of T_{EX}, such as inhibitory receptors PD-1, 2B4, Lag-3, TIGIT, or transcription factor Eomes. Interestingly, CD38 and CD39, which are also frequently used as activation markers due to their induction on T_{EFF} cells, displayed further exhaustion-specific up-regulation and enhancer changes compared with functional T cell populations. These observations suggest that the interpretation as activation markers indicative for T_{EFF} cells may need to be reevaluated. Furthermore, this analytic approach also identified additional exhaustion markers induced on T_{EX}, such as surface proteins CD7, CXCR5, cytotoxic molecule granzyme K or transcription factors Helios and TOX, many of which are also found enriched

TABLE 1 | Exhaustion markers for T_{EX} profiling.

Exhaustion markers	Predicted expression vs. T_N T_{EFF} T_{MEM}	Functional role	Minimal exhaustion panel
2B4	UP	Co-regulatory receptor	X
Amphiregulin	UP	Cytokine	
CCL3	UP	Chemokine	
CCR7	DN	Chemokine receptor	
CD38	UP	Ectoenzyme	
CD39	UP	Ectoenzyme	X
CD7	UP	Co-regulatory receptor	
CD73	DN	Ectoenzyme	
CD127	DN	Interleukin receptor	X
CTLA-4	UP	Co-regulatory receptor	X
CXCL10	UP	Chemokine	
CXCR5	UP	Chemokine receptor	X
Eomes	UP	Transcription factor	X
Granzyme K	UP	Cytotoxic molecule	
Helios	UP	Transcription factor	
IFN-γ	ns	Cytokine	
IL-2	DN	Cytokine	
IL-10	UP	Cytokine	
IL-21	UP	Cytokine	
Lag-3	UP	Co-regulatory receptor	
PD-1	UP	Co-regulatory receptor	X
Ptger2	UP	Prostaglandin receptor	
TCF1	DN	Transcription factor	X
TIGIT	UP	Co-regulatory receptor	X
TNF	ns	Cytokine	X
TOX	UP	Transcription factor	X
XCL-1	UP	Chemokine	

Markers were selected based on exhaustion-specific expression patterns using transcriptomic and epigenomic profiling and validated using mass cytometry. Markers associated with T cell exhaustion, their predicted expression on T_{EX} compared to other cell populations, their functional role as well as their utility for a minimal exhaustion panel is noted. Moreover, cytokines required for the assessment of T_{EX} function are included.

in tumor-infiltrating lymphocytes by single-cell transcriptomics (46, 47). In agreement with the high levels of TOX on exhausted T cell populations, TOX was recently identified as a master regulator of exhaustion required for the longevity and persistence of exhausted T cells that acts via epigenetic mechanisms facilitating the expression of exhaustion-related gene programs (48, 49). In addition to these novel markers of T_{EX}, it has to be noted that other molecules which are also frequently expressed by T_{EX} were not identified as exhaustion-specific candidates by this approach, including inhibitory receptors Tim-3, KLRG1, CD160, or transcription factor T-bet. This was due to lack of significant differences to canonical T cell subsets at the level of gene expression or associated enhancer changes. Similarly, additional immunoregulatory molecules such as CD72 and CD100 which have been previously described as linked to T cell exhaustion have not been identified by this pipeline, suggesting reduced specificity across T cell populations or context-dependent roles (50). It has to be noted that in this analysis of the specific expression patterns on exhausted cells, individual "exhaustion-specific" molecules can still be expressed to some degree on other T cell subsets (although with a significantly different expression level). Moreover, this strategy also predicted down-regulation of markers associated with naïve and/or memory T cells, such as CCR7, CD73, CD127 and transcription factor TCF-1 on T_{EX} (**Table 1**). The integration of a high number of phenotypic "exhaustion-specific" markers into mass cytometry analysis is expected to allow a better discrimination of T_{EX} populations from T_N, T_{EFF}, or T_{MEM}.

FUNCTIONAL ASSESSMENT OF T_{EX} ON A SINGLE-CELL OR POPULATION LEVEL

Functional impairment is a key characteristic of exhausted T cells. Indeed, the term exhaustion was initially used to describe complete loss of effector function and disappearance of the antigen-specific $CD8^+$ T cell response (5, 51). However, it has since become clear that in comparison to functional effector and memory T cells, T_{EX} frequently experience a more gradual loss of effector function that can range from mild impairments in antiviral cytokine production to complete deletion. Typically, mildly exhausted cells exhibit impaired ability to produce IL-2, followed by loss of TNF production in more severe exhaustion, while the ability to produce IFN-γ is frequently maintained and lost usually only in severe exhaustion (52). Reduced expression of anti-apoptotic molecules (i.e., Bcl2) and higher levels of pro-apoptotic Bim have been reported in T_{EX} and might be linked to a pre-apoptotic phenotype in more severely exhausted cells (53–55). Moreover, reduced cytotoxicity and impaired proliferation have been announced for T_{EX}, and successful reinvigoration by checkpoint blockade is frequently measured using metrics of cell cycle activity and proliferation (7). However, it has to be noted that T cell exhaustion is not simply a "loss-of-function" phenotype affecting all T cell functions. On the contrary, higher induction of some chemokines, such as CCL3 and XCL-1, and higher message of other cytokines, such as IL-10 or IL-21, by T_{EX} has been reported (8, 45, 56).

Mass cytometry has been instrumental in the comprehensive characterization of T_{EX} function. For example, differences in the cytotoxic program of T_{EX} with an increased expression of granzyme K, but reduced granzyme B and perforin can be readily assessed in combination with phenotypic profiling (57). Similarly, cell cycle activity assessed by Ki-67 combined with exhaustion marker phenotyping has been pivotal in mass cytometry analysis of responding T_{EX} during checkpoint therapies (3). Nevertheless, the unbiased per-cell assessment of complex exhaustion-related patterns of impaired cytokine production with phenotypic analysis has remained challenging. For example, analyses focusing on the ability of T cells to express effector cytokines frequently struggle to differentiate between cells that never expressed those molecules (i.e., antigen-naïve T cells) or those that lost expression (including T_{EX}). To address these challenges, the characteristic impairment of polyfunctionality with regards to cytokine (e.g., IFN-γ, TNF, IL-2) but increased chemokine production (e.g., CCL3/4, XCL-1) can be used to rate individual T cells for their functional chemokine/cytokine exhaustion profile on a single-cell level using a function-passed exhaustion score. Combined with a comprehensive phenotypic exhaustion profiling possible through the use of mass cytometry, the integration of T_{EX} function as a separate metric of T cell exhaustion was able to reliably discriminate T_{EX} from T_{EFF}, T_N, and T_{MEM} (45). The combination of high-parametric functional and phenotypic exhaustion profiling may thus represent a helpful tool for the assessment of individual T_{EX} populations but also for the general degree of $CD8^+$ T cell immune dysfunction in chronic disease.

IDENTIFICATION OF CLINICALLY RELEVANT HIGH-DIMENSIONAL T_{EX} PHENOTYPES USING MASS CYTOMETRY

The integration of a larger set of exhaustion markers in mass cytometry panels creates novel challenges in data evaluation. In flow cytometry-based studies with few exhaustion markers, data evaluation relies heavily on manual gating and boolean analysis of inhibitory receptor co-expression or polyfunctionality (e.g., using SPICE software analysis) (29, 58, 59). These approaches remain valuable for the assessment of T_{EX} using mass cytometry, but have disadvantages compared to bioinformatics algorithm-aided pipelines suitable for the higher data dimensionality generated by mass cytometry. Several bioinformatic strategies have been developed that allow more intuitive visualization of the high-dimensional data using dimension reduction approaches [most prominently based on visualization of "t stochastic neighborhood embedding," tSNE (60)], and cluster identification strategies in high-dimensional data [e.g., SPADE (61), FlowSOM (62), PhenoGraph (63) and many more] or trajectory inferences that are reviewed elsewhere (64–66). For example, tSNE can be used to generate an "exhaustion map" by calculating a two-dimensional representation of the high-dimensional complexity of T_{EX} phenotypes based on exhaustion marker expression (**Figure 2**). This approach helps in the identification of T_{EX} heterogeneity and points toward differences of the exhaustion landscape in clinical settings (**Figure 2**), including the detection of specific populations of exhausted T cells enriched in the tumor microenvironment (45). Moreover, one-dimensional tSNE implementation ("OneSense") has been used to reduce high-dimensional exhaustion phenotypes to a single parameter and compare them with other sets of marker categories (such as "function") (67, 68). However, despite the advantages of tSNE-based analysis and high accuracy regarding local neighborhood relationships, tSNE performs different transformations on different regions of a map, resulting in possible challenges regarding interpretation of distance relationships on a tSNE map. Thus, use of tSNE for the discovery of discrete high-dimensional clusters as a crucial correlate of subsets with distinct biology is challenging. Other dimension reduction strategies with manifold approximation, such as uMAP, may address some of these limitations, but loss of information inherent to dimension-reduction strategies cannot be completely avoided (69). As a consequence, cluster identification based on the complete high-dimensional data is often preferred. For example, 25 high-dimensional clusters of $CD8^+$ T cells were identified using PhenoGraph analysis based on the analysis of exhaustion markers in a large and diverse cohort of patients with chronic HIV infection, lung cancer and healthy controls (45). These clusters often projected to discrete regions of a tSNE exhaustion map that was calculated using the same exhaustion parameters but also displayed cluster affiliations that were not obvious from a tSNE map (**Figure 2**). Clearly, such an exhaustion marker-based clustering approach will also identify functional T cells, such as T_N, T_{EFF}, or T_{MEM} cells, but will have increased granularity for T_{EX} subset identification.

The characterization of discrete T cell clusters in high-dimensional "exhaustion data space" thus serves as a foundation that requires further detailed analysis of their functional and clinical role. In particular, a combination with functional profiling following short term stimulation is valuable to assess the extent of cellular exhaustion and can be used to determine the single-cell chemokine or cytokine pattern necessary for calculation of a "functional exhaustion score" discussed above. Such a functional profiling combined with a scaffold of phenotypic markers allowed appropriate mapping of chemokine/cytokine functionality to the high-dimensional exhaustion clusters, suggesting that 9–12 of the 25 phenotypically defined discrete $CD8^+$ T cell subpopulations fit functional properties of T cell exhaustion (45).

Several of the identified exhausted clusters enriched in severe disease contexts, such as severe HIV infection with possible AIDS, or in the tumor microenvironment of lung cancer patients. Phenotypically, these disease-associated exhausted T cells displayed co-expression of exhaustion-specific receptors such as PD-1, CD38 and a transcription factor signature characterized by high Eomes and TOX but low TCF-1 expression (**Figure 3**). Interestingly, disease-associated T_{EX} in chronic infection were further characterized by co-expression of inhibitory receptors TIGIT and 2B4 (as well as some KLRG1 and CD160) while in cancer, T_{EX} more frequently exhibited higher expression of CTLA-4, Lag-3, and CD39. These data suggest a conserved biology of exhausted T cells in chronic infection and cancer but also highlight specific differences in exhaustion programs with potentially large translational relevance. For example, the altered co-expression patterns of immuno-regulatory molecules on different T_{EX} populations across different disease entities or even across different stages of disease suggest that the therapeutic efficacy of combination therapies (i.e., combined

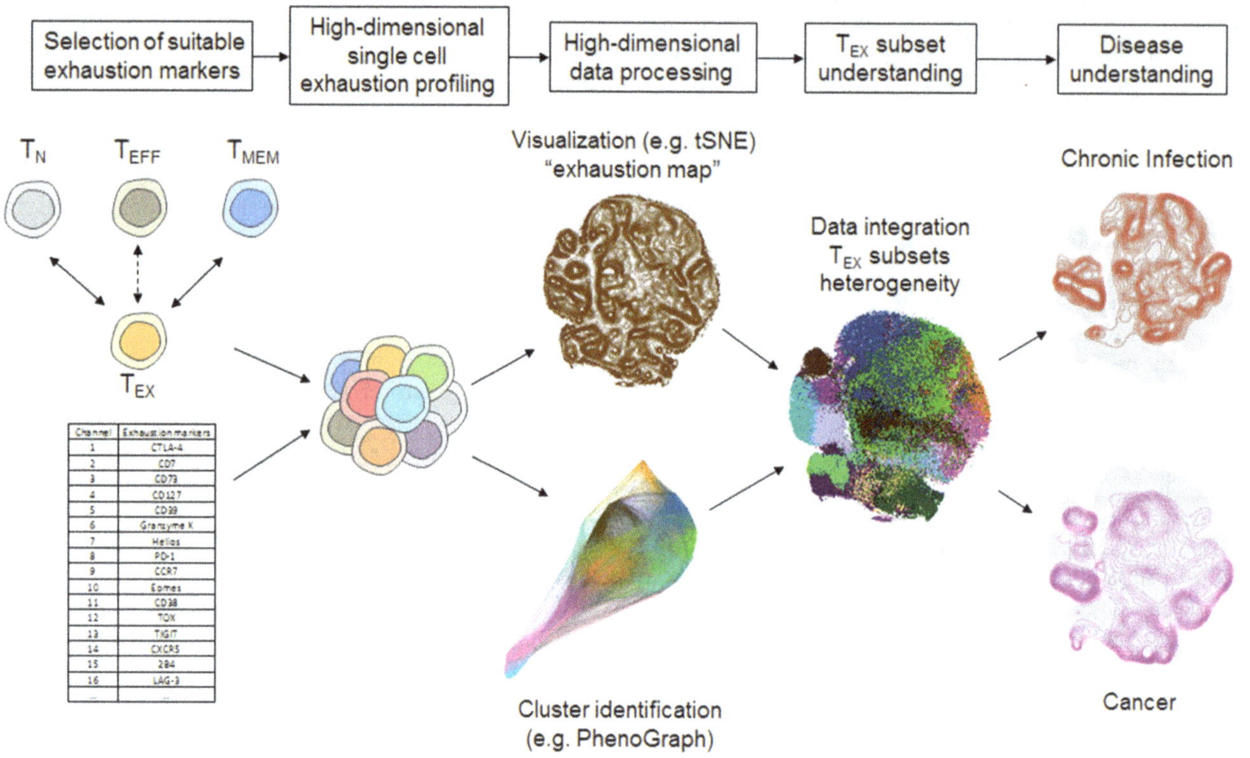

FIGURE 2 | Systems immunology approach for T_{EX} characterization using mass cytometry. Selection of suitable exhaustion markers able to differentiate T_{EX} from T_{EFF} and T_{MEM} such as by transcriptomic or epigenomic profiling is a critical step for T_{EX}-directed immune profiling using mass cytometry. High-dimensional analysis of T_{EX} provides further insights into the heterogeneity of T_{EX} that can be unraveled by a bioinformatics pipeline including cluster identification and dimension reduction strategies (i.e., tSNE, Phenograph) that provide detailed overview about the exhaustion landscape. Detailed T_{EX} subset profiling provides the basis for understanding the heterogeneity of T_{EX} and their involvement in different disease settings, such as chronic infection and cancer. Data-driven visualizations in this figure were computed based on a dataset published in Bengsch et al. (12).

targeting of PD-1 and CTLA-4) could vary according to the T_{EX} subset composition. Importantly, not all subsets of functionally exhausted T cells enrich with disease progression. For example, subsets with expression of PD-1 and co-expression of CD127, TCF-1, and CXCR5 were found enriched in HIV patients with relatively good disease control (i.e., high CD4 counts, CD4/CD8 ratio and low viral load) and these "health-associated" T_{EX} subsets were also detected in large amounts in tumor-surrounding macroscopically non-infiltrated lung compared to the tumor tissue.

These T_{EX} subpopulations identified by high-dimensional analysis using mass cytometry are in agreement with reports about severely exhausted T cells co-expressing several inhibitory receptors being linked to severe disease in chronic infection and cancer in HIV, HCV, HBV, and melanoma patients (29–32, 70–75). They are also in agreement with findings of progenitor and progeny relationships within exhausted T cell populations based on PD-1, Eomes and T-bet expression and the enrichment of T_{EX} populations with high homeostatic potential expressing TCF-1 and CD127 in scenarios of disease control (e.g., clearance of HCV infection) (40, 44, 76). Moreover, T_{EX} expressing CXCR5 have been linked to better control of HIV infection and are thought to constitute a major subset responding to checkpoint therapy (41, 42, 77). Precursor populations of exhausted tumor-infiltrating T cells with higher TCF-1 and CXCR5 expression were also identified to be linked to better clinical outcomes after checkpoint blockade therapy (78).

Thus, mass cytometry is perfectly suited for the interrogation of the clinically significant T_{EX} heterogeneity. A model of T_{EX} heterogeneity including potential lineage relationships and the suggested markers required for minimal T_{EX} immunoprofiling via mass cytometry is displayed in **Figure 3** and **Table 1**.

T_{EX} PROFILING BY MASS CYTOMETRY: INSIGHTS FOR CHECKPOINT THERAPY MONITORING

T_{EX} are emerging as a central correlate and useful biomarker of successful immune checkpoint blockade therapies. In clinical trials with patients receiving checkpoint therapies, special attention has to be directed to immune-profiling panels, as therapeutic antibodies and staining reagents may compete for the same epitope. While combination stainings with secondary antibodies against the checkpoint reagents are established, these remain to provide challenges for bioinformatic analysis. Moreover, transient permeabilization protocols frequently used for intracellular barcoding in mass cytometry trials can reduce

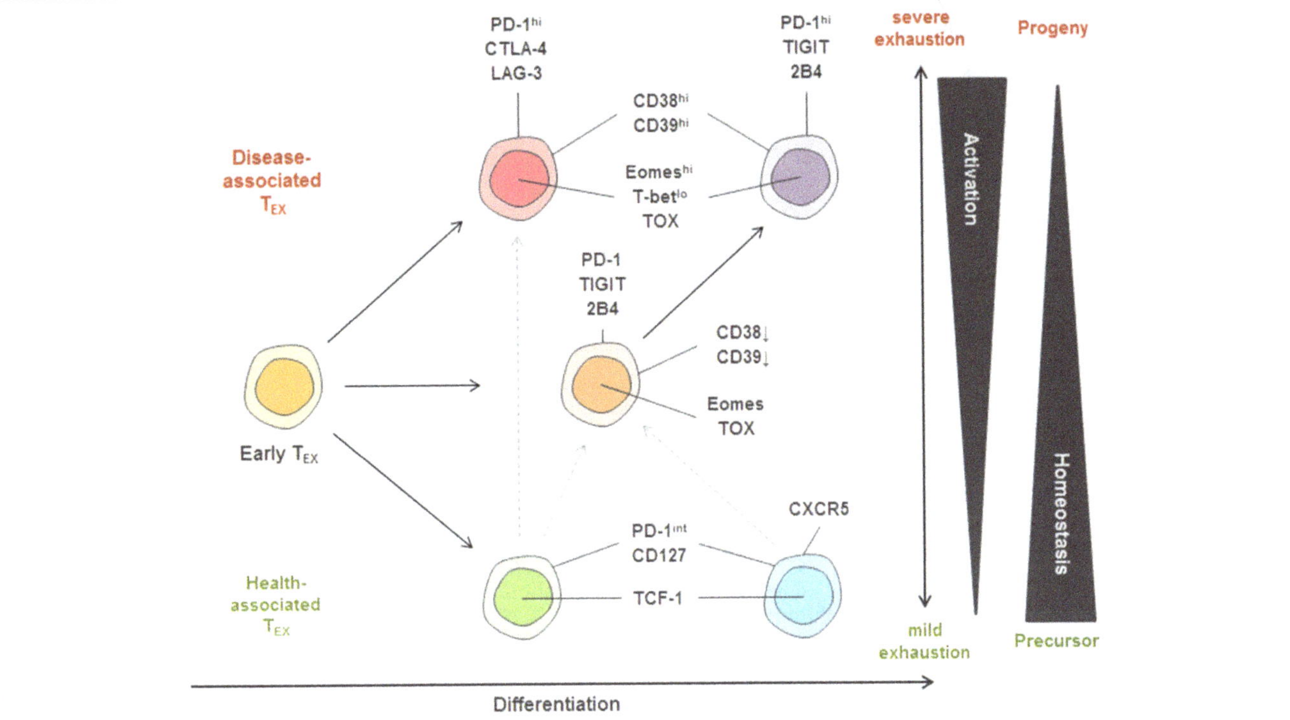

FIGURE 3 | Model of T_{EX} heterogeneity and key markers linked to individual subsets. Within the pool of exhausted T cells, three major trajectories of T_{EX} subsets are proposed. Early T_{EX} can give rise to a pool of disease-associated or health-associated T_{EX} that massively differ in their activation program as well as in their transcriptional signature, while between both extremes, a balanced pool of differentiated T_{EX} can be observed. One differentiation trajectory leads to populations with high homeostatic potential that are identified in settings of disease control ("health-associated T_{EX}") and can have memory-like features such as high TCF-1 and CD127 expression. Strong expression of activation markers also found on T_{EFF} cells (e.g., CD38, CD39) and co-expression of many inhibitory receptors (IRs) is a key feature of T_{EX} populations identified in progressive disease in chronic infection and cancer. According to this model, T_{EX} with recent history of activation and severe exhaustion after priming express a different set of IRs (e.g., PD-1, CTLA-4, Lag-3) more frequently observed in cancer compared to highly activated T cells arising in many chronic infections. These highly activated T cells in chronic infection are thought to arise from an intermediate trajectory of T_{EX} (expressing e.g., PD-1, 2B4, TIGIT) after encountering additional antigen stimulation and inhibitory signals. Furthermore, a precursor-progenitor relationship between health- and disease-associated T_{EX} important for cancer immunotherapy has been described, and is indicated by the dotted lines. The different T_{EX} trajectories also reflect differential transcriptional programming by varying T-bet, TCF-1, TOX and Eomes expression.

anti-PD-1 staining. Despite these challenges, mass cytometry has been successfully applied in multiple studies profiling $CD8^+$ T cells. Reinvigoration of T_{EX} compared to tumor mass was identified as a major correlate of the clinical response of patients with malign melanoma receiving checkpoint therapy with anti-PD-1 antibodies (3). Similar observations have been made using flow cytometry and in patients with non-small cell lung cancer (4). In a study comparing the differential effects of PD-1 and CTLA-4 checkpoint therapies, PD-1 blockade was found to preferentially induce a response in the $CD8^+$ T_{EX} compartment, while anti-CTLA-4 therapy caused more profound changes in $CD4^+$ T cells (79). These reports also highlight the utility of combining T_{EX}-directed panels with markers focusing on other immune cell populations. Indeed, further evidence for the on-treatment role of T_{EX} reinvigoration during anti-PD-1 checkpoint blockade therapies came from a study that also identified a pre-treatment biomarker for checkpoint response on the level of a $CD14^+$ $CD16^-$ $HLA\text{-}DR^+$ monocyte population (80). However, improved and more focused exhaustion-directed profiling of the heterogeneity of T_{EX} subsets will be required for a detailed understanding of T_{EX} dynamics during checkpoint therapies and personalized medicine approaches for combination therapies.

SUMMARY AND OUTLOOK

The inability to discriminate T_{EX} from T_{EFF} and T_{MEM} using conventional phenotyping approaches has been a longstanding problem, preventing optimal monitoring and understanding of the relevance of T_{EX} in disease. The use of high-parametric mass cytometry has been instrumental in addressing this issue and advanced the characterization of T_{EX}. The combinatorial information from several exhaustion markers is required to distinguish T_{EX} from T_{EFF} and T_{MEM} and has also informed our understanding of the heterogeneity of T_{EX}. One advantage of mass cytometry—the ability to integrate the higher parametric expression profile of T_{EX} with readouts for functional profiling allows the fine characterization of T_{EX} subpopulations and their involvement in human diseases. Induction of several molecular programs linked to recent T cell activation remains a shared feature of many T_{EX} populations with effector T cells (e.g., CD38, CD39, PD-1), while programs of homeostasis and access to anatomic niches can be shared by other T_{EX} populations (including those linked to disease control) with memory T cells. Heterogeneous T_{EX} subsets with different clinical roles have now been described in several translational settings of human chronic infection and cancer and are implied in differential responsiveness to immune checkpoint blockade.

Other strategies that allow an in-depth profiling of the heterogeneity of exhausted T cell populations have been described, such as scRNA-Seq, which allows the analysis of T cell transcriptomes with single cell resolution. However, currently, these approaches have several limitations over the described mass cytometry approach as they are limited by the limited sensitivity for lowly expressed genes; low cell numbers that can be practically analyzed and therefore limited ability to identify rare populations and limited scaling toward cohort analysis; lack of information on protein expression missing potential post-transcriptional regulation; and, importantly, lack of testing for T cell function. It is further unclear whether excessively larger datasets of mRNA transcripts on a single cell level will reveal more relevant heterogeneity of T_{EX} populations, as the profiling approach outlined above already was designed to maximize utilization of markers informative for differences between T_{EX} and functional T cell subsets. Of note, the combinatorial complexity of high dimensional data generated during immunome analysis by mass cytometry is different from other omics approaches. For example, simultaneous analysis of mass cytometric immune profiling together with transcriptome, microbiome, proteome and metabolome analysis during pregnancy indicated that the mass cytometry dataset was more informative based on modularity analysis (as measured by the number of principal components needed to account for 90% variance of each dataset) compared to the other omics datasets assessing significantly larger numbers of parameters (81).

To date the most detailed profiling of T_{EX} has been performed in murine models of chronic infection or cancer. With detailed resolution of T_{EX} heterogeneity in humans now accessible through the use of specialized mass cytometry analysis, more detailed identification of T_{EX} features associated with specific types of diseases and anatomical locations that will guide understanding of changes in T_{EX} cell populations in chronic infections, cancer and even autoimmunity is expected. The expression of many exhaustion-related proteins involved in many immuno-regulatory pathways amenable to therapeutic intervention also suggests that T_{EX} profiling might be required for adequate selection of combination therapies and could become indispensable for the rational design of personalized therapeutic treatments.

In sum, deep immune profiling of T_{EX} using mass cytometry is expected to provide further insights into the biology underlying this special T cell differentiation stage and its role in pathogenesis and response to immune therapies in cancer, viral infection and autoimmunity.

AUTHOR CONTRIBUTIONS

FW and BB conceived and wrote the manuscript, revising it critically for important intellectual content.

ACKNOWLEDGMENTS

We thank the members of the Bengsch, Thimme, and Wherry labs for the fruitful discussions. We thank F. Gherardini for the help with Phenograph visualization.

REFERENCES

1. Ahn E, Araki K, Hashimoto M, Li W, Riley JL, Cheung J, et al. Role of PD-1 during effector CD8 T cell differentiation. *Proc Natl Acad Sci USA.* (2018) 115:4749–54. doi: 10.1073/pnas.1718217115
2. Alfei F, Kanev K, Hofmann M, Wu M, Ghoneim HE, Roelli P, et al. TOX reinforces the phenotype and longevity of exhausted T cells in chronic viral infection. *Nature.* (2019) 571:265–9. doi: 10.1038/s41586-019-1326-9
3. Amir El AD, Davis KL, Tadmor MD, Simonds EF, Levine JH, Bendall SC, et al. viSNE enables visualization of high dimensional single-cell data and reveals phenotypic heterogeneity of leukemia. *Nat Biotechnol.* (2013) 31:545–52. doi: 10.1038/nbt.2594
4. Angelosanto JM, Blackburn SD, Crawford A, Wherry EJ. Progressive loss of memory T cell potential and commitment to exhaustion during chronic viral infection. *J Virol.* (2012) 86:8161–70. doi: 10.1128/JVI.00889-12
5. Appay V, Van Lier RA, Sallusto F, Roederer M. Phenotype and function of human T lymphocyte subsets: consensus and issues. *Cytometry A.* (2008) 73:975–83. doi: 10.1002/cyto.a.20643
6. Baitsch L, Baumgaertner P, Devevre E, Raghav SK, Legat A, Barba L, et al. Exhaustion of tumor-specific CD8(+) T cells in metastases from melanoma patients. *J Clin Invest.* (2011) 121:2350–60. doi: 10.1172/JCI46102
7. Barber DL, Wherry EJ, Masopust D, Zhu B, Allison JP, Sharpe AH, et al. Restoring function in exhausted CD8 T cells during chronic viral infection. *Nature.* (2006) 439:682–7. doi: 10.1038/nature04444
8. Becht E, Mcinnes L, Healy J, Dutertre CA, Kwok IWH, Ng LG, et al. Dimensionality reduction for visualizing single-cell data using UMAP. *Nat Biotechnol.* (2018) 37:38–44. doi: 10.1038/nbt.4314
9. Bengsch B, Johnson AL, Kurachi M, Odorizzi PM, Pauken KE, Attanasio J, et al. Bioenergetic insufficiencies due to metabolic alterations regulated by the inhibitory receptor PD-1 are an early driver of CD8(+) T cell exhaustion. *Immunity.* (2016) 45:358–73. doi: 10.1016/j.immuni.2016.07.008
10. Bengsch B, Martin B, Thimme R. Restoration of HBV-specific CD8+ T cell function by PD-1 blockade in inactive carrier patients is linked to T cell differentiation. *J Hepatol.* (2014) 61:1212–9. doi: 10.1016/j.jhep.2014.07.005
11. Bengsch B, Ohtani T, Herati RS, Bovenschen N, Chang KM, Wherry EJ. Deep immune profiling by mass cytometry links human T and NK cell differentiation and cytotoxic molecule expression patterns. *J Immunol Methods.* (2018) 453:3–10. doi: 10.1016/j.jim.2017.03.009

12. Bengsch B, Ohtani T, Khan O, Setty M, Manne S, O'brien S, et al. (2018). Epigenomic-guided mass cytometry profiling reveals disease-specific features of exhausted CD8 T cells. *Immunity.* 48, 1029–45.e1025. doi: 10.1016/j.immuni.2018.04.026
13. Bengsch B, Seigel B, Ruhl M, Timm J, Kuntz M, Blum HE, et al. Coexpression of PD-1, 2B4, CD160 and KLRG1 on exhausted HCV-specific CD8+ T cells is linked to antigen recognition and T cell differentiation. *PLoS Pathog.* (2010) 6:e1000947. doi: 10.1371/journal.ppat.1000947
14. Betts MR, Nason MC, West SM, De Rosa SC, Migueles SA, Abraham J, et al. HIV nonprogressors preferentially maintain highly functional HIV-specific CD8+ T cells. *Blood.* (2006) 107:4781–9. doi: 10.1182/blood-2005-12-4818
15. Blackburn SD, Shin H, Haining WN, Zou T, Workman CJ, Polley A, et al. Coregulation of CD8+ T cell exhaustion by multiple inhibitory receptors during chronic viral infection. *Nat Immunol.* (2009) 10:29–37. doi: 10.1038/ni.1679
16. Boni C, Fisicaro P, Valdatta C, Amadei B, Di Vincenzo P, Giuberti T, et al. Characterization of hepatitis B virus (HBV)-specific T-cell dysfunction in chronic HBV infection. *J Virol.* (2007) 81:4215–25. doi: 10.1128/JVI.02844-06
17. Brooks DG, Ha SJ, Elsaesser H, Sharpe AH, Freeman GJ, Oldstone MB. IL-10 and PD-L1 operate through distinct pathways to suppress T-cell activity during persistent viral infection. *Proc Natl Acad Sci USA.* (2008) 105:20428–33. doi: 10.1073/pnas.0811139106
18. Buggert M, Tauriainen J, Yamamoto T, Frederiksen J, Ivarsson MA, Michaelsson J, et al. T-bet and Eomes are differentially linked to the exhausted phenotype of CD8+ T cells in HIV infection. *PLoS Pathog.* (2014) 10:e1004251. doi: 10.1371/journal.ppat.1004251
19. Cheng Y, Wong MT, Van Der Maaten L, Newell EW. Categorical analysis of human T cell heterogeneity with one-dimensional soli-expression by nonlinear stochastic embedding. *J Immunol.* (2016) 196:924–32. doi: 10.4049/jimmunol.1501928
20. Cheng Y, Zhu YO, Becht E, Aw P, Chen J, Poidinger M, et al. Multifactorial heterogeneity of virus-specific T cells and association with the progression of human chronic hepatitis B infection. *Sci Immunol.* (2019) 4:eaau6905. doi: 10.1126/sciimmunol.aau6905
21. Chevrier S, Levine JH, Zanotelli VRT, Silina K, Schulz D, Bacac M, et al. An immune atlas of clear cell renal cell carcinoma. *Cell.* (2017) 169:736–49.e718. doi: 10.1016/j.cell.2017.04.016
22. Correa-Rocha R, Lopez-Abente J, Gutierrez C, Perez-Fernandez VA, Prieto-Sanchez A, Moreno-Guillen S, et al. CD72/CD100 and PD-1/PD-L1 markers are increased on T and B cells in HIV-1+ viremic individuals, and CD72/CD100 axis is correlated with T-cell exhaustion. *PLoS ONE.* (2018) 13:e0203419. doi: 10.1371/journal.pone.0203419
23. Day CL, Kaufmann DE, Kiepiela P, Brown JA, Moodley ES, Reddy S, et al. PD-1 expression on HIV-specific T cells is associated with T-cell exhaustion and disease progression. *Nature.* (2006) 443:350–4. doi: 10.1038/nature05115
24. Doering TA, Crawford A, Angelosanto JM, Paley MA, Ziegler CG, Wherry EJ. Network analysis reveals centrally connected genes and pathways involved in CD8+ T cell exhaustion versus memory. *Immunity.* (2012) 37:1130–44. doi: 10.1016/j.immuni.2012.08.021
25. Duraiswamy J, Ibegbu CC, Masopust D, Miller JD, Araki K, Doho GH, et al. Phenotype, function, and gene expression profiles of programmed death-1(hi) CD8 T cells in healthy human adults. *J Immunol.* (2011) 186:4200–12. doi: 10.4049/jimmunol.1001783
26. Fourcade J, Sun Z, Benallaoua M, Guillaume P, Luescher IF, Sander C, et al. Upregulation of Tim-3 and PD-1 expression is associated with tumor antigen-specific CD8+ T cell dysfunction in melanoma patients. *J Exp Med.* (2010) 207:2175–86. doi: 10.1084/jem.20100637
27. Fuller MJ, Zajac AJ. Ablation of CD8 and CD4 T cell responses by high viral loads. *J Immunol.* (2003) 170:477–86. doi: 10.4049/jimmunol.170.1.477
28. Gehring AJ, Ho ZZ, Tan AT, Aung MO, Lee KH, Tan KC, et al. Profile of tumor antigen-specific CD8 T cells in patients with hepatitis B virus-related hepatocellular carcinoma. *Gastroenterology.* (2009) 137:682–90. doi: 10.1053/j.gastro.2009.04.045
29. Ghaemi MS, Digiulio DB, Contrepois K, Callahan B, Ngo TTM, Lee-Mcmullen B, et al. Multiomics modeling of the immunome, transcriptome, microbiome, proteome and metabolome adaptations during human pregnancy. *Bioinformatics.* (2019) 35:95–103. doi: 10.1093/bioinformatics/bty537
30. Ghoneim HE, Fan Y, Moustaki A, Abdelsamed HA, Dash P, Dogra P, et al. *De novo* epigenetic programs inhibit PD-1 blockade-mediated T cell rejuvenation. *Cell.* (2017) 170:142–57.e19. doi: 10.1016/j.cell.2017.06.007
31. Grayson JM, Weant AE, Holbrook BC, Hildeman D. Role of Bim in regulating CD8+ T-cell responses during chronic viral infection. *J Virol.* (2006) 80:8627–38. doi: 10.1128/JVI.00855-06
32. He R, Hou S, Liu C, Zhang A, Bai Q, Han M, et al. Follicular CXCR5-expressing CD8+ T cells curtail chronic viral infection. *Nature.* (2016) 537:412–28. doi: 10.1038/nature19317
33. Hoffmann M, Pantazis N, Martin GE, Hickling S, Hurst J, Meyerowitz J, et al. Exhaustion of activated CD8 T cells predicts disease progression in primary HIV-1 infection. *PLoS Pathog.* (2016) 12:e1005661. doi: 10.1371/journal.ppat.1005661
34. Huang AC, Postow MA, Orlowski RJ, Mick R, Bengsch B, Manne S, et al. T-cell invigoration to tumour burden ratio associated with anti-PD-1 response. *Nature.* (2017) 545:60–5. doi: 10.1038/nature22079
35. Im SJ, Hashimoto M, Gerner MY, Lee J, Kissick HT, Burger MC, et al. Defining CD8+ T cells that provide the proliferative burst after PD-1 therapy. *Nature.* (2016) 537:417–21. doi: 10.1038/nature19330
36. Kaech SM, Tan JT, Wherry EJ, Konieczny BT, Surh CD, Ahmed R. Selective expression of the interleukin 7 receptor identifies effector CD8 T cells that give rise to long-lived memory cells. *Nat Immunol.* (2003) 4:1191–8. doi: 10.1038/ni1009
37. Kamphorst AO, Pillai RN, Yang S, Nasti TH, Akondy RS, Wieland A, et al. Proliferation of PD-1+ CD8 T cells in peripheral blood after PD-1-targeted therapy in lung cancer patients. *Proc Natl Acad Sci USA.* (2017) 114:4993–8. doi: 10.1073/pnas.1705327114
38. Khan O, Giles JR, Mcdonald S, Manne S, Ngiow SF, Patel KP, et al. TOX transcriptionally and epigenetically programs CD8(+) T cell exhaustion. *Nature.* (2019) 571:211–8. doi: 10.1038/s41586-019-1325-x
39. Krieg C, Nowicka M, Guglietta S, Schindler S, Hartmann FJ, Weber LM, et al. High-dimensional single-cell analysis predicts response to anti-PD-1 immunotherapy. *Nat Med.* (2018) 24:144–53. doi: 10.1038/nm.4466
40. Legat A, Speiser DE, Pircher H, Zehn D, Fuertes Marraco SA. Inhibitory receptor expression depends more dominantly on differentiation and activation than "exhaustion" of human CD8 T cells. *Front Immunol.* (2013) 4:455. doi: 10.3389/fimmu.2013.00455
41. Levine JH, Simonds EF, Bendall SC, Davis KL, Amir El AD, Tadmor MD, et al. Data-driven phenotypic dissection of AML reveals progenitor-like cells that correlate with prognosis. *Cell.* (2015) 162:184–97. doi: 10.1016/j.cell.2015.05.047
42. Lopes AR, Kellam P, Das A, Dunn C, Kwan A, Turner J, et al. Bim-mediated deletion of antigen-specific CD8 T cells in patients unable to control HBV infection. *J Clin Invest.* (2008) 118:1835–45. doi: 10.1172/JCI33402
43. Mclane LM, Abdel-Hakeem MS, Wherry EJ. CD8 T Cell Exhaustion during chronic viral infection and cancer. *Annu Rev Immunol.* (2019) 37:457–95. doi: 10.1146/annurev-immunol-041015-055318
44. Miller BC, Sen DR, Al Abosy R, Bi K, Virkud YV, Lafleur MW, et al. Subsets of exhausted CD8(+) T cells differentially mediate tumor control and respond to checkpoint blockade. *Nat Immunol.* (2019) 20:326–36. doi: 10.1038/s41590-019-0312-6
45. Moskophidis D, Lechner F, Pircher H, Zinkernagel RM. Virus persistence in acutely infected immunocompetent mice by exhaustion of antiviral cytotoxic effector T cells. *Nature.* (1993) 362:758–61. doi: 10.1038/362758a0
46. Nakamoto N, Cho H, Shaked A, Olthoff K, Valiga ME, Kaminski M, et al. Synergistic reversal of intrahepatic HCV-specific CD8 T cell exhaustion by combined PD-1/CTLA-4 blockade. *PLoS Pathog.* (2009) 5:e1000313. doi: 10.1371/journal.ppat.1000313
47. Nakamoto N, Kaplan DE, Coleclough J, Li Y, Valiga ME, Kaminski M, et al. Functional restoration of HCV-specific CD8 T cells by PD-1 blockade is defined by PD-1 expression and compartmentalization. *Gastroenterology.* (2008) 134:1927–1937, 1937.e1–2. doi: 10.1053/j.gastro.2008.02.033
48. Newell EW, Sigal N, Bendall SC, Nolan GP, Davis MM. Cytometry by time-of-flight shows combinatorial cytokine expression and virus-specific cell niches within a continuum of CD8+ T cell phenotypes. *Immunity.* (2012) 36:142–52. doi: 10.1016/j.immuni.2012.01.002

49. Olsen LR, Leipold MD, Pedersen CB, Maecker HT. The anatomy of single cell mass cytometry data. *Cytometry A.* (2019) 95:156–72. doi: 10.1002/cyto.a.23621
50. Paley MA, Kroy DC, Odorizzi PM, Johnnidis JB, Dolfi DV, Barnett BE, et al. Progenitor and terminal subsets of CD8+ T cells cooperate to contain chronic viral infection. *Science.* (2012) 338:1220–5. doi: 10.1126/science.1229620
51. Pauken KE, Sammons MA, Odorizzi PM, Manne S, Godec J, Khan O, et al. Epigenetic stability of exhausted T cells limits durability of reinvigoration by PD-1 blockade. *Science.* (2016) 354:1160–1165. doi: 10.1126/science.aaf2807
52. Penna A, Pilli M, Zerbini A, Orlandini A, Mezzadri S, Sacchelli L, et al. Dysfunction and functional restoration of HCV-specific CD8 responses in chronic hepatitis C virus infection. *Hepatology.* (2007) 45:588–601. doi: 10.1002/hep.21541
53. Petrovas C, Chaon B, Ambrozak DR, Price DA, Melenhorst JJ, Hill BJ, et al. Differential association of programmed death-1 and CD57 with *ex vivo* survival of CD8+ T cells in HIV infection. *J Immunol.* (2009) 183:1120–32. doi: 10.4049/jimmunol.0900182
54. Petrovas C, Ferrando-Martinez S, Gerner MY, Casazza JP, Pegu A, Deleage C, et al. Follicular CD8 T cells accumulate in HIV infection and can kill infected cells *in vitro* via bispecific antibodies. *Sci Transl Med.* (2017) 9:eaag2285. doi: 10.1126/scitranslmed.aag2285
55. Philip M, Fairchild L, Sun L, Horste EL, Camara S, Shakiba M, et al. Chromatin states define tumour-specific T cell dysfunction and reprogramming. *Nature.* (2017) 545:452–6. doi: 10.1038/nature22367
56. Qiu P, Simonds EF, Bendall SC, Gibbs KD Jr, Bruggner RV, Linderman MD, et al. Extracting a cellular hierarchy from high-dimensional cytometry data with SPADE. *Nat Biotechnol.* (2011) 29:886–91. doi: 10.1038/nbt.1991
57. Radziewicz H, Ibegbu CC, Fernandez ML, Workowski KA, Obideen K, Wehbi M, et al. Liver-infiltrating lymphocytes in chronic human hepatitis C virus infection display an exhausted phenotype with high levels of PD-1 and low levels of CD127 expression. *J Virol.* (2007) 81:2545–53. doi: 10.1128/JVI.02021-06
58. Roederer M, Nozzi JL, Nason MC. SPICE: exploration and analysis of post-cytometric complex multivariate datasets. *Cytometry A.* (2011) 79:167–74. doi: 10.1002/cyto.a.21015
59. Saelens W, Cannoodt R, Todorov H, Saeys Y. A comparison of single-cell trajectory inference methods. *Nat Biotechnol.* (2019) 37:547–54. doi: 10.1038/s41587-019-0071-9
60. Sauce D, Almeida JR, Larsen M, Haro L, Autran B, Freeman GJ, et al. PD-1 expression on human CD8 T cells depends on both state of differentiation and activation status. *AIDS.* (2007) 21:2005–13. doi: 10.1097/QAD.0b013e3282eee548
61. Schietinger A, Philip M, Krisnawan VE, Chiu EY, Delrow JJ, Basom RS, et al. Tumor-specific T cell dysfunction is a dynamic antigen-driven differentiation program initiated early during tumorigenesis. *Immunity.* (2016) 45:389–401. doi: 10.1016/j.immuni.2016.07.011
62. Sen DR, Kaminski J, Barnitz RA, Kurachi M, Gerdemann U, Yates KB, et al. The epigenetic landscape of T cell exhaustion. *Science.* (2016) 354:1165–9. doi: 10.1126/science.aae0491
63. Simoni Y, Fehlings M, Newell EW. Multiplex MHC class I tetramer combined with intranuclear staining by mass cytometry. *Methods Mol Biol.* (2019) 1989:147–58. doi: 10.1007/978-1-4939-9454-0_11
64. Staron MM, Gray SM, Marshall HD, Parish IA, Chen JH, Perry CJ, et al. The transcription factor FoxO1 sustains expression of the inhibitory receptor PD-1 and survival of antiviral CD8(+) T cells during chronic infection. *Immunity.* (2014) 41:802–14. doi: 10.1016/j.immuni.2014.10.013
65. Tirosh I, Izar B, Prakadan SM, Wadsworth MH II, Treacy D, Trombetta JJ, et al. Dissecting the multicellular ecosystem of metastatic melanoma by single-cell RNA-seq. *Science.* (2016) 352, 189–196. doi: 10.1126/science.aad0501
66. Trautmann L, Janbazian L, Chomont N, Said EA, Gimmig S, Bessette B, et al. Upregulation of PD-1 expression on HIV-specific CD8+ T cells leads to reversible immune dysfunction. *Nat Med.* (2006) 12:1198–202. doi: 10.1038/nm1482
67. Urbani S, Amadei B, Tola D, Massari M, Schivazappa S, Missale G, et al. PD-1 expression in acute hepatitis C virus (HCV) infection is associated with HCV-specific CD8 exhaustion. *J Virol.* (2006) 80:11398–403. doi: 10.1128/JVI.01177-06
68. Utzschneider DT, Charmoy M, Chennupati V, Pousse L, Ferreira DP, Calderon-Copete S, et al. T Cell factor 1-expressing memory-like CD8(+) T cells sustain the immune response to chronic viral infections. *Immunity.* (2016) 45:415–27. doi: 10.1016/j.immuni.2016.07.021
69. Utzschneider DT, Legat A, Fuertes Marraco SA, Carrie L, Luescher I, Speiser DE, et al. T cells maintain an exhausted phenotype after antigen withdrawal and population reexpansion. *Nat Immunol.* (2013) 14:603–10. doi: 10.1038/ni.2606
70. Van Gassen S, Callebaut B, Van Helden MJ, Lambrecht BN, Demeester P, Dhaene T, et al. FlowSOM: using self-organizing maps for visualization and interpretation of cytometry data. *Cytometry A.* (2015) 87:636–45. doi: 10.1002/cyto.a.22625
71. Weber LM, Robinson MD. Comparison of clustering methods for high-dimensional single-cell flow and mass cytometry data. *Cytometry A.* (2016) 89:1084–96. doi: 10.1002/cyto.a.23030
72. Wei SC, Levine JH, Cogdill AP, Zhao Y, Anang NAS, et al. Distinct cellular mechanisms underlie anti-CTLA-4 and anti-PD-1 checkpoint blockade. *Cell.* (2017) 170:1120–33.e1117. doi: 10.1016/j.cell.2017.07.024
73. Wherry EJ, Ahmed R. Memory CD8 T-cell differentiation during viral infection. *J Virol.* (2004) 78:5535–45. doi: 10.1128/JVI.78.11.5535-5545.2004
74. Wherry EJ, Blattman JN, Murali-Krishna K, Van Der Most R, Ahmed R. Viral persistence alters CD8 T-cell immunodominance and tissue distribution and results in distinct stages of functional impairment. *J Virol.* (2003) 77:4911–27. doi: 10.1128/JVI.77.8.4911-4927.2003
75. Wherry EJ, Ha SJ, Kaech SM, Haining WN, Sarkar S, Kalia V, et al. Molecular signature of CD8+ T cell exhaustion during chronic viral infection. *Immunity.* (2007) 27:670–84. doi: 10.1016/j.immuni.2007.09.006
76. Wieland D, Kemming J, Schuch A, Emmerich F, Knolle P, Neumann-Haefelin C, et al. TCF1(+) hepatitis C virus-specific CD8(+) T cells are maintained after cessation of chronic antigen stimulation. *Nat Commun.* (2017) 8:15050. doi: 10.1038/ncomms15050
77. Yamamoto T, Price DA, Casazza JP, Ferrari G, Nason M, Chattopadhyay PK, et al. Surface expression patterns of negative regulatory molecules identify determinants of virus-specific CD8+ T-cell exhaustion in HIV infection. *Blood.* (2011) 117:4805–15. doi: 10.1182/blood-2010-11-317297
78. Youngblood B, Hale JS, Kissick HT, Ahn E, Xu X, Wieland A, et al. Effector CD8 T cells dedifferentiate into long-lived memory cells. *Nature.* (2017) 552:404–9. doi: 10.1038/nature25144
79. Zajac AJ, Blattman JN, Murali-Krishna K, Sourdive DJ, Suresh M, Altman JD, et al. Viral immune evasion due to persistence of activated T cells without effector function. *J Exp Med.* (1998) 188:2205–13. doi: 10.1084/jem.188.12.2205
80. Zhang Z, Zhang JY, Wherry EJ, Jin B, Xu B, Zou ZS, et al. Dynamic programmed death 1 expression by virus-specific CD8 T cells correlates with the outcome of acute hepatitis B. *Gastroenterology.* (2008) 134:1938–49, 1949.e1–3. doi: 10.1053/j.gastro.2008.03.037
81. Zheng C, Zheng L, Yoo JK, Guo H, Zhang Y, Guo X, et al. Landscape of infiltrating T cells in liver cancer revealed by single-cell sequencing. *Cell.* (2017) 169:1342–56.e1316. doi: 10.1016/j.cell.2017.05.035

10

Quantitative Comparison of Conventional and t-SNE-guided Gating Analyses

Shadi Toghi Eshghi[1†], *Amelia Au-Yeung*[1†], *Chikara Takahashi*[1], *Christopher R. Bolen*[2], *Maclean N. Nyachienga*[1], *Sean P. Lear*[1], *Cherie Green*[1], *W. Rodney Mathews*[1] and *William E. O'Gorman*[1*]

[1] OMNI Biomarker Development, Genentech Inc., South San Francisco, CA, United States, [2] Bioinformatics, Genentech Inc., South San Francisco, CA, United States

***Correspondence:**
William E. O'Gorman
ogormanw@gene.com

† These authors have contributed equally to this work

Dimensionality reduction using the t-Distributed Stochastic Neighbor Embedding (t-SNE) algorithm has emerged as a popular tool for visualizing high-parameter single-cell data. While this approach has obvious potential for data visualization it remains unclear how t-SNE analysis compares to conventional manual hand-gating in stratifying and quantitating the frequency of diverse immune cell populations. We applied a comprehensive 38-parameter mass cytometry panel to human blood and compared the frequencies of 28 immune cell subsets using both conventional bivariate and t-SNE-guided manual gating. t-SNE analysis was capable of stratifying every general cellular lineage and most sub-lineages with high correlation between conventional and t-SNE-guided cell frequency calculations. However, specific immune cell subsets delineated by the manual gating of continuous variables were not fully separated in t-SNE space thus causing discrepancies in subset identification and quantification between these analytical approaches. Overall, these studies highlight the consistency between t-SNE and conventional hand-gating in stratifying general immune cell lineages while demonstrating that particular cell subsets defined by conventional manual gating may be intermingled in t-SNE space.

Keywords: cyTOF, t-SNE, cytometry informatics, dimensionality reduction, immunophenotyping, high-dimensional cytometry

INTRODUCTION

The analysis of cytometry data through manual "hand-gating" has progressively become more and more impractical as cytometry data sets continue to increase in dimensionality and size (1). The sequential inspection and gating of more than 20 bivariate plots is now necessary to conduct even a basic immunophenotyping analysis of 40-parameter data. The primary problems with conventional cytometric analysis are the subjectivity of operator-defined gating thresholds and the low throughput of manual gating (2, 3). Frequency quantitation of cell subsets defined by the subjective discretization of continuously distributed markers, such as CCR7 and CD45RA in defining T cell subsets, are particularly subject to inter-analyst variability. The goal of cytometry informatics is to automate, or at least augment, the objective stratification of cell populations in cytometry data sets. Although an overwhelming variety of computational tools have been developed as potential alternatives to manual hand-gated analyses (4), the field has yet to unite around a single computational approach.

Clustering and dimensionality reduction are algorithmic methods that have frequently been applied to cytometry data. Over the past decade, clustering algorithms have been critically assessed through comparison to expert manual analysis as well as through the cross-validation of clustering results between different clustering algorithms (5, 6). In contrast, there have been very few critical assessments of dimensionality reduction as a cytometric analytical tool or even as a tool that simply enables the visualization of single-cell data (7, 8).

Recently, the dimensionality reduction algorithm, t-distributed stochastic neighbor embedding (t-SNE) (9), has gained popularity as a means to visualize high dimensional single-cell data (10–12). While t-SNE produces bivariate dot-plot based visualizations that are inherently intuitive for cytometrists to comprehend, there is still an important need to assess the strengths and limitations of this approach, especially in respect to how t-SNE relates to expert manual hand-gated analysis which has historically been the gold standard.

Currently, in cytometric analysis t-SNE is typically used as a visualization tool to qualitatively assess cell population diversity, rather than as a quantitative analytical tool for calculating the frequency of specific cell populations. In these studies, we sought to quantitatively compare cell population frequencies determined by both conventional bivariate plot-based and t-SNE-guided manual gating. Our goal was not to definitively validate dimensionality reduction as a quantitative analytical approach, but simply to understand the relationship between dimensionality reduction and conventional manual gating in defining canonical cell populations. Given that t-SNE analysis is primarily being used to explore novel cellular landscapes, the ability of this approach to accurately represent well-characterized and defined populations is important for establishing its general validity. Alternatively, t-SNE mapping could reveal flaws in conventional gating strategies.

We found that immune populations stratified by divergent and discrete marker expression in a conventional analysis were also well separated by t-SNE dimensionality reduction. As expected, the projection of general cell lineages identified via conventional gating onto the t-SNE map demonstrated congruence in the cell populations distinguished by these analytical approaches. In contrast, particular T cell subsets defined by continuous markers were often not well separated in t-SNE space. In these cases, the projection of hand-gated T cell populations onto the t-SNE map showed high levels of interspersion between subsets. Isolation and t-SNE analysis of only the CD4+ T cell lineage produced only marginally better separation between canonical subsets than in the global analysis. In summary, cell populations that are well stratified by conventional bivariate plot-based gating will also be separated via t-SNE-based dimensionality reduction; however, subsets defined by the gating of continuous markers on a bivariate plot will not be fully separated in t-SNE space unless discrete orthogonal markers are included that facilitate further stratification.

MATERIALS AND METHODS

PBMC Isolation

Healthy human donors ($N = 10$) peripheral blood mononuclear cells (PBMCs) were isolated using 50 mL Leucosep™ tubes (Greiner Bio-One International, Germany) and Ficoll-Paque™ PLUS (GE Healthcare, Sweden). Whole blood was drawn into sodium heparin anticoagulant collection tubes and diluted with phosphate-buffered saline (PBS) without calcium or magnesium (Lonza, Walkersville, Maryland). Whole blood was centrifuged for 15 min at 800x g at room temperature (RT). PBMCs were then harvested and washed with PBS and centrifuged for 10 min at 250x g at RT before preparation for cell staining.

Source of mAb-Isotope Conjugates

See **Table S1** for a list of the metal conjugated mAbs used in these studies. In-house conjugations were performed using Multi-Metal Maxpar® Kits (Fluidigm, South San Francisco, California). 115In was purchased from Trace Sciences International Corporation.

Staining of Cells

Washed PBMCs were re-suspended at a cell concentration of 10^7 cells/mL with PBS. Cells were then incubated with a viability reagent, Cell-ID™ Cisplatin (Fluidigm, South San Francisco, California) at a final concentration of 5 μM for 5 min on ice. Viability staining was quenched with a 5x volume of MaxPar® Cell Staining Buffer (Fluidigm, South San Francisco, California) and centrifuged at 300x g, then re-suspended to a final concentration of 30 million cells/mL in staining buffer. For antibody labeling, 3 million cells were transferred to Falcon® 5 mL 12 × 75 mm tubes (Corning, New York). To block Fc receptor binding, cells were incubated with 5 μL of Human TruStain FcX™ (BioLegend, San Diego, California) for 10 min on ice. A master mAb cocktail containing all metal-conjugated surface antibodies (50 μL of total staining reagent volume) was added to samples for cell-surface staining and incubated for 30 min on ice. See **Table S1** for a list of the metal conjugated mAbs used in these studies. Cells were then washed once with 4 mL cell staining buffer to prepare for intracellular staining. Briefly, cells were re-suspended in 1 mL of fixation/permeabilization solution by using the FoxP3 Staining Buffer Set (eBioscience, San Diego, California) for 45 min on ice, washed with 3 mL of permeabilization buffer at 800x g for 5 min, and re-suspended in 50 μL of permeabilization buffer. Cells were then stained for intracellular targets by addition of 50 μL antibody cocktail. After 30 min incubation on ice, the cells were washed with 4 mL cell staining buffer and fixed overnight at 4°C in a 1 mL solution containing Cell-ID™ Intercalator-Ir in 1.6% EMS Fix (Electron Microscopy Sciences, Hatfield, Pennsylvania).

For flow cytometry, 20 μL of the TBNK cocktail from BD Biosciences was added into each of the 10 TruCount FACS tubes. 100 μL of each donor's blood was reverse pipetted into the TruCount tubes and incubated for 30 min. After incubation, 450 μL of 1x BD FACS Lysing solution was added and incubated for 15 min. Samples were then acquired within an hour from lysing on a FACS Canto II (BD Biosciences, San Jose, CA).

Acquisition on CyTOF® Instrument

Cells were washed with 3 mL of MaxPar® cell staining buffer and centrifugated at 800x g for 5 min followed by a 2x wash with 4 mL MaxPar® Water (Fluidigm, South San Francisco, California). Before introduction into the Helios™, a CyTOF® System (Fluidigm, South San Francisco, California), pelleted cells were re-suspended with MaxPar® Water containing EQ™ Four Element Calibration Beads (Fluidigm, South San Francisco, California) and filtered using a 12 × 75 mm tube with a 35 μm nylon mesh cell-strainer cap (Corning, New York).

Data Processing and Analysis

All FCS files were normalized using the MATLAB® (MathWorks®, Natick, Massachusetts) normalizer and analyzed using FlowJo® software (Flowjo, Ashland, Oregon).

Dimensionality Reduction (t-SNE) Analysis

Individual donor fcs files were imported into R and their expression matrices containing measured intensities for each marker at single-cell level were extracted using functions from the flowCore package (13). A subset of 50,000 cells were selected for each donor at random and merged into a single expression matrix prior to t-SNE analysis. The following channels were removed from the expression matrix to only include protein markers in t-SNE analysis: beads, event length, intercalator, viability, center, offset, residual, and time. Marker intensities were transformed using the inverse hyperbolic sine (arcsinh) function. A total of 500,000 cells and 38 markers (**Table S1**) were used to create a t-SNE map of the peripheral human immune system.

The Barnes-Hut implementation of t-SNE by the Rtsne package (14) with 1,000 iterations, a perplexity parameter of 30, and a trade-off θ of 0.5 (9, 15), was used for applying the dimensionality reduction algorithm. The output was in the form of a matrix with 500,000 rows and 2 columns corresponding to t-SNE dimension 1 and dimension 2. t-SNE maps were generated by plotting each event by its t-SNE dimensions in a dot-plot. Intensities for markers of interest were overlaid on the dot-plot to show the expression of those markers on different cell islands and facilitate assignment of cell subsets to these islands. The t-SNE dimensions were appended to the original expression matrix as derived parameters and exported as an fcs file, which could subsequently be opened and analyzed using FlowJo (Ashland, Oregon). For flow cytometry data FCS Express (Glendale, California) was used to conduct t-SNE analysis.

To evaluate the impact of modulating pre-specified parameters on t-SNE map generation, a subset of the 10-donor data (50,000 cells) was analyzed using varying perplexity, iteration number and trade-off θ values. Perplexity of 5, 30, and 100, iteration number of 1,000 and 10,000 and trade-off θ of 0.2, 0.5, and 0.8 were compared. The impact of limiting the markers used to construct a global t-SNE map to only general lineage markers was examined by running t-SNE with only the following markers: CD45, CD3, CD4, CD8, γδTCR, IgD, CD19, CD20, HLA-DR, CD14, CD11c, CD66, CD56, CD16, CD1c, CD38, and CD11b (data not shown).

Concordance between manually hand gated populations projected onto t-SNE space and computationally defined clusters was qualitatively assessed for Phenograph (16), DensVM (17), and FlowSOM (18) clustering methods. Clustering and overlay with t-SNE maps was performed using the cytofkit package in R (19).

Comparison of Hand-gated and t-SNE-guided Gated Subsets at Single-cell Level

To evaluate the concordance between hand-gating and t-SNE-guided gating at single-cell level, the FlowJo workspace file (tsp) of the aggregated and t-SNE appended fcs file was imported into R. For each population, the cells captured in the corresponding subset using hand-gating or t-SNE-guided gating were extracted and compared between the two methods. t-SNE-guided manual gates were drawn based on observed boundaries of canonical phenotypic marker expression rather than on cell subset density. The ability of the t-SNE-guided gating to match the hand-gating results was quantified by the fraction of cells in the hand-gated population that matched with the t-SNE-guided population. This was calculated by dividing the number of cells in the overlap between the two gates by the total number of cells in the hand-gated population. The fraction of cells in the t-SNE-guided gated population that matched with the hand-gated population was similarly calculated by dividing the number of cells in the overlap between the gates by the total number of cells in the t-SNE-guided gate (Supporting Information **Figure S5**). The flowWorkspace package (2) was used for analysis of wsp file in R.

RESULTS

Conventional Bivariate Plot-based Gating Strategy Defining the Peripheral Human Immune System

In order to define the relationship between cell populations stratified by a global t-SNE map of the peripheral immune system and a conventional hand-gating analysis, a diverse 38-parameter cytometry panel was applied to identify 28 distinct immune cell populations in human blood (**Table S1**). Peripheral blood mononuclear cells (PBMCs) from 10 healthy donors were isolated and processed for mass cytometric analysis. **Figure 1** shows the conventional manual gating strategy used to define these populations. Neutrophils and Eosinophils were identified based on CD66 positivity and further subsetted based on CD16 and CD49d expression (20). CD3, CD4, CD8, CCR7, CD45RA, CD25, and Foxp3 were used to identify regulatory, naïve, central, effector, and effector memory T cells expressing CD45RA (TEMRA) (21). γδ TCR, Vα7.2 TCR, and CD161 expression defined γδ and mucosal associated invariant TCR (MAIT) T cells (22). CD19+ B cell subsets were defined based on the differential expression of CD27, CD38, and IgD into plasmablast, naïve, memory, transitional, and double-negative subsets (23). Following the exclusion of

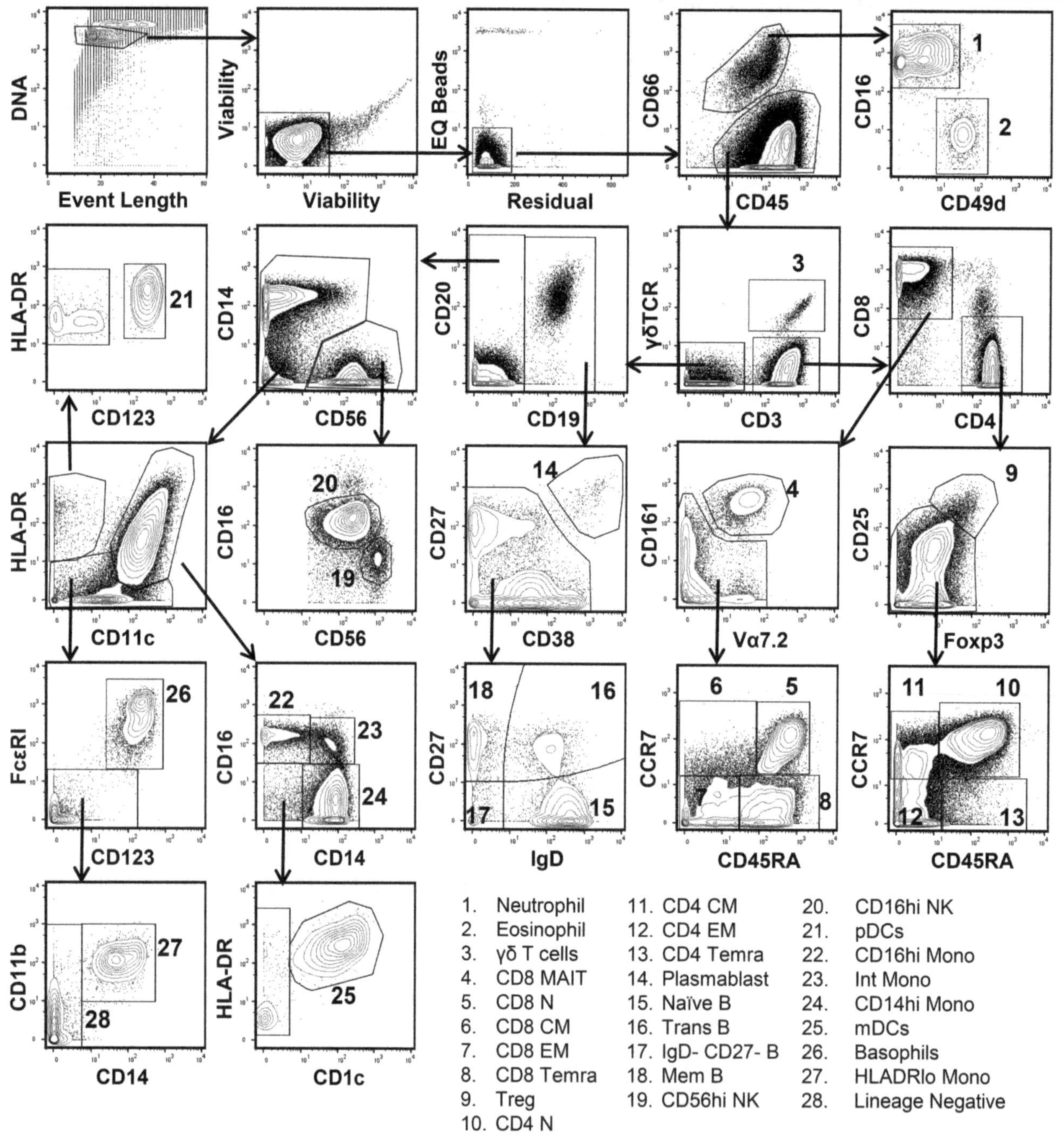

FIGURE 1 | Conventional manual gating strategy for 38-parameter human immunophenotyping. Human PBMCs were isolated and prepared for mass cytometry analysis as described in Materials and Methods section. Data shown are from the merger of 10 donor samples (50,000 cells per donor) into a single fcs file. Single living cells were identified based on intercalator 193Ir, event length, cisplatin 192 & 195Pt, EQ Bead (140Ce), and residual signal intensity. Differential expression of CD66, CD16, and CD49d was used to discern Neutrophils and Eosinophils from other immune cell populations. CD3, CD4, CD8, CD25, CD45RA, CD161, Vα7.2, CCR7, Foxp3, and γδ-TCR expression were used to define 11 T cell subsets. CD19, CD20, CD27, CD38, and IgD were used to define 5 B cell subsets. Two NK cell subsets were defined based on CD56 and CD16 expression. Plasmacytoid dendritic cells (pDCs) were CD11clo, HLADRhi, and expressed high levels of CD123. Monocyte and myeloid dendritic cell subsets (mDCs) were identified based on the differential expression of HLADR, CD11c, CD14, CD16, CD11b, and CD1c. Basophils co-express high levels of CD123 and FcεR1.

the lineages described above, two NK cell populations were identified based on the expression of CD56 and CD16 (24). Monocytes and dendritic cell subsets were identified based on the differential expression of CD11c, CD11b, HLADR, CD14, CD1c, and CD123 (25). Lastly, FcεRI and CD123 co-expression identified basophils.

Comparison of Conventional and t-SNE-guided Manual Analysis Across General Immune Cell Lineages

For t-SNE analysis singlet and viability gating was performed manually prior to data export for downstream computation (see **Figure S1** for a workflow schematic and Materials and Methods section for details on t-SNE analysis). Due to the stochastic nature of t-SNE, analyzing each donor independently would yield maps in which the same cell populations would be in different locations. Data merger was therefore conducted to ensure spatial alignment of the same cell populations between donors in t-SNE space. 50,000 cells were randomly sampled per donor to create a final file containing 500,000 total cells. Specific donor identifiers were integrated prior to data merger to enable deconvolution of the merged t-SNE map into individual maps specific to each donor. Following dimensionality reduction, coordinates for each t-SNE dimension (i.e., t-SNE1 and t-SNE2) were determined for every cell and were integrated into a new appended fcs file as novel parameters.

In contrast to conventional sequential biaxial plot-based analysis, t-SNE analysis generates a single map in which the complex multi-dimensional geometric relationships between single cells are represented in a two-dimensional space. A third dimension using a color-based representation of the expression levels of a single parameter is then used in order to facilitate the identification of specific cellular lineages (10) (**Figure 2A**). Islands of cells can usually be deciphered on the t-SNE map, which often uniformly express lineage specific markers such as CD3, CD19, and CD14. *A priori* knowledge of immunophenotyping can subsequently be applied to a series of these single-parameter maps in order to facilitate the supervised annotation of different cellular lineages. In this manner, on the global t-SNE map, 8 general cell populations were manually gated in t-SNE space and putatively identified as: basophils, neutrophils, eosinophils, plasmacytoid dendritic cells (pDCs), NK cells, monocytes and conventional dendritic cells (cDCs), B cells, and T cells. A small fraction of cells (0.24% of total) was left unidentified.

The overlap between cell populations identified via conventional and t-SNE-guided gating was qualitatively assessed by projecting hand-gated cell populations onto t-SNE space (**Figure 2B**). This approach showed minimal intermingling of cell populations between the different islands of cells stratified by dimensionality reduction. Subsequently, more quantitative methods to assess the relationship between conventional and t-SNE-guided gating were also applied both on a population level as well as single-cell level. Specifically, the frequencies (as % of total CD45+ cells) of each general cell population for each of the individual ten donors and the aggregated data (11 total data points) were determined and correlated between each analysis method (**Figure S2A**). This population-based analysis was highly correlated between both methods. The reproducibility of t-SNE-guided analysis across multiple independent t-SNE runs was also evaluated (**Figure S3A**). Due to the stochastic nature of t-SNE, the same cell populations fell in different parts of each map; however, the overall quantitation of the 8 general lineages was nearly identical between different runs (**Figure S3B**). A comparison of these analytical approaches also showed high correlation in the analysis of a 6-parameter flow cytometry data set demonstrating that high dimensional data is not required for separating distinct cell population in t-SNE space (**Figure S4**).

In order to assess overlap between conventional and t-SNE-guided analysis at the single-cell level, the cells that were captured by either analytical method for the aggregated donor data were compared for each cell subset. The fraction of cells captured by conventional gating that overlapped with those captured by t-SNE-guided gating were calculated to quantify the sensitivity of the t-SNE-guided gating method for replicating results from the conventional analysis. Analogously, the fraction of cells captured by t-SNE-guided gating matching those in the hand-gated population was also calculated (see Materials and Methods and **Figure S5** for more details). **Figure 2C** shows that for the 8 general cell populations identified, 97% or more of the cells that were conventionally hand-gated were matched with the t-SNE-guided analysis. Cell populations identified based on t-SNE stratification were matched with hand-gated populations at slightly lower levels but still above 93% matching for these 8 populations. Similar results were obtained for manually segregating general T cell lineages in t-SNE space based on CD3, CD4, CD8, γδ TCR, Vα7.2 TCR, and CD161 expression (**Figures S6, S2B**).

Comparison of Conventional and t-SNE-guided Manual Analysis Across Immune Cell Subsets

Subsequently, we evaluated the ability of t-SNE mapping to stratify the deeper subsets of lymphocytes, monocytes, and mDCs which we identified via conventional gating in **Figure 1**. Specifically, the differential expression of the markers shown in **Figure S7** were used to manually gate these general populations into sub lineages. Importantly, in contrast to the t-SNE-guided gating used to identify more general cell lineages, which leveraged the intrinsic topography of clearly separated cellular islands, for some subsets clear separation in t-SNE space was not observed. Thus, manual gates were drawn based on marker expression levels (analogous to the approach used in conventional gating in **Figure 1**) in the absence of topographic features that informed more objective boundaries (**Figure 3A**). **Figure 3B** demonstrates that certain subsets, especially central and effector memory T cell subsets, defined by conventional hand-gating were often commingled in t-SNE space.

While some cell subpopulations were well matched (>90%) by both manual and t-SNE-guided gating others were only matched at low levels (<30%) (**Figure 4**). Naïve lymphocytes were matched most concordantly (>80%) most likely due to redundancy between markers specific to the naïve state such as CD45RA, CCR7, CD27, and IgD. In contrast, central and effector memory T cell subsets defined even in high dimensional space by the expression of continuous markers were not well matched. Overall, when t-SNE map topography inherently defined discrete boundaries between cellular islands there was a higher likelihood for overlap between both gating approaches.

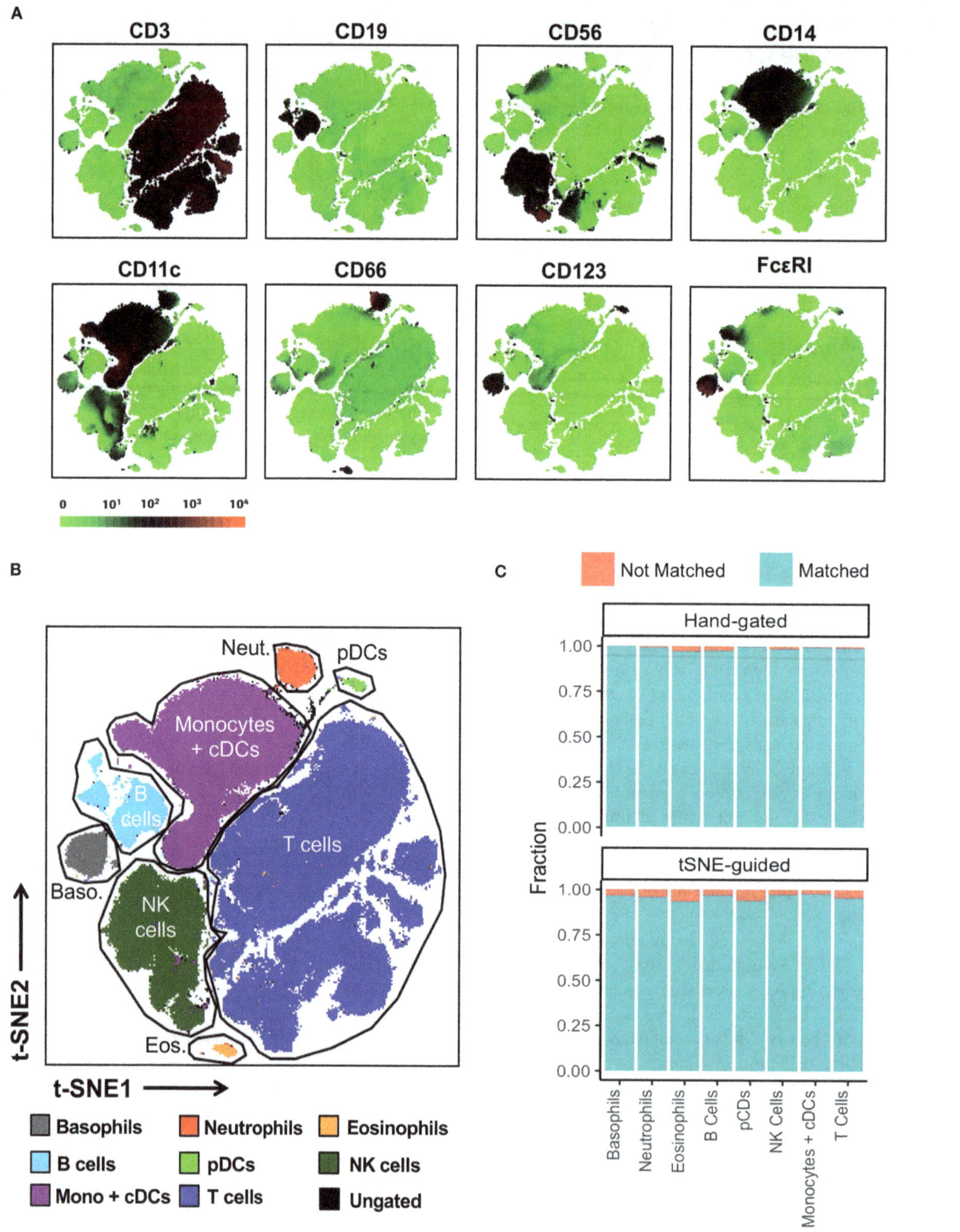

FIGURE 2 | t-SNE-guided manual gating analysis of general immune lineages. **(A)** 10 healthy donor PBMC samples were merged to create a single t-SNE map with the signal strength of key phenotypic markers defining specific cellular lineages expressed with a green-black-red continuous color scale. t-SNE analysis was performed using 1,000 iterations, a perplexity of 30, a trade-off θ of 0.5, and all 38 of the phenotypic markers listed in **Table S1**. **(B)** Cell populations defined by the manual gating strategy in **Figure 1** were projected onto t-SNE space and assigned specific colors. **(C)** The level of overlap or matching between conventional and t-SNE-guided manual gating analyses was calculated for every general cellular lineage. See Materials and Methods and **Figure S5** for details on how the level of matching between analytical strategies was calculated. The proportion of cells that were not matched is shown in red while the proportion of cells that were matched is shown in blue.

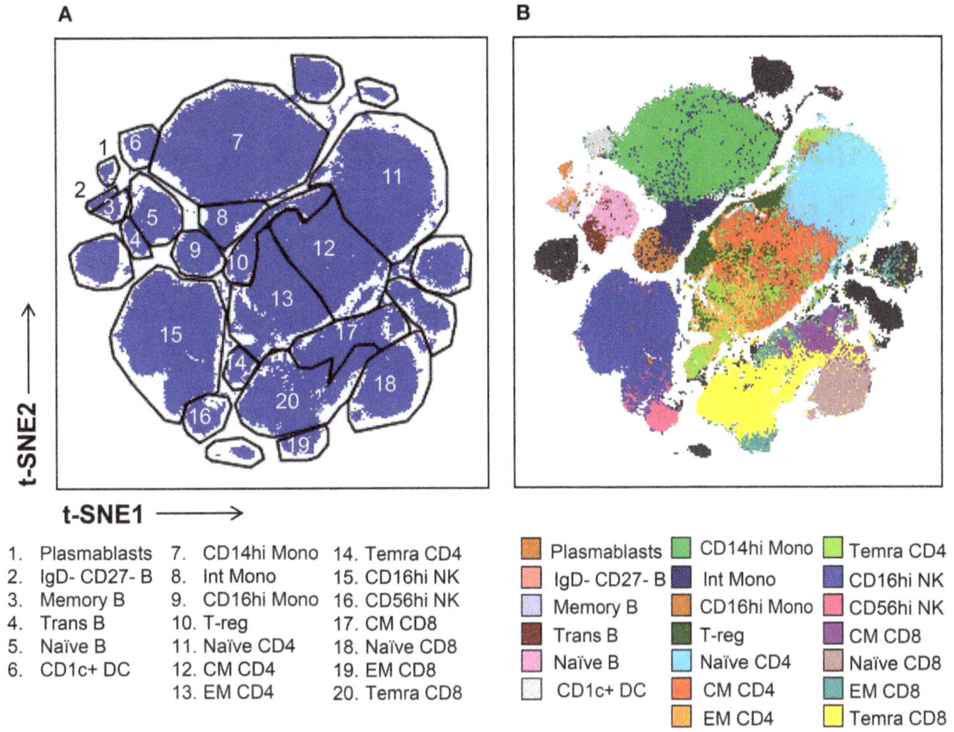

FIGURE 3 | t-SNE-guided manual gating analysis of immune cell subsets. **(A)** Immune cell subsets were identified and manually gated in t-SNE space based on the signal intensity of the phenotypic markers shown in **Figure S7A** in order to correspond to the subsets defined in **Figure 1**. **(B)** Cell subsets defined by conventional manual analysis were projected into t-SNE space and assigned different colors.

Isolated t-SNE Analysis of the CD4 T Cell Lineage

We next sought to determine whether t-SNE mapping of a single lineage that exhibited interspersion between manually defined canonical subsets in our global t-SNE map, could be better stratified with more discrete topographies when mapped as an individual lineage (**Figure 5**). To address this question, we isolated only the CD4+ T cell lineage (25,0000 cells from each of 10 donors) and ran t-SNE on this general population alone (with the entire 38 marker panel). **Figure 5A** shows the expression levels of markers relevant to the CD4 T cell lineage. While this approach led to more separation of minor T cell islands which became more distant from the main population in the CD4 T cell restricted analysis, it did not achieve clear resolution between general CD4+ T cell subsets other than the naïve subset (**Figure 5B**, left panel).

We hypothesized that parameters that were common to all CD4 T cells such as CD3 and CD4 were potentially restricting the ability of t-SNE to segregate CD4 T cell subsets. We compared t-SNE analysis of the CD4 T cell lineage with and without including markers either universally present or absent within this lineage and found little effect of constraining the markers used by t-SNE on the segregation of CD4 T cell subsets (data not shown).

Alternatively, it is possible that our inability to clearly delineate these populations in t-SNE space was the result of merging of different donors within a single map. This is because the conventional hand-gating performed on the merged file might not have been sufficiently tailored to the individual differences in marker expression which could vary between donors for either technical or biological reasons. To address this question t-SNE analysis was performed on individual donors with manual gating being tailored to each individual's particular expression patterns of CD25, Foxp3, CCR7, and CD45RA (**Figure 5B**, right panel). Again, we observed that while the naïve population is reproducibly segregated to one side of the map and shows little commingling with memory subsets, the other subsets are not clearly stratified within the t-SNE map. Thus, the lack of separation between memory T cell populations in t-SNE space was not due to the merger of different donors into a single t-SNE map.

Subsequently, we asked whether the application of a variety of clustering algorithms [Phenograph (16), DensVM (17), and FlowSOM (18)] could at least qualitatively stratify the 5 specific hand-gated T-cell populations we projected onto t-SNE space in **Figure 5B**; **Figure S8**. Naïve T-cells and a subset of T-regulatory cells were captured by one or a few clusters by each algorithm in a manner that was congruent with t-SNE map topography as well as manual hand gating. In contrast, the 3 other subsets of CD4 memory T-cells were not as clearly related to projected hand gates.

To further examine the effect of continuous markers on separation of phenotypes in t-SNE space, synthetic datasets containing two markers, M1 and M2 were created. Marker expressions for these channels were sampled from distributions

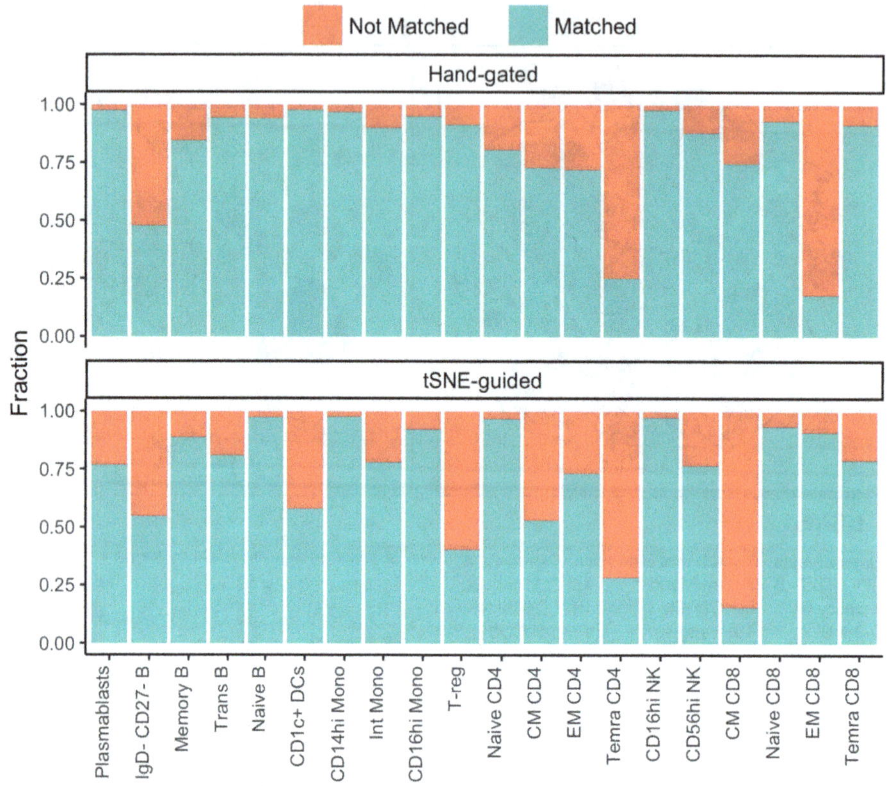

FIGURE 4 | Correspondence between conventional and t-SNE-guided manual gating analyses for immune cell subsets. The level of overlap or matching between conventional and t-SNE-guided manual gating analyses was calculated for every general cellular lineage as in **Figure 2C**. The proportion of cells that were not matched is shown in red while the proportion of cells that were matched is shown in blue.

with varying levels of continuity, including discrete bimodal, continuous bimodal, and unimodal (**Figure S9**). This was achieved by sampling two normal distributions with fixed mean values at negative and positive expression and variable standard deviation values to tune the level of continuity across these two levels. Dimensionality reduction using t-SNE was applied to these datasets to generate 2-dimensional projection of the data onto the t-SNE space. We observed that in the absence of a marker with discrete distribution, t-SNE is unable to fully resolve populations with continuous marker expression. This suggests that the distribution of marker expression is a contributing factor in the separation or intermingling of cells in t-SNE space.

Modulation of t-SNE Parameters Does Not Fully Separate Cell Populations Defined by Continuous Variables

The pre-specification of iteration number, perplexity, and trade-off θ can potentially impact cell stratification in t-SNE space and we qualitatively assessed whether the modulation of these parameters could lead to more concordance between t-SNE-guided and manual gating (**Figure S10**). Increasing perplexity and iteration number and decreasing the trade-off θ resulted in more separation between distinct cellular lineages with discrete marker distribution (**Figure S10A**). In contrast, modulating these parameters only marginally impacted the analysis of memory T-cell populations with continuous marker distributions (**Figure S10B**). Barnes-hut approximation through introduction of trade-off parameter θ enables practical application of t-SNE on large datasets. Importantly, increasing the trade-off parameter θ to 0.8, thus moving away from exact t-SNE, resulted in the inability of t-SNE-based mapping to resolve pDCs, a rare cell population (**Figure S10A**).

DISCUSSION

The inability of t-SNE to clearly separate canonical memory T cell subsets defined by a priori knowledge is not an inherent defect in dimensionality reduction as an analytical approach. Our analysis revealed that the information in our data set was insufficient to fully separate central and effector memory T cell subsets using t-SNE most likely because the parameters we expected to fully differentiate memory T cells were continuously distributed. In contrast, conventional bivariate gating arbitrarily discretizes cell populations based on operator defined areas of low density between largely continuous underlying data distributions as in the case for CCR7, CD45RA, and CD45RO. In contrast, the t-SNE maps we examined did not arbitrarily separate cell populations with similar patterns and levels of cell surface marker expression. This does not mean that these observations call into question the existence of the central and effector memory T

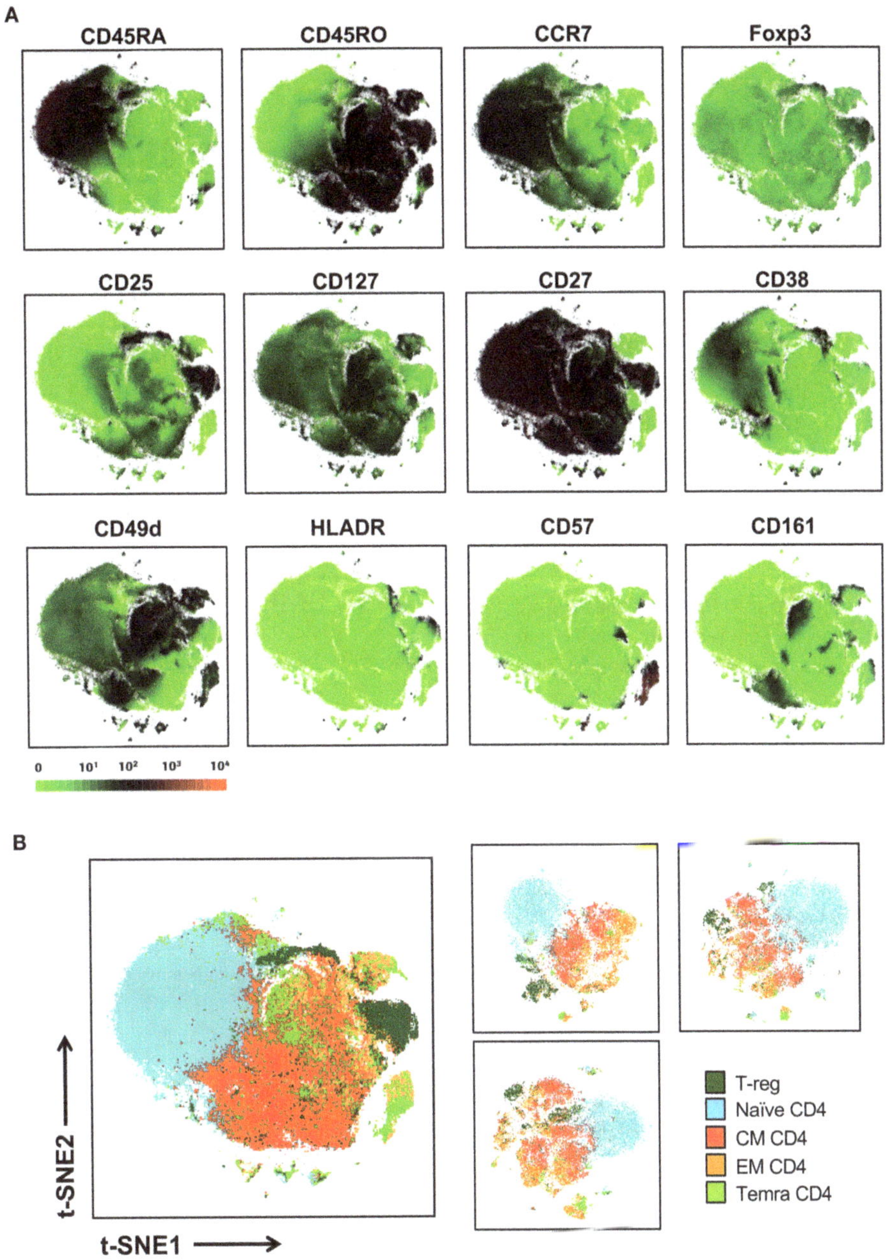

FIGURE 5 | Local t-SNE mapping of only the CD4 T cell lineage does not clearly separate memory subsets defined by conventional manual analysis. **(A)** 250,000 CD4 T cells were extracted from the 10-donor data set and were reanalyzed using t-SNE as an isolated lineage using the entire panel as in **Figure 2**. Signal intensity for individual markers involved in defining various T cell subsets are shown. **(B)** Projection of hand-gated CD4 T cell subsets from 10 donor data set into t-SNE space (left panel). CD4 T cell t-SNE maps were independently generated for 3 individual donors (25,000 cells per donor right panel).

cell subsets, but that our data set did not provide sufficient information to clearly differentiate memory T cell populations in t-SNE space. We found this to be true both in the context of a global as well as local t-SNE map in which only the CD4 T cell lineage was visualized (**Figure 5**). Lineage extraction and local t-SNE map generation was also performed for the monocyte & dendritic cell lineage (data not shown). We found that in global t-SNE maps dendritic cells typically formed a peninsular structure jutting out from the "mainland" of classical CD14hi monocytes, and in at least one local map we generated, DCs did achieve full separation from the major monocyte population (data not shown). Thus, finer resolution can be achieved in a local map; however, this did not seem to significantly alter the interpretation of the topography of a global t-SNE map. A hierarchical approach to t-SNE has been described (26), and the field should continue to evaluate the relative value of global t-SNE analyses vs. local analyses in which only specific lineages are isolated and visualized.

It is becoming convention for dimensionality reduction and clustering algorithms to be applied in tandem to single-cell data sets with populations defined by clustering algorithms being projected onto t-SNE space (16). This approach is undoubtedly more objective and reproducible than performing t-SNE-guided manual gating to segregate populations with continuous marker distributions, which recapitulates the "original sin" of manual hand gating.

It is currently unclear whether the use of t-SNE derived coordinates as part of a clustering approach is preferable to using these tools independently. Distance in t-SNE space should not be overinterpreted since distinct cell populations that are close in one t-SNE analysis can be distant in a second analysis of the same data set (**Figure S3**). Thus, it is questionable whether t-SNE coordinates should be included in defining cellular clusters. Regardless, a comparison of how clusters projected onto t-SNE space compare to conventional manual analysis is outside the scope of these studies and would be redundant with publications that have already performed this comparison without t-SNE visualization (6).

Going forward, an essential question for visualizing single-cell data with both dimensionality reduction and clustering is whether these approaches can deliver messages that are contradictory about the same data set. For example, what does an analyst conclude if a t-SNE map does not display distinct and well separated cellular islands but a clustering algorithm applied to the map parses out a variety of clusters that are only continuously differentiated in t-SNE space (as in **Figure S8**)? The biological relevance of poorly differentiated clusters should be assessed with orthogonal functional assays or additional markers providing more robust phenotypic stratification.

The application of t-SNE to single cell analysis probably provides the most value in efforts to survey the cellular heterogeneity of complex tissues and to characterize novel or poorly defined cell populations. In these studies, we tested the ability of the t-SNE approach to stratify familiar cell populations in an extremely well characterized sample matrix. If our studies had identified profound discrepancies between our "ground truth" conventional analysis of canonical subsets and the t-SNE-guided analysis, we may have questioned whether this approach is appropriate for the characterization of poorly defined cell populations or whether our ground truth assumptions were incorrect. Instead, a high degree of overlap in the general cellular lineages defined by these approaches was found, and the identified discrepancies led us to revisit the logic of subjectively discretizing continuous variables rather than the validity of dimensionality reduction.

ETHICS STATEMENT

This study was carried out in accordance with the recommendations of the Western Institutional Review Board (WIRB) as part of the Genentech Employee Blood donation program with written informed consent from all subjects. All subjects gave written informed consent in accordance with the Declaration of Helsinki. The protocol was approved by the WIRB.

AUTHOR CONTRIBUTIONS

WO oversaw research, designed experiments, and wrote manuscript. ST analyzed data, generated t-SNE plots, and adapted an R based t-SNE package created by CB who also aided in these activities. AA-Y, CT, MN, and SL generated and analyzed data. CG and WM oversaw research and aided in manuscript preparation.

ACKNOWLEDGMENTS

We would like to acknowledge the contributions of the Genentech Core Biophysical Characterization and Reagent Facility including Mehraban Kosraviani, Bartek Bossak, Justin Low, Paul Vu, Jose Diaz, Minh Michael Phan, Hanjo Lim, Jihong Yang, and Valerie Quarmby. We would also like to thank Evan Newell and Erin Simonds for many helpful discussions.

SUPPLEMENTARY MATERIAL

Figure S1 | Overview of t-SNE-guided analysis strategy. PBMCs were prepared from 10 healthy donors and analyzed via mass cytometry. Live singlet cells were manually gated using FlowJo software and individually exported as fcs files. Following file merger t-SNE analysis was conducted as described in Materials and Methods. A new fcs file was written for the merged data set as well as each individual donor with appended t-SNE parameters, which was then manually gated in t-SNE space using Flowjo. t-SNE-guided gates were then copied from the merged data to each individual donor.

Figure S2 | Correlation of cell subset frequencies. Cell frequencies were obtained from conventional and t-SNE-guided gating of individual donors and the aggregated data for **(A)** general immune lineages, **(B)** general T cell lineages, and **(C)** immune cell subsets.

Figure S3 | The stochastic nature of the t-SNE algorithm results in different maps in multiple runs. **(A)** Hand-gated subsets were projected onto t-SNE maps generated from 3 independent t-SNE runs. **(B)** Cell frequencies of general immune subsets obtained from t-SNE-guided gating of multiple runs are not affected by the topological changes of the maps.

Figure S4 | t-SNE analysis of PBMCs analyzed by a 6-parameter flow cytometry assay. **(A)** t-SNE map overlaid with expression of phenotypic markers. **(B)** Cell populations defined by the manual gating strategy in **Figure 1** were projected onto t-SNE space and assigned specific colors. **(C)** Correlation of cell population frequencies obtained from conventional and t-SNE-guided gating.

Figure S5 | Comparison of hand-gated vs. t-SNE-guided analysis at the single-cell level**.** Concordance between the two gating strategies was quantified by the fraction of cells present in both gates. For every cell population A_h represents the number of cells included in hand-drawn conventional gate and excluded from the t-SNE-guided gate, A_t is the number of cells included in t-SNE-guided gate and excluded from the hand-gated conventional gate and B is the number of cells that were present in both gating strategies.

Figure S6 | t-SNE-guided manual gating analysis of T cell lineages. **(A)** t-SNE map overlaid with signal intensities of key phenotypic markers. **(B)** Cell populations defined by the manual gating strategy in **Figure 1** were projected onto t-SNE space and assigned specific colors. **(C)** Level of overlap between conventional and t-SNE-guided manual gating is shown in blue.

Figure S7 | Additional t-SNE maps of aggregated 10-donor data. **(A)** Markers used for t-SNE-guided analysis of immune cells subsets. **(B)** Additional markers included in the generation of the t-SNE map but not for t-SNE-guided subsetting.

Figure S8 | Computationally defined CD4 T-cell clusters projected onto t-SNE space. Data from **Figure 5** were clustered with 3 different computational algorithms: Phenograph **(A)**, DensVM **(B)**, and FlowSOM with k = 20 **(C)**.

Figure S9 | Impact of marker expression distribution on separation of subsets in t-SNE space in synthetic datasets with 1,000 data points and 2 markers. **(A)** Markers have a bimodal and discrete distribution. Data points are fully separated in the t-SNE space. **(B)** Markers have a bimodal, yet continuous distribution. Although some structure is seen on the t-SNE map that distinguishes double positive, double negative, M1hi M2lo and M1lo M2hi groups, the data subsets are not fully separated. **(C)** Markers have a unimodal distribution. t-SNE is unable to resolve any subsets. t-SNE was run with perplexity parameter of 30 and trade-off θ of 0.5.

Figure S10 | Evaluation of the impact of algorithm parameters (iteration number, perplexity, and trade-off θ values) on t-SNE. 50,000 cells were analyzed using iteration number of 1,000 and 10,000, perplexity of 5, 30, and 100, and trade off θ values of 0.2, 0.5, and 0.8 for all PBMC lineages **(A)** and only CD4 T cells **(B)**.

Table S1 | List of metal conjugated mAbs and their targets used in the 38-parameter cytometry panel.

REFERENCES

1. Mair F, Hartmann FJ, Mrdjen D, Tosevski V, Krieg C, Becher B. The end of gating? An introduction to automated analysis of high dimensional cytometry data. *Eur J Immunol.* (2015) 46:34–43. doi: 10.1002/eji.201545774
2. Finak G, Frelinger J, Jiang W, Newell EW, Ramey J, Davis MM, et al. OpenCyto: an open source infrastructure for scalable, robust, reproducible, and automated, end-to-end flow cytometry data analysis. *PLoS Comput Biol.* (2014) 10:e1003806. doi: 10.1371/journal.pcbi.1003806
3. Finak G, Langweiler M, Jaimes M, Malek M, Taghiyar J, Korin Y, et al. Standardizing flow cytometry immunophenotyping analysis from the human immunophenotyping consortium. *Nat Publish Group.* (2016) 2016:1–11. doi: 10.1038/srep20686
4. Saeys Y, Gassen SV, Lambrecht BN. Computational flow cytometry: helping to make sense of high-dimensional immunology data. *Nat Rev Immunol.* (2016) 16:449–62. doi: 10.1038/nri.2016.56
5. Weber LM, Robinson MD. Comparison of clustering methods for high-dimensional single-cell flow and mass cytometry data. *Cytometry.* (2016) 89:1084–96. doi: 10.1002/cyto.a.23030
6. Aghaeepour N, Finak G, Dougall D, Khodabakhshi AH, Mah P, Obermoser G, et al. Critical assessment of automated flow cytometry data analysis techniques. *Nat Methods.* (2013) 10:228–38. doi: 10.1038/nmeth.2365
7. Becht E, Dutertre C-A, Kwok IWH, Ng LG, Ginhoux F, Newell EW. Evaluation of UMAP as an alternative to t-SNE for single-cell data. *bioRxiv.* (2018) 2018:1–10. doi: 10.1101/298430
8. Konstorum A, Vidal E, Jekel N, Laubenbacher R. Comparative analysis of linear and nonlinear dimension reduction techniques on mass cytometry data. *bioRxiv.* (2018) 2018:1–15. doi: 10.1101/273862
9. Van Der Maaten L, Res GHJML. Visualizing high-dimensional data using t-SNE. *J Mach Learn Res.* (2008) 9:2579–605. Available online at: http://www.jmlr.org/papers/v9/vandermaaten08a.html
10. Amir E-AD, Davis KL, Tadmor MD, Simonds EF, Levine JH, Bendall SC, et al. viSNE enables visualization of high dimensional single-cell data and reveals phenotypic heterogeneity of leukemia. *Nat Biotechnol.* (2013) 31:545–52. doi: 10.1038/nbt.2594
11. Guilliams M, Dutertre C-A, Scott CL, McGovern N, Sichien D, Chakarov S, et al. Unsupervised high-dimensional analysis aligns dendritic cells across tissues and species. *Immuni.* (2016) 45:669–84. doi: 10.1016/j.immuni.2016.08.015
12. Wong MT, Ong DEH, Lim FSH, Teng KWW, McGovern N, Narayanan S, et al. A high-dimensional atlas of human T cell diversity reveals tissue-specific trafficking and cytokine signatures. *Immuni.* (2016) 45:442–56. doi: 10.1016/j.immuni.2016.07.007
13. Hahne F, LeMeur N, Brinkman RR, Ellis B, Haaland P, Sarkar D, et al. flowCore: a Bioconductor package for high throughput flow cytometry. *BMC Bioinformatics.* (2009) 10:106. doi: 10.1186/1471-2105-10-106
14. Software JKC. *Rtsne: T-Distributed Stochastic Neighbor Embedding using Barnes-Hut Implementation (R package version 0.10)* (2015).
15. Van Der Maaten. Accelerating t-SNE using tree-based algorithms. *J Mach Learn Res L.* (2014) 15:3221–45. Available online at: http://jmlr.org/papers/v15/vandermaaten14a.html
16. Levine JH, Simonds EF, Bendall SC, Davis KL, Amir E-AD, Tadmor MD, et al. Data-driven phenotypic dissection of AML reveals progenitor-like cells that correlate with prognosis. *Cell.* (2015) 2015:47. doi: 10.1016/j.cell.2015.05.047
17. Vazquez J, Chavarria M, Li Y, Lopez GE, Stanic AK. Computational flow cytometry analysis reveals a unique immune signature of the human maternal-fetal interface. *Am J Reprod Immunol.* (2017) 79:e12774-15. doi: 10.1111/aji.12774
18. Van Gassen S, Callebaut B, Van Helden MJ, Lambrecht BN, Demeester P, Dhaene T, et al. FlowSOM: using self-organizing maps for visualization and interpretation of cytometry data. *Cytometry.* (2015) 2015:22625. doi: 10.1002/cyto.a.22625
19. Chen H, Lau MC, Wong MT, Newell EW, Poidinger M, Chen J. Cytofkit: a bioconductor package for an integrated mass cytometry data analysis pipeline. *PLoS Comput Biol.* (2016) 12:e1005112-17. doi: 10.1371/journal.pcbi.1005112
20. Thurau AM, Schylz U, Wolf V, Krug N, Schauer U. Identification of eosinophils by flow cytometry. *Cytometry.* (1996) 23:150–8. doi: 10.1002/(SICI)1097-0320(19960201)23:2<150::AID-CYTO8>3.0.CO;2-O
21. Mahnke YD, Beddall MH, Roederer M. OMIP-013: differentiation of human T-cells. *Cytometry.* (2012) 81A:935–6. doi: 10.1002/cyto.a.22201
22. Fergusson JR, Smith KE, Fleming VM, Rajoriya N, Newell EW, Simmons R, et al. CD161 defines a transcriptional and functional phenotype across distinct human T cell lineages. *Cell Rep.* (2014) 9:1075–88. doi: 10.1016/j.celrep.2014.09.045
23. Wei C, Jung J, Sanz I. OMIP-003: phenotypic analysis of human memory B cells. *Cytometry.* (2011) 79A:894–6. doi: 10.1002/cyto.a.21112
24. Mahnke YD, Beddall MH, Roederer M. OMIP-029: human NK-cell phenotypization. *Cytometry.* (2015) 87:986–8. doi: 10.1002/cyto.a.22728
25. O'Gorman WE, Hsieh EWY, Savig ES, Gherardini PF, Hernandez JD, Hansmann L, et al. Single-cell systems-level analysis of human Toll-like receptor activation defines a chemokine signature in patients with systemic lupus erythematosus. *J Allergy Clin Immunol.* (2015) 136:1326–36. doi: 10.1016/j.jaci.2015.04.008
26. Unen V, Höllt T, Pezzotti N, Li N, Reinders MJT, Eisemann E, et al. Visual analysis of mass cytometry data by hierarchical stochastic neighbour embedding reveals rare cell types. *Nat Commun.* (2017) 2017:1–9. doi: 10.1038/s41467-017-01689-9

11

Candidate Markers for Stratification and Classification in Rheumatoid Arthritis

Lucius Bader[1,2*], *Stein-Erik Gullaksen*[3,4], *Nello Blaser*[5], *Morten Brun*[5], *Gerd Haga Bringeland*[6,7], *André Sulen*[1,6], *Clara Gram Gjesdal*[1,2], *Christian Vedeler*[6,7] and *Sonia Gavasso*[1,6,7*]

[1] Bergen Group of Epidemiology and Biomarkers in Rheumatic Disease, Department of Rheumatology, Haukeland University Hospital, Bergen, Norway, [2] Department of Clinical Science, University of Bergen, Bergen, Norway, [3] Center of Cancer Biomarkers, University of Bergen, Bergen, Norway, [4] Department of Internal Medicine, Hematology Section, Haukeland University Hospital, Bergen, Norway, [5] Department of Mathematics, University of Bergen, Bergen, Norway, [6] Department of Neurology, Haukeland University Hospital, Bergen, Norway, [7] Department of Clinical Medicine, University of Bergen, Bergen, Norway

***Correspondence:**
Lucius Bader
lucius.bader@helse-bergen.no
Sonia Gavasso
sonia.gavasso@helse-bergen.no*

Rheumatoid arthritis (RA) is a chronic autoimmune, inflammatory disease, characterized by synovitis in small- and medium-sized joints and, if not treated early and efficiently, joint damage, and destruction. RA is a heterogeneous disease with a plethora of treatment options. The pro-inflammatory cytokine tumor necrosis factor (TNF) plays a central role in the pathogenesis of RA, and TNF inhibitors effectively repress inflammatory activity in RA. Currently, treatment decisions are primarily based on empirics and economic considerations. However, the considerable interpatient variability in response to treatment is a challenge. Markers for a more exact patient classification and stratification are lacking. The objective of this study was to identify markers in immune cell populations that distinguish RA patients from healthy donors with an emphasis on TNF signaling. We employed mass cytometry (CyTOF) with a panel of 13 phenotyping and 10 functional markers to explore signaling in unstimulated and TNF-stimulated peripheral blood mononuclear cells from 20 newly diagnosed, untreated RA patients and 20 healthy donors. The resulting high-dimensional data were analyzed in three independent analysis pipelines, characterized by differences in both data clean-up, identification of cell subsets/clustering and statistical approaches. All three analysis pipelines identified p-p38, IkBa, p-cJun, p-NFkB, and CD86 in cells of both the innate arm (myeloid dendritic cells and classical monocytes) and the adaptive arm (memory CD4$^+$ T cells) of the immune system as markers for differentiation between RA patients and healthy donors. Inclusion of the markers p-Akt and CD120b resulted in the correct classification of 18 of 20 RA patients and 17 of 20 healthy donors in regression modeling based on a combined model of basal and TNF-induced signal. Expression patterns in a set of functional markers and specific immune cell subsets were distinct in RA patients compared to healthy individuals. These signatures may support studies of disease pathogenesis, provide candidate markers for response, and non-response to TNF inhibitor treatment, and aid the identification of future therapeutic targets.

Keywords: rheumatoid arthritis, patient stratification, tumor necrosis factor, tumor necrosis factor inhibitors, mass cytometry

INTRODUCTION

Rheumatoid arthritis (RA) is a chronic autoimmune disease characterized by synovial inflammation that, if not treated early and efficiently, causes joint damage. The pro-inflammatory cytokine tumor necrosis factor (TNF) plays a central role in the pathogenesis of RA and is the target of treatment with TNF inhibitors. TNF inhibitors are generally effective and well-tolerated (1, 2); however, up to one-third of patients are primary non-responders, and responses in up to one-third of initial responders abate over time (3, 4).

Currently, only a few markers for diagnostic and stratification purposes are used in daily clinical practice in patients with RA. Anti-citrullinated peptide antibodies are a highly disease-specific biomarker with an impact mostly on diagnosis and classification (5). TNF inhibitor drug levels and anti-drug antibodies are indicative of treatment responses; however, these markers are not standardized for clinical application (3, 6, 7). Several candidate biomarkers for prediction of treatment responses have been suggested based on gene, cytokine, and immune cell profiles, but none have added significant value to patient stratification in a clinical setting (8). Previous studies have indicated the potential of single-cell profiling by flow or mass cytometry in patient stratification in RA and in other autoimmune conditions (9, 10). Distinct signaling patterns have been found in RA patients before and during treatment with TNF inhibitors in exploratory and proof-of-principle studies (11, 12).

We hypothesize that signaling patterns in RA are distinct from those of healthy donors. The unbiased identification of RA-specific signaling patterns in immune cell subsets before treatment may improve diagnosis, therapeutic stratification, and monitoring, and may also facilitate studies of disease pathogenesis and the development of drugs that target dysfunctional pathways with high precision.

In this study, we used mass cytometry to explore signaling responses to TNF in single immune cells of RA patients and healthy donors. In mass cytometry metal-tagged antibodies serve as markers with a read-out in a mass spectrometry time-of-flight chamber (13). Using mass cytometry, up to 50 markers can be simultaneously analyzed with single cell resolution with relatively little signal overlap and very low background noise (14, 15). Here we used a panel of 13 phenotyping and 10 functional markers for an in-depth characterization of peripheral blood mononuclear cells (PBMCs) from patients and controls with and without stimulation with TNF. Based on results from three different analysis pipelines, we suggest a smaller set of phenotyping and functional markers, which strongly correlate with disease status for future use in e.g., flow cytometry.

MATERIALS AND METHODS

In-depth information on material, methods and results is provided in the **Supplementary Material** in the same order and with the same headings/sub-headings as in the main article.

Healthy Donors and RA Patients

Twenty healthy donors (HD, 4 male, 16 female, ages 39–67) and 20 RA patients (4 male, 16 female, ages 31–76) were included in this study (**Table 1**). All RA patients were included at the time of diagnosis and fulfilled the ACR/EULAR 2010 criteria for RA. None of the patients had received synthetic or biologic disease-modifying anti-rheumatic drugs, but five had been prescribed low to moderate dosages of prednisolone by their general practitioners prior to the first consultation with a rheumatologist. Despite ongoing prednisolone-treatment at inclusion (range 2.5–15 mg), these patients had high disease activity with a mean disease activity score (DAS28) of 6.1 (range 5.4–7).

All donors and patients gave written informed consent for inclusion into the Norwegian Arthritis Registry (NorArtritt) and the Research Biobank for Rheumatic Diseases in Western Norway (approval REK 2012/1689). Utilization of registry data and biobank material for this study was approved by the Regional Ethics Committee (approval REK 2014/317).

Peripheral Blood Mononuclear Cells (PBMCs)

PBMCs were chosen due to the possibility of culturing and application of standardized and simultaneous conditions (such as e.g., cytokine stimulation) after cryo-preservation.

PBMCs were harvested by density gradient centrifugation (BD Vacutainer® CPT™ Mononuclear Cell Preparation Tube—Sodium Citrate), processed for cryo-preservation within 4 h and stored in liquid nitrogen in 50% hematopoietic cell medium (X-VIVO™, Lonza), 42.5% freezing medium (ProFreeze™, Lonza), and 7.5% dimethyl sulfoxide (Sigma-Aldrich).

TABLE 1 | Patient and healthy donor characteristics.

Healthy donors (HD)	
Female/male	16/4
Median age (range)	49 (34–67) years
RA patients (RA)	
Female/male	16/4
Median age (range)	63.5 (31–76)
Disease characteristics	
RF+	14
ACPA+	11
RF+ ACPA+	9
RF- ACPA-	4
Mean DAS28 (range)	5.37 (3–7.6)
Mean DAS28–CRP (range)	4.86 (2.5–7.2)
Mean CRP (range)	25.3 (1–156)
Mean ESR (range)	36.6 (6–104)
Medication	
Prednisolone	5 of 20 patients
Prednisolone daily dose	2.5-15 mg (2.5, 2.5, 12.5, 12.5, 15 mg)

RF, rheumatoid factor; ACPA, anti-citrullinated peptide antibodies; DAS28, disease activity score with 28 joint count; CRP, C-reactive protein; ESR, erythrocyte sedimentation rate.

Antibody Panel

All antibodies used in this study (**Table 2**) were titrated on PBMCs from one healthy donor. Titrations were performed on unstimulated PBMCs and cells stimulated with TNF and phorbol myristate acetate (PMA) for optimization of pathway activation markers. The antibodies against CD120a, CD120b, and p-cJun were conjugated to metals in our laboratory (conjugation kits and protocols by Fluidigm), all other antibodies were pre-conjugated (Fluidigm).

Thirteen markers were applied to define common PBMC subsets; these were used in both automated clustering and manual gating. Functional markers for TNF signaling were the cleaved caspase 3 as a marker for apoptosis signaling; p-p38 [T180/Y182] and p-Erk1/2 [T202/Y204] as markers for the MAPK-pathway activation; IkBa and p-NFkB p65 [S529] for the NFkB canonical pathway; p-Akt [S473] for the PI3K-Akt pathway; and p-cJun [S73] for the SAPK/JNK signaling pathway. CD86 was added as a marker of T cell regulation and analyzed as functional marker, although signaling through this pathway is not directly related to TNF.

Treatment with PMA resulted in significant increases in Erk1/2 phosphorylation, whereas TNF treatment did not have significant effects on Erk1/2 phosphorylation. This marker was therefore omitted from experiments after panel titration.

TABLE 2 | Antibody panel with epitopes, antibody clones, conjugated metals, and target cell populations or signaling pathways.

Epitope	Clone	Metal	Target/Function	Abbrev.
PHENOTYPING				
CD20	2H7	^{147}Sm	B lymphocytes	Bc
CD3	UCHT1	^{170}Er	T lymphocytes	
CD4	RPA-T4	^{145}Nd	CD4+ T lymphocytes	CD4 Tc
CD8a	RPA-T8	^{146}Nd	CD8+ T lymphocytes	CD8 Tc
CD45RA	HI100	^{169}Tm	Naïve/effector vs. memory	Naïve, mem
CD56	NCAM16.2	^{176}Yb	Natural killer cells	NKc
CD16	3G8	^{148}Nd	NK T cells	NK Tc
CD14	M5E2	^{160}Gd	Classical monocytes	cM
CD61	VI-PL2	^{209}Bi	Monocytes	cM
CD11c	Bu15	^{159}Tb	Myeloid dendritic cells	mDc
CD123 (IL-3R)	6H6	^{151}Eu	Plasmacytoid dendritic cells	pDc
HLA-DR	L243	^{174}Yb	MHCII, antigen presentation	
CD45	HI30	^{89}Y	Leukocyte Common Antigen	
FUNCTIONAL				
Cleaved Caspase 3	D3E9	^{142}Nd	Apoptotic signaling	Caspase3
p-p38 [T180/Y182]	D3F9	^{156}Gd	MAPK pathway	p-p38
p-Erk1/2 [T202/Y204]*	D13.14.4E	^{171}Yb	MAPK pathway	p-Erk
p-Akt [S473]	D9E	^{152}Sm	PI3K-Akt pathway	p-Akt
p-cJun [S73]**	D47G9	^{167}Er	SAPK/JNK signaling	p-cJun
p-NFkB p65 [S529]	K10-895.12.50	^{166}Er	NFkB canonical pathway	p-NFkB
IkBa	L35A5	^{164}Dy	with IkBa degradation	IkBa
CD120a**	MABTNFR1-B1	^{155}Gd	TNF receptor 1	TNFR1
CD120b**	hTNR-M1	^{165}Ho	TNF receptor 2	TNFR2
CD86	IT2.2	^{150}Nd	Regulation of T cell activity	CD86

**p-Erk1/2 was omitted from the panel after TNF titration experiments, since TNF stimulation did not alter p-Erk1/2 expression.*

***Metal-conjugation carried out at our laboratory (all other antibodies were purchased pre-conjugated).*

Experimental Workflow

Cryopreserved PBMCs were thawed, rapidly transferred to warm X-VIVO™ containing a nuclease (Benzonase® Nuclease, Merck Millipore, 25 U/mL), followed by centrifugation and resting in X-VIVO™ for 4 h at 37°C, 5% CO_2. The resting time was optimized in set-up experiments (data not shown). Viability staining was performed according to the manufacturer's instructions with Cell-ID™ cisplatin (Fluidigm). PBMCs from each individual were split into two aliquots; one was not stimulated, and the other was stimulated with 50 ng/mL TNF for 12 min. Stimulation time and dose had been defined after a series of TNF time and dose titrations. Cells in both samples were fixed in proteomic stabilizer (Smart Tubes Inc.) for 10 min and stored at −80°C until barcoding and staining. All cells were barcoded simultaneously with 20-plex Cell-ID™ barcoding kits (Fluidigm) as recommended by the manufacturer. After pooling, surface staining, methanol-permeabilization, and intracellular staining were carried out. PBMCs were then stained with MaxPar DNA intercalator overnight (Fluidigm) and analyzed the following day on a Helios mass cytometer (Fluidigm) after addition of normalization beads (Fluidigm). Raw FCS-files were bead-normalized, concatenated, and debarcoded with software tools from Fluidigm before subsequent analysis.

Data Analysis Workflow

Three independent analysis pipelines were performed to test and share different approaches as well as to validate our in-house NM2B algorithm (pipeline 1).

Pipeline 1: NM2B Algorithm

This algorithm consisted of three main steps: preprocessing (A), finding cell types (B) and classification (C).

A. Preprocessing: We fitted a mixture of two Gaussian distributions to mean-variance scaled "Event_length," "Center," "Offset," "Width," "Residual," "191Ir_DNA1," "193Ir_DNA2" markers for cleanup and discarded data belonging to the smaller cluster as doublets and debris (16, 17).
B. Finding cell types: We used the following phenotyping markers to detect cell types: "147Sm_CD20," "170Er_CD3," "145Nd_CD4," "146Nd_CD8a," "169Tm_CD45RA," "176Yb_CD56," "148Nd_CD16," "160Gd_CD14," "209Bi_CD61," "159Tb_CD11c," "151Eu_CD123," and

"174Yb_HLA-DR." We performed farthest point sampling to find 49 clusters. Farthest point sampling is an approximation to k-means clustering, which can be calculated for large datasets. Clusters of size less than 1/100,000 of the total data size were discarded. We then employed complete linkage meta-clustering of the farthest points with 15 meta-clusters and discarded all meta-clusters of less than 0.5% of the total data size. The final 12 meta-clusters contained a total of 18,374,011 cell events (**Supplementary Figure 3**).

C. Classification: We used the following functional markers as features for classification of individuals as patients or controls: "142Nd_Caspase3," "156Gd_p-p38," "152Sm_p-Akt," "167Er_p-cJun," "166Er_p-NFkB," "164Dy_IkBa," "155Gd_CD120a," "165Ho_CD120b," "150Nd_CD86." For each meta-cluster we calculated the median and 90% quantile of each of the functional markers for all basal cells. In addition, we calculated the arcsinh ratios of the expression of functional markers in stimulated and basal cells. We tested three models, based on either only basal variables (basal), or only arcsinh ratios between stimulated and basal variables (ratio) or both basal and arcsinh ratios (combined). We fitted a logistic lasso regression model, that is a logistic regression model with automatic variable selection, using double leave-one-out cross validation. For details of how double leave-one-out cross-validation was performed we refer to the **Supplementary Material**. We report cross-validation accuracy, area under the ROC curve (AUC), and all non-zero coefficients.

Pipeline 2: CITRUS Algorithm

Normalized, concatenated and debarcoded files were imported in Cytobank for downstream analysis (18). Data were cleaned for doublets, debris and dead cells by biaxial gating and analyzed with the cluster identification, characterization, and regression tool CITRUS in cytobank.org, applying the predictive regression model Nearest Shrunken Centroid/PAMR (19). CITRUS was run on the same data set, but with independent downsampling, with 3 repetitions.

Pipeline 3: Manual Analysis

Normalized, concatenated, and debarcoded files were imported in Cytobank. Data were cleaned for doublets, debris, and dead cells by biaxial gating. viSNE analysis based on t-distributed stochastic neighbor embedding was performed for each donor and patient after downsampling to 50,000 cell events per individual and condition (20), and cell subsets were gated on individual viSNE plots (**Supplementary Figure 6**). Expression of functional markers was compared in all cell subsets, both unstimulated and TNF-stimulated, by applying non-parametric Mann-Whitney U tests using GraphPad prism version 7.0c for Mac OS X. A correction for multiple comparisons was not conducted due to the explorative character of this study.

RESULTS

Pipeline 1: NM2B Algorithm

Single-cell data from all 40 individuals were clustered and meta-clustered, and different numbers of clusters and meta-clusters were tested. The model used provided the best translation of meta-clusters into common immune cell subsets. The numbers of clusters and meta-clusters influenced cross-validation accuracy for the classification of RA patients and healthy donors, but when higher numbers of meta-clusters were used, the results were more difficult to interpret with regards to common cell subsets (data not shown).

Results presented here are based on 49 clusters and 12 meta-clusters; the latter include one B cell meta-cluster (4.3%), four of T cells (75.3%), two of natural killer cells (5%), one of classical monocytes (5.7%), three of myeloid dendritic cells (8.8%) and one of plasmacytoid dendritic cells (1%). Phenotyping markers are differentially expressed in the meta-clusters (**Figure 1A**); differences in expression of phenotyping markers in healthy donors vs. RA patients were not significant (**Supplementary Figure 10**).

A regression model based on both basal expression of functional markers and arcsinh ratios ("combined model") provided the best predictive TNF signaling patterns for healthy donors and RA patients. In this model seven functional markers (IkBa, CD120b, CD86, p-cJun, p-NFkB, p-p38, and p-Akt) in five cell subsets (memory $CD4^+$ T cells, CD11c+HLA-DR+$CD14^{low}CD61^{low}$ myeloid dendritic cells, naïve $CD4^+CD45RA^+CD11c^{low}$ T cells, classical monocytes, and $CD11c^{high}$HLA-$DR^{high}CD61^{low}$ myeloid dendritic cells) were identified as predictive markers (**Figure 1B**). Applying these markers, the combined model correctly classified 18 of 20 RA patients and 17 of 20 healthy donors (**Figure 1C**). The two patients who were not classified correctly were both females older than 67 years with high disease activity (DAS28 5.3/6.4). One was seronegative and one was being treated with prednisolone at 12.5 mg per day. Principle component analysis (PCA) of features identified by the Lasso-regression showed a good separation of HD vs. RA in the combined (**Figure 1D**) and basal model, but to a lesser degree in the ratio model (**Supplementary Figures 7–9**).

Pipeline 2: CITRUS Algorithm

We performed four repetitive CITRUS analyses of basal expression of functional markers. p-p38, IkBa, p-cJun, p-NFkB, and CD86 were identified as predictive markers by CITRUS, with memory $CD4^+$ T cells being the most relevant cell subset for both p-p38, IkBa, and p-cJun, while clusters within myeloid dendritic cell subets (mDc) and classical monocytes (cM) were the most relevant for p-NFkB and CD86 (**Supplementary Figure 11** and **Supplementary Table 10**). There was not always a clear distinction between myeloid dendritic cells and classical monocytes in hierarchical clustering in CITRUS, and both these cell subsets were relevant for the markers p-NFkB and CD86 (**Figure 1E** and **Supplementary Table 10**).

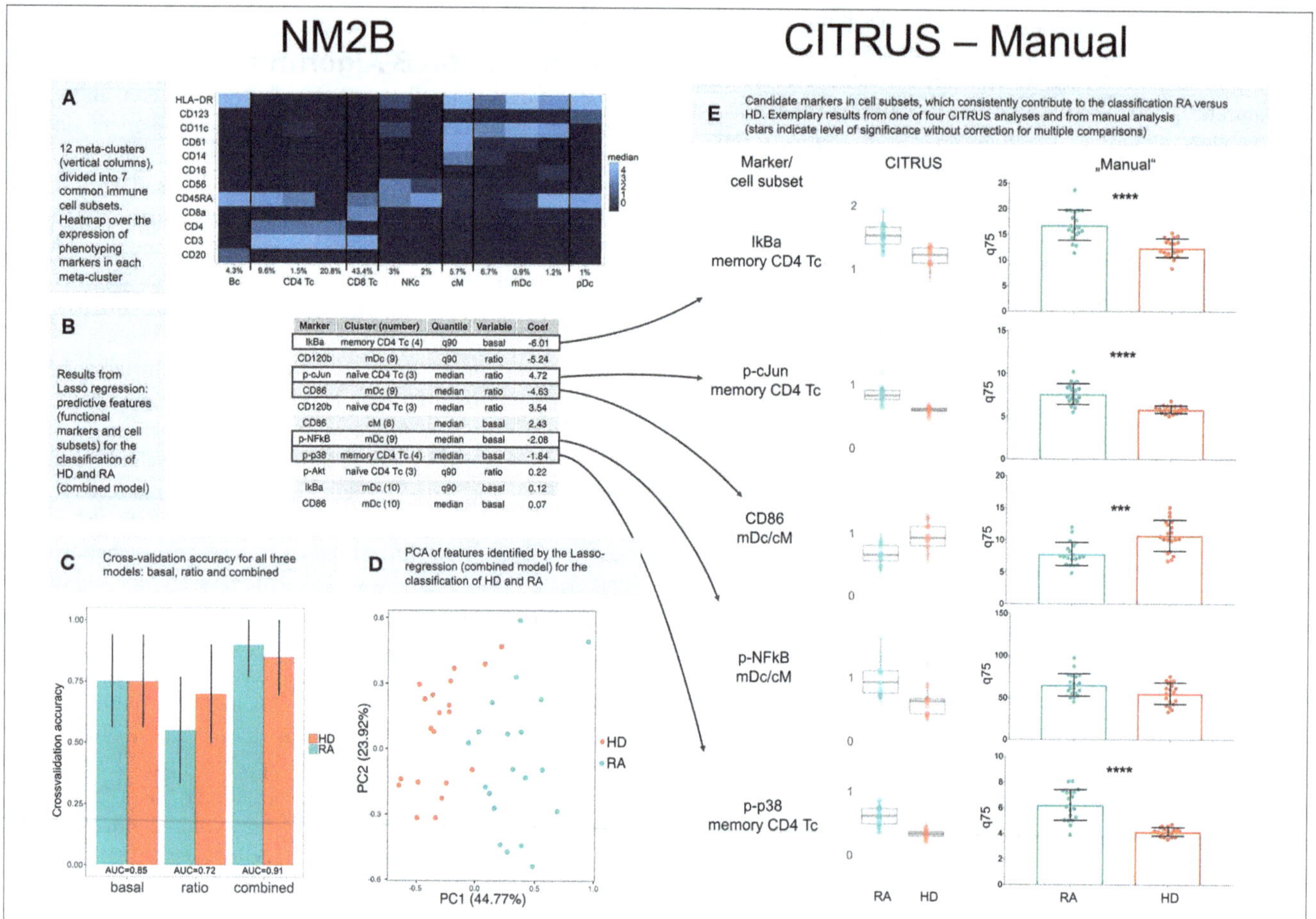

FIGURE 1 | Results. **(A)** Heatmap over the expression of phenotyping markers in 12 meta-clusters (columns). Meta-clusters were identified as B cells (Bc), CD4$^+$ T cells (CD4 Tc), CD8$^+$ T cells (CD8 Tc), natural killer cells (NKc), classical monocytes (cM), myeloid dendritic cells (mDc), and plasmacytoid dendritic cells (pDc). Relative abundance is given for each cell subset in percent. **(B)** Results from Lasso regression: predictive features (functional markers and cell subsets) and their contribution to the classification of healthy donors (HD) and RA patients (RA). Only nonzero coefficients are shown. Coefficients for CD86 and p-cJun are based on ratios and therefore inverted compared to CITRUS and manual comparisons of basal marker expression. **(C)** Cross-validation accuracy for all three NM2B analyses ("basal," "ratio," and "combined"), with area-under-the-curve (AUC) values for ROC analysis. **(D)** Principle component analysis (PCA) of features identified by Lasso-regression (combined model) for the classification of RA patients and healthy donors. **(E)** Cluster identification, characterization, and regression algorithm (CITRUS) and non-parametric testing (Manual). CITRUS results are presented in boxplots, as provided by the algorithm. Results from manual analysis are presented in scatter dot plots. Medians (CITRUS) and 75th percentiles (manual) are plotted for each RA patient (blue) and healthy donor (red); median, and upper and lower quartile. Asterisks indicate level of significance without correction for multiple comparisons (***$p < 0.001$, ****$p < 0.0001$).

Compared to the NM2B and manual analysis, there were slight differences in the weighting of cell subsets for p-cJun (**Figure 1E**). In four CITRUS analyses, memory CD4$^+$ T cells were the primary cell subset of interest for p-cJun, whereas automated analysis pointed to naïve CD4$^+$ T cells as the most significant cell subset. In manual analysis, p-cJun expression was significantly different between HD and RA in both naïve and memory CD4 Tc.

Exemplary CITRUS results and cross validation model error rates can be found in **Supplementary Figures 11, 12**.

Pipeline 3: Manual Analysis

The manual analysis generally confirmed results from regression data modeling (**Figure 1E**). For the p-NFkB, regression tools had suggested significant differences in myeloid dendritic cell and classical monocyte subsets. However, in non-parametric testing, p-NFkB expression was not significantly different in myeloid dendritic cell and classical monocyte subsets of healthy donors vs. RA patients, but there were differences in p-NFkB in memory CD4$^+$ T cells. Complete results from manual analysis are shown in **Supplementary Figures 13–15**.

In summary, and based on all three analysis pipelines, we suggest that the phenotyping markers CD4, CD45RA, and CD11c (to identify CD4 naïve and memory CD4$^+$ T cells, and myeloid dendritic cells) and the functional markers p-p38, IkBa, p-cJun, p-NFkB, and CD86 may be candidate markers for a simplified setup, e.g., in confirmatory studies by flow cytometry.

DISCUSSION

In this study, comprehensive investigation of signaling patterns in unstimulated and TNF-stimulated immune cells by mass cytometry revealed cell type specific differences in RA patients compared to healthy donors of the same gender and with similar ages. Applying predictive regression models, we found that the basal expression of p-p38 and IkBa in memory CD4$^+$ T cells, p-cJun in naïve, and memory CD4$^+$ T cells, and p-NFkB and CD86 in myeloid dendritic cells and classical monocytes differentiated between healthy donors and RA patients. We want to emphasize the explorative character of our study and the role of mass cytometry in this setting. Mass cytometry and related analysis tools are currently not used in routine clinical practice. However, in this study we suggest a smaller set of markers for the distinction between HD and RA. These markers could make our approach applicable and feasible in future research e.g., on a flow cytometry platform. Our data indicate that phenotyping markers CD4, CD45RA, CD11c for the identification of CD4$^+$ T cell subsets and myeloid dendritic cells, and p-p38, IkBa, p-cJun, p-NFkB, and CD86 as relevant functional markers could be used to analyze unstimulated PBMCs by flow cytometry for diagnosis and stratification in RA.

Studies of signaling pathways in arthritis are often limited to one or two distinct cell subsets and a few functional markers and are frequently carried out in animal arthritis models. Comprehensive investigation of signaling in immune cell subsets in patients and healthy individuals has been challenging due to technical limitations. High-dimensional mass cytometry can fill a gap as it enables the simultaneous investigation of many markers in millions of heterogeneous cells with a single-cell resolution. Our study utilized a total of 34 channels (including barcoding and beads) and only partially exploited the potential of the technology.

In an analysis of a single RA patient and one healthy donor Nair et al. demonstrated that a complex mass cytometry setup distinguished between health and disease and was able to detect changes after TNF inhibitor treatment (12). Due to the illustrational character of their study, differences in signaling were not quantified, but both p-p38 and p-NFkB were differentiating markers in several cell subsets. Their data pointed to granulocytes as a cell population altered by TNF pathway activation. In support of this, another study had previously shown that granulocytes express high levels of TNF receptors (21). Unfortunately, our study did not include granulocytes as we studied PBMCs. PBMCs were selected to provide a detailed insight into non-granulocyte white blood cell populations, allowing for simultaneous stimulation of cells from the entire cohort under standardized conditions after cryo-preservation.

The use of cryo-preserved PBMCs introduces several potential contributors to variation, and deprives cells from their individual surroundings by the removal of plasma (22–26). We reduced variation through stringent use of standard operating procedures for the handling of live cells from the time of collection to cryo-preservation to resting and stimulation. Moreover, the experimental steps were conducted simultaneously on cells from all donors whenever feasible. However, for future study we would recommend the use of peripheral blood leukocytes with immediate fixation after sample acquisition from patient and donor.

Galligan et al. performed a phospho-flow analysis on PBMCs on a less homogeneous RA population than our cohort. The Galligan et al. cohort included RA patients at different disease stages treated with different medications and patients with osteoarthritis and healthy donors (11). In agreement with our results, they found elevated levels of several phospho-epitopes in CD4$^+$ T cell subsets in RA patients compared to healthy donors, and, to a lesser degree, to osteoarthritis patients. Interestingly, there were not significant differences in p38 phosphorylation levels between RA patients and healthy controls in the Galligan et al. study. Unfortunately, markers for the canonical NFkB-signaling pathway were not included.

To identify differences between "healthy" and "sick" representative cohorts of both groups are required. However, the number of simultaneously applicable barcodes, parallel handling of all samples, read-out time on the mass cytometer, and analysis of multi-dimensional data on millions of events set currently limits on cohort sizes. Based on a total of 40 individuals, our study is primarily of explorative character. Our cohorts were sex-matched. We aimed to achieve an age match between patients and healthy donors, although immune status has been shown to be rather stable over time in healthy adults (27). Our experimental setup allowed for a high degree of simultaneous analysis, running 80 samples (20HD+20RA in two conditions) at the same time. For future studies with more samples, it is important to assure that results are robust across different cytometry runs, e.g., through the use of a reference sample.

We only included newly diagnosed patients in whom disease related immune status was unaffected by immune-modulatory or immune-suppressive treatment with the exception of low-to-moderate dosages of prednisolone in five of the 20 patients. While prednisolone treatment may introduce an unwanted heterogeneity, this reflects the real-life situation at rheumatology outpatient clinics, with some patients being referred after pre-treatment. In a sub-group analysis with CITRUS we couldn't identify factors that differentiated prednisolone-treated from prednisolone-naïve patients.

RA is an inflammatory condition, and untreated patients are expected to express signs of inflammation on a cellular level compared to healthy donors. In our RA cohort, 15 patients had elevated levels of CRP, including all five patients treated with prednisolone. The higher levels of markers known to be involved in inflammatory signaling pathways, such as the canonical NFkB and the MAPK signaling pathways, in patients compared to healthy donors in this cohort was, therefore, not a surprise. We did not include patients with different inflammatory conditions in our study, hence the specificity of the observed signaling signatures for RA compared to other inflammatory conditions is not known. For future studies, cohorts with other TNF-driven conditions such as e.g., inflammatory bowel diseases should be added as disease controls.

That CD86 was consistently expressed to a lesser degree on classical monocytes and myeloid dendritic cells of RA patients compared to healthy donors is likely relevant to the pathogenesis of RA. CD86 is highly expressed on antigen-presenting cells in synovial fluid and synovia of RA patients, whereas CD28, the T cell counterpart of CD86, is expressed at lower levels in patients with active RA compared to healthy donors (28).

In conclusion, this study provided insight into TNF-mediated signaling patterns, which are distinct for RA patients compared to healthy individuals. A comprehensive understanding of signaling signatures may facilitate more accurate diagnosis, better stratification of patients to guide treatment decisions, and the identification of candidate treatment targets in RA patients.

ETHICS STATEMENT

All donors and patients gave written informed consent for inclusion into the Norwegian Arthritis Registry (NorArtritt) and the Research Biobank for Rheumatic Diseases in Western Norway (approval REK 2012/1689). Utilization of registry data and biobank material for this study was approved by the Regional Ethics Committee (approval REK 2014/317).

AUTHOR'S NOTE

A summary of this work was presented in poster form at Cyto2018 in Prague, abstract B13 156.

AUTHOR CONTRIBUTIONS

All authors have contributed to manuscript review. LB has contributed with experiment design, collection of samples and clinical data, cytokine and antibody titration, all laboratory work, data analysis pipeline 1 and 2, manuscript writing. S-EG has contributed to cytokine and antibody titrations, followed critically through especially the data analysis part of this study. NB and MB have contributed with data analysis pipeline 3 and manuscript writing. GB has contributed with laboratory work, ciritical follow-up through all stages of this study. AS has contributed with initial experiments for TNF stimulation and background work on TNF receptors/TNF receptor antibodies. CG has contributed to experiment design and facilitated collection of samples and clinical data. CV has contributed to experiment design and facilitated sample collection, laboratory work, and mass cytometry experiments. SG has contributed to experiment design and critical supervision throughout all parts of this study.

ACKNOWLEDGMENTS

The authors want to thank all patients and healthy donors for their contributions to this work.

REFERENCES

1. Klareskog L, Catrina AI, Paget S. Rheumatoid arthritis. *Lancet.* (2009) 373:659–72. doi: 10.1016/s0140-6736(09)60008-8
2. Scott DL, Wolfe F, Huizinga TWJ. Rheumatoid arthritis. *Lancet.* (2010) 376:1094–108. doi: 10.1016/s0140-6736(10)60826-4
3. Bendtzen K. Personalized medicine: theranostics (therapeutics diagnostics) essential for rational use of tumor necrosis factor-alpha antagonists. *Discov Med.* (2013) 15:201–11.
4. Singh JA, Christensen R, Wells GA, Suarez-Almazor ME, Buchbinder R, Lopez-Olivo MA, et al. A network meta-analysis of randomized controlled trials of biologics for rheumatoid arthritis: a Cochrane overview. *Can Med Assoc J.* (2009) 181:787–96. doi: 10.1503/cmaj.091391
5. Aletaha D, Neogi T, Silman AJ, Funovits J, Felson DT, Bingham CO, III, et al. 2010 rheumatoid arthritis classification criteria: an american college of rheumatology/european league against rheumatism collaborative initiative. *Ann Rheum Diseases.* (2010) 69:1580–8. doi: 10.1136/ard.2010.138461
6. Bader LI, Solberg SM, Kaada SH, Bolstad N, Warren DJ, Gavasso S, et al. Assays for infliximab drug levels and antibodies: a matter of scales and categories. *Scand J Immunol.* (2017) 86:165–70. doi: 10.1111/sji.12572
7. Steenholdt C, Brynskov J, Thomsen OO, Munck LK, Fallingborg J, Christensen LA, et al. Individualised therapy is more cost-effective than dose intensification in patients with Crohn's disease who lose response to anti-TNF treatment: a randomised, controlled trial. *Gut.* (2013). doi: 10.1136/gutjnl-2013-305279
8. Cuppen BV, Welsing PM, Sprengers JJ, Bijlsma JW, Marijnissen AC, van Laar JM, et al. Personalized biological treatment for rheumatoid arthritis: a systematic review with a focus on clinical applicability. *Rheumatology.* (2016) 55:826–39. doi: 10.1093/rheumatology/kev421
9. Ermann J, Rao DA, Teslovich NC, Brenner MB, Raychaudhuri S. Immune cell profiling to guide therapeutic decisions in rheumatic diseases. *Nat Rev Rheumatol.* (2015) 11:541–51. doi: 10.1038/nrrheum.2015.71
10. Gavasso S, Gjertsen B, Anderssen E, Myhr K, Vedeler C. Immunogenic effects of recombinant interferon-beta therapy disrupt the JAK/STAT pathway in primary immune cells from patients with multiple sclerosis. *Multiple Sclerosis.* (2012) 18:1116–24. doi: 10.1177/1352458511434066
11. Galligan CL, Siebert JC, Siminovitch KA, Keystone EC, Bykerk V, Perez OD, et al. Multiparameter phospho-flow analysis of lymphocytes in early rheumatoid arthritis: implications for diagnosis and monitoring drug therapy. *PLoS ONE.* (2009) 4:e6703. doi: 10.1371/journal.pone.0006703
12. Nair N, Mei HE, Chen SY, Hale M, Nolan GP, Maecker HT, et al. Mass cytometry as a platform for the discovery of cellular biomarkers to guide effective rheumatic disease therapy. *Arthritis Res Ther.* (2015) 17:127. doi: 10.1186%2Fs13075-015-0644-z
13. Ornatsky O, Baranov VI, Bandura DR, Tanner SD, Dick J. Multiple cellular antigen detection by ICP-MS. *J Immunol Methods.* (2006) 308:68–76. doi: 10.1016/j.jim.2005.09.020
14. Ornatsky O, Bandura D, Baranov V, Nitz M, Winnik MA, Tanner S. Highly multiparametric analysis by mass cytometry. *J Immunol Methods.* (2010) 361:1–20. doi: 10.1016/j.jim.2010.07.002
15. Spitzer MH, Nolan GP. Mass cytometry: single cells, many features. *Cell.* (2016) 165:780–91. doi: 10.1016/j.cell.2016.04.019
16. Bagwell B. *A New Analytic Approach for Live Singlet Identification*. (2017). Available online at: https://www.fluidigm.com/articles/mass-cyto-summit-videos?mkt__tok=eyJpIjoiT0RVeU5ERTBNbU5oWW1GbSIsInQiOiJ4U3NDdUZjbVoyRCt6UThrWXg4b3M3RUNick5ZK0lsekJZQzU3VFZyU0QwYW5UaHdaQUxwbDh3ZHJzbTRcLzg3MlhIWkh5bEFDMUdWSFk0NWpiTmhueGVXQ3IzQzI4K0Q5a015cGM1bFdrVHl2elpNY2JGUERqb2I3MEk0RW9FemgifQ%3D%3D#bagwell (accessed June 09, 2017).

17. Fluidigm. *Maxpar Human Immune Monitoring Panel Kit Validation Studies.* (2018).
18. Kotecha N, Krutzik PO, Irish JM. Web-based analysis and publication of flow cytometry experiments. *Curr Protocols Cytometry.* (2010) Chapter 10:Unit10.7. doi: 10.1002/0471142956.cy1017s53
19. Bruggner RV, Bodenmiller B, Dill DL, Tibshirani RJ, Nolan GP. Automated identification of stratifying signatures in cellular subpopulations. *Proc Natl Acad Sci USA.* (2014) 111:E2770–7. doi: 10.1073/pnas.1408792111
20. Amir el AD, Davis KL, Tadmor MD, Simonds EF, Levine JH, Bendall SC, et al. viSNE enables visualization of high dimensional single-cell data and reveals phenotypic heterogeneity of leukemia. *Nat Biotechnol.* (2013) 31:545–52. doi: 10.1038/nbt.2594
21. Liu C, Tang J. Expression levels of tumor necrosis factor-α and the corresponding receptors are correlated with trauma severity. *Oncol Lett.* (2014) 8:2747–51. doi: 10.3892/ol.2014.2575
22. Corkum CP, Ings DP, Burgess C, Karwowska S, Kroll W, Michalak TI. Immune cell subsets and their gene expression profiles from human PBMC isolated by Vacutainer Cell Preparation Tube (CPT) and standard density gradient. *BMC Immunol.* (2015) 16:48. doi: 10.1186/s12865-015-0113-0
23. Grievink HW, Luisman T, Kluft C, Moerland M, Malone KE. Comparison of three isolation techniques for human peripheral blood mononuclear cells: cell recovery and viability, population composition, and cell functionality. *Biopreserv Biobank.* (2016) 14:410–5. doi: 10.1089/bio.2015.0104
24. Kadic E, Moniz RJ, Huo Y, Chi A, Kariv I. Effect of cryopreservation on delineation of immune cell subpopulations in tumor specimens as determinated by multiparametric single cell mass cytometry analysis. *BMC Immunol.* (2017) 18:6. doi: 10.1186/s12865-017-0192-1
25. Lemieux J, Jobin C, Simard C, Neron S. A global look into human T cell subsets before and after cryopreservation using multiparametric flow cytometry and two-dimensional visualization analysis. *J Immunol Methods.* (2016) 434:73–82. doi: 10.1016/j.jim.2016.04.010
26. Rahmanian N, Bozorgmehr M, Torabi M, Akbari A, Zarnani AH. Cell separation: potentials and pitfalls. *Preparat Biochem Biotechnol.* (2017) 47:38–51. doi: 10.1080/10826068.2016.1163579
27. Brodin P, Davis MM. Human immune system variation. *Nat Rev Immunol.* (2017) 17:21–9. doi: 10.1038/nri.2016.125
28. Sfikakis PP, Via CS. Expression of CD28, CTLA4, CD80, and CD86 molecules in patients with autoimmune rheumatic diseases: implications for immunotherapy. *Clin Immunol Immunopathol.* (1997) 83:195–8.

12

Mass Cytometry Discovers Two Discrete Subsets of CD39^{-}Treg Which Discriminate MGUS From Multiple Myeloma

*Felix Marsh-Wakefield[1,2†], Annabel Kruzins[3†], Helen M. McGuire[4,5,6], Shihong Yang[7], Christian Bryant[7], Barbara Fazekas de St. Groth[4,5,6], Najah Nassif[3], Scott N. Byrne[1], John Gibson[7,8], Christina Brown[7,8], Stephen Larsen[7,8], Derek McCulloch[7,8], Richard Boyle[9], Georgina Clark[10], Douglas Joshua[7,8], Phoebe Joy Ho[7,8] and Slavica Vuckovic[7,11]**

[1] Discipline of Infectious Diseases and Immunology, Faculty of Medicine and Health, Central Clinical School, The University of Sydney, Sydney, NSW, Australia, [2] Discipline of Pathology, Faculty of Medicine and Health, School of Medical Science, The University of Sydney, Sydney, NSW, Australia, [3] School of Life Sciences, University of Technology Sydney, Sydney, NSW, Australia, [4] Ramaciotti Facility for Human Systems Biology, The University of Sydney, Sydney, NSW, Australia, [5] Discipline of Pathology, Sydney Medical School, The University of Sydney, Sydney, NSW, Australia, [6] Charles Perkins Centre, The University of Sydney, Sydney, NSW, Australia, [7] Royal Prince Alfred Hospital, Institute of Haematology, Sydney, NSW, Australia, [8] Sydney Medical School, The University of Sydney, Sydney, NSW, Australia, [9] Orthopaedics Department, Royal Prince Alfred Hospital, Sydney, NSW, Australia, [10] Concord Repatriation General Hospital, ANZAC Research Institute, Concord, NSW, Australia, [11] Faculty of Medicine, University of Queensland, Brisbane, QLD, Australia

***Correspondence:**
Slavica Vuckovic
slavica.vuckovic@health.nsw.gov.au

† These authors have contributed equally to this work

Multiple Myeloma (MM) is preceded by the clinically stable condition monoclonal gammopathy of undetermined significance (MGUS). Critical immune events that discriminate MGUS from newly diagnosed MM (ND)MM patients remain unknown, but may involve changes in the regulatory T cell (Treg) compartment that favor myeloma growth. To address this possibility, we used mass cytometry and the unsupervised clustering algorithm Flow self-organizing map (FlowSOM) to interrogate the distribution of multiple subsets within CD25^{+}CD127$^{low/neg}$Treg in matched bone marrow (BM) and peripheral blood (PB) of MGUS and NDMM patients. Both mass cytometry and flow cytometry confirmed a trend toward prevalence of CD39^{-}Treg within the Treg compartment in BM and PB of NDMM patients compared to CD39^{-}Treg in MGUS patients. FlowSOM clustering displayed a phenotypic organization of Treg into 25 metaclusters that confirmed Treg heterogeneity. It identified two subsets which emerged within CD39^{-}Treg of NDMM patients that were negligible or absent in CD39^{-}Treg of MGUS patients. One subset was found in both BM and PB which phenotypically resembled activated Treg based on CD45RO, CD49d, and CD62L expression; another subset resembled BM-resident Treg based on its tissue-resident CD69^{+}CD62L^{-}CD49d^{-} phenotype and restricted location within the BM. Both subsets co-expressed PD-1 and TIGIT, but PD-1 was expressed at higher levels on BM-resident Treg than on activated Treg. Within BM, both subsets had limited Perforin and Granzyme B production, whilst activated Treg in PB acquired high Perforin and Granzyme B production. In conclusion, the use of mass cytometry and FlowSOM clustering discovered two discrete subsets of $CD39^{-}$Treg which are discordant in MGUS and NDMM patients and may be permissive of myeloma growth which warrants further study. Understanding the regulatory properties of these subsets may also advance MGUS and MM diagnosis, prognosis, and therapeutic implications for MM patients.

Keywords: MGUS, multiple myeloma, mass cytometry, FlowSom, Treg

INTRODUCTION

Multiple Myeloma (MM) is characterized by clonal expansion of malignant plasma cells in the bone marrow (BM). It is preceded by the clinically stable condition monoclonal gammopathy of undetermined significance (MGUS), which is defined by the presence of a monoclonal protein and <10% malignant plasma cell infiltration in the BM. The underlining immunological mechanism preventing malignant plasma cell expansion in MGUS compared to the permissive expansion of malignant plasma cells in MM patients is poorly understood and remains under active investigation (1). However, an accepted concept has been that the immune system in MM patients is tipped in favor of myeloma growth by initiating immunosuppressive mechanisms mediated by different regulatory immune cells, particularly regulatory T cells (Treg) (2).

Suppressive Treg are a subset of $CD4^{+}$T lymphocytes driven by the expression of transcription factor forkhead box P3 (FoxP3), and play an important role in the maintenance of self-tolerance and the control of immune homeostasis (3). In humans, the Treg compartment encompasses multiple subsets which delineate different developmental stages and their associated regulatory functions (4). Based on CD45RA and FoxP3 expression Treg were divided into three subsets: resting Treg ($CD45RA^{+}FoxP3^{lo}$), activated Treg ($CD45RA^{-}FoxP3^{hi}$) and non-suppressive Treg ($CD45RA^{-}FoxP3^{lo}$) which secrete IL-10 as well as TGF-β (5). Additional phenotypic features of these defined Treg subsets include CD49d expression on activated Treg (6) and ICOS expression on IL-10 and TGF-β secreting Treg (7). In addition specific combinations of chemokine receptor expression (CCR6, CXCR3, CCR4, CCR10) can be used to define Treg subsets capable of regulating Th cell responses (8). Expression of ectonucleotidase CD39 defines a subset of Treg involved in the CD39/CD73 adenosine pathway, a key immunosuppressive mechanism operating in tumor microenvironments (9, 10).

Heterogeneity within the human Treg compartment has usually been defined by classical flow cytometry which may underestimate the complexity due to a limited multiplexing capacity as well as limitations associated with classical biaxial gating. The recent introduction of mass cytometry provides multiparametric analyses (11), combined with high-dimensional data analysis allowing the identification of 22 phenotypically distinct subsets based on 26 analyzed parameters within the Treg compartment in peripheral blood (PB) samples of healthy adults (12).

Previous studies demonstrated the ability of myeloma cells to induce activation and expansion of functional Treg in either myeloma-infiltrated BM or *in vitro* cultures (13, 14). We considered that in a growth permissive BM environment, myeloma cells may change pre-existing heterogeneity within the Treg compartment by inducing discrete Treg subsets which facilitate its progression. The emergence of these Treg subsets may support critical initiating events indicative of clinically active myeloma and potentially discriminate between MGUS and newly diagnosed (ND)MM patients. In this study we used mass cytometry and the unsupervised clustering algorithm Flow self-organizing map (FlowSOM) to interrogate at a high resolution the heterogeneity within the Treg compartment in matched BM and PB of MGUS and NDMM patients, and discovered two discrete subsets of $CD39^{-}$Treg which are able to discriminate between these two clinical entities.

MATERIALS AND METHODS

Patient and Healthy Donor Samples

MGUS and MM patients were recruited at the Royal Prince Alfred Hospital and diagnosed based on clinical symptoms and biopsies. Age-matched healthy donors (HD) included healthy blood donors and patients without diagnosed malignancy, autoimmune disease (including diabetes), or active infection undergoing hip arthroplasty at the Department of Orthopedic Surgery at the Royal Prince Alfred Hospital. A total of 22 patients, MGUS ($n = 6$) and NDMM ($n = 16$) and 15 HD (blood donors $n = 6$; patient $n = 9$) donated either blood, BM or both for this study. Matched BM and PB samples were always analyzed in the same experiment. Due to sampling restrictions, it was not possible to obtain matched BM and PB samples from all patients and HD or to analyze all samples by both mass cytometry and flow cytometry, so an assay selection was based on sample availability. Patient and HD characteristics and assay usage are displayed in **Table S1**. BM-mononuclear cells (BM-MNC) and PB-MNC were isolated by Ficoll-Hypaque (GE Healthcare) density gradient and cryopreserved prior to experimentation. The study was approved by the institutional Human Ethics Committee (X15-0357, X16-0291, X18-0096, HREC/11/CRGH/61). All patients gave written informed consent in accordance with the amended Declaration of Helsinki.

Flow Cytometry

Antibodies used for flow cytometry analysis were: V500-CD3 (clone UCHT1, BD), APC-H7-CD8 (clone SK1, BD), V450-CD4 (clone RPA-T4, BD), PerCy5.5-CD4 (clone SK3), PE-CD25 (clone 2A3, BD), FITC-CD127 (clone HIL-7R-M21, BD), APC-CD39 (clone B249211, BioLegend), PE-Cy7-CD73 (clone AD2, BD), IgG1-APC (clone MOPC-21, BD), IgG1-PerCP-Cy5.5 (clone X40, BD), IgG1-PE-Cy7 (clone X40, BD),

AF647-Foxp3 (clone 206D, Biolegend). Intranuclear FoxP3 staining was conducted using eBiosciences FoxP3 buffer kit (San Diego, CA, USA) according to the manufacturers' protocol. The LIVE/DEAD™ Fixable Violet dead cell stain kit (L34955, Invitrogen) was used to exclude dead cells. Stained cells were acquired using the BD FACSCanto II and analyzed using FlowJo software 10.4.2. Treg were defined as $CD25^{+}CD127^{low/neg}$ or $CD4^{+}FoxP3^{+}$ events.

Mass Cytometry Staining and Data Acquisition

Three million BM-MNC or PB-MNC were stained for mass cytometry with metal-conjugated monoclonal antibodies (mAb) as listed in **Table S2**. Briefly, cells were stained with 1.25 μM cisplatin in RPMI for 3 min at room temperature and quenched with FACS buffer (PBS, 0.02% Sodium Azide, 0.5% BSA, and 2 mM EDTA). Cells were incubated at 4°C for 30 min initially with AF647-labeled CD160. Following a FACS wash step cells were subsequently incubated at 4°C for 30 min with a cocktail of metal-conjugated mAb targeting surface proteins. Metal-conjugated mAb were purchased from Fluidigm (Toronto, Canada) or purchased in a carrier-protein-free format and conjugated with the respective metal isotope using the MaxPAR antibody conjugation kit (Fluidigm) according to the manufacturer's recommended protocol by the Ramaciotti Facility for Human Systems Biology, Sydney, Australia. Following wash with FACS buffer, cells were fixed and permeabilized for 45 min using the eBioscience's FoxP3 buffer kit, then incubated for 30 min at 4°C with a cocktail of metal-conjugated mAb targeting intracellular proteins. Cells were subsequently washed with Perm buffer then FACS buffer, and fixed overnight in 4% paraformaldehyde containing DNA intercalator (0.125 μM iridium-191; Fluidigm). After multiple washes with FACS buffer and MilliQ water, cell concentration was adjusted to 0.8×10^{6} cells/mL in MilliQ water with EQ beads (Fluidigm) diluted 1 in 10 and filtered through a 35 μm nylon mesh. Cells were acquired at a rate of 200–400 cells/s using a CyTOF 2 Helios upgraded mass cytometer (Fluidigm, Toronto, Canada). Data collected in .fcs file format were normalized for signal intensity of EQ beads using the Helios software.

Mass Cytometry Data Analysis

FlowJo 10.4.2 software (FlowJo, LLC, Ashland, OR, USA) was used to gate Treg. Our gating strategy excluded calibration beads by gating on 140 Ce^{-} events and cell aggregates using DNA signal (191Ir) and event length. $CD38^{+}CD3^{-}$ (myeloma cells), $CD19^{+}$ (B cells), and $CD56^{+}$ (NK cells) were excluded prior to Treg gating. Treg were identified within gated $CD3^{+}CD8^{-}CD4^{+}$ T cells as $CD25^{+}CD127^{low/neg}$. All Treg with channel numbers for all markers across all samples were imported into R studio (v1.1.456). To assist in mass cytometry data analysis, the script Cytometry Analysis Pipeline for large and compleX datasets (CAPX) was utilized (15). CAPX includes both the clustering algorithm FlowSOM (16) and dimensionality reduction algorithm t-SNE (17) in a single script (https://github.sydney.edu.au/fmar5916/FMW-2019-TReg). For these algorithms, each sample contributed the same number of Treg (2,550 cells) to minimize any bias. Thirteen markers associated with Treg identification and activation were used for both clustering and dimensionality reduction. This included CD122, CD27, CD39, CD62L, CD127, CD45RA, CD69, CD49d, CD28, CD45RO, CD197, CD25, and CD38 (**Table S2**). FlowSOM was first run to create 25 metaclusters (MC), using two different seeds: seed A (FlowSOM_seed = 42) and seed B (FlowSOM_seed = 204) to confirm reproducibility. After this, the concatenated data were down-sampled to a total of 35,000 cells. t-SNE plots were generated on these data using the same 13 markers with the following parameters: perplexity = 30, theta = 0.5, and 1,000 iterations. Further details can be found at the CAPX script used above. Due to the limitation in patient sample availability, we were not able to accommodate all patients' samples in the computational analysis. To find a robust solution for this limitation, we ran FlowSOM and t-SNE algorithms using mass cytometry data with minimal batch fluctuation, using BM and PB of MGUS ($n = 3$) and NDMM patients ($n = 4$). Based on these results, MC of interest were further interrogated by manual gating to validate these observed changes, utilizing all available patient data from paired BM and PB of total MGUS ($n = 4$) and NDMM ($n = 8$) patients.

Statistical Analysis

Non-parametric Mann–Whitney and Wilcoxon matched-pairs signed rank test for two samples, or Kruskal–Wallis with Dunn's multiple comparison tests for multiple samples were performed as appropriate. All statistical tests were performed at the $p < 0.05$ significance level. Statistical analyses were performed using GraphPad Prism 7 (San Diego, USA).

RESULTS

Flow Cytometry Defines a Trend Toward Prevalence of $CD39^{-}$ Cells Within the Treg Compartment of NDMM Patients

Our initial analysis of Treg by flow cytometry confirmed a comparable size of $CD25^{+}CD127^{low/neg}$Treg in both BM and PB of HD, MGUS, and NDMM patients (**Figure 1A**). Treg represented higher proportion of $CD4^{+}$T cells in BM then in PB of HD and NDMM patients (**Figure 1A**). Considering the well-established role of $CD39^{+}$Treg in adenosine production within a suppressive tumor environment (9, 10, 18), we analyzed CD39 expression on Treg in matched BM and PB of MGUS and NDMM patients. Based on current knowledge, we expected a shift toward $CD39^{+}$ cells within the Treg compartment of NDMM patients. In contrast to our initial hypothesis, we found a trend toward prevalence of $CD39^{-}$Treg within both the BM and PB of NDMM compared to MGUS patients (**Figures 1B,C**). It appeared that $CD39^{-}$Treg were more frequent in BM than in PB of individual MGUS and NDMM patients (**Figure 1D**). The increasing trend of $CD39^{-}$Treg in NDMM patients did not affect FoxP3 expression within the Treg compartment, as Treg of NDMM and MGUS patients maintained comparable levels of FoxP3 expression (**Figure S1A**). We also analyzed expression of CD73 (another

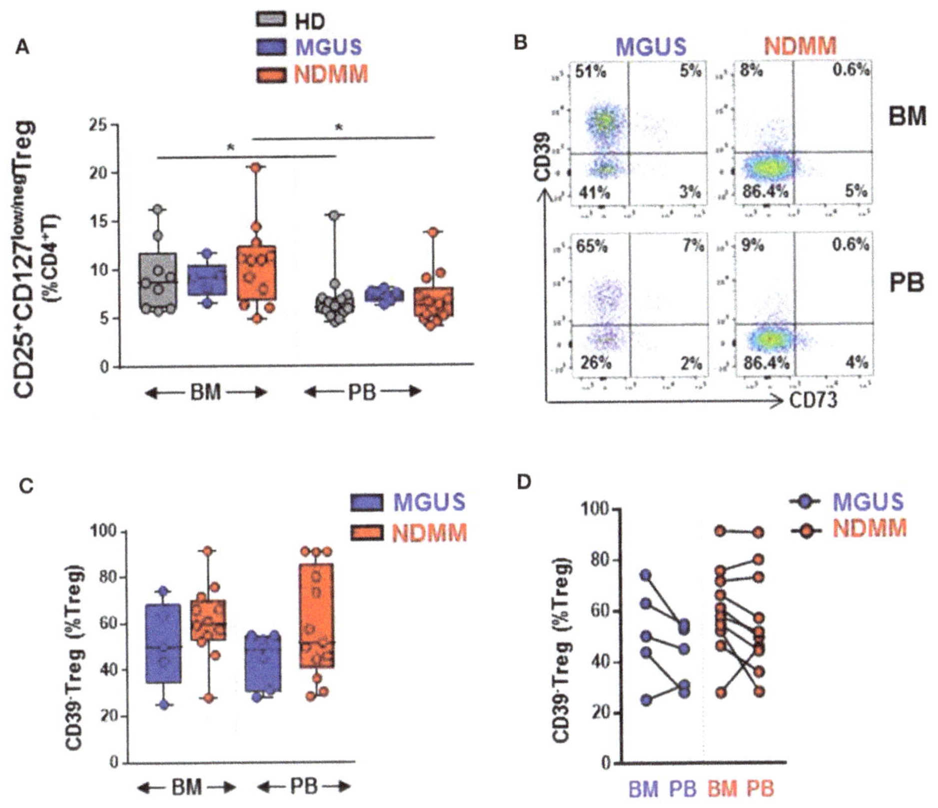

FIGURE 1 | CD39$^-$Treg are prevalent within the Treg compartment of NDMM patients. Flow cytometry data: **(A)** Frequency of Treg in BM and PB of HD (BM = 9, PB = 14), MGUS (BM = 5, PB = 6), and NDMM (BM = 12, PB = 13) patients. **(B)** Representative biaxial plot of CD39 vs. CD73 expression on Treg. Numbers indicate percentage of cells in each quadrant. **(C)** Frequency of CD39$^-$Treg within the Treg compartment in BM and PB of MGUS (BM = 5, PB = 6) and NDMM (BM = 12, PB = 13) patients. **(D)** Frequency of CD39$^-$Treg in paired BM and PB of MGUS (n = 5) and NDMM (n = 10) patients. Box and whisker plots show min and max, with median and individual data points. Multiple independent variables were analyzed using the Kruskal-Wallis test with Dunn's multiple comparison tests and 2 independent variables with the Mann-Whitney-*U*-test and Wilcoxon matched-pairs signed rank test; $^*p < 0.05$.

ectonucleotidase required for adenosine production), finding a low frequency of CD73$^+$Treg across patients (**Figure 1B; Figure S1B**), consistent with reported low expression of CD73 on Treg in humans (19). These data suggest CD39$^-$Treg although highly variable between MGUS and NDMM patients are more dominant within the Treg compartments of NDMM patients.

Mass Cytometry Reveals That Phenotypic Organization of CD39$^-$Treg Differs Between MGUS and NDMM Patients

Since flow cytometry data suggested that CD39$^-$Treg can be differently represented between MGUS and NDMM patients, mass cytometry was then used to interrogate at a high resolution the phenotypic organization of the Treg compartment in BM and PB of MGUS and NDMM patients. We assembled a panel of 35 metal isotope-conjugated antibodies to simultaneously measure the expression of surface and intracellular proteins known to define stages of Treg activation, effector/suppressor function and senescence (**Table S2**). In non-overlapping patient cohorts, mass cytometry and flow cytometry detected a comparable frequency of Treg in the BM and PB of MGUS and NDMM patients (**Figure 1A; Figure S1C**).

Overall, a heatmap of the mass cytometry data revealed lower expression of CD39 on Treg within the BM and PB of NDMM patients compared to Treg of MGUS patients (**Figure 2A**). There was noticeable heterogeneity in the level of CD39 expression within NDMM patients (BM1, PB1, BM3-4, PB3-4 vs. BM2, PB2; **Figure 2A**). Consistent with flow cytometry data, mass cytometry confirmed the prevalence of CD39$^-$Treg in both the BM and PB of NDMM patients compared to MGUS patients (**Figures 2B,C**). Also in line with flow cytometry data, CD39$^-$Treg were more frequent in BM than in PB samples of individual MGUS and NDMM patients by mass cytometry (**Figure 2D**).

To assist in our phenotypic analysis of CD39$^-$Treg, t-SNE plots were generated to visualize marker expression by pooling Treg from either BM or PB of MGUS and NDMM patients. As expected, based on the prevalence of CD39$^-$Treg in NDMM, CD39$^-$Treg occupied a larger area of Treg in NDMM patients compared to corresponding plots of MGUS patients (**Figure 2E,**

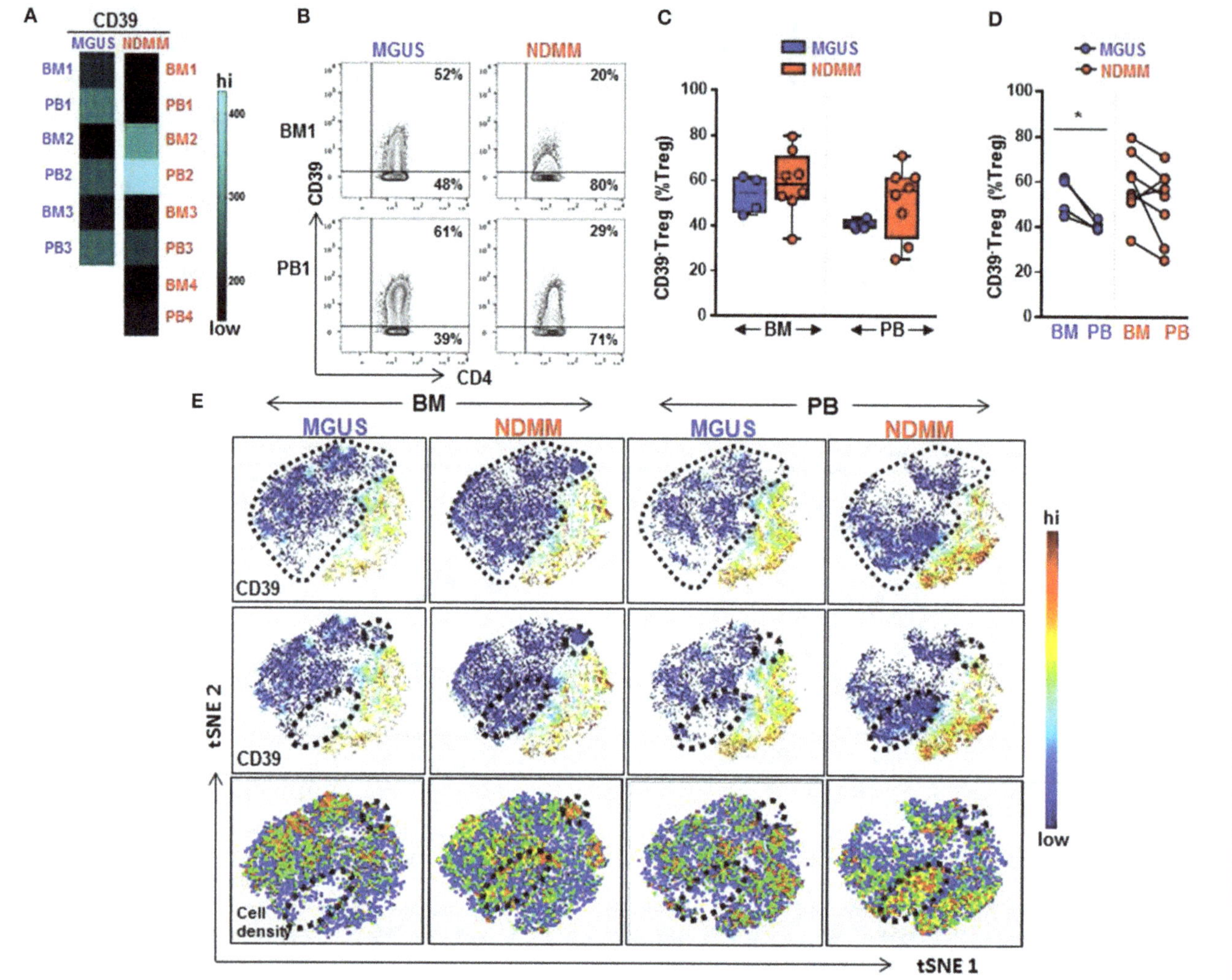

FIGURE 2 | Frequency of CD39$^-$Treg increases in NDMM compared to MGUS patients. Mass Cytometry data: **(A)** Heatmap of median signal intensity of CD39 expression on Treg in matched PB and BM from MGUS ($n = 3$) and NDMM ($n = 4$) patients. **(B)** Representative biaxial plots of CD39 vs. CD4 expression in the Treg compartment (CD25$^+$CD127$^{low/neg}$). Numbers indicate percentage of CD39$^+$ and CD39$^-$Treg. **(C)** Frequency of CD39$^-$Treg in BM and PB of MGUS ($n = 4$) and NDMM ($n = 8$) patients obtained by biaxial gating shown in **(B)**. Box and whisker plots show min and max, with median and individual data points. **(D)** Frequency of CD39$^-$Treg in paired BM and PB of MGUS ($n = 4$) and NDMM ($n = 8$) patients. Mann-Whitney-*U*-test and Wilcoxon matched-pairs signed rank test; $^*p < 0.05$. **(E)** t-SNE plots of the Treg compartment in pooled BM and PB of MGUS ($n = 3$) and NDMM ($n = 4$) patients. t-SNE plots show clustering patterns of CD39$^+$Treg (top, middle panels) and cell density (bottom panels). Area occupied by CD39$^-$Treg (top panel) and distinct regions which are occupied differently by CD39$^-$Treg (middle, bottom panels) are indicated.

t-SNE top panel). Interestingly, t-SNE plots displayed two distinct regions which were occupied differently by CD39$^-$Treg dependent on their patient or tissue origin. In NDMM patients, CD39$^-$Treg from BM occupied both, while CD39$^-$Treg from PB only one of these two distinct regions. Overall, these two distinct regions occupied sparsely by CD39$^-$Treg originated either from BM or PB of MGUS patients (**Figure 2E**, t-SNE middle panel). These CD39$^-$Treg had differential cell distribution between the tissues and patients, as shown by the cell density (**Figure 2E**, t-SNE bottom panel). These data reveal two exciting novel points: (i) CD39$^-$Treg of NDMM patients encompassed discrete subsets localized within a distinct regions of t-SNE plot which are obscured in CD39$^-$Treg of MGUS patients and (ii) these discrete subsets within CD39$^-$Treg are differently distributed between BM and PB of NDMM patients.

Unsupervised FlowSOM Clustering Reveals Activated CD39$^-$Treg and BM-Resident CD39$^-$Treg Which Emerge in NDMM Patients

To interrogate the phenotypic organization of the Treg compartment and further define the phenotype of two discrete subsets of CD39$^-$Treg which emerged in NDMM patients, we performed unsupervised clustering analysis of mass cytometry data using FlowSOM (16). FlowSOM was performed using the

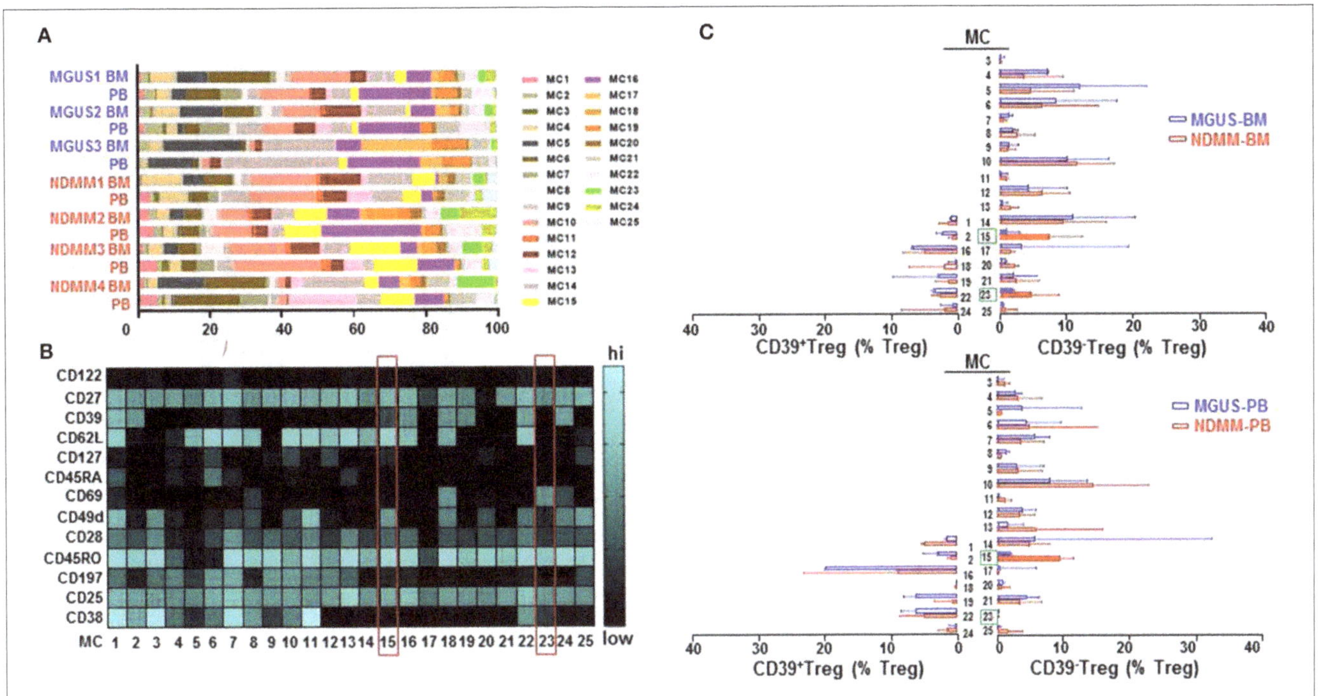

FIGURE 3 | Treg compartment of MGUS and NDMM patients displayed in 25 phenotypically different MC generated by the FlowSOM. **(A)** Inter-patient heterogeneity for each sample is represented by a horizontal bar in which segment lengths represent the frequency of the Treg assigned to each MC, colored according to the accompanying legend. **(B)** Heatmap of median signal intensity of indicated surface markers (rows) and MC (columns) summarizing the 25 different phenotypes within the Treg compartment generated by FlowSOM (seed A). The phenotypes of Treg in MC15 and MC23 are indicated on the heatmap (red rectangles). **(C)** Horizontal bars are frequency of Treg in each MC. MC occupied by CD39$^+$Treg (left) and by CD39$^-$Treg (right); MC15 and MC23 are indicated (closed bars, green rectangles). Bars are medians with interquartile range.

same number of CD25$^+$CD127$^{low/neg}$Treg from each BM and PB samples of MGUS (n = 3) and NDMM (n = 4) patients and 13 parameters (**Table S2**) associated with Treg identification and activation (4). We decided to split the Treg compartment into 25 phenotypically different MC (**Figure 3**), based on the recently reported number of 22 MC using 26 parameters in the Treg compartment in PB of HD (12). To evaluate the robustness of these MC, we used two different FlowSOM seeds (seed A, B) and observed high reproducibility in term of MC size and phenotype (**Figure 3**; **Figure S2**). We evaluated each patient sample quantitatively in term of its MC distribution and demonstrated each sample was unique in terms of the Treg frequency assigned to each MC (**Figure 3A**; **Figure S2A**), reflecting inter-patient differences within and between MGUS and NDMM cohorts.

We found that CD39$^-$Treg encompassed a majority of MC, and were more heterogeneous compared to their CD39$^+$Treg counterparts (18 vs. 7 MC, respectively, **Figures 3B,C**; **Figures S2B,C**). MC occupied by CD39$^+$Treg were consistently present across tissues and patients (**Figure 3C**; **Figure S2C**), suggesting that tissue residency or patient specificity was not embedded to CD39$^+$Treg. Among all MC displaying CD39$^-$Treg in BM and PB of MGUS and NDMM patients, the occupancy of MC15 and MC23 appeared to be consistently different between patients and tissues (**Figures 4A,B**). CD39$^-$Treg in MC15 represented 7% and 9.7% of Treg in BM and PB, respectively of NDMM patients. CD39$^-$Treg in MC23 was found exclusively in the BM of NDMM patients and represented 5% of Treg. In MGUS patients, both MC15 and MC23 were almost undetectable (**Figures 4A,B**). MC15 phenotypically resembled activated Treg based on CD45RO, CD49d, and CD62L expression (**Figure 4C**). Interestingly, MC23 had a core signature defining tissue residency, including CD69 expression, a lack of CD62L and CD49d expression and exclusive detection in the BM (**Figures 4A–C**).

To assist in data visualization, t-SNE plots were generated showing MC location. These t-SNE plots revealed that MC15 and MC23 overlapped with two previously defined regions within the CD39$^-$Treg that differed between patients and tissues (**Figures 2E, 4D**). Two different FlowSOM seeds produced similar results (Seed A in **Figures 3, 4**; Seed B in **Figures S2, S3**). This concludes that two discrete subsets defined as activated CD39$^-$Treg and BM-resident CD39$^-$Treg emerge in NDMM and discriminate MGUS from clinically active myeloma.

Activated CD39$^-$Treg and BM-Resident CD39$^-$Treg Can Be Matched by Classical Biaxial Gating of Mass Cytometry Data

Distinct clusters produced by computational clustering of mass cytometry data have to be matched in multiple samples to demonstrate their biological reality. Therefore, we next analyzed

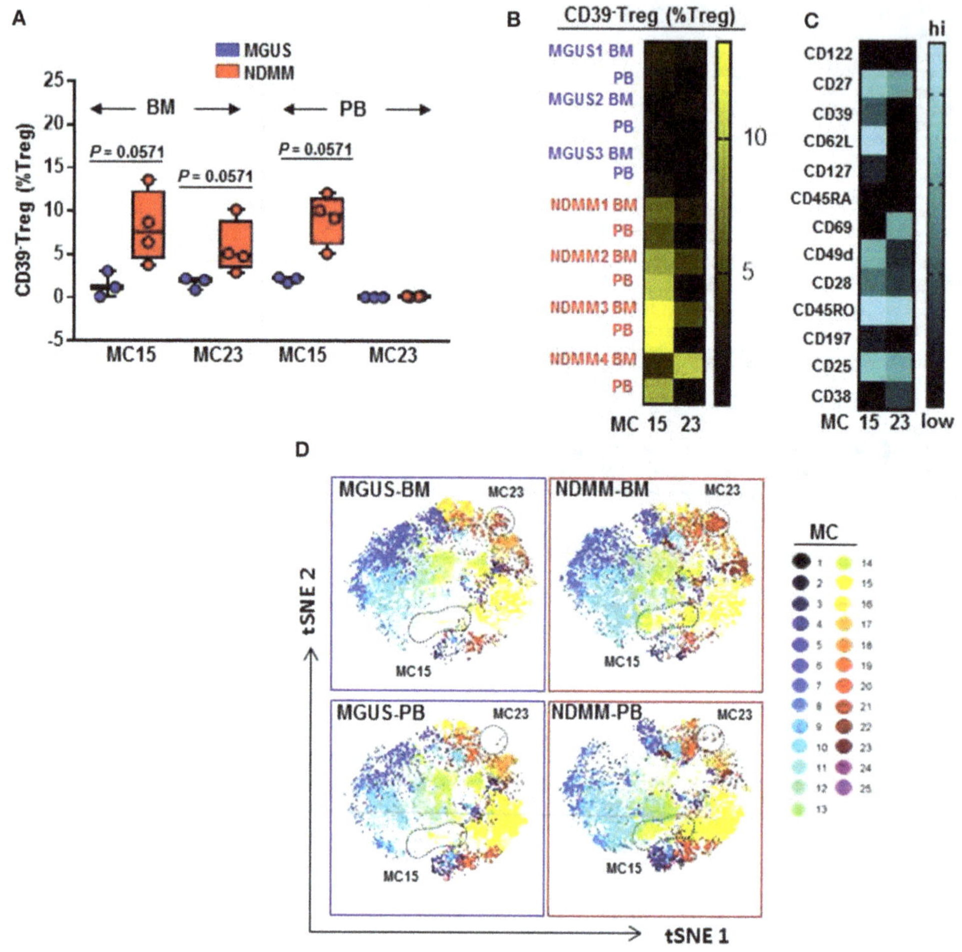

FIGURE 4 | Activated CD39⁻Treg and BM-resident CD39⁻Treg emerge in NDMM patients. **(A)** Frequency of Treg in MC15 and MC23 in BM and PB of MGUS ($n = 3$) and NDMM ($n = 4$) patients. Box and whisker plots show min and max, with median and individual data points. **(B)** Heatmap of Treg frequency in MC15 and MC23 in individual BM and PB from MGUS ($n = 3$) and NDMM patients ($n = 4$). **(C)** Phenotype of Treg in MC15 and MC23. **(D)** t-SNE plots display MC in pooled BM and PB of MGUS ($n = 3$) and NDMM ($n = 4$) patients colored according to the accompanying legend. MC15 and MC23 are indicated by dotted lines.

whether activated $CD39^-$Treg and BM-resident $CD39^-$Treg defined by FlowSOM clustering can be matched, quantified, and compared between samples by classical biaxial gating of mass cytometry data. We developed a biaxial gating strategy to fit the MC phenotype defined by automated FlowSOM clustering, and applied this same gating strategy to BM and PB samples of MGUS ($n = 4$) and NDMM ($n = 8$) patients (**Figure 5**). It is worth noting that one of the total 4 MGUS and 4 of the total 8 NDMM patients did not contribute to the MC phenotypes defined in the original FlowSOM clustering (**Figure 3B**). However, by classical biaxial gating activated $CD39^-$Treg and BM-resident $CD39^-$Treg were well-separated from the other $CD45RO^+CD38^-$Treg (**Figures 5A,B**). Activated $CD39^-$Treg phenotypically resembled MC15 defined by gating on $CD27^+CD69^-CD62L^+CD197^-CD49d^+$Treg (**Figures 5B,C**). BM-resident $CD39^-$Treg phenotypically resembled MC23 defined by gating on $CD27^+CD69^+CD62L^-CD197^-CD49d^-$Treg (**Figures 5B,D**). Although frequency of activated $CD39^-$Treg and BM-resident $CD39^-$Treg were generally smaller by biaxial gating than by FlowSOM clustering, these subsets were prevalent in NDMM and obscured or absent in MGUS samples by biaxial gating (**Figure 5E**). This proves biaxial gating analysis effective in matching activated $CD39^-$Treg and BM-resident $CD39^-$Treg, and overlap between the biaxial gating and the clustered analysis for these Treg subsets.

Both $CD39^-$Treg Subsets Co-expressed PD-1 and TIGIT But PD-1 Was Expressed at Higher Levels on BM-Resident Treg Then on Activated Treg

We considered that activated $CD39^-$Treg and BM-resident $CD39^-$Treg which develop in the stage of active disease in NDMM patients may acquire inhibitory check point molecules, or markers of effector/senescent cells, that are associated with enhanced Treg-mediated suppression in the tumor environment

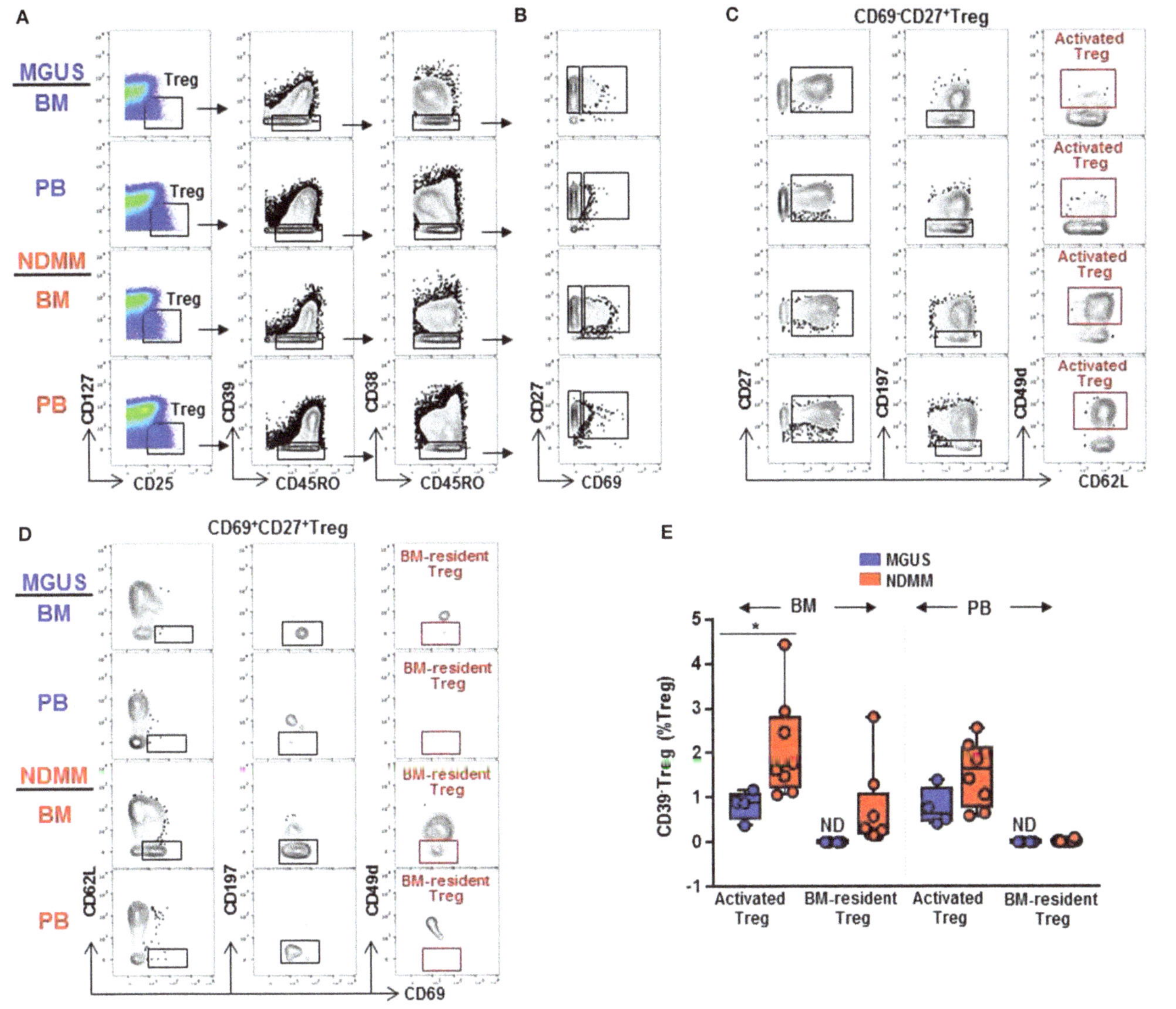

FIGURE 5 | Biaxial gating of mass cytometry data to match activated CD39$^-$Treg (MC15) and BM-resident CD39$^-$Treg (MC23) in MGUS and NDMM samples. **(A)** Representative biaxial gating of CD45RO$^+$CD39$^-$CD38$^-$Treg displayed in a plot of CD27 vs. CD69 in **(B)**. Representative gating strategy to match **(C)** activated CD39$^-$Treg (MC15) within CD69$^-$CD27$^+$Treg and **(D)** BM-resident CD39$^-$Treg (MC23) within CD69$^+$CD27$^+$Treg. **(E)** Frequency of activated CD39$^-$Treg and BM-resident CD39$^-$Treg in matched BM and PB samples of MGUS ($n = 4$) and NDMM ($n = 8$) patients. $^*p < 0.05$. ND, not defined.

(20). Thus, we compared expression levels of 13 markers on total Treg, activated CD39$^-$Treg and BM-resident CD39$^-$Treg in MGUS and NDMM patients by biaxial gating (**Figure 6**, data not shown). PD-1 and TIGIT were expressed at higher levels on activated CD39$^-$Treg in both BM and PB then on total Treg population. In the majority of patients, PD-1 and TIGIT expression was comparable on activated CD39$^-$Treg in the BM and PB (**Figure 6A**). PD-1 was expressed at greater levels but TIGIT was at lower levels on BM-resident Treg then on activated CD39$^-$Treg (**Figures 6A,B**). Both CD39$^-$Treg subsets co-expressed PD-1 and TIGIT (**Figure 6B**). Other inhibitory checkpoint molecules PD-L1, Lag3, Tim3, CD160, CXCR3 [a chemokine receptor associated with effector/memory cells (21)], KLRG1 [a marker of replicative senescence (22)], marker of proliferation Ki67, transcription factors Tbet and Eomes [regulators of T cell-mediated cytotoxicity (23)] had low-intensity staining undistinguishable from background (data not shown), consistent with reported low expression of these molecules on human Treg (24). Despite the lack of Tbet and Eomes expression, both activated CD39$^-$Treg and BM-resident CD39$^-$Treg produced Perforin and Granzyme B at levels similar to the total Treg population. There was an obvious difference in Perforin and Granzyme B production by Treg in BM and PB, such as Treg in PB (including activated CD39$^-$Treg) were major producers of both Perforin and Granzyme B (**Figures 6A,B**). There was noticeable inter-patient heterogeneity in the levels

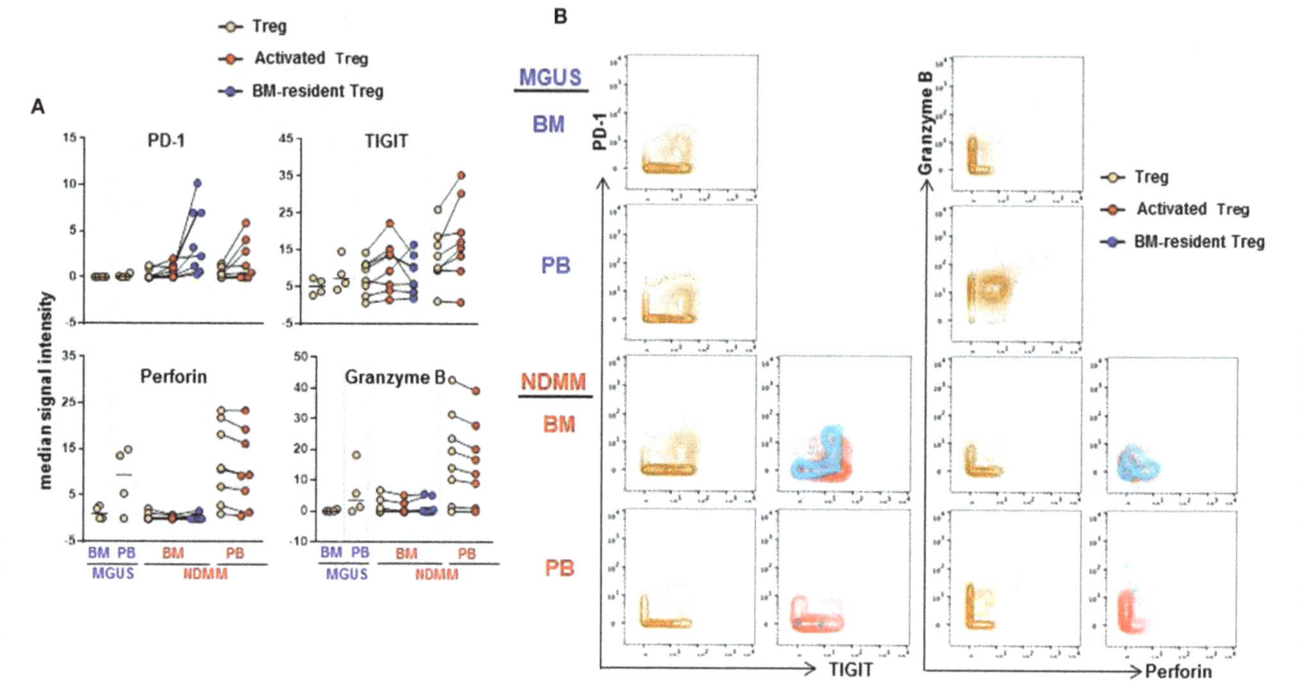

FIGURE 6 | Expression of PD-1, TIGIT, Perforin and Granzyme B on activated CD39^{-}Treg and BM-resident CD39^{-}Treg **(A)**. Median signal intensity of PD-1, TIGIT, Perforin. and Granzyme B defined by biaxial gating in total Treg, activated CD39^{-}Treg and BM-resident CD39^{-}Treg in BM and PB of MGUS ($n = 4$) and NDMM ($n = 8$) patients. Total Treg, activated CD39^{-}Treg and BM-resident CD39^{-}Treg from individual NDMM patients were connected. **(B)** Representative biaxial plots of PD-1 vs. TIGIT and Granzyme B vs. Perforin expression in total Treg, activated CD39^{-}Treg and BM-resident CD39^{-}Treg in matched BM and PB of individual MGUS and NDMM patient.

of Perforin and Granzyme B expression by total Treg within MGUS and NDMM cohorts, thus more data are required to interpret Perforin and Granzyme B expression by Treg across patient cohorts with confidence. Nevertheless, these data revealed important novel attributes associated with Treg in NDMM patients, including co-expression of PD-1 and TIGIT on both Treg subsets and higher levels of PD-1 expression on BM-resident CD39^{-}Treg than on activated Treg.

DISCUSSION

One of the challenges in the field of plasma cell dyscrasia and myeloma is to understand which factors keep MGUS clinically stable, and what critical events allow permissive expansion of malignant plasma cells to lead to the progression of clinical MM. This is particularly perplexing as MGUS patients have already been shown to have increased infiltration of T cells within the BM, as well as frequent TCR-Vβ expansions indicative of ongoing immune responses, and genetic changes similar to MM patients (25–28). Here, we provide an exciting novel discovery which may help to resolve this mystery. We discovered that two discrete subsets: activated CD39^{-}Treg and BM-resident CD39^{-}Treg emerge in NDMM, thus allowing discrimination between MGUS and NDMM patients. The availability and use of mass cytometry which allows interrogation of the Treg compartment of MGUS and NDMM patients at high resolution has facilitated the discovery of these two discrete subsets of CD39^{-}Treg.

Treg have been implicated in myeloma progression based on their contribution to the complex immunosuppressive environment through secretion of cytokines IL-10 and TGF-β (29), as well as direct inhibition of effector T cell responses (30). An additional important suppressive mechanism mediated by Treg involves the CD39/CD73 adenosine pathway. In this pathway, Treg expressing the ectonucleotidase CD39 in conjunction with CD73-expressing cells hydrolyse extracellular ATP and generate adenosine. Extracellularly produced adenosine following the engagement with its cognate receptors suppress effector T cell responses and induces myeloid-derived suppressor cells (18). Besides its immunosuppressive function, adenosine is also a growth factor for osteoblasts and osteoclasts (31), further implicating the importance of the CD39/CD73 adenosine pathway in MM pathogenesis. Expression of CD39 is upregulated on several solid tumors (including colorectal, pancreatic, head and neck cancer), implicating the CD39/CD73 adenosine pathway in the pathogenesis of a number of malignancies (32).

Based on all preceding observations, it is reasonable to expect that CD39^{+}Treg can be maintained or even increased in malignant MM when compared to the premalignant MGUS setting. In humans, CD39^{+}Treg are defined as activated effector memory cells (33) and are implicated in the suppression of Th17 responses and the control of autoimmunity (34). Unexpectedly, we found a trend toward prevalence of CD39^{-}Treg along with preserved FoxP3 expression within the Treg compartment of NDMM patients. CD39^{-}Treg with a preserved suppressor function pertinent to Treg have been reported as crucial effector/pathogenic cells that produce IL-17 in patients with multiple sclerosis (34). A role for CD39$^-$Treg in MM has never been described before, but it may be speculated that these cells can serve as IL-17-producing myeloma-promoting cells, particularly in the myeloma-permissive BM environment (35, 36). It is interesting that both IL-17 and now the prevalence of CD39$^-$Treg are common in the pathology of MM and autoimmunity. We observed noticeable heterogeneity between NDMM patients in the frequency of CD39$^-$Treg. The inclusion of increased numbers of patients in future studies than presented in this preliminary study will support our observation and establishment of potential dissimilarity between CD39$^-$Treg in MGUS and NDMM patients.

Previous studies have reported the production of IL-17 and IL-10 by a small proportion of CD39$^-$Treg (34), however the phenotype and function of the remaining major portion of CD39$^-$Treg remains uncertain. Using the advantages afforded by mass cytometry, we interrogated at a high resolution the phenotypic organization of CD39$^-$Treg in matched BM and PB of MGUS and NDMM patients. From our knowledge, this report represents the first description of a phenotypic organization of CD39$^-$Treg that provides some novel and exciting findings relevant to MGUS and NDMM patients. We found that CD39$^-$Treg in both MGUS and NDMM patients encompass multiple MC, suggesting that they are undergoing an intensive continuum of differentiation that involves multiple stages. In contrast, their CD39$^+$Treg counterpart appeared to be less dynamic and encompass a limited number of MC. We discovered subsets of activated CD39$^-$Treg and BM-resident CD39$^-$Treg that emerge in NDMM, and are thus able to discriminate between MGUS and NDMM patients. These two subsets are likely resistant to anti-CD38 monoclonal antibody therapy (37) based on their low/lack of CD38 expression. Based on their TIGIT and PD-1 co-expression, they may represent recently activated Treg. Remarkably, BM-resident CD39$^-$Treg have higher PD-1 expression than activated Treg and may represent exhausted Treg with the highest suppressive activity (38) induced in myeloma-infiltrated BM.

Our data suggest the compelling possibility that MGUS and NDMM patients can be discriminated based on the presence of activated CD39$^-$Treg and BM-resident CD39$^-$Treg. These Treg subsets differently presented between MGUS and NDMM patients initially revealed by automated FlowSOM clustering and subsequently matched and quantified in an expanded panel of MGUS and NDMM patients by classical biaxial gating of mass cytometry data. Thus, activated CD39$^-$Treg and BM-resident CD39$^-$Treg represent distinct biologically-relevant cell types and as such need to be matched, quantified and compared in a larger cohort of patients in different phases of disease.

Our data also raises several outstanding questions which will inspire further studies. Does myeloma directly or indirectly (through changes to myeloma-infiltrated BM) induce activated CD39$^-$Treg and BM-resident CD39$^-$Treg? What is the ontological origin of these two subsets of CD39$^-$Treg? Are they a result of CD39 downregulation, precursors of CD39$^+$Treg cells or are they developmentally independent of CD39$^+$Treg? Are they clonal Treg with myeloma antigen specificity? Do they relate to the currently established categories of human Treg, or do they represent a novel type of Treg? Are BM-resident CD39$^-$Treg responsible for maintenance of the myeloma niches and how do they relate to Treg being implicated in the maintenance of the haematopoietic stem cell and plasma cell niches (39, 40)?

Emergence of activated CD39$^-$Treg and BM-resident CD39$^-$Treg may represent necessary early changes in normal physiological Treg biology adopted by malignant myeloma cells to allow progression from MGUS to clinical MM. These changes in the Treg compartment of NDMM patients have real potential to improve our understanding of the clinical stability in MGUS and disease progression into MM, to further advance clinical diagnosis, prognosis, and therapeutic implications for MM.

ETHICS STATEMENT

This study was carried out in accordance with the recommendation of Royal Prince Alfred Hospital (X15-0357, X16-0291, X18-0096) and ANZAC Research Institute (HREC/11/CRGH/61) Ethics committee. All subjects gave written informed consent in accordance with the Declaration of Helsinki.

AUTHOR CONTRIBUTIONS

FM-W and AK performed the research, analyzed the data, and wrote the paper. HM designed and performed mass cytometry assays and wrote the paper. SY performed the research and analyzed the data. CBry reviewed patients, wrote the Human Ethics and analyzed the data. BF designed research and assisted in mass cytometry assays. NN, DJ, and PH designed research and wrote the paper. SB assisted Flow/CAPX approach, analyzed FLowSOM data and wrote the paper. JG, CBro, SL, and DM reviewed patients and designed research. RB reviewed patients undergoing hip arthroplasty and designed research. GC assisted collection of the healthy donor samples, designed research, analyzed data. SV designed research, performed experiments, analyzed data, and wrote the paper.

ACKNOWLEDGMENTS

The authors thank Dr. Alberto Catalano for excellent research management support, Royal Prince Alfred Hospital Medical Registrars for collection of patients samples and informed consent, patients, and their families for donating samples for research.

SUPPLEMENTARY MATERIAL

Figure S1 | Treg detection by flow cytometry and mass cytometry in the BM and PB of MGUS and NDMM patients. **(A,B)** Treg detection by flow cytometry: **(A)** Representative biaxial plot of Treg defined as FoxP3^{+} events. Numbers indicate percentage of FoxP3^{+}Treg. Representative histograms of the FoxP3 intensity in the Treg compartment in matched BM and PB of MGUS ($n = 2$) and NDMM ($n = 3$) patients. **(B)** Representative biaxial plot of Treg defined as CD25^{+}CD127$^{low/neg}$. Numbers indicate percentage of CD25^{+}CD127$^{low/neg}$ Treg. Frequency of CD73^{+}Treg within the Treg compartment in BM and PB of MGUS (BM = 5, PB = 6) and NDMM (BM = 12, PB = 13) patients.
(C) Representative biaxial plot of Treg defined as CD25+CD127$^{low/neg}$ by mass cytometry. Numbers indicate percentage of CD25^{+}CD127$^{low/neg}$ Treg. Frequency of Treg in BM and PB of MGUS ($n = 4$) and NDMM ($n = 8$) patients. Box and whisker plots show min and max, with median and individual data points.

Figure S2 | Treg compartment of MGUS and NDMM patients displayed in 25 phenotypically different MC generated by the FlowSOM (seed B). Data presented as in **Figure 3 (A–C)** (FlowSom seed A) demonstrating reproducibility in terms of MC size and phenotype across seed changes (Seed A vs. seed B). MC15 and MC23 depicted in Seed A (**Figure 3**) correspond to MC21 and MC1 depicted in Seed B, respectively.

Figure S3 | Activated CD39^{-}Treg and BM-resident CD39^{-}Treg emerge in NDMM patients (seed B). Data presented as in **Figure 4 (A–D)** (FlowSom seed A) demonstrating reproducibility in terms of MC size and phenotype across seed changes (Seed A vs. seed B). MC15 and MC23 depicted in Seed A (**Figure 4**) correspond to MC21 and MC1 depicted in Seed B, respectively.

Table S1 | Patients and HD characteristics and assay used for each subject included in study.

Table S2 | List of antibodies, clones, and conjugates used for mass cytometry staining and data analysis.

REFERENCES

1. Dhodapkar MV. MGUS to myeloma: a mysterious gammopathy of underexplored significance. *Blood.* (2016) 128:2599–606. doi: 10.1182/blood-2016-09-692954
2. Raja KR, Hajek R. Contribution of regulatory T cells to immunosuppression and disease progression in multiple myeloma patients. *Oncoimmunology.* (2013) 2:e25619. doi: 10.4161/onci.25619
3. Allan SE, Broady R, Gregori S, Himmel ME, Locke N, Roncarolo MG, et al. CD4^{+} T-regulatory cells: toward therapy for human diseases. *Immunol Rev.* (2008) 223:391–421. doi: 10.1111/j.1600-065X.2008.00634.x
4. Sakaguchi S, Miyara M, Costantino CM, Hafler DA. FOXP3+ regulatory T cells in the human immune system. *Nat Rev Immunol.* (2010) 10:490–500. doi: 10.1038/nri2785
5. Miyara M, Yoshioka Y, Kitoh A, Shima T, Wing K, Niwa A, et al. Functional delineation and differentiation dynamics of human CD4+ T cells expressing the FoxP3 transcription factor. *Immunity.* (2009) 30:899–911. doi: 10.1016/j.immuni.2009.03.019
6. Kleinewietfeld M, Starke M, Di Mitri D, Borsellino G, Battistini L, Rötzschke O, et al. CD49d provides access to "untouched" human Foxp3+ Treg free of contaminating effector cells. *Blood.* (2009) 113:827–36. doi: 10.1182/blood-2008-04-150524
7. Chen Q, Mo L, Cai X, Wei L, Xie Z, Li H, et al. ICOS signal facilitates Foxp3 transcription to favor suppressive function of regulatory T cells. *Int J Med Sci.* (2018) 15:666–73. doi: 10.7150/ijms.23940
8. Duhen T, Duhen R, Lanzavecchia A, Sallusto F, Campbell DJ. Functionally distinct subsets of human FOXP3+ Treg cells that phenotypically mirror effector Th cells. *Blood.* (2012) 119:4430–40. doi: 10.1182/blood-2011-11-392324
9. Borsellino G, Kleinewietfeld M, Di Mitri D, Sternjak A, Diamantini A, Giometto R, et al. Expression of ectonucleotidase CD39 by Foxp3+ Treg cells: hydrolysis of extracellular ATP and immune suppression. *Blood.* (2007) 110:1225–32. doi: 10.1182/blood-2006-12-064527
10. Chillemi A, Quarona V, Antonioli L, Ferrari D, Horenstein AL, Malavasi F. Roles and modalities of ectonucleotidases in remodeling the multiple myeloma niche. *Front Immunol.* (2017) 8:305. doi: 10.3389/fimmu.2017.00305
11. Bendall SC, Simonds EF, Qiu P, Amir el-AD, Krutzik PO, Finck R, et al. Single-cell mass cytometry of differential immune and drug responses across a human hematopoietic continuum. *Science.* (2011) 332:687–96. doi: 10.1126/science.1198704
12. Mason GM, Lowe K, Melchiotti R, Ellis R, de Rinaldis E, Peakman M, et al. Phenotypic complexity of the human regulatory T cell compartment revealed by mass cytometry. *J Immunol.* (2015) 195:2030–7. doi: 10.4049/jimmunol.1500703
13. Kawano Y, Zavidij O, Park J, Moschetta M, Kokubun K, Mouhieddine TH, et al. Blocking IFNAR1 inhibits multiple myeloma-driven Treg expansion and immunosuppression. *J Clin Invest.* (2018) 128:2487–99. doi: 10.1172/JCI88169
14. Feyler S, Scott GB, Parrish C, Jarmin S, Evans P, Short M, et al. Tumour cell generation of inducible regulatory T-cells in multiple myeloma is contact-dependent and antigen-presenting cell-independent. *PLOS ONE.* (2012) 7:e35981. doi: 10.1371/journal.pone.0035981
15. Ashhurst TM. Cytometry analysis pipeline for large and complex datasets v2.5. GitHub repository. (2018). doi: 10.5281/zenodo.3273252
16. Van Gassen S, Callebaut B, Van Helden MJ, Lambrecht BN, Demeester P, Dhaene T, et al. FlowSOM: using self-organizing maps for visualization and interpretation of cytometry data. *Cytometry A.* (2015) 87:636–45. doi: 10.1002/cyto.a.22625
17. van der Maaten L, Hinton G. Visualizing data using t-SNE. *J Mach Learn Res.* (2008) 9:2579–605.
18. Antonioli L, Blandizzi C, Pacher P, Haskó G. Immunity, inflammation and cancer: a leading role for adenosine. *Nat Rev Cancer.* (2013) 13:842–57. doi: 10.1038/nrc3613
19. Dwyer KM, Hanidziar D, Putheti P, Hill PA, Pommey S, McRae JL, et al. Expression of CD39 by human peripheral blood CD4+ CD25+ T cells denotes a regulatory memory phenotype. *Am J Transplant.* (2010) 10:2410–20. doi: 10.1111/j.1600-6143.2010.03291.x
20. Marin-Acevedo JA, Dholaria B, Soyano AE, Knutson KL, Chumsri S, Lou Y. Next generation of immune checkpoint therapy in cancer: new developments and challenges. *J Hematol Oncol.* (2018) 11:39. doi: 10.1186/s13045-018-0582-8
21. Kurachi M, Kurachi J, Suenaga F, Tsukui T, Abe J, Ueha S, et al. Chemokine receptor CXCR3 facilitates CD8(+) T cell differentiation into short-lived effector cells leading to memory degeneration. *J Exp Med.* (2011) 208:1605–20. doi: 10.1084/jem.20102101
22. Xu W, Larbi A. Markers of T cell senescence in humans. *Int J Mol Sci.* (2017) 18:E1742. doi: 10.3390/ijms18081742
23. Hamilton SE, Jameson SC. CD8(+) T cell differentiation: choosing a path through T-bet. *Immunity.* (2007) 27:180–2. doi: 10.1016/j.immuni.2007.08.003
24. Kunicki MA, Amaya Hernandez LC, Davis KL, Bacchetta R, Roncarolo MG. Identity and diversity of human peripheral Th and T regulatory cells defined by single-cell mass cytometry. *J Immunol.* (2018) 200:336–46. doi: 10.4049/jimmunol.1701025
25. Pérez-Andres M, Almeida J, Martin-Ayuso M, Moro MJ, Martin-Nuñez G, Galende J, et al. Characterization of bone marrow T cells in monoclonal gammopathy of undetermined significance, multiple myeloma, and plasma cell leukemia demonstrates increased infiltration by cytotoxic/Th1 T cells demonstrating a squed TCR-Vbeta repertoire. *Cancer.* (2006) 106:1296–305. doi: 10.1002/cncr.21746

26. Walker BA, Wardell CP, Melchor L, Brioli A, Johnson DC, Kaiser MF, et al. Intraclonal heterogeneity is a critical early event in the development of myeloma and precedes the development of clinical symptoms. *Leukemia.* (2014) 28:384–90. doi: 10.1038/leu.2013.199
27. Dutta AK, Fink JL, Grady JP, Morgan GJ, Mullighan CG, To LB, et al. Subclonal evolution in disease progression from MGUS/SMM to multiple myeloma is characterised by clonal stability. *Leukemia.* (2019) 33:457–68. doi: 10.1038/s41375-018-0206-x
28. Bolli N, Maura F, Minvielle S, Gloznik D, Szalat R, Fullam A, et al. Genomic patterns of progression in smoldering multiple myeloma. *Nat Commun.* (2018) 9:3363. doi: 10.1038/s41467-018-05058-y
29. Strauss L, Bergmann C, Szczepanski M, Gooding W, Johnson JT, Whiteside TL. A unique subset of CD4+CD25highFoxp3+ T cells secreting interleukin-10 and transforming growth factor-beta1 mediates suppression in the tumor microenvironment. *Clin Cancer Res.* (2007) 13:4345–54. doi: 10.1158/1078-0432.CCR-07-0472
30. Cao X, Cai SF, Fehniger TA, Song J, Collins LI, Piwnica-Worms DR, et al. Granzyme B and perforin are important for regulatory T cell-mediated suppression of tumor clearance. *Immunity.* (2007) 27:635–46. doi: 10.1016/j.immuni.2007.08.014
31. Ham J, Evans BA. An emerging role for adenosine and its receptors in bone homeostasis. *Front Endocrinol.* (2012) 3:113. doi: 10.3389/fendo.2012.00113
32. Bastid J, Cottalorda-Regairaz A, Alberici G, Bonnefoy N, Eliaou JF, Bensussan A. ENTPD1/CD39 is a promising therapeutic target in oncology. *Oncogene.* (2013) 32:1743–51. doi: 10.1038/onc.2012.269
33. Kleinewietfeld M, Puentes F, Borsellino G, Battistini L, Rötzschke O, Falk K. CCR6 expression defines regulatory effector/memory-like cells within the CD25(+)CD4+ T-cell subset. *Blood.* (2005) 105:2877–86. doi: 10.1182/blood-2004-07-2505
34. Fletcher JM, Lonergan R, Costelloe L, Kinsella K, Moran B, O'Farrelly C, et al. CD39+Foxp3+ regulatory T Cells suppress pathogenic Th17 cells and are impaired in multiple sclerosis. *J Immunol.* (2009) 183:7602–10. doi: 10.4049/jimmunol.0901881
35. Vuckovic S, Minnie SA, Smith D, Gartlan KH, Watkins TS, Markey KA, et al. Bone marrow transplantation generates T cell-dependent control of myeloma in mice. *J Clin Invest.* (2019) 129:106–21. doi: 10.1172/JCI98888
36. Prabhala RH, Pelluru D, Fulciniti M, Prabhala HK, Nanjappa P, Song W, et al. Elevated IL-17 produced by TH17 cells promotes myeloma cell growth and inhibits immune function in multiple myeloma. *Blood.* (2010) 115:5385–92. doi: 10.1182/blood-2009-10-246660
37. Lokhorst HM, Plesner T, Laubach JP, Nahi H, Gimsing P, Hansson M, et al. Targeting CD38 with daratumumab monotherapy in multiple myeloma. *N Engl J Med.* (2015) 373:1207–19. doi: 10.1056/NEJMoa1506348
38. Sasidharan Nair V, Elkord E. Immune checkpoint inhibitors in cancer therapy: a focus on T-regulatory cells. *Immunol Cell Biol.* (2018) 96:21–33. doi: 10.1111/imcb.1003
39. Fujisaki J, Wu J, Carlson AL, Silberstein L, Putheti P, Larocca R, et al. *In vivo* imaging of Treg cells providing immune privilege to the haematopoietic stem-cell niche. *Nature.* (2011) 474:216–9.
40. Glatman Zaretsky A, Konradt C, Dépis F, Wing JB, Goenka R, Atria DG, et al. T regulatory cells support plasma cell populations in the bone marrow. *Cell Rep.* (2017) 18:1906–16. doi: 10.1016/j.celrep.2017.01.067

13

Immunocyte Profiling Using Single-Cell Mass Cytometry Reveals EpCAM$^+$ CD4$^+$ T Cells Abnormal in Colon Cancer

Ting Zhang [1], Junwei Lv [1], Ziyang Tan [1], Boqian Wang [1], Antony R. Warden [1], Yiyang Li [1], Hui Jiang [1], Hao Li [2] and Xianting Ding [1]**

[1] State Key Laboratory of Oncogenes and Related Genes, School of Biomedical Engineering, Institute for Personalized Medicine, Shanghai Jiao Tong University, Shanghai, China, [2] Department of General Surgery, Affiliated First People's Hospital, Shanghai Jiao Tong University, Shanghai, China

***Correspondence:**
Hao Li
lihao6656@163.com
Xianting Ding
dingxianting@sjtu.edu.cn

Colon cancer (CC) is one of the leading causes of cancer related mortality. Research over past decades have profoundly enhanced our understanding of immunotherapy, a major clinical accomplishment, and its potential role toward treating CC. However, studies investigating the expression of these immune checkpoints, such as epithelial cell adhesion molecule (EpCAM), programmed death-1 (PD-1), and programmed death-ligand 1 (PD-L1), by peripheral blood mononuclear cells (PBMCs) is lacking. Here, high-dimensional mass cytometry (CyTOF) is used to investigate immune alterations and promising immunotherapeutic targets expression by PBMCs of CC patients. Results reveal that expression of EpCAM and PD-L1 on CD4$^+$ T cells significantly increased in patients with CC, compared with age- and sex- matching healthy controls and patients with colonic polyps. These differences are also validated in an independent patient cohort using flow cytometry. Further analysis revealed that EpCAM$^+$ CD4$^+$ T cells are PD-L1$^+$ CCR5$^+$ CCR6$^+$. Immunofluorescence staining results demonstrate that the increase of EpCAM$^+$ CD4$^+$ T cells is also observed in tumor tissues, rather than para-cancerous tissues. To ascertain the functional disorders of the identified cell subset, phosphorylated signaling protein levels are assessed using imaging mass cytometry. Increases in pp38 MAPK and pMAPKAPK2 are observable, indicating abnormal activation of pp38 MAPK-pMAPKAPK2 signaling pathway. Results in this study indicate that EpCAM$^+$ CD4$^+$ T cells may play a role in CC development. Detailed knowledge on the functionality of EpCAM$^+$ CD4$^+$ T cells is of high translational relevance.

Keywords: colon cancer, EpCAM, T cell immunity, mass cytometry, p38 MAPK

INTRODUCTION

Colon cancer (CC) is one of the main causes of cancer death worldwide (1, 2), with high incidence and mortality rates for all genders. Age-adjusted incidence rate is reported at 46.3 per 100,000 individuals per year worldwide, with only 12% 5-year survival rate for late-stage colorectal cancer patients (3). The prognosis of CC is generally unfavorable with high recurrence and metastasis rates. Immunotherapy, in combination with chemotherapy and anti-angiogenic agents, is gaining support as an effective approach to battle CC (4).

The epithelial cellular adhesion molecule (EpCAM), which overexpresses in epithelial cancer associated with enhanced malignant potential, is regarded as a desirable target for CC therapy (5). EpCAM-specific monoclonal antibodies have been used to treat human CC since the 1990s. Programmed death-1 (PD-1), an inhibitory receptor expressed on activated T cells, is regarded as a promising target protein for cancer therapy. Patient safety, clinical activity, and tolerability of PD-1 blockade were subsequently determined (6). However, the therapeutic efficacy of blocking these immune pathways is limited. Immunotherapeutic drugs targeting EpCAM have been developed by utilizing monoclonal antibodies (7, 8), bispecific antibodies (9), or conjugates with other agents, such as toxins (10). Data from clinical trials of EpCAM blockade suggest limited anti-tumor effects and low immune-activating efficacy. Reports of the therapeutic effects of PD-1 blockade in melanomas, non-small cell lung cancer, and renal-cell cancer patients are promising, however, exhibiting only a 3% treatment response rate with CC patients (11). Examining the role of EpCAM and PD-1 in carcinogenesis and malignant progression would aid the development of more efficacious immunotherapeutic schemes.

The importance of T cells in CC is well-established and fully illustrated by checkpoint blockade approaches (12, 13). Therefore, in addition to investigating the pool of functionally diverse T cell subsets, it is crucial to determine the expression levels of checkpoint-related molecules, such as EpCAM, PD-1, and programmed death-ligand 1 (PD-L1). Expression analyses of these checkpoints would help define the relative contributions of these molecules toward the immunotherapy responsiveness of CC patients. Although these suppressive markers have been widely investigated in tumor microenvironments, research on their expression by human immune cells and relevant importance in the peripheral blood remains scarce. Few studies characterize the importance of these molecules in circulating immune cells. Chevolet and colleges found that PD-L1 expression occurs in circulating cytotoxic T cells, which confers a worsen prognosis on overall survival rates (14). There is an urgent need for systemic and comprehensive profiling of immune checkpoint expressions.

Mass cytometry, also known as cytometry by time-of-flight (CyTOF), combines the high throughput of flow cytometry and the fine resolution of mass spectrometry (15, 16). In CyTOF, fluorophore reporters are substituted with rare metal isotope-conjugated antibodies (17, 18), circumventing the spectral overlap limitation in flow cytometric analysis and allows for a simultaneous determination of over 40 parameters at the single-cell level. Advances in data visualization and interpretation (19, 20) widens the application of CyTOF to various fields, including cellular reprogramming (21), phenotype heterogeneity mapping (22), and cell development analysis (23). Using this platform, we aim to investigate the checkpoints expression profile by specific T cell subsets and examine the underlying functional pathway mechanisms in these checkpoint expressed cell subsets (workflow presented in **Supplementary Figure 1**).

MATERIALS AND METHODS

Subjects

This study is approved by the Ethical Committee and Institutional Review Board of Shanghai Jiao Tong University. Human peripheral blood specimens, obtained from patients diagnosed with either colon polyps or stage I-IV CC, were sampled from the First People's Hospital (Shanghai, China) between May 2016 and August 2018. Exclusion criteria included: (1) age over 70; (2) the presence of systemic disease or medication that could compromise the immune system; (3) having autoimmune disease or pregnancy; (4) having infectious disease, history of alcohol abuse, or other inflammatory conditions that could induce immunological impairments. Each patient was assigned to a stage based on the American Joint Committee on Cancer's (AJCC) staging system. Healthy subjects were recruited from the Medical Examination Center of the First People's Hospital. These individuals did not have a previous history or signs of increased blood pressure nor diabetes. In addition, they did not experience any fever within a defined period prior to the initiation of the study. All blood tests and imaging analyses, including computed tomography (CT) and X-rays were within normal ranges. Demographic characteristics are listed in **Supplementary Table 1**.

PBMC Sample Collection, Pretreatment, and Preservation

Peripheral blood mononuclear cells (PBMCs) were obtained through a Ficoll-Paque density-gradient centrifugation of freshly drawn (within 4 h) EDTA-anticoagulated blood. After washing the extracted PBMCs once, the cells were stained with cisplatin for 5 min at 37°C to discriminate live-dead cells. Staining was terminated by adding cell-staining buffer (CSB) followed by centrifugation. Immediately after discarding the supernatants, the cells were fixed at room temperature in a paraformaldehyde solution at a final working concentration of 1.6% for 10 min. Cells were cryopreserved in DMSO-containing CSB at −80°C after washing.

Antibody Staining and Data Acquisition by CyTOF

Cryopreserved PBMCs were thawed in a water bath pre-warmed to 37°C in 5 min. 3×10^6 cells were then transferred into CSB for antibody staining. Mass cytometry antibody staining was implemented following previous study (24). The staining panel is listed in **Supplementary Table 2**. Stained cells were washed twice with 2 mL CSB, then incubated overnight at 4°C with 1 mL DNA Intercalator (Fluidigm, CA, USA), which was diluted in a Fix and Perm Buffer (Fluidigm) at a final concentration of 125 nM, which facilitated the discrimination between singlets, doublets, and triplets. Prior to data acquisition, cell pellets were resuspended in distilled water containing 10% EQ Four Element Calibration Beads (Fluidigm), and the cells were filtered through a 35-μm membrane. The cells were analyzed with Helios (Fluidigm) through several runs at an acquisition rate of ~500 events per second (25). Following the manufacturer's instructions, settings were on default.

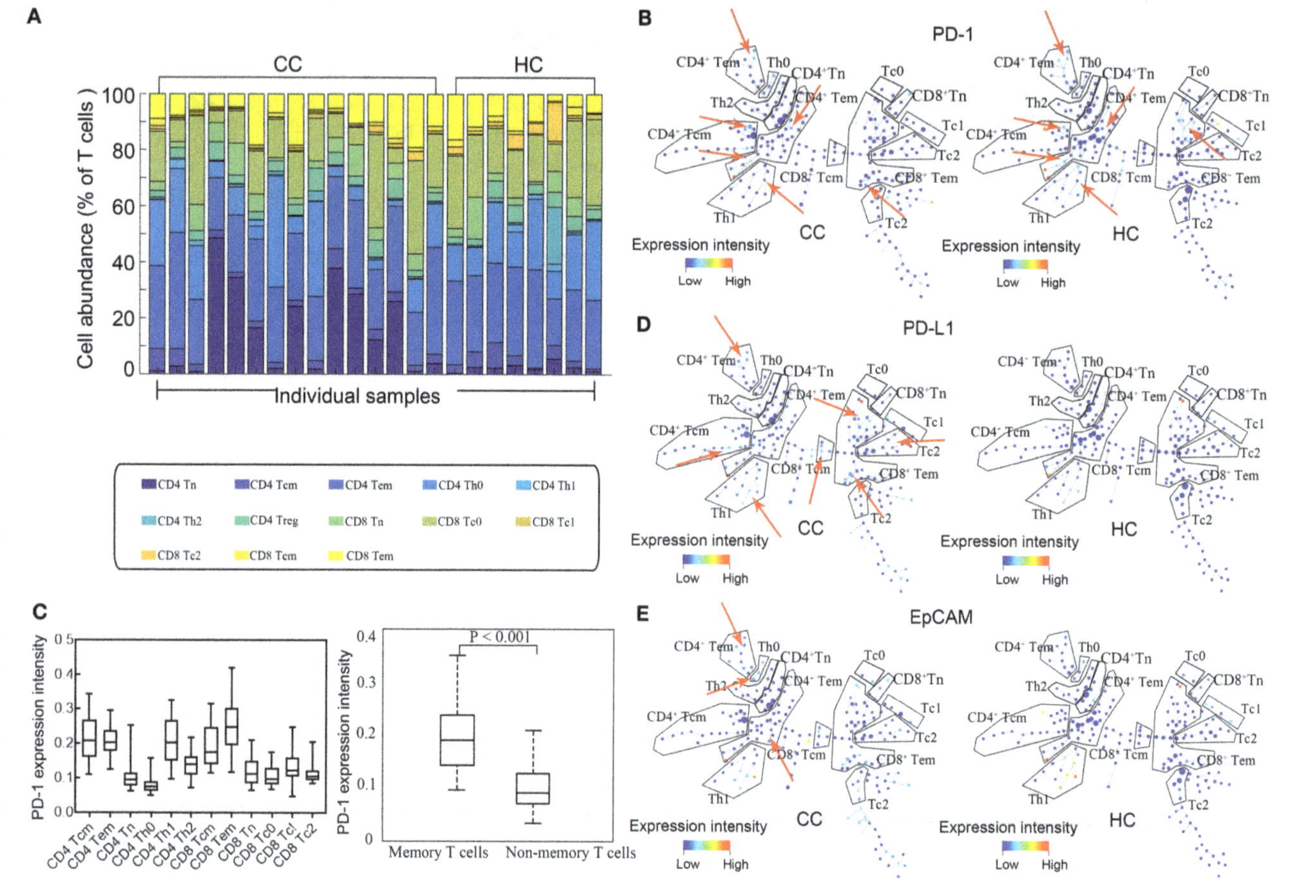

FIGURE 1 | Expression profiles of EpCAM, PD-1, and PD-L1 by T cells. **(A)** Stacked bars of T cell subtypes in each individual sample. Cell abundance is expressed as percentage of total T cells. **(B)** Representative SPADE plot of PD-1 expression profile by T cells for colon cancer patients (CC) and healthy controls (HC). Color coding indicates the signified marker expression. Red arrows mark the extensive PD-1 expression by memory T cells. **(C)** Comparison of PD-1 in all T cell subtypes (left) and between memory and non-memory T cells (right). PD-1 is mainly expressed by memory T cells. **(D,E)** Representative SPADE plot of the expression profiles of PD-L1 **(D)** and EpCAM **(E)** by T cells. Color coding indicate the expression intensity of the corresponding markers. Red arrows indicate the abundant and heterogeneous patterns of PD-L1 and EpCAM expression in CC patients.

Data Processing and Analysis

The short-term signal fluctuations of Helios was normalized with EQ bead signals prior to data export and analysis (26). Abundance values obtained by mass cytometry were transformed using a scaled arcsinh with a factor of 5, which diminished near-zero noise values in the measurements. Surface marker expression in each channel was normalized based on the signal intensity at the 99.5th percentile across all samples, thus yielding expression values as x-fold of the 99.5th percentile values (27). To avoid debris and doublets, events recorded were gated based on DNA contents and cell length. Gating, viSNE plots (19), and spanning-tree progression analysis of density-normalized events (SPADE) analysis (28) were performed using the Cytobank platform (www.cytobank.org) as previously described (29). The following markers were used for SPADE and viSNE analysis: EpCAM, CD45RA, CCR5, CD4, CD8a, PD-L1, CD45RO, CCR6, PD-1, CD161, CTLA-4, CCR4, LAG3, CCR7, CD127, and CD25. Major cell subpopulations were annotated in the viSNE and SPADE maps based on prior knowledge of expected marker expression in various cell types. PhenoGraph clustering (27) was performed using all markers on a combined sample of 115,000 cells (subsampling of 5,000 cells per sample) using the cytofkit R package (30). A series of gates for T cell subpopulations (31) are presented in **Supplementary Figure 2**. Data plots and histograms were generated using MATLAB (MathWorks, R2018a).

Flow Cytometry Validation

An independent cohort ($N = 14$, 7 CC patients, and 7 healthy controls) was included for validation (**Supplementary Table 3**). PE-conjugated EpCAM mAb (Invitrogen, CA, USA) and APC-conjugated CD4 mAb (Tonbo Biosciences, CA, USA) were purchased for flow cytometric analysis. Briefly, 100 μL freshly collected peripheral blood was blocked with Fc block (BioLegend, CA, USA) in the staining buffer for 10 min and incubated with antibodies for another 15 min at room temperature, then treated with red blood cell lysing buffer (BD Biosciences, CA, USA). The samples were washed with PBS and re-suspended in 300 μL PBS and analyzed with flow cytometry in a Canto II analyzer

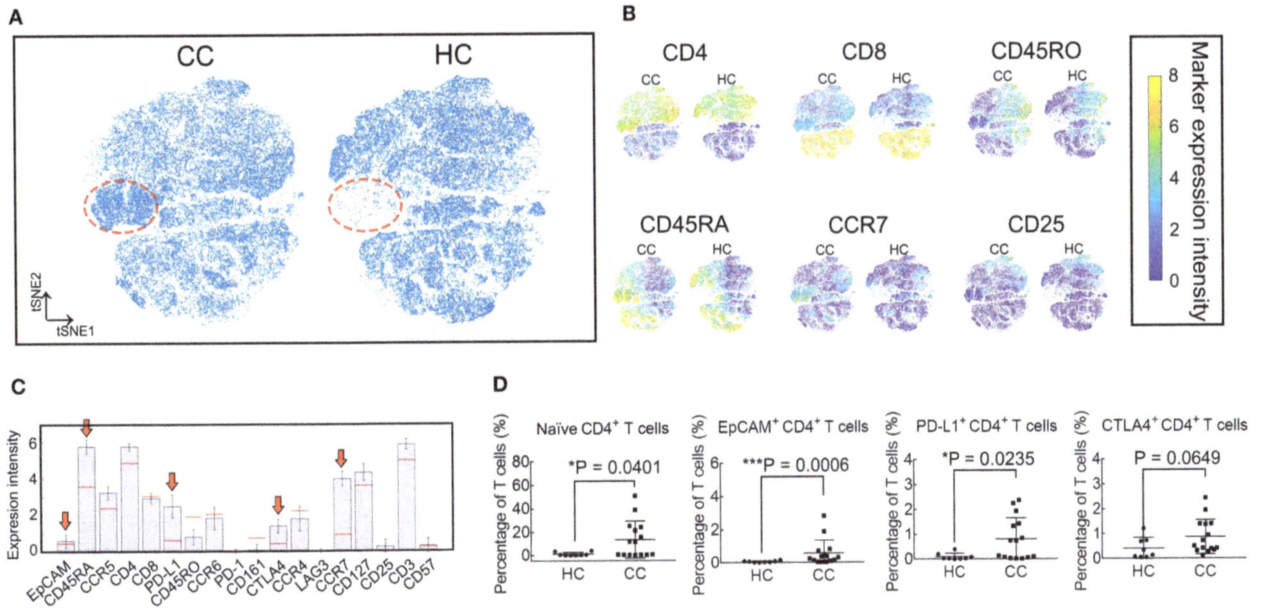

FIGURE 2 | viSNE analysis revealed that EpCAM$^+$ CD4$^+$ T cells increased in CC patients. **(A)** Synthetic t-SNE maps depicting T cell subtypes in colon cancer patients (CC, $N = 15$) and healthy controls (HC, $N = 8$). Suspect populations that compose almost entirely of cells from CC patients are marked in the red dotted regions. **(B)** viSNE maps of T cells in CC and HC illustrating the expression of CD4, CD8, CD45RA, CD45RO, CCR7, and CD25. Color scale indicates the signified marker expression intensity. **(C)** Expression signatures of the identified subpopulations in **(A)**. Bar height indicates the median expression of each marker within a subpopulation. The horizontal line for each marker corresponds to median expression across all cells. Red arrows indicate positive immune blockade marker expressions. **(D)** Comparison of percentages in T cells of naïve (CD45RA$^+$ and CCR7$^+$), EpCAM$^+$, PD-L1$^+$, and CTLA4$^+$ CD4$^+$ T cells between CC and HC. Error bars indicate standard deviation (SD). Statistical differences are annotated with asterisk (*) and P (p-value) or ns, not significant. $^*P < 0.05$, $^{**}P < 0.01$, $^{***}P < 0.001$.

(BD Biosciences). The FlowJo X10 software (Treestar, CA, USA) was employed for data analysis. Cells were sequentially gated on lymphocytes (based on FFC vs. SSC), single cells (based on FSC-A vs. FSC-H), and CD4$^+$ cells (indiscriminating live/dead) for the assessment of EpCAM expression.

Immunofluorescence (IF) Staining

The tumor or para-cancerous tissues of the studied patients were sectioned by a pathologist who was blind to the patient group but aware of the study design. Sections were stained and examined under light microscope to assess the positivity for EpCAM (red) and CD4 (green). Ten regions of interests (ROIs) were randomly selected per sample. The average marker expression area (measured using ImageJ© software) or cell counts of ten ROIs were used for subsequent statistical analysis.

Imaging Mass Cytometry (IMC)

To assess the spatial distribution of EpCAM$^+$ CD4$^+$ T cell subpopulations in CC tissues, IMC (Hyperion, Fluidigm) (32) was employed to analyze tumor sections. Sections including para-cancerous and carcinoma tissues were collected and prepared as previously described (33). The antibody staining panel is listed in **Supplementary Table 4**. Image acquisition after daily tuning was carried out following manufacturer's instruction at a laser frequency of 200 Hz. Approximately 500 × 500 μm regions were selected based on bright field images. Two to five ROIs were selected per slide, which are dependent on the section size (**Supplementary Table 5**). The marker expression intensity associated with individual ROI were used as input for further analysis.

Statistical Analysis

Data is expressed as mean ± standard deviation (SD) or as medians with interquartile ranges. Statistical significance between two groups was calculated using non-parametric Mann-Witney test. Rejection of the null hypothesis with a p value < 0.05 was considered as significant.

RESULTS

Expression Profiles of EpCAM, PD-1, and PD-L1 by T Cells

The eligibility of the volunteer CC patients and healthy controls (HCs) is screened as described in the Materials and Methods section. Only untreated patients that have a biopsy-proven diagnosis, along with clinical and pathologic assessments, are enrolled. Based on the combinations of surface markers, we simultaneously analyze expression of EpCAM, PD-1, and PD-L1 by CD4$^+$/CD8$^+$ naïve (Tn), CD4$^+$/CD8$^+$ central memory (Tcm), CD4$^+$/CD8$^+$ effective memory (Tem), subsets of CD4$^+$ helper (Th0, Th1, Th2, & Treg), and CD8$^+$ cytotoxic T cells (Tc0, Tc1, & Tc2). No significant difference is found between CC patients and HCs in the percentages of total T cells, CD4$^+$ T cells, and CD8$^+$ T cells (**Figure 1A**). In order to build a comprehensive landscape of immune blockade marker expressions, we employ the SPADE plot to sketch the profiles (**Figure 1B**).The results show that PD-1 is mainly expressed by memory T cells for both Tcm and Tem, irrespective of $CD4^+$, and $CD8^+$ (**Figure 1C**, left panel). Statistically significant difference in PD-1 expression is observable between memory and non-memory T cells ($P < 0.001$, **Figure 1C**, right panel). There is no difference in PD-1 expression by T cells between CC patients and HCs. PD-L1 expressions across all T cell subtypes are shown in **Figure 1D** and they exhibit increased expressions in CC patients. **Figure 1E** displays the representative SPADE plot of EpCAM expression landscape on T cell subsets.

viSNE Analysis Shows an Increase of $EpCAM^+$ $CD4^+$ T Cells in CC Patients

Given the high dimensionality of the mass cytometry data, we employ viSNE maps to visualize and search for high dimensional cell phenotypes that distinguish these groups (**Figures 2A,B**). A population, marked in the red dotted circles, is more abundant in CC patients. This population mainly contains $CD4^+$ T cells expressing EpCAM, CD45RA, PD-L1, CTLA4, and CCR7 (**Figure 2C**). Results of viSNE analysis are reproduced with random event sampling (**Supplementary Figures 3A,B**), and PhenoGraph clustering is applied to the tSNE map (**Supplementary Figure 3C**). The subset marked in black polygon in **Supplementary Figure 3B** is subdivided into 4 clusters: S1, S8, S12, and S23. From the clustergram in **Supplementary Figure 3D**, we can tell that S12 and S23, two small clusters, are $EpCAM^+$ $CD4^+$ T cells, while S1 and S8 are $EpCAM^-$ $CD4^+$ Tn cells. Therefore, we further compare the frequencies of $CD4^+$ Tn cells ($CD45RA^+$ and $CCR7^+$), PD-$L1^+$ $CD4^+$, $EpCAM^+$ $CD4^+$, and $CTLA4^+$ $CD4^+$ T cells between CC patients and HCs. $CD4^+$ Tn cell increases are observable in CC patients ($P = 0.0401$, **Figure 2D**). Despite its low frequency, EpCAM and PD-L1 expression by $CD4^+$ T cells are clinically relevant ($P = 0.0006$ and 0.0235, respectively, **Figure 2D**). CC patients had higher levels of $EpCAM^+$ $CD4^+$ T cells at the time of inclusion. No statistical difference is found in the percentages of $CTLA4^+$ $CD4^+$ T cells.

Phenotypic Characterization of $EpCAM^+$ $CD4^+$ T Cells

Figure 3A demonstrates the EpCAM expression profile using the viSNE map. The EpCAM expression is prominent in $CD4^+$ T cells, while no difference is observable in the relative levels of $EpCAM^+$ $CD8^+$ T cells or $EpCAM^+$ T cells (**Figure 3B**). We further define whether differences exist among traditional $CD4^+$ T cell subsets. There are significant differences in frequencies of $EpCAM^+$ memory $CD4^+$ T cells (both Tcm and Tem) and $EpCAM^+$ $CD4^+$ Tn cells between CC patients and HCs. However, this difference is not observable in the $CD4^+$ TEMRA cells ($CD45RA^+$ and $CCR7^-$), as displayed in **Figure 3C**. To investigate other possible phenotypic alterations associated with EpCAM expression, we characterize $EpCAM^+$ $CD4^+$ T cells and compare the phenotype with $EpCAM^-$ $CD4^+$ T cells (**Figure 3D**). In contrast to $EpCAM^-$ $CD4^+$, $EpCAM^+$ $CD4^+$ T cells show higher levels of PD-L1, CCR5, and CCR6. We proceed to determine the functional marker expression intensities by $EpCAM^+$ $CD4^+$ T cells in CC patients, compared with HCs (**Figure 3E**). $EpCAM^+$ $CD4^+$ T cells exhibit higher levels of CD127 (**Figure 3E**, upper panel), the Interleukin-7 receptor (IL-7R), which might be involved in the maturation and aging of this subset. The expression of PD-L1 by $EpCAM^+$ $CD4^+$ T cells exhibits great heterogeneity in CC patients (**Figure 3E**, lower panel). The percentages of PD-$L1^+$ $EpCAM^+$ $CD4^+$ T cells in $EpCAM^+$ $CD4^+$ T cells range from 2.38 to 99.39% in CC patients, and no significant difference is observed between CC and HC groups in the expression of PD-L1 by $EpCAM^+$ $CD4^+$ T cells.

High Frequency of $EpCAM^+$ $CD4^+$ T Cell Subsets in the Tumor Microenvironment

Differences of EpCAM expression by $CD4^+$ T cells in CC patients and HCs are further validated using conventional flow cytometry in an independent, untreated patient cohort (**Figures 4A,B**). Patient cohort characteristics of this confirmation study are listed in **Supplementary Table 3**. Patients with CC have higher frequencies of $EpCAM^+$ $CD4^+$ T cells, as compared to HCs ($P = 0.006$, **Figure 4B**). Considering the higher expression of chemokines, including CCR5 and CCR6, which might attract $EpCAM^+$ $CD4^+$ T cells to the tumor sites, we determine whether $EpCAM^+$ $CD4^+$ T cells are present in the tumor microenvironment within CC patients using light microscopy. The results of IF staining (**Figures 4C,D**) show the EpCAM expression and $CD4^+$ T cells distribution in tumor tissues and their para-cancerous tissues of CC patients. Magnified views with arrow-marked $EpCAM^+$ $CD4^+$ T cells in para-cancerous and carcinoma tissues are displayed in the lower panel of **Figures 4C,D**. EpCAM expression in tumor tissues is significantly higher than that in para-cancerous tissues (**Figure 4E**), which is in accord with former publications (34, 35). A higher number of $EpCAM^+$ $CD4^+$ T cells are observable in the carcinoma tissue images (**Figure 4F**). These results highlight a potential role of $EpCAM^+$ $CD4^+$ T cells in the course of CC development.

Frequency of $EpCAM^+$ $CD4^+$ T Cells in Colonic Polyp Patients

To verify whether the identified population $EpCAM^+$ $CD4^+$ T cells increased in patients with benign polyps, we examine a cohort of patients with colonic polyps (CP) and determine their T cell subset landscape using the same mass cytometry staining panel above (**Supplementary Table 2**). viSNE maps in **Figures 5A,B** show similar subpopulation deficiency pattern comparing CP and CC patients with the identified subset marked in red dotted circle. The phenotype characterization of the identified population is displayed in **Figure 5C**, showing similar expression pattern to the subsets identified in **Figure 2**. We further compare the frequencies of $EpCAM^+$ T cells, $EpCAM^+$ $CD8^+$ T cells, and $EpCAM^+$ $CD4^+$ T cells between the CC and CP groups (**Figures 5D,E**). Only the $EpCAM^+$ $CD4^+$ T cells frequency is significantly different. To the best of our knowledge,

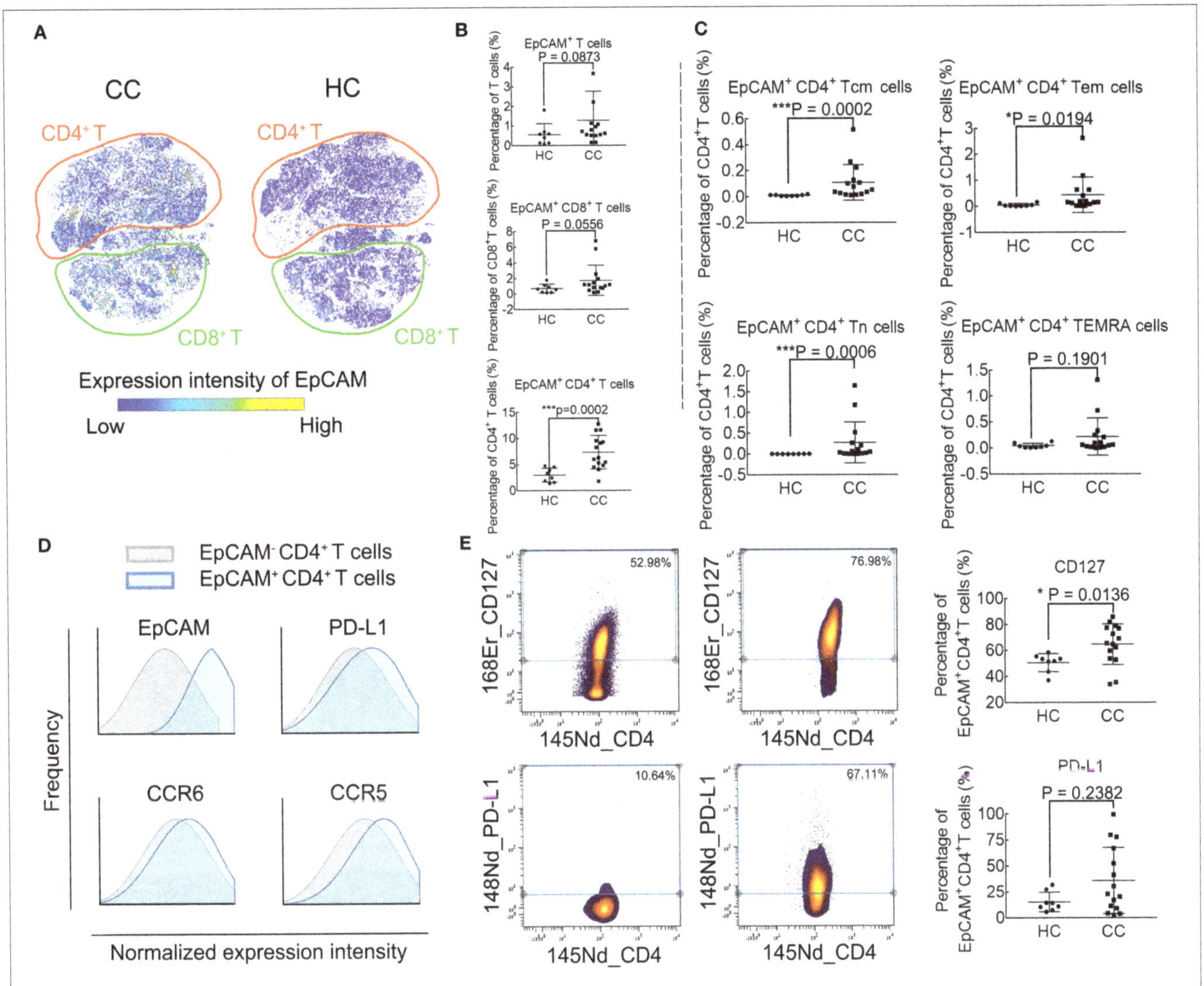

FIGURE 3 | Phenotype profiling of EpCAM+ CD4+ T cells. **(A)** viSNE maps illustrating the expression profiles of EpCAM in T cell subsets in colon cancer patients (CC) and healthy controls (HC), with color-coding representing the expression intensity of EpCAM. The relative location of CD4+ (red) and CD8+ (cyan) T cells are marked through manual gating. **(B)** EpCAM expression in T cells and CD8+ T cells. **(C)** EpCAM expression in CD4+ T cell subpopulations. **(D)** Histograms comparing marker expression of PD-L1, CCR6, CCR5 in EpCAM+ and EpCAM− CD4+ T cells. **(E)** Comparison of CD127 and PD-L1 expression in EpCAM+ CD4+ T cells in CC and HC groups. Statistically significant differences are annotated with asterisk (*) and *P* (*p*-value) or ns, not significant. *$P < 0.05$, **$P < 0.01$, ***$P < 0.001$.

this is the first documented study to demonstrate increased frequencies of EpCAM+ CD4+ T cells in the PBMC of CC patients, but not in CP patients or HCs.

Activation of p38 MAPK Pathway in EpCAM+ CD4+ T Cells in the Tumor Microenvironment

To assess the functional impact of EpCAM+ CD4+ T cells, we perform IMC on paired CC tissues and para-cancerous tissues. IMC utilizes laser ablation to generate particle plumes carried to time-of-flight detector via a stream of inert gas. IMC has a resolution comparable to light microscope and boasts simultaneous highly multiplex measurements through the use of isotopically labeled probes (33). Three tumor tissue samples and its corresponding para-cancerous tissues are obtained and stained for this experiment. In total, 29 markers are measured per cell in per slide, including markers that distinguish subpopulations and markers that characterize proliferative, signaling, and activation status (**Supplementary Table 4**). Two to five regions of interests were selected per slide (**Supplementary Table 5**). **Figure 6A** shows that predominantly EpCAM+ CD4+ T cells infiltrate is present in the tumor tissues, consistent with the results using IF. We also determine the distribution pattern of PD-L1, CD25, and CTLA4 in **Figure 6B**. Higher expression of PD-L1 by EpCAM+ CD4+ T cells is further validated. Furthermore, **Figure 6C** exhibits overlay images of expression profile of pp38 MAPK, pMAPKAPK2, pAkt, and DNA. **Figure 6D** displays overlay images of pRb, pStat1, pStat3, and DNA expression. We employ the tSNE

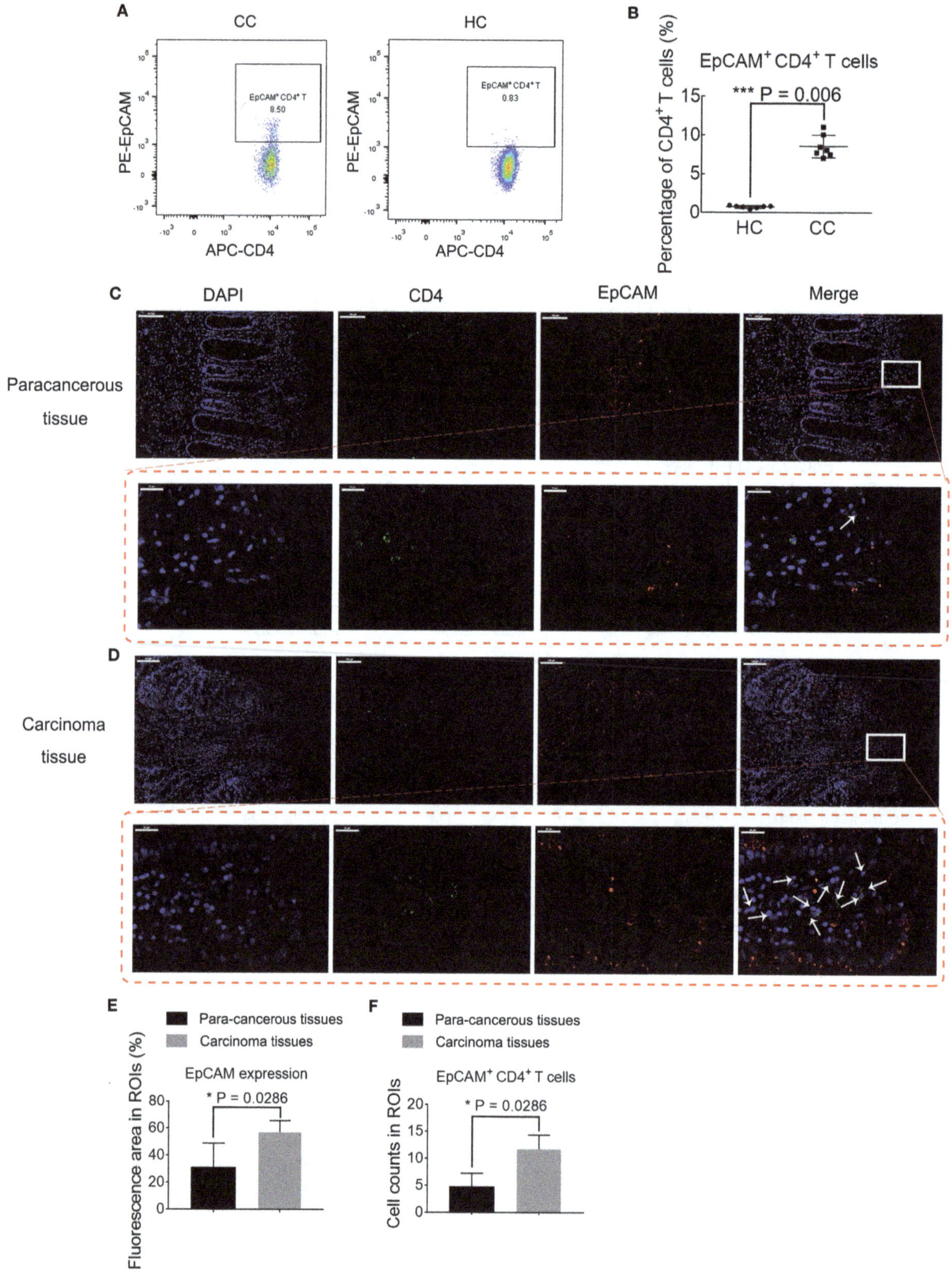

FIGURE 4 | Validation of disparity in percentages of EpCAM+ CD4+ T cells. **(A)** Biaxial plots comparing percentages of EpCAM+ CD4+ T cells in colon cancer patients (CC) and healthy controls (HC). **(B)** Percentages of EpCAM+ CD4+ T cell subsets in PBMCs in CC and HC. The data is illustrated as the mean ± SD. **(C,D)** Immunofluorescence staining of para-cancerous **(C)** or carcinoma tissues **(D)** from CC. Data is representative result of four experiments. Scale bar = 100 μm.

(Continued)

FIGURE 4 | Lower panel in red dotted box represent magnified views of arrow-marked EpCAM$^+$ CD4$^+$ T cells in para-cancerous **(C)** or carcinoma tissues **(D)**. Scale bar = 20 μm. **(E)** Bar plot comparing the EpCAM expression area in carcinoma tissues and para-cancerous tissues. $N = 4$ for each group. Data is expressed as mean ± SD. **(F)** Bar plot depicting the differences in EpCAM$^+$ CD4$^+$ T cell abundance in carcinoma tissues and para-cancerous tissues. $N = 4$ for each group. Data is expressed as mean ± SD. Statistically significant differences are annotated with asterisk (*) and P (p-value) or ns, not significant. $^*P < 0.05$, $^{**}P < 0.01$, $^{***}P < 0.001$.

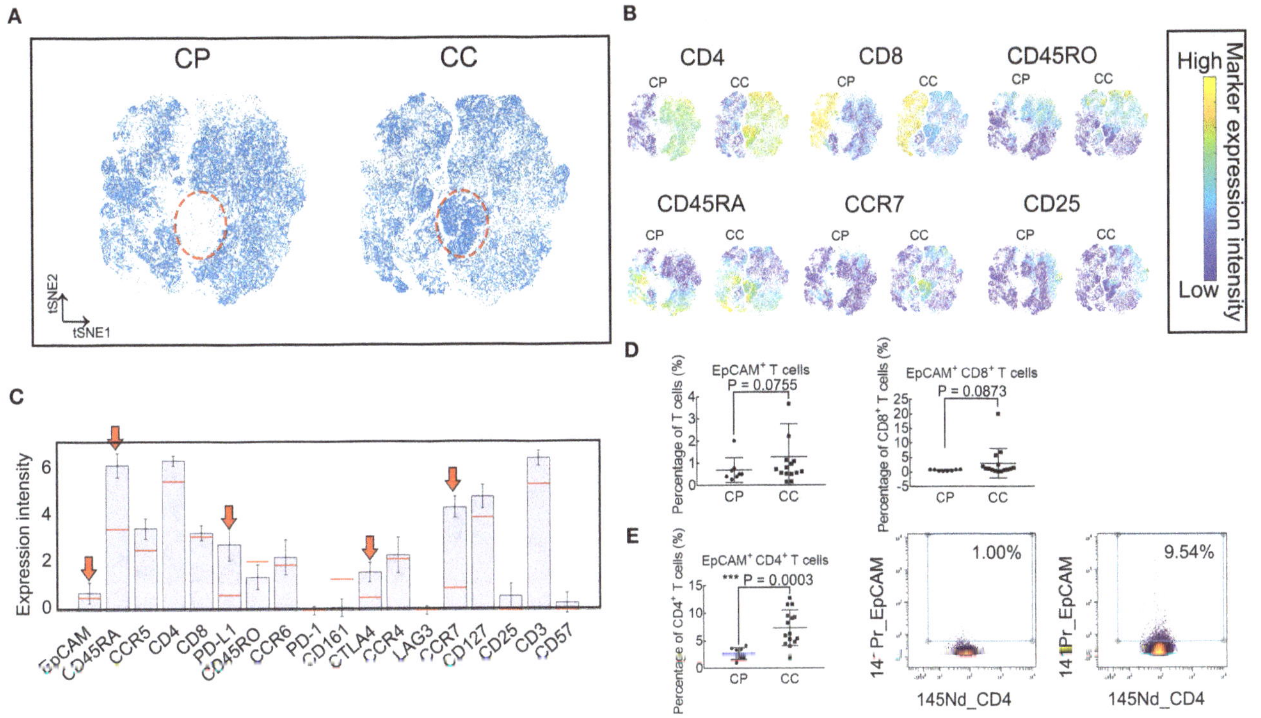

FIGURE 5 | Frequency of EpCAM$^+$ CD4$^+$ T cells were elevated in PBMC of patients with CC, but not CP. **(A)** Synthetic t-SNE maps depicting T cell subsets in colonic polyp (CP, $N = 8$) and colon cancer (CC, $N = 15$) patient groups. Suspect populations that compose almost entirely of cells from CC patients are marked in the red dotted ellipse region. **(B)** viSNE maps of T cells in CP and CC illustrating the expression of CD4, CD8, CD45RA, CD45RO, CCR7, and CD25. Color coding indicates the signified marker expression intensity. **(C)** Expression signatures of the identified subpopulations in **(A)**. Bar height indicates the median expression of each marker within a subpopulation. The horizontal line for each marker corresponds to its median expression across all cells. Red arrow indicates three positive immune blockade marker expression. **(D)** Comparison of percentages in T cells of EpCAM$^+$ and EpCAM$^+$ CD8$^+$ T cells between CP and CC. Error bar indicates standard deviation (SD). **(E)** Comparison of percentages of EpCAM$^+$ CD4$^+$ T cells in CD4$^+$ T cells between CP and CC (left panel). Biaxial plots showing higher frequency of EpCAM$^+$ CD4$^+$ T cells in CC than in CP (right panel). Statistically significant differences are annotated with asterisk (*) and P (p-value) or ns, not significant. $^*P < 0.05$, $^{**}P < 0.01$, $^{***}P < 0.001$.

algorithm to analyze the distributions and characteristics of cells extracted from these images and identify a subset of EpCAM$^+$ CD4$^+$ T cells marked in red dotted circle, in the upper panel in **Figure 6E**. Considering the small number of samples assessed by IMC, the cell percentages and marker expression intensity associated with individual ROI were used as input for statistical analysis. A significant increase of EpCAM$^+$ CD4$^+$ T cells is observed in tumor tissues. Increased expression of pp38 MAPK and pMAPKAPK2 by EpCAM$^+$ CD4$^+$ T cells is observed in the tumor tissues images, compared with para-cancerous tissues ($P = 0.0229$ and $P = 0.0068$, respectively, **Figure 6F**), suggesting that pp38 MAPK-pMAPKAPK2 signaling is up regulated. At the same time, no significant difference is detected in expression of pAkt, pRb, pStat1, and pStat3 by EpCAM$^+$ CD4$^+$ T cells between para-cancerous tissues and tumor tissues (**Figure 6F**), which suggests that complex upstream mechanisms might be involved in the development of CC.

DISCUSSION

Even though the immune checkpoints such as EpCAM and PD-1 are common targets for immunotherapy in various types of cancer, there is limited data recording their expression by human immune cells and relevant importance in the peripheral blood. In this study, we demonstrate, for the first time, the systemic and comprehensive expression profile of EpCAM, PD-1, and PD-L1 by T cells and their various subsets. Our results indicate the frequency of CD4$^+$ Tn cells, PD-L1 levels, and EpCAM expressed by CD4$^+$ T cells are higher in CC patients, in comparison to HCs. It is worth drawing attention to EpCAM$^+$ CD4$^+$ T cells since this

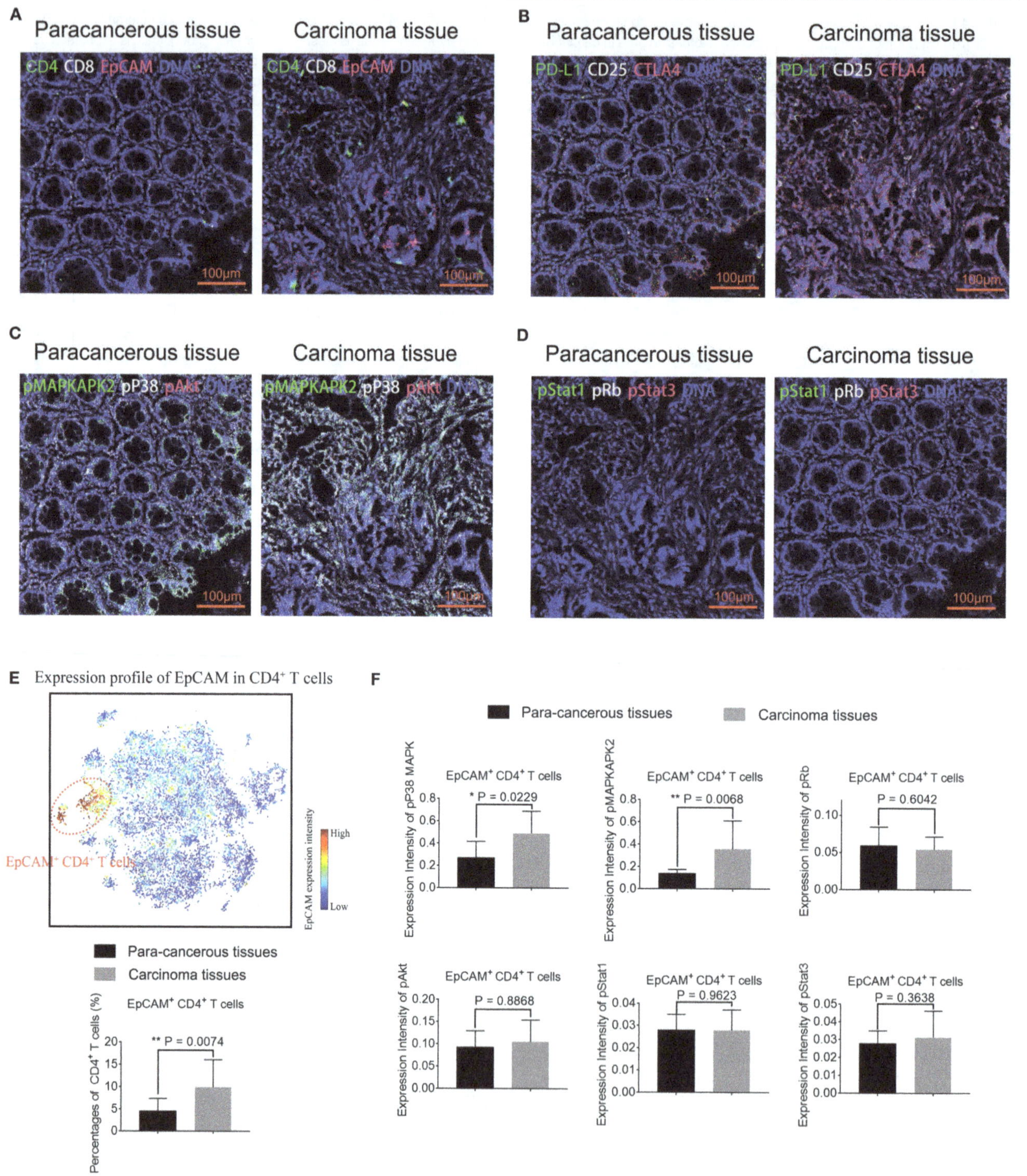

FIGURE 6 | Representative mass cytometry images of para-cancerous and carcinoma tissue samples from colon cancer patients. EpCAM$^+$ CD4$^+$ T cells in carcinoma tissues display activated pp38 MAPK/pMAPKAPK2 pathway. **(A–D)** Representative IMC images of para-cancerous or tumor tissues from CC patients. Data is representative of results of three experiments. Scale bar = 100 µm. **(A)** Overlay of EpCAM (red), CD4 (green), CD8 (white), and DNA (blue). **(B)** Overlay of CTLA4 (red), PD-L1 (green), CD25 (white), and DNA (blue). **(C)** Overlay of pAkt (red), pMAPKAPK2 (green), pp38 MAPK (white), and DNA (blue). **(D)** Overlay of pStat3 (red), pStat1 (green), pRb (white), and DNA (blue). **(E)** viSNE map of cells extracted from IMC images (upper panel) with EpCAM$^+$ CD4$^+$ T cells marked in red dotted circles. Percentages of EpCAM$^+$ CD4$^+$ T cells in para-cancerous and tumor tissues are compared and displayed in the lower panel. **(F)** Expression of phosphorylated signaling proteins including pMAPKAPK2, pp38 MAPK, pAkt, pRb, pStat1, and pStat3 by EpCAM$^+$ CD4$^+$ T cells in para-cancerous and tumor tissues are compared. $N = 11$ for tumor tissue group and $n = 9$ for para-cancerous tissue group. The data is illustrated as the mean ± SD. Statistically significant differences are annotated with asterisk (*) and P (p-value) or ns, not significant. $^*P < 0.05$, $^{**}P < 0.01$, $^{***}P < 0.001$.

subset increase only in CC patients but not in CP patients nor HCs. We characterize the phenotype of EpCAM$^+$ CD4$^+$ T cells as PD-L1$^+$ CCR5$^+$ CCR6$^+$ and further confirm that this subset also increases in tumor microenvironments with irregulated p38 MAPK signaling pathway.

Previous studies demonstrate that a balanced loss and replacement of CD4$^+$ Tn cells exists in the periphery during T cell maturation and differentiation (36, 37). Alterations in CD4$^+$ Tn cells may likely affect T cell homeostasis and functionality. Previous study illustrates that Tn cells are prone to undergo apoptosis and lose quiescence in ovarian cancer patients, providing an insight into tumor-immune evasion mechanisms (38). Results in this study reveal that the frequency of CD4$^+$ Tn cells is significantly higher in CC patients, in comparison to HCs, indicating compromised Tn cell priming and responses. However, the alterations in CD4$^+$ Tn cells should be validated in an independent cohort study to further explore the underlying mechanisms.

With regard to PD-L1, Meniawy (39) and Arrieta (40) demonstrate higher proportions of PD-L1$^+$ CD3$^+$ T cells in patients with non-small cell lung cancer (NSCLC) and a correlation between PD-L1 expression on peripheral T cells and clinical outcomes in EGFR-TKI-treated NSCLC. Results in this study, to some extent, corroborate, and expand the findings of previous works. We demonstrate that PD-L1 is expressed by multiple circulating T cell subsets. Significant differences are found in frequencies of PD-L1$^+$ CD4$^+$ T cells, but not in PD-L1$^+$ CD3$^+$ T cells in CC patients, compared to HCs. Further studies should focus on the prognostic value of assessing the expression of PD-1 and PD-L1 on the surface of peripheral T cells in CC patients that are receiving PD-1 blockade treatments.

EpCAM, a 40-kDa transmembrane glycoprotein, is a promising therapeutic target for antitumor schemes for its tumor-specific overexpression (41, 42). To the best of our knowledge, this paper is the first investigative report of EpCAM expression on circulating immunocytes and the first study to reveal the phenotypic characteristics and the intracellular signaling protein expression profile of EpCAM$^+$ CD4$^+$ T cells. EpCAM expression is demonstrated to correlate with proliferation and low differentiation (43). Recent research confirms that therapeutic strategies, using EpCAM/CD3 bispecific antibody, are significantly effective in tumor elimination (44). One of the explanation might be that the bi-functional antibody has the ability to bind EpCAM expressing cancer cells as well as cytotoxic T cells (45). Here, we propose that this treatment might influence the compositions or functions of EpCAM$^+$ CD4$^+$ T cells. These are promising prospects to investigate the effect of EpCAM/CD4-bispecific antibody, as part of combination strategies with other immunotherapies, for CC patients.

In this study, we further characterize EpCAM$^+$ CD4$^+$ T cells as PD-L1$^+$ CCR5$^+$ CCR6$^+$. It is widely accepted that ligation of PD-1 and PD-L1 leads to T cell dysfunction, exhaustion, and tolerance (8). High expression of PD-L1 by EpCAM$^+$ CD4$^+$ T cells indicates inhibited antitumor function or ineffective immune response. Expressions of chemokines, including CCR5 and CCR6, suggest that EpCAM$^+$ CD4$^+$ T cells are directed to the tumor sites, which is corroborated in this study through IF and IMC, as shown in **Figures 4C, 6A**. All these results show that EpCAM$^+$ CD4$^+$ T cells play an immune suppressive role in CC.

Many researchers explore the role of MAPK signal pathways in EpCAM$^+$ cells (11, 46). The p38 MAPK, one serine/threonine kinases of the MAPK family [namely ERK, p38 MAPK, and c-junctional N-terminal kinases (JNK)], play a central role in long-term self-renewal, survival growth, differentiation, and apoptosis (47). Activated p38 MAPK can phosphorylate and activate MAPKAPK2 and is associated with tumor initiation and development (9). We reveal excessively activated pp38 MAPK-pMAPKAPK2 signaling expressed by EpCAM$^+$ CD4$^+$ T cells in tumor tissues in CC patients, indicating that the p38 MAPK pathway might be a potential therapeutic target in EpCAM$^+$ CD4$^+$ T cell-rich CC patients. These findings should be further validated, however, considering the actual number assessed by IMC was small and that the functional investigation was preliminary and exploratory.

Future work could concentrate on clinical responses and prognosis prediction values of proportions and functions of EpCAM$^+$ CD4$^+$ T cells, as well as the therapeutic values of this subset. Further understanding of the role of EpCAM in the regulation of immune functions in any given subtype of immunocytes is in great demand.

After stringent exclusion criteria, patient groups in this study are homogeneous, treatment-naïve, and compatible with statistical requirements. Yet, the results here require prospective validation in an independent and larger patient cohort, together with the identification of the mechanisms underlying the observable increase of EpCAM$^+$ CD4$^+$ T cells. Nonetheless, this pilot study demonstrates the EpCAM$^+$ CD4$^+$ T cells abnormal in CC patients and provides an insight in immunotherapy decisions and prognosis for CC patients.

ETHICS STATEMENT

The study was approved by the Ethical Committee and Institutional Review Board of Shanghai Jiao Tong University. All participants provided written informed consent.

AUTHOR CONTRIBUTIONS

TZ and JL: conceptualization and methodology. TZ, ZT, and BW: analysis. TZ, YL, HJ, and AW: manuscript writing. HL and XD: resources and supervision.

REFERENCES

1. Siegel RL, Miller KD, Jemal A. Cancer statistics, 2016. *CA Cancer J Clin.* (2016) 66:7–30. doi: 10.3322/caac.21332
2. Chen W, Zheng R, Baade PD, Zhang S, Zeng H, Bray F, et al. Cancer statistics in China, 2015. *CA Cancer J Clin.* (2016) 66:115–32. doi: 10.3322/caac.21338
3. Society AC. *Cancer Facts and Figures.* (2012). Availabal online at: https://www.cancer.org/research/cancer-facts-statistics/all-cancer-facts-figures/cancer-facts-figures-2012.html
4. Lin X, Zhang H, Dai J, Zhang W, Zhang J, Xue G, et al. TFF3 Contributes to Epithelial-Mesenchymal Transition (EMT) in papillary thyroid carcinoma cells via the MAPK/ERK signaling pathway. *J Cancer.* (2018) 9:4430–9. doi: 10.7150/jca.24361
5. Zuo L, Du Y, Lu M, Gao J, Hu R, Zhang S, et al. Atorvastatin inhibits hyperglycemia-induced expression of osteopontin in the diabetic rat kidney via the p38 MAPK pathway. *Mol Biol Rep.* (2014) 41:2551–8. doi: 10.1007/s11033-014-3113-x
6. Liang KH, Tso HC, Hung SH, Kuan, II, Lai JK, Ke FY, et al. Extracellular domain of EpCAM enhances tumor progression through EGFR signaling in colon cancer cells. *Cancer Lett.* (2018) 433:165–75. doi: 10.1016/j.canlet.2018.06.040
7. Meniawy TM, Lake RA, McDonnell AM, Millward MJ, Nowak AK. PD-L1 on peripheral blood T lymphocytes is prognostic in patients with non-small cell lung cancer (NSCLC) treated with EGFR inhibitors. *Lung Cancer.* (2016) 93:9–16. doi: 10.1016/j.lungcan.2015.12.006
8. Xu-Monette ZY, Zhang M, Li J, Young KH. PD-1/PD-L1 blockade: have we found the key to unleash the antitumor immune response? *Front Immunol.* (2017) 8:1597. doi: 10.3389/fimmu.2017.01597
9. Alam R, Schultz CR, Golembieski WA, Poisson LM, Rempel SA. PTEN suppresses SPARC-induced pMAPKAPK2 and inhibits SPARC-induced Ser78 HSP27 phosphorylation in glioma. *Neuro Oncol.* (2013) 15:451–61. doi: 10.1093/neuonc/nos326
10. Liao MY, Lai JK, Kuo MY, Lu RM, Lin CW, Cheng PC, et al. An anti-EpCAM antibody EpAb2-6 for the treatment of colon cancer. *Oncotarget.* (2015) 6:24947–68. doi: 10.18632/oncotarget.4453
11. Chiba T, Suzuki E, Yuki K, Zen Y, Oshima M, Miyagi S, et al. Disulfiram eradicates tumor-initiating hepatocellular carcinoma cells in ROS-p38 MAPK pathway-dependent and -independent manners. *PLoS ONE.* (2014) 9:e84807. doi: 10.1371/journal.pone.0084807
12. Lee JH, Park MS, Chung IJ. Induction of 90K-specific cytotoxic T lymphocytes for colon cancer immunotherapy. *Immune Netw.* (2010) 10:206–11. doi: 10.4110/in.2010.10.6.206
13. Moore PA, Shah K, Yang Y, Alderson R, Roberts P, Long V, et al. Development of MGD007, a gpA33 x CD3-bispecific DART protein for T-cell immunotherapy of metastatic colorectal cancer. *Mol Cancer Ther.* (2018) 17:1761–72. doi: 10.1158/1535-7163.MCT-17-1086
14. Chevolet I, Speeckaert R, Schreuer M, Neyns B, Krysko O, Bachert C, et al. Characterization of the *in vivo* immune network of IDO, tryptophan metabolism, PD-L1, and CTLA-4 in circulating immune cells in melanoma. *Oncoimmunology.* (2015) 4:e982382. doi: 10.4161/2162402X.2014.982382
15. Coindre S, Tchitchek N, Alaoui L, Vaslin B, Bourgeois C, Goujard C, et al. Mass cytometry analysis reveals the landscape and dynamics of CD32a(+) CD4(+) T cells from early HIV infection to effective cART. *Front Immunol.* (2018) 9:1217. doi: 10.3389/fimmu.2018.01217
16. Stern L, McGuire H, Avdic S, Rizzetto S, Fazekas de St Groth B, Luciani F, et al. Mass cytometry for the assessment of immune reconstitution after hematopoietic stem cell transplantation. *Front Immunol.* (2018) 9:1672. doi: 10.3389/fimmu.2018.01672
17. Spitzer MH, Gherardini PF, Fragiadakis GK, Bhattacharya N, Yuan RT, Hotson AN, et al. An interactive reference framework for modeling a dynamic immune system. *Science.* (2015) 349:1259425. doi: 10.1126/science.1259425
18. Kaiser Y, Lakshmikanth T, Chen Y, Mikes J, Eklund A, Brodin P, et al. Mass cytometry identifies distinct lung CD4+ T cell patterns in lofgren's syndrome and non-lofgren's syndrome sarcoidosis. *Front Immunol.* (2017) 8:1130. doi: 10.3389/fimmu.2017.01130
19. Amir el AD, Davis KL, Tadmor MD, Simonds EF, Levine JH, Bendall SC, et al. viSNE enables visualization of high dimensional single-cell data and reveals phenotypic heterogeneity of leukemia. *Nat Biotechnol.* (2013) 31:545–52. doi: 10.1038/nbt.2594
20. Gautreau G, Pejoski D, Le Grand R, Cosma A, Beignon AS, Tchitchek N. SPADEVizR: an R package for visualization, analysis and integration of SPADE results. *Bioinformatics.* (2017) 33:779–81. doi: 10.1093/bioinformatics/btw708
21. Zunder ER, Lujan E, Goltsev Y, Wernig M, Nolan GP. A continuous molecular roadmap to iPSC reprogramming through progression analysis of single-cell mass cytometry. *Cell Stem Cell.* (2015) 16:323–37. doi: 10.1016/j.stem.2015.01.015
22. Ramskold D, Parodis I, Lakshmikanth T, Sippl N, Khademi M, Chen Y, et al. B cell alterations during BAFF inhibition with belimumab in SLE. *EBioMedicine.* (2018) 40:517–27. doi: 10.1016/j.ebiom.2018.12.035
23. Setty M, Tadmor MD, Reich-Zeliger S, Angel O, Salame TM, Kathail P, et al. Wishbone identifies bifurcating developmental trajectories from single-cell data. *Nat Biotechnol.* (2016) 34:637–45. doi: 10.1038/nbt.3569
24. Bendall SC, Simonds EF, Qiu P, Amir el AD, Krutzik PO, Finck R, et al. Single-cell mass cytometry of differential immune and drug responses across a human hematopoietic continuum. *Science.* (2011) 332:687–96. doi: 10.1126/science.1198704
25. Ornatsky OI, Kinach R, Bandura DR, Lou X, Tanner SD, Baranov VI, et al. Development of analytical methods for multiplex bio-assay with inductively coupled plasma mass spectrometry. *J Analyt Atomic Spectrometry.* (2008) 23:463–9. doi: 10.1039/b710510j
26. Finck R, Simonds EF, Jager A, Krishnaswamy S, Sachs K, Fantl W, et al. Normalization of mass cytometry data with bead standards. *Cytometry Part A.* (2013) 83:483–94. doi: 10.1002/cyto.a.22271
27. Levine JH, Simonds EF, Bendall SC, Davis KL, Amir el AD, Tadmor MD, et al. Data-driven phenotypic dissection of AML reveals progenitor-like cells that correlate with prognosis. *Cell.* (2015) 162:184–97. doi: 10.1016/j.cell.2015.05.047
28. Qiu P, Simonds EF, Bendall SC, Gibbs KD Jr, Bruggner RV, Linderman MD, et al. Extracting a cellular hierarchy from high-dimensional cytometry data with SPADE. *Nat Biotechnol.* (2011) 29:886–91. doi: 10.1038/nbt.1991
29. Gaudilliere B, Fragiadakis GK, Bruggner RV, Nicolau M, Finck R, Tingle M, et al. Clinical recovery from surgery correlates with single-cell immune signatures. *Sci Transl Med.* (2014) 6:255ra131. doi: 10.1126/scitranslmed.3009701
30. Chen H, Lau MC, Wong MT, Newell EW, Poidinger M, Chen J. Cytofkit: A Bioconductor package for an integrated mass cytometry data analysis pipeline. *PLoS Comput Biol.* (2016) 12:e1005112. doi: 10.1371/journal.pcbi.1005112
31. Nakayamada S, Takahashi H, Kanno Y, O'Shea JJ. Helper T cell diversity and plasticity. *Curr Opin Immunol.* (2012) 24:297–302. doi: 10.1016/j.coi.2012.01.014
32. Giesen C, Wang HA, Schapiro D, Zivanovic N, Jacobs A, Hattendorf B, et al. Highly multiplexed imaging of tumor tissues with subcellular resolution by mass cytometry. *Nat Methods.* (2014) 11:417–22. doi: 10.1038/nmeth.2869
33. Guo RR, Zhang T, Meng XY, Lin Z, Lin JR, Gong Y, et al. Lymphocyte mass cytometry identifies a CD3(-)CD4(+) cell subset with a potential role in psoriasis. *JCI Insight.* (2019) 4:e125306. doi: 10.1172/jci.insight.125306

34. Brahmer JR, Drake CG, Wollner I, Powderly JD, Picus J, Sharfman WH, et al. Phase I study of single-agent anti-programmed death-1 (MDX-1106) in refractory solid tumors: safety, clinical activity, pharmacodynamics, and immunologic correlates. *J Clin Oncol.* (2010) 28:3167–75. doi: 10.1200/JCO.2009.26.7609
35. Herr AE, Singh AK. Photopolymerized cross-linked polyacrylamide gels for on-chip protein sizing. *Anal Chem.* (2004) 76:4727–33. doi: 10.1021/ac049686u
36. Takada K, Jameson SC. Naive T cell homeostasis: from awareness of space to a sense of place. *Nat Rev Immunol.* (2009) 9:823–32. doi: 10.1038/nri2657
37. Appay V, Sauce D. Naive T cells: the crux of cellular immune aging? *Exp Gerontol.* (2014) 54:90–3. doi: 10.1016/j.exger.2014.01.003
38. Xia H, Wang W, Crespo J, Kryczek I, Li W, Wei S, et al. Suppression of FIP200 and autophagy by tumor-derived lactate promotes naive T cell apoptosis and affects tumor immunity. *Sci Immunol.* (2017) 2:eaan4631. doi: 10.1126/sciimmunol.aan4631
39. Irrazabal T, Martin A. T Regulatory cells gone bad: an oncogenic immune response against enterotoxigenic *B. fragilis* infection leads to colon cancer. *Cancer Discov.* (2015) 5:1021–3. doi: 10.1158/2159-8290.CD-15-0987
40. Arrieta O, Montes-Servin E, Hernandez-Martinez JM, Cardona AF, Casas-Ruiz E, Crispin JC, et al. Expression of PD-1/PD-L1 and PD-L2 in peripheral T-cells from non-small cell lung cancer patients. *Oncotargetology.* (2017) 8:101994–2005. doi: 10.18632/oncotarget.22025
41. Ang WX, Li Z, Chi Z, Du SH, Chen C, Tay JC, et al. Intraperitoneal immunotherapy with T cells stably and transiently expressing anti-EpCAM CAR in xenograft models of peritoneal carcinomatosis. *Oncotargetology.* (2017) 8:13545–59. doi: 10.18632/oncotarget.14592
42. Cioffi M, Dorado J, Baeuerle PA, Heeschen C. EpCAM/CD3-Bispecific T-cell engaging antibody MT110 eliminates primary human pancreatic cancer stem cells. *Clin Cancer Res.* (2012) 18:465–74. doi: 10.1158/1078-0432.CCR-11-1270
43. Martowicz A, Rainer J, Lelong J, Spizzo G, Gastl G, Untergasser G. EpCAM overexpression prolongs proliferative capacity of primary human breast epithelial cells and supports hyperplastic growth. *Mol Cancer.* (2013) 12:56. doi: 10.1186/1476-4598-12-56
44. Herrmann I, Baeuerle PA, Friedrich M, Murr A, Filusch S, Ruttinger D, et al. Highly efficient elimination of colorectal tumor-initiating cells by an EpCAM/CD3-bispecific antibody engaging human T cells. *PLoS ONE.* (2010) 5:e13474. doi: 10.1371/journal.pone.0013474
45. Imrich S, Hachmeister M, Gires O. EpCAM and its potential role in tumor-initiating cells. *Cell Adh Migr.* (2012) 6:30–8. doi: 10.4161/cam.18953
46. Yip NC, Fombon IS, Liu P, Brown S, Kannappan V, Armesilla AL, et al. Disulfiram modulated ROS-MAPK and NFkappaB pathways and targeted breast cancer cells with cancer stem cell-like properties. *Br J Cancer.* (2011) 104:1564–74. doi: 10.1038/bjc.2011.126
47. Lakshmanan AP, Thandavarayan RA, Watanabe K, Sari FR, Meilei H, Giridharan VV, et al. Modulation of AT-1R/MAPK cascade by an olmesartan treatment attenuates diabetic nephropathy in streptozotocin-induced diabetic mice. *Mol Cell Endocrinol.* (2012) 348:104–11. doi: 10.1016/j.mce.2011.07.041

14

Characterization of Leukocytes From HIV-ART Patients Using Combined Cytometric Profiles of 72 Cell Markers

Adrien Leite Pereira [1†], *Nicolas Tchitchek* [1*†], *Olivier Lambotte* [1,2,3], *Roger Le Grand* [1] *and Antonio Cosma* [1]

[1] *CEA–Université Paris Sud 11–INSERM U1184, Immunology of Viral Infections and Autoimmune Diseases, IDMIT Infrastructure, Fontenay-aux-Roses, France,* [2] *APHP, Service de Médecine Interne-Immunologie Clinique, Hôpitaux Universitaires Paris Sud, Le Kremlin-Bicêtre, France,* [3] *Université Paris Sud, Le Kremlin-Bicêtre, France*

***Correspondence:**
Nicolas Tchitchek
nicolas.tchitchek@gmail.com

[†] *These authors have contributed equally to this work*

Motivation: Mass cytometry is a technique used to measure the intensity levels of proteins expressed by cells, at a single cell resolution. This technique is essential to characterize the phenotypes and functions of immune cell populations, but is currently limited to the measurement of 40 cell markers that restricts the characterization of complex diseases. However, algorithms and multi-tube cytometry techniques have been designed for combining phenotypic information obtained from different cytometric panels. The characterization of chronic HIV infection represents a good study case for multi-tube mass cytometry as this disease triggers a complex interactions network of more than 70 cell markers.

Method: We collected whole blood from non-viremic HIV-infected patients on combined antiretroviral therapies and healthy donors. Leukocytes from each individual were stained using three different mass cytometry panels, which consisted of 35, 32, and 33 cell markers. For each patient and using the CytoBackBone algorithm, we combined phenotypic information from three different antibody panels into a single cytometric profile, reaching a phenotypic resolution of 72 markers. These high-resolution cytometric profiles were analyzed using SPADE and viSNE algorithms to decipher the immune response to HIV.

Results: We detected an upregulation of several proteins in HIV-infected patients relative to healthy donors using our profiling of 72 cell markers. Among them, CD11a and CD11b were upregulated in PMNs, monocytes, mDCs, NK cells, and T cells. CD11b was also upregulated on pDCs. Other upregulated proteins included: CD38 on PMNs, monocytes, NK cells, basophils, B cells, and T cells; CD83 on monocytes, mDCs, B cells, and T cells; and TLR2, CD32, and CD64 on PMNs and monocytes. These results were validated using a mass cytometry panel of 25 cells markers.

Impacts: We demonstrate here that multi-tube cytometry can be applied to mass cytometry for exploring, at an unprecedented level of details, cell populations impacted by complex diseases. We showed that the monocyte and PMN populations were strongly affected by the HIV infection, as CD11a, CD11b, CD32, CD38, CD64, CD83, CD86, and TLR2 were upregulated in these populations. Overall, these results demonstrate that HIV induced a specific environment that similarly affected multiple immune cells.

Keywords: high-dimensional cytometry, cytometric profiles merging, HIV infection, chronic inflammation, biomarkers

INTRODUCTION

Cytometry is an experimental technique used to measure the intensity levels of proteins expressed by cells, at a single cell resolution. However, none of these technologies can currently handle the simultaneous study of more than 50 markers (1). This restriction is particularly limiting to deeply characterize immune cell populations in complex inflammatory diseases, such as HIV infection.

Bioinformatics approaches have been successfully developed and applied to extend the number of observable cell markers per cytometric profiles through the merging of phenotypic information obtained from different cytometry profiles (generated from different cytometry panels). In such approaches, phenotypic information from the different profiles is combined into a single profile based on the expression of a common set of shared markers (2–4). Especially, the CytoBackBone algorithm, which is based on a Nearest Neighbor technique, can be used to extend our vision of complex immune diseases (5). However, no application of these bioinformatics approaches was performed in the context of infectious diseases using mass cytometry data.

HIV infection is still a major sexually transmissible disease. Although detected by different immune receptors, HIV is not cleared by the immune system. A global overview of the cell interaction network triggered in HIV infections is required to understand the immune system dysfunctions and to set up new therapeutic treatments.

HIV preferentially infects $CD4^+$ T cells. In the long term, HIV induces a decrease of T cells number both in the blood and in the lymphoid organs. This situation then triggers a severe immune deficiency, that leads to Acquired Immunodeficiency Syndrome (AIDS) (6, 7). The monocyte compartment is also heavily impacted by HIV-infection. Indeed, this disease leads to an increase in the number of $CD14^{low}$ $CD16^{high}$ circulating monocytes (called non-classical monocytes), which is to the detriment of $CD14^{high}$ $CD16^{low}$ monocytes (8). Non-classical monocytes have been characterized as pro-inflammatory cells, as they are able to produce TNF-α, IL-1α, IL1-β, and IP-10 (9–11). In addition, they also overexpress costimulatory molecules such as CD80 and CD86, which again characterizes their activation state (12). Furthermore, the persistence of the virus in the organism results in chronic inflammation, which is also observed in treated HIV-infected patients (13, 14). Interestingly, the persistence of chronic inflammation could lead to an exhaustion of leukocytes (15). This exhaustion is characterized by a delay in the TLR4- or TLR7/8-dependent cytokine productions in monocytes and dendritic cells, as well as by the loss of functional and proliferative capacities of effector T cells. Moreover, several negative regulators of immune activation, such as PD-1, LAG-3, Tim-3, and CTLA-4, are preferentially upregulated on T cells during HIV infection (16–18). Overall, a large set of immune cell populations are involved in this disease.

Many proteins involved in chronic inflammation in HIV-infected subjects have been described (19, 20). Indeed, the literature provides more than 70 cell markers involved in this disease (19, 20). Nonetheless, it is likely that a large number of cell markers are yet to be discovered. Also, a single-cell technology able to simultaneously monitor the expression of a complex network of proteins, involving more than 70 cell markers, is needed to better understand the inflammatory processes generated by HIV infection.

Here, we used the CytoBackBone algorithm (5) to characterize innate and adaptive immune cells obtained from treated HIV-infected patients and healthy donors using combined mass cytometric profiles of 72 cell markers. CytoBackBone is multi-tube cytometry algorithm based on a nearest neighbor approach. Especially, this algorithm uses the notion of acceptable and non-ambiguous neighbors to optimize the quality of the merging of cytometric profiles. Thanks to this notion, the merging performed by CytoBackBone are more stringent and noise-free compared to other approaches. Using this innovative multi-tube cytometry approach, we observed important phenotypic differences between treated HIV-infected patients and healthy donors in the whole leukocyte populations. Especially, we show that monocytes and polymorphonuclear cells (PMNs) are deeply impacted in treated HIV-infected patients. We confirmed these findings using cytometric profiles obtained from a single mass cytometry panel.

MATERIALS AND METHODS

Ethics

This experiment was approved by the Comité de Protection des Personnes (CPP) Ile de France VII, under protocol number PP 14-003. All subjects gave written informed consent to participate in this study.

Whole Blood Collection

Whole blood from healthy ($n = 3$) and HIV-1 ART-treated non-viremic donors (undetectable plasma RNA, $n = 3$) was collected in lithium heparin tubes by the Etablissement Français du Sang (EFS, Hôpital Saint Louis, Paris, France) and Hôpital du Kremlin Bicêtre, respectively. Information concerning the gender, current age, contamination pathway, viral load, year of detection of the HIV infection, starting year of ARV treatment, and the type and the duration of treatment is provided for each HIV-infected

TABLE 1 | Characteristics of HIV-infected patients and healthy donors.

Individuals	Gender	Current age	Contamination	Number of CD4+ T cells (cells/mm^3)	CD4+ T cells nadir (cells/mm^3)	Viral load (copie/ml)	Detection (age of patient)	Treatment started - Updated treatment	Current treatment	HCV co-infection
PAT-1	Male	54	Sexual (Homo)	543	204	<40	1994 (32 years)	1997 – 2015	Tivicay Truvada	No
PAT-2	Female	54	Sexual (Hetero)	1376	167	<40	1991 (26 years)	1994 – 2014	Isentress Kivexa	No
PAT-3	Female	70	Sexual (Hetero)	404	170	<40	2001 (55 years)	2008 – 2010	Isentress Truvada	No
PAT-4	Male	51	Sexual (Homo)	1,451	130	<40	1990 (24 years)	1997 – 2013	Kivexa Norvir Reyataz	No
PAT-5	Male	58	Sexual (Hetero)	324	13	<40	2002 (43 years)	2002 – 2016	Kivexa Norvir Reyataz	No
PAT-6	Male	48	Sexual (Homo)	744	243	<40	1991 (22 years)	1998 – 2015	Eviplera	No
HEA-1	Male	48								
HEA-2	Male	63								
HEA-3	Female	28								
HEA-4	Male	59								
HEA-5	Male	56								
HEA-6	Male	56								
HEA-7	Female	59								
HEA-8	Female	25								
HEA-9	Male	27								

Information about the gender, current age, contamination pathway, viral load, year of detection of the HIV infection, starting year of the ARV treatment, updated year of the ARV treatment, type treatment, the duration of treatments, and the HCV co-infection status were provided for each HIV-infected patient. Information about the gender and the age were provided for each healthy donor. Information presented in this table corresponds to information obtained at the time of the blood samplings.

patient in **Table 1**. The gender and current age of each healthy donor are also provided.

To validate the results with a single cytometric panel, blood from the three previous HIV-infected subjects, three new HIV-infected patients ($n = 6$), and six new healthy subjects ($n = 6$) was collected. Information concerning the gender and the current age is provided for each HIV-infected patient and each healthy donor in **Table 1**. In addition, information concerning contamination pathway, viral load, year of detection of the HIV infection, starting year of ARV treatment, and type and duration of treatment is also provided for each HIV-infected patient.

Sample Processing for Mass Cytometry Data

Blood samples were processed according to a previously described protocol (21). The cells (from 1 ml blood) were mixed with 10 ml fixation mixture (FM) in 50-ml plastic tubes and incubated for 10 min at 4°C. After centrifugation at 800 x g for 5 min at room temperature (RT), red cells were lysed by adding 10 ml Milli-Q water at RT for 20 min, without agitation. After two washes with 1X DPBS, cells were counted and stored at −80°C in FM at a final concentration of 15×10^6 cells/ml and distributed into aliquots containing 3×10^6 cells. FM used to fix and store the cells was prepared the day before the experiments and conserved at 4°C. The 5% formaldehyde FM solution was prepared from 36% paraformaldehyde (VWR BDH Prolabo, Fontenay-sous-Bois) and contained 18.5% glycerol (Sigma-Aldrich, Lyon, France) in 1X-Dulbecco's phosphate buffered saline (DPBS), without $CaCl_2$ or $MgCl_2$, pH 7.4 (Gibco by life Technologies, Villebon-Sur-Yvette, France). This solution allowed freezing and recovery of all blood leukocytes, especially polymorphonuclear cells, which are highly labile and cryopreservation-sensitive. Healthy and HIV-infected samples used for the multi-tube 72-marker experiment were cryopreserved for a maximum of 12 days.

Staining Protocols for Mass Cytometry Data

For each sample, 3×10^6 cryopreserved fixed cells were washed twice with staining buffer [PBS/0.5% BSA, prepared by mixing

1X DPBS modified (Gibco by Life Technologies) with 0.5% BSA (Sigma-Aldrich, Lyon, France)] and labeled with conjugated antibodies according to the following procedure. Cells were incubated at 4°C for 30 min with a mix of the metal-labeled surface antibodies (Abs) in staining buffer. After two washes with 1X DPBS, cells were incubated in fixation solution (PBS/1.6% PFA, prepared by diluting 16% paraformaldehyde (PFA; Electron Microscopy Sciences Hartfield, USA) in DPBS 10X and Milli-Q water) at RT for 20 min and permeabilized with 1X Perm/wash (BD) buffer at RT for 10 min. Staining with metal-labeled intracellular Abs and an iridium nucleic acid intercalator in 1X Perm/Wash was carried out as for extracellular staining, but without a new permeabilization step. Cells were stored overnight with 0.1 μM iridium nucleic acid intercalator in fixation mixture. The following day, cells were washed with Milli-Q water, resuspended in 1 ml Milli-Q water and filtered using a 35-μm nylon mesh cell strainer (BD Biosciences), before the addition of EQ Four-Element Calibration Beads (Fluidigm, San Francisco, USA), according to the manufacturer's instructions. Acquisition of each sample was performed two times in succession on a CyTOF or Helios instrument (Fluidigm). No autosampler was used for sample acquisition. Moreover, the dual sample loop system was used for sample acquisition performed on the CyTOF. CyTOF settings were parametrized following the quality control of the instrument.

Processing of Mass Cytometry Data

Data were acquired using EQ™ Four-Element Calibration Beads, normalized using Rachel Finck's MATLAB normalizer, and concatenated using the FCS file concatenation tool (Cytobank, Mountain View, CA). Cytometric profiles were manually gated to exclude the EQ™ Four-Element Calibration Beads, select singlets, and gate out non-specific background generated by metal-conjugated Ab binding to eosinophils (22), as represented in **Supplementary Figure 1**. The arcsinh (cofactor = 5) transformation was applied on marker expressions.

Merging of Cytometry Profiles Using CytoBackBone

The CytoBackBone algorithm (5) was used to merge cytometric profiles from the different panels. In details, CytoBackBone is an nearest neighbor-based algorithm that combines phenotypic information of different cytometric profiles obtained from different cytometry panels. In our approach, CytoBackBone combines marker expression information of two cells from different cytometric profiles if, and only if, these two cells are *acceptable* and *non-ambiguous* nearest neighbors. In details, each time two cells from different cytometric profiles are identified as acceptable and non-ambiguous nearest neighbors, CytoBackBone merges them and a new cell with a combined phenotype is created. This new cell is added to the resulting cytometric profile and its phenotype corresponds to the average marker expression for the set of common markers. For the non-common markers (i.e., markers that do not belong to the backbone composition), the phenotype of this cell corresponds to the specific marker expression. CytoBackBone is implemented in R and the source code can be found at: https://github.com/tchitchek-lab/CytoBackBone. Each merge realized by CytoBackBone was calculated based on the set of common markers between the cytometric profiles to be merged (CD1c, CD3, CD11c, CD14, CD16, CD19, CD32, CD64, CD66, CD86, CD123, CD141, Granzyme B, and HLADR). A distance threshold of 3 was used for all merging.

Analysis of Merged Mass Cytometric Profiles

SPADE analyses were generated using the public version of the SPADE R package. viSNE representations were generated based on the Barnes-Hut implementation of the t-SNE algorithm. Dot-plot visualizations were performed using Cytobank software (Mountain View, CA). SPADE analyses were set up and carried out with a down-sampling parameter of 5%. A random pre-downsampling was used to select 67,000 cells from each sample (67,000 corresponded to the number of cells contained in the smallest sample) before the SPADE analysis. Full upsampling was eventually performed after the cell cluster identification by SPADE. Categorical marker heatmaps were generated using the SPADEVizR package (23). Marker expression categories represented in the heatmap were generated based on the intensity expression range of each marker. Marker expression ranges were calculated based on the 5 and 95th percentiles of marker expression. Then, each range was divided into five uniform categories. The categorization of marker expression was computed based on the means of the individual SPADE-expression medians of each marker. These categories represented negative, low, medium, high, and very high marker expression using a color scale from white to dark red, which was used to produce the heatmap. Cell clusters with <50 cells (for the whole dataset) were annotated as unassigned and were colored in gray in the categorical heatmap representation. Indeed, the phenotypes of these clusters cannot be evaluated based on the mean expression of marker expressions. Hierarchical clustering of markers and clusters was performed using the Euclidian distance and was based on the complete linkage method. Statistical analyses of cell cluster abundances were obtained using a non-parametric permutation test (available in the Deducer R package).

RESULTS

Phenotypic Characterization of Leukocytes From HIV-Infected Patients and Healthy Donor Using Merged Cytometric Profiles of 72 Cell Markers

To characterize the phenotypes of leukocytes obtained from HIV-infected patients and healthy donors, we used three different mass cytometry panels. Phenotypic information from the different cytometry profiles was combined using the CytoBackBone algorithm. Such multidimensional phenotype characterization was performed based on the simultaneous expression of 72 markers.

We collected whole blood from three non-viremic HIV-infected patients on combined antiretroviral therapies (named

TABLE 2 | Antibodies and cell markers used to create combined mass cytometry profiles including 72 cell markers.

	Panel #A		Panel #B		Panel #C	
Metals	**Antibodies**	**Clones**	**Antibodies**	**Clones**	**Antibodies**	**Clones**
Pr141	**CD66**	TET2	**CD66**	TET2	**CD66**	TET2
Nd142	**HLADR**	L243 (G46-6)	**HLADR**	L243 (G46-6)	**HLADR**	L243 (G46-6)
Nd143	**CD3**	UCHT1	**CD3**	UCHT1	**CD3**	UCHT1
Nd144	**CD64**	10.1.1	**CD64**	10.1.1	**CD64**	10.1.1
Nd145	CD8a	37006	CCR7	150503	CD209	DCN47.5
Nd146	IL-6	MQ2-13A5	NF-ATC	.7A6	CD62L	DREG-56
Sm147	Granzyme A	CTLA-3	CD335	9 E 2	CD45	D058-1283
Nd148	IL-1β	H1b-98	IL-4	7A3-3	CD137	4B4-1
Sm149	**CD14**	M5E2	**CD14**	M5E2	**CD14**	M5E2
Nd150	**CD123**	7G3	**CD123**	7G3	**CD123**	7G3
Eu151	IL-8	NAPII	CD107a	H4A3	-	-
Sm152	**CD16**	B73.1	**CD16**	B73.1	**CD16**	B73.1
Eu153	CD23	M-L233	CD154	TRAP1	CXCR3 (CD183)	1C6
Sm154	**CD86**	2,331 (FUN-1)	**CD86**	2,331 (FUN-1)	**CD86**	2331 (FUN-1)
Gd155	**CD32**	2 E1	**CD32**	2 E1	**CD32**	2 E1
Gd156	MIP-1β	D21-1351	CD54	LB-2	CD56	AF12-7H3
Gd158	IP-10	6D4	IL-2	N7.48A	ITGβ7	FIB504
Tb159	TNF-α	MAb11	-	-	Bcl-6	K112-91
Gd160	IL-1α	364/3B3-14	CD69	FN50	CD83	HB15E
Dy161	**CD141**	MAB3947	**CD141**	MAB3947	**CD141**	MAB3947
Dy162	IL-12	C8,6	Ki67	B56	CD279	MIH4
Dy163	**CD1c**	AF5916	**CD1c**	AF5916	**CD1c**	AF5916
Dy164	CXCR4	12G5	CD25	BC96	CD127	HIL-7R-M21
Ho165	TLR2	REA109	CD11a	HI111	IL-10R	3F9
Er166	CCR5	3A9	CD11b	ICRF44	CD27	M-T271
Er167	CD28	CD28.2	CD38	AT1	IgG2c	A23-1
Er168	**CD11c**	B-ly6	**CD11c**	B-ly6	**CD11c**	B-ly6
Tm169	IFN-α	LT27:295	-	-	-	-
Er170	CD45RA	T6D11	IgG2b	27-35	CCL5	2D5
Yb171	IFN-γ	25723	IL-10	JES3-9D7	IgG1 K	MOPC-21
Yb172	CD4	L200	MyD88	RB2101	IL-2RA	24212
Yb173	**Granzyme B**	GB11	**Granzyme B**	GB11	**Granzyme B**	GB11
Yb174	**CD19**	HIB19	**CD19**	HIB19	**CD19**	HIB19
Yb175	IL-1RA	AS17	-	-	IgG2a	R35-95
Yb176	MCP-1	5D3-F7	Perforin	dG9-DTAG9	nfKB	K10-892.12.50
Ir191	-	-	-	-	-	-
Ir193	-	-	-	-	-	-

The metal isotopes, markers, and antibody clones are indicated for each panel. Backbone markers are indicated in bold.

PAT-1 to PAT-3) and three healthy donors (named HEA-1 to HEA-3), as indicated in **Table 1**. Following red cell lysis, cells from each sample were stained using three mass cytometry panels, named #A, #B, #C, which consisted of 35, 32, and 33 markers, respectively (**Table 2**). These three panels shared 14 common markers.

For each patient, phenotypic information from various mass cytometry panels was merged using the CytoBackBone algorithm. Thus, for each of the six subjects, we generated a merged cytometric profile of 72 cell markers.

For each cytometric profile, the number of cells obtained before and after merging is shown in **Table 3**. The average of cells present in merged files was 142,265 cells. Furthermore, cytometric profiles related to healthy subjects were composed of 157,083 merged cells (ranging from 103,088 to 229,058 cells), whereas cytometric profiles related to HIV patients were composed of 127,446 merged cells (ranging from 67,280 to 211,223 cells). Among the three cytometric profiles to combine for each individual, more of 97% of cells included in cytometric profiles having the lowest number of cells

TABLE 3 | Number of events and cells obtained, before and after cell merging, for samples used to characterize specific cell populations from healthy subjects and HIV-infected patients.

Sample ID	Stimulation	Profile	Number of events	Number of cells	Number of excluded cells
HEA-1	CTRL	#A	443,527	237,039	-
HEA-1	CTRL	#B	321,545	192,201	-
HEA-1	CTRL	#C	245,550	139,218	-
HEA-1	CTRL	#A+B+C	-	139,104	151,146
HEA-2	CTRL	#A	464,263	249,773	
HEA-2	CTRL	#B	463,584	249,003	-
HEA-2	CTRL	#C	413,188	229,388	-
HEA-2	CTRL	#A+B+C	-	229,058	40,990
HEA-3	CTRL	#A	304,750	128,604	-
HEA-3	CTRL	#B	243,011	112,246	-
HEA-3	CTRL	#C	219,468	103,360	-
HEA-3	CTRL	#A+B+C	-	103,088	34,946
PAT-1	CTRL	#A	395,659	221,756	-
PAT-1	CTRL	#B	275,968	162,754	-
PAT-1	CTRL	#C	177,213	104,389	-
PAT-1	CTRL	#A+B+C	-	103,834	177,397
PAT-2	CTRL	#A	424,726	254,188	-
PAT-2	CTRL	#B	380,247	229,615	-
PAT-2	CTRL	#C	333,418	211,915	-
PAT-2	CTRL	#A+B+C	-	211,223	62,049
PAT-3	CTRL	#A	132,587	77,907	-
PAT-3	CTRL	#B	108,431	68,757	
PAT-3	CTRL	#C	110,803	68,749	-
PAT-3	CTRL	#A+B+C	-	67,280	13,573

The number of cells obtained for each profile before and after cells merging was indicated. The profile #A+B+C represents the combined cytometric profiles obtained by the merging of profiles #A, #B, and #C. For each combined profile, the number of cells excluded during the merging was indicated. Samples with names starting with HEA correspond to healthy subjects, and samples with names starting with PAT correspond to HIV-infected patients.

have were merged. Thus, the processes of merging were thus efficient.

HIV-Infection Induces Deep Phenotypic Modifications in Leukocytes

The SPADE algorithm was then used to identify 500 cell populations in the whole dataset of the six merged cytometric profiles. The 72 markers were used as clustering markers to capture the maximal cell diversity (**Supplementary Figure 2A**). For each cluster, the expression of CD3, CD11c, CD14, CD16, CD19, CD64, CD66, CD123, Granzyme B, and HLADR was represented (**Supplementary Figure 2B**).

We then generated a categorical heatmap representing the relative marker expression for each cluster to interpret the cell-cluster phenotypes (**Figure 1**). T cell, B cell, PMN, NK cell, monocyte, and dendritic cell clusters were directly annotated on the heatmap according to the expression of CD3, CD11c, CD14, CD16, CD19, CD66, CD123, Granzyme B, and HLADR (**Figure 1A**). Clusters annotated as unassigned in the heatmap correspond to cell clusters having <50 cells from the whole dataset. In these situations, the number of associated cells is not enough to properly define an MSI for each marker and to associate a population to these cell clusters. The PMN population had the highest diversity and represented more than 50% of the cell clusters. In contrast, the pDC population represented only 0.4% of the cell clusters.

The 500 identified clusters were classified into two categories according to their cell abundance. The first category, named Enrichment Trend Clusters (ETCs), corresponded to clusters for which the cell abundance was specific to either HIV patients or healthy donors (cell abundance fold-change >4). The second category corresponded to other cell clusters (clusters without a specific enrichment trend). The trends of cell-cluster abundance are displayed at the bottom of the heatmap (**Figure 1B**). The sum of the associated cells from HIV-infected patients or healthy donors is also indicated for each cluster (**Figure 1C**).

The localization of the ETCs in the heatmap revealed groups of T cell, B cell, PMN, NK cell, and monocyte clusters that were homogeneously enriched either in HIV-infected patients or healthy donors. ETCs specific to the HIV condition were almost exclusively composed of cells from HIV-infected patients, whereas the number of cells from healthy subjects was negligible. Inversely, the enriched clusters for the healthy (HEA) condition were almost exclusively composed of cells from healthy donors,

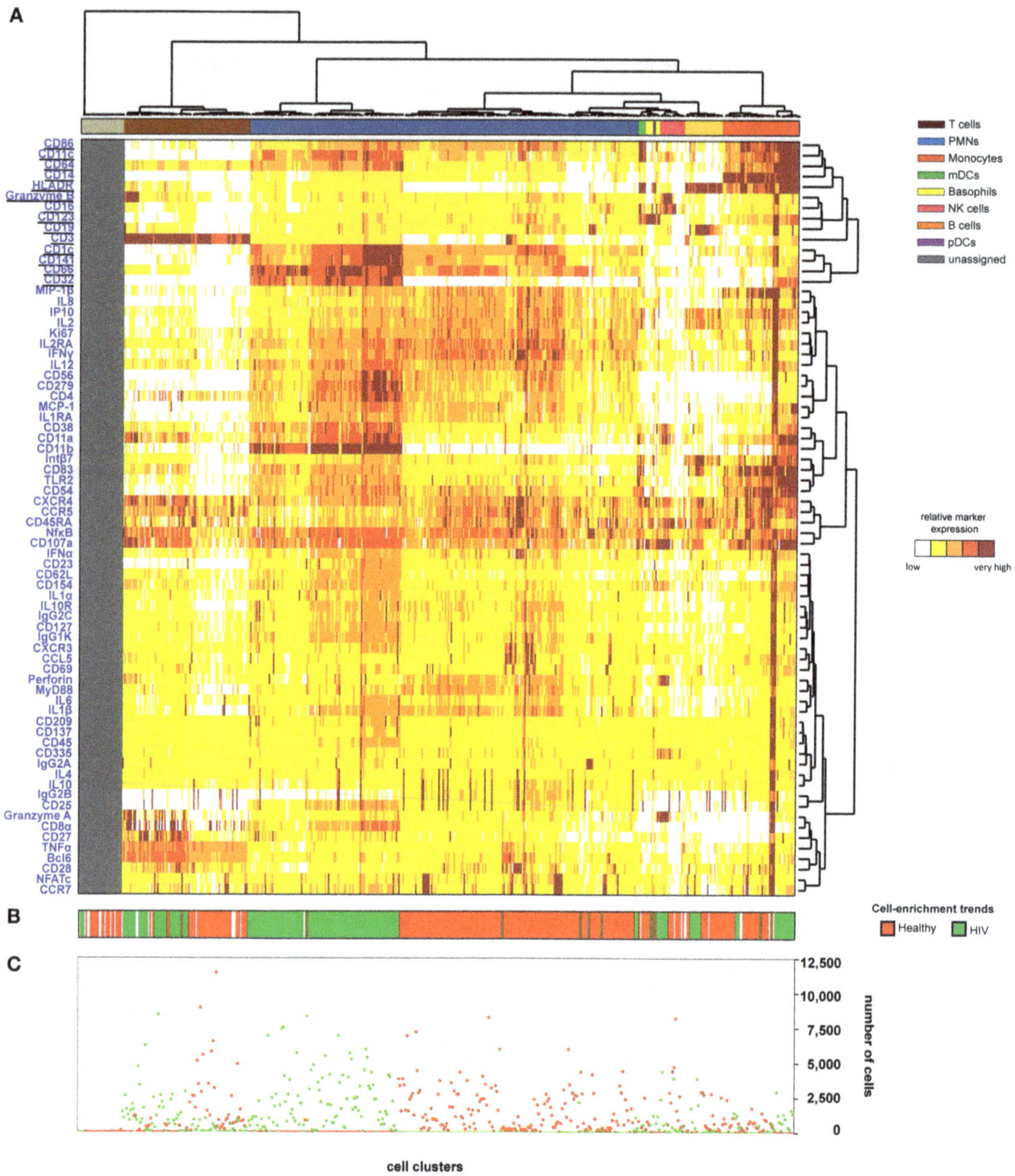

FIGURE 1 | Heatmap representing immune cells from healthy and HIV-infected individuals. Whole blood was collected from three non-viremic HIV-infected patients and three healthy subjects. Following red blood cell lysis, leukocytes of each sample were stained using three mass cytometry panels consisting of 35, 32, and 33 markers. Fourteen markers were shared between the three panels. CytoBackBone was used to generate a merged cytometric profile at the cellular level for each of the six individuals. SPADE analysis was performed to identify 500 cell clusters. The SPADE clustering was generated based on the expression levels of the whole set of 72 cell markers. **(A)** A categorical heatmap representing the relative marker expression for each cluster was generated. Marker expression ranges were calculated based on the 5 and 95th percentile of marker expression. Then, each range was divided into five uniform categories. The categorization of marker expression was computed based on the means of the individual SPADE expression medians of each marker. The categories represent negative, low, medium, high, and bright relative marker expression using a color scale from white to dark red. Hierarchical clustering was performed to visualize clusters with similar expression patterns. Two additional hierarchical clusterings were performed to visualize markers with similar expression patterns: one for common markers and one for non-common markers. Underlined markers correspond to the backbone markers (i.e., markers present in all cytometric panels). Cell clusters were manually annotated on the heatmap. Colors correspond to cell populations. **(B)** The cell-enrichment trend, toward HIV or healthy profiles, is indicated for each cluster. **(C)** The sum of the cells for all individuals and each condition is indicated for each cluster.

whereas the number of cells from HIV-infected patients was negligible. We identified two pDC clusters: one enriched in the HEA condition, and another in the HIV condition. We compared the phenotypes of CD4 T cells, CD8 T cells, B cells, PMNs, NK cells, monocytes, and pDCs of HIV-infected patients and healthy donors using this heatmap representing

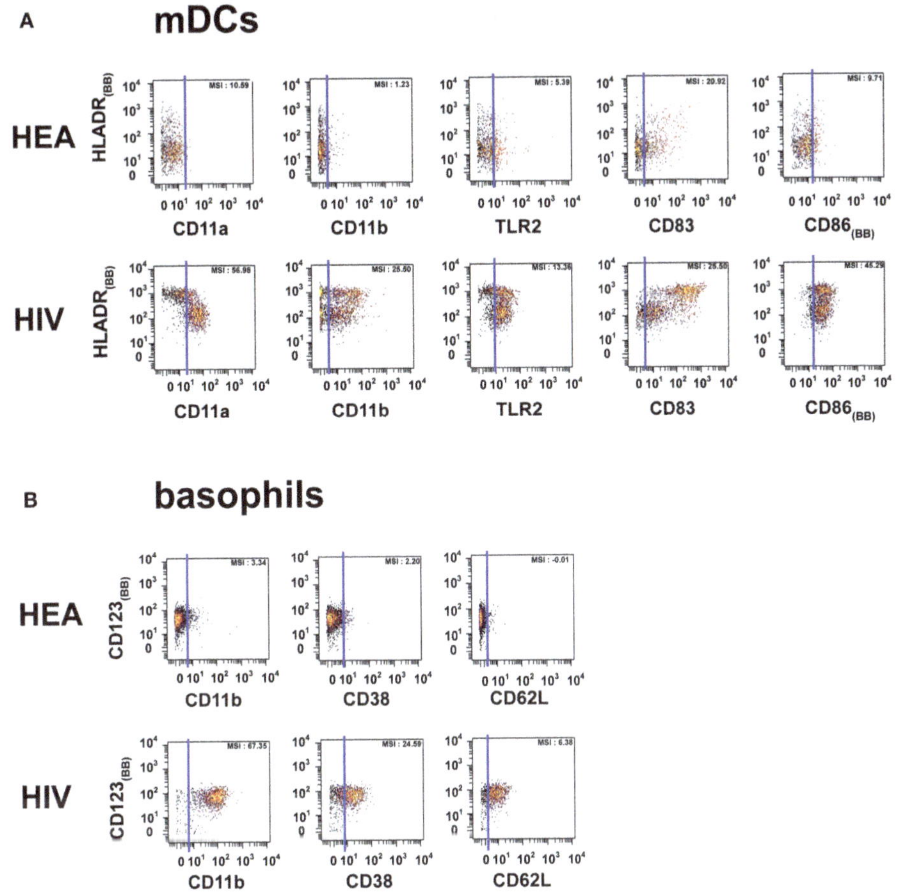

FIGURE 2 | Dot plots representing the phenotypes of mDCs and basophils from HIV-infected patients and healthy donors. Cell clusters corresponding to mDCs were isolated based on the same SPADE analysis presented in **Figure 1**. The same approach was used to isolate basophils. **(A)** Biplot representations showing the co-expression of HLADR and either CD11a, CD11b, CD83, CD86, or TLR2 by mDC populations. **(B)** Biplot representations showing the co-expression of CD123 and either CD11b, CD38, or CD62L by basophil populations. Blue lines were added to better visualize the difference in marker expression between healthy donors and HIV-infected patients. MSI represents the mean (MSI) of the markers in the X axes. "BB" in subscript indicates backbone markers.

the level of 72 cell markers. No specific groups of basophils or mDCs were associated with a specific individual group. The cell clusters of these populations were thus annotated on the SPADE tree and the cells directly analyzed using biplot representations (**Figures 2A,B**). The CytoBackBone algorithm enabled to observe with a high level of detail differences in the levels of several cell markers. The results and statistical analyses performed here are summarized in **Supplementary Table 1**.

Most CD8 T cells from healthy subjects were CXCR4^{mid}, CD11a^{low}, CD11b^{neg}, CD27^{low}, CD38^{neg}, CD83^{neg}, Granzyme A^{neg}, and Granzyme B$^{neg/low}$. In contrast, CD8 T cells from HIV-infected patients were CXCR4^{high}, CD11a^{high}, CD11b^{mid}, CD27^{mid}, CD38^{mid}, CD83^{mid}, Granzyme A^{high}, and Granzyme B^{high} or CXCR4^{high}, CD11a^{mid}, CD11b^{mid}, CD27^{high}, CD38^{mid}, CD83^{mid}, Granzyme A^{mid}, and Granzyme B^{mid}. Although low in abundance, we observed a CD32^{+} subpopulation in HIV-infected patients. Additionally, CD8 T cells from HIV-infected and healthy individuals were mainly CCR7^{neg}, although a set was CCR7^{high} in healthy subjects.

CD4 T cells from healthy subjects were CD11a^{low}, CD27^{low}, CD38^{neg}, CD83^{neg}, and Granzyme B$^{neg/low}$. In contrast, CD4 T cells from HIV-infected patients were CD11a^{mid}, CD27^{mid}, CD38^{mid}, CD83^{mid}, and Granzyme B^{mid}. Although low in abundance, we observed a CD32^{+} subpopulation in HIV-infected patients.

B cells from HIV-infected patients had higher expression of CXCR4, HLADR, CD38, and CD83 than healthy subjects. Indeed, B cells from HIV-infected patients were CXCR4^{high}, HLADR^{bright}, CD38^{mid}, and CD83^{high}, whereas B cells from healthy individuals were CXCR4^{mid}, HLADR$^{mid/high}$, CD38^{neg}, and CD83^{neg}.

NK cells from healthy donors were CXCR4^{mid}, CD11a^{low}, CD11b^{neg}, CD38^{neg}, Granzyme A^{neg}, Granzyme B^{neg}, and Perforin^{neg}, whereas they were CXCR4^{high}, CD11a^{high}, CD11b^{mid}, CD38^{high}, Granzyme A^{high}, Granzyme B^{high}, and Perforin^{high} in HIV-infected patients.

PMNs from HIV-infected patients were CD11a^{high}, CD11b^{high}, CD32^{high}, CD38^{high}, CD64^{high}, and TLR2^{mid}.

However, PMNs from healthy donors were CD11a^{low}, CD11b^{low}, CD32^{neg}, CD38^{neg}, CD64^{neg}, and TLR2^{low}. PMNs from healthy donors also exhibited a set of CCR7^{high} clusters. Basophils from HIV patients were CD11b^{high}, CD38^{mid}, CD62L^{high}, whereas they were CD11b^{neg}, CD38^{neg}, and CD62L^{neg} in healthy donors.

Monocytes from healthy donors were CD11a^{mid}, CD11b^{neg}, CD11c^{mid}, CD32^{neg}, CD38^{neg}, TLR2^{mid}, and MCP1^{neg}, whereas they were CD11a^{high}, CD11b^{high}, CD11c^{high}, CD32^{high}, CD38^{high}, TLR2^{high}, and MCP1$^{mid/high}$ in HIV-infected patients. Although CD64, CD83, CD86, and HLADR were highly expressed by both HIV-infected patients and healthy donors, their levels were higher in HIV-infected patients.

The mDC population can be split into two parts based on the expression of HLADR. However, the modifications of protein expression levels in HIV-infected patients were similar for the two mDC populations. mDCs from HIV-infected patients were CD11a^{mid}, CD11b^{mid}, CD83^{bright}, CD86^{bright}, TLR2^{high}, and HLADR^{bright}, whereas those from healthy donors were CD11a^{low}, CD11b^{neg}, CD83^{mid}, CD86^{mid}, TLR2^{mid}, and HLADR^{high}.

pDCs from HIV-infected patients were CD11b^{mid} and Granzyme B^{mid}, unlike pDCs from healthy donors which were CD11b^{neg} and Granzyme B^{neg}. Although HLADR was highly expressed in both HIV-infected patients and healthy donors, its level was higher in HIV-infected individuals.

Here, we have described HIV infection-dependent phenotypic changes in T cells, B cells, NK cells, PMNs, monocytes, dendritic cells, and basophils. Overall, the monocyte and PMN populations appeared to be the cell populations most highly affected by HIV infection.

Confirmation of HIV Infection-Dependent Phenotypic Changes Observed in Monocytes

We next intended to confirm several phenotypic changes obtained with the combined cytometry profiles of 72 markers. To do so, we designed a single mass cytometry panel of 25 cell markers targeting the monocyte population, which was used to stain six new healthy donors (named HEA-4 to HEA-9), three previously used HIV-ART patients (named PAT-1 to PAT-3) and three new HIV-ART patients (named PAT-4 to PAT-6).

The monocyte population was used for validation based on two main reasons. First, monocytes were the most impacted population by HIV and were thus of strong relevance in term of disease characterization. Second, we previously predicted the upregulation of CD11b, CD32, CD64, CD83, CD86, and TLR2 in monocytes from HIV-infected patients. However, these markers were located on different panels. CD32, CD64, and CD86 were present in the backbone, whereas TLR2 was present in panel #A, CD11b in panel #B, and CD83 in panel #C (**Table 2**). Therefore, the monocyte population represented a good opportunity to validate our results, as these cells expressed these six markers. Thus, we created a single mass cytometry panel of 25 markers that contained these six specific markers (**Supplementary Table 2**).

Leukocytes from the original three HIV-infected patients (named PAT-1 to PAT-3), three new HIV-infected patients (named PAT-4 to PAT-6), and six new healthy donors (named HEA-4 to HEA-9) (**Table 1**) were stained using this panel (**Supplementary Table 2**). After the acquisition of the whole dataset, SPADE analysis was performed. The SPADE analysis was parameterized to obtain 100 clusters using 5% down-sampling, and the clustering based on the levels of CD1c, CD3, CD4, CD8, CD11c, CD14, CD16, CD19, CD32, CD64, CD66, CD86, CD123, CD141, HLADR, and Granzyme B. Then, we annotated the SPADE cell clusters based on the levels of HLADR, CD3, CD11c, CD14, CD16, CD19, CD64, CD66, and CD123. Thereafter, monocytes were computationally isolated. Finally, we visualized the upregulation and co-expression of CD11b, CD32, CD64, CD83, CD86, and TLR2 on monocytes by performing a viSNE analysis (24).

The viSNE visualization, based on the expression of CD11b, CD32, CD64, CD83, CD86, and TLR2, allowed the perfect separation of monocytes from healthy and HIV-infected individuals (**Figure 3A**). This result demonstrates that the phenotype of monocytes from healthy donors was different from that from HIV-infected individuals. The use of statistical comparisons based on permutation tests allowed us to show that monocytes from HIV-infected patients significantly upregulated (MSI) CD11b ($p = 0.0011$), CD32 ($p \leq 0.0001$), CD64 ($p = 0.0028$), CD83 ($p = 0.0016$), CD86 ($p = 0.0410$), and TLR2 ($p = 0.0008$) (**Figure 3B**). In addition, the viSNE visualization allowed us to show that most monocytes from HIV-infected patients were CD11b^{high}, CD32^{high}, CD64^{bright}, CD83^{bright}, CD86^{bright}, and TLR2^{high}. However, there was a subpopulation of monocytes with a CD64^{bright} and TLR2^{neg} phenotype.

Results from the validation experiment were compared to those obtained from the combined mass cytometry profiles using classical dot plots (**Figures 4A,B**). We observed the same trends of co-expression but no statistical analyses were performed, as these two sets of data were obtained using different panels and were unbalanced in terms of the number of samples.

DISCUSSION

So far, multi-tube cytometry approaches have not been used in the context of chronic inflammation characterization. In addition to the technical difficulties to perform these experiments using mass cytometry panels, the analysis of such complex data requires further bioinformatics approaches. Here, we addressed these analysis challenges using the SPADE and SPADEVizR pipelines. Even if this study is based on a restricted number of samples from HIV-infected patients, the methodology that we describe here demonstrates that multi-tube cytometry can be applied for characterizing complex diseases.

Here, we characterized the HIV inflammation at an unprocessed phenotypical resolution of 72 cell marker. We detected the upregulation of several proteins in HIV-infected patients. Among them, CD11a and CD11b were upregulated in PMNs, monocytes, mDCs, NK cells, and T cells. CD11b was also upregulated on pDCs. Other upregulated proteins included: CD38 on PMNs, monocytes, NK cells, basophils, B cells, and T cells; CD83 on monocytes, mDCs, B cells, and T cells; and TLR2,

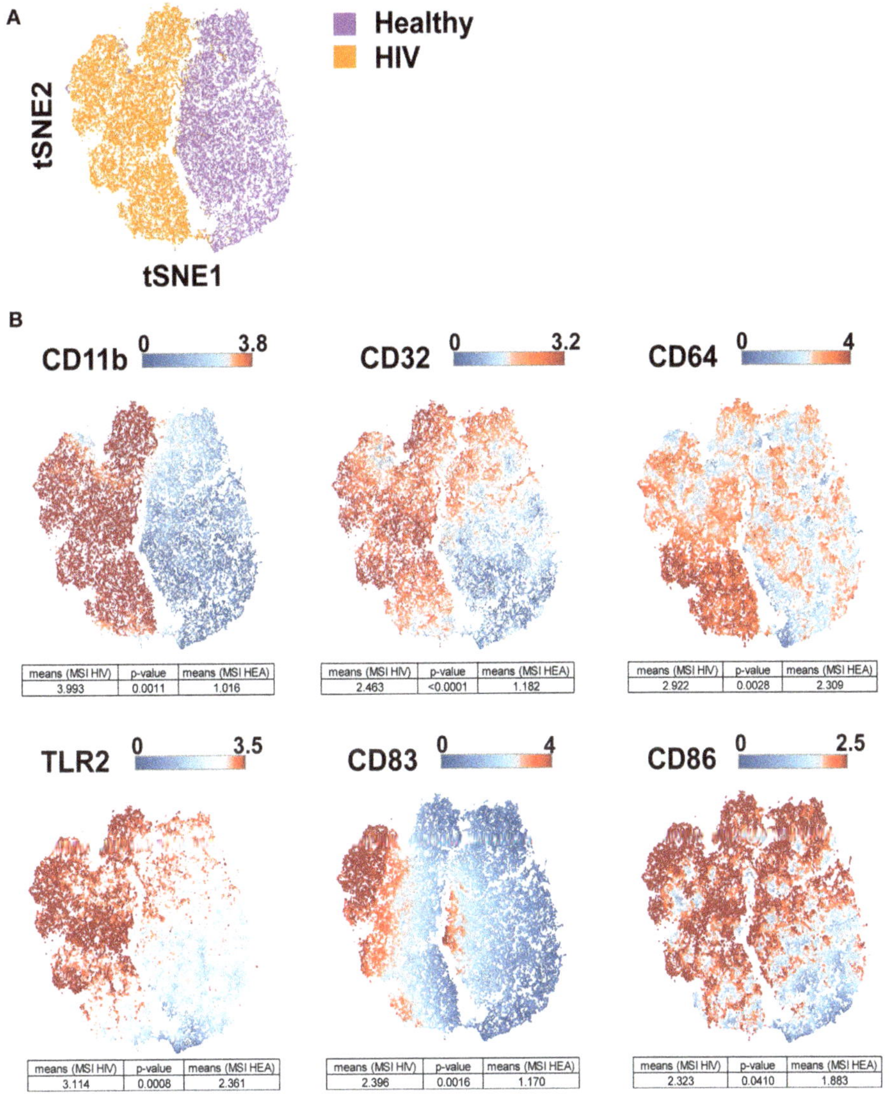

FIGURE 3 | viSNE map representing the phenotype of leukocytes from HIV-infected patients and healthy donors using a single antibody panel. Leukocytes from the three original HIV-infected subjects, three new HIV-infected patients, and six new healthy subjects were collected. SPADE analysis was performed to isolate monocytes. Monocyte cells were computationaly distributed into a two-dimensional space using the viSNE algorithm. Such viSNE representations were generated based on the expressions of CD11b, CD32, CD64, CD83, CD86, and TLR2. **(A)** The viSNE map is colored to represent cells from HIV-infected patients in orange and those from healthy individuals in purple. **(B)** The viSNE map is colored to represent the mean marker expression (MSI) of CD11b, CD32, CD64, CD83, CD86, and TLR2 for each cell. Comparisons of the MSIs from the individual groups were performed using non-parametric permutation tests.

CD32, and CD64 on PMNs and monocytes. The monocyte and PMN population appeared to be strongly affected by the HIV infection, as CD11a, CD11b, CD32, CD38, CD64, CD83, CD86, and TLR2 were upregulated in these populations. Overall, these results show that HIV infection induced a specific environment that similarly affected various immune cells in these patients.

Following the detection of Pathogen Associated Molecular Patterns (PAMP) in tissues by cell populations expressing pattern recognition receptors (PRRs), different cytokines and chemokines are produced. The release of these inflammatory proteins leads to the recruitment of innate immune cells, such as neutrophils, monocytes, dendritic cells, and NK cells (25, 26). Whereas, IL-8 and MIP-1β upregulate expression level of adhesion molecules on innate immune cells, cytokines such as IL-1α, IL-6, and TNF-α upregulate the expression levels of selectin molecules on endothelial cells. Interactions between adhesion molecules and selectin molecules trigger the diapedesis mechanism (27–29). In our study, we found that the HIV infection induced an overexpression of adhesion molecules CD11a or CD11b on the surface of neutrophils, monocytes, and dendritic cells. An overexpression of CD11a in NK cells was also detected. Thus, these results suggest that immune cells could be more easily recruited on inflammatory sites.

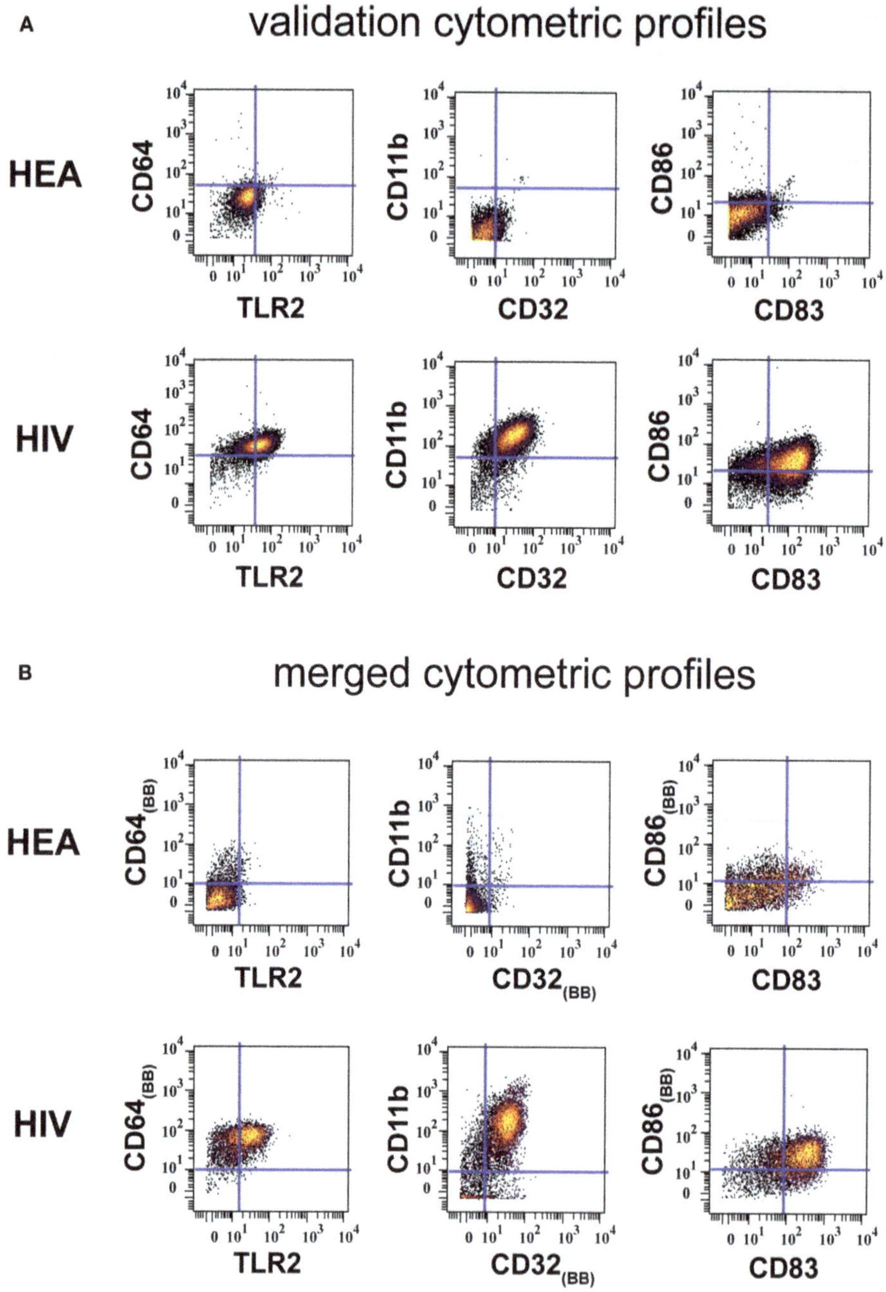

FIGURE 4 | Confirmation of results generated by CytoBackBone. **(A)** Leukocytes were collected from HIV-infected patients and healthy subjects. Cells were stained with a single antibody panel and SPADE analysis was performed to isolate monocytes. The biplot representations show the co-expression of CD64 and TLR2, CD11b and CD32, and CD86 and CD83 in monocytes from patient PAT-1. **(B)** Leukocytes were collected from HIV-infected patients and healthy subjects. Cells were stained with three different antibody panels. Then, CytoBacBone was used to merge the different cytometry profiles. SPADE analysis was then performed to isolate monocytes. The biplot representations show the co-expression of CD64 and TLR2, CD11b and CD32, and CD86 and CD83 in monocytes from patient PAT-1.

The HIV infection induces an exhaustion of different innate immune cells, such as neutrophils, monocytes, and dendritic cells. Indeed, we demonstrated that the production of IL-1α, IL-6, and TNF-α were delayed following different TLR stimulations in HIV-infected patients (15). These proteins are essential for the induction of selectin molecules on the surface of endothelial cells. Without these cytokines, leukocytes expressing high levels of CD11a and CD11b cannot adhere to endothelial cells (27–29), which greatly limits the recruitment of immune cells to inflammatory sites.

Innate immunity is strongly activated in primary infection as depicted by the cytokine storm present in the first weeks of HIV infection (30). Numerous types of immune cells are involved in the acute inflammation seen in primary infection.

Additionally, these cells are involved in the persistence of the chronic inflammation observed in treated HIV-infected patients. Moreover, a low neutrophil count is associated with the disease progression, a $CD4^+$ T cells loss, and a high HIV viral load (31).

Neutrophils contribute to an anti-HIV response through the production of α-defensins, myeloperoxidase, and reactive oxygen species. Neutrophils also participate in the elimination of HIV-infected cells using antibody-dependent cell-mediated cytotoxic processes (ADCC) but are less effective than monocytes and NK cells. Finally, neutrophils and monocytes can perform antibody-dependent cellular phagocytosis of infected cells and immune complexes (32). Thus, phenotype impairment related to PMN and monocytes could be severely harmful. In our study, we observed strong upregulations of CD32 and CD64 on PMN and monocyte populations. CD32 and CD64 are two Fc receptors playing a major role in antibody-mediated processes such as phagocytosis. As phagocytosis is known to be affected by the HIV infection (33, 34), upregulation of these proteins could compensate for this impairment.

CD32 and CD64 also mediate ADCC, which is important in the response against HIV. ADCC is mostly performed by NK cells, but we did not observe an upregulation of Fc receptors on this population. However, monocytes and PMNs also carry out ADCC (35–37). The upregulation of CD32 and CD64 could suggest an increase of ADCC by these cells. Additionally, the increase of expression level of Fc receptors could facilitate the development and maintenance of chronic inflammation. Indeed, the engagement of these receptors leads to the production of cytokines, chemokines, and inflammatory mediators. Consequently, due to the increased expression of these Fc-receptors, associated signaling pathways are probably more expressed. Therefore, this increased expression would result in a greater release of inflammatory molecules, which would promote the maintenance of chronic inflammation.

We also detected an overexpression of MCP-1 on monocytes. MCP-1 is a chemokine that attracts monocytes, lymphocytes, and polymorphonuclear cells. The HIV-NEF protein is known to upregulate the expression of MCP-1 in astrocytes, the most abundant cell type in the brain (38). The detection of MCP-1 on monocytes can be explained by the fact that MCP-1 binds to the CCR2 receptor expressed on monocytes. This could lead to the recruitment of monocytes to the brain through the blood-brain barrier, which could subsequently enhance both the generation of the viral reservoir and neurological complications (39).

Alterations in cytokine expression profiles have reported in treated and non-treated HIV-infected individuals. Here, several cytokines were included in our antibody panels, such as IL-1α, IL-1β, IL-1RA, IL2, IL4, IL6, IL8, IL10, IL12, IP-10, IFN-α, IFN-γ, MIP-1β, TNF-α, and MCP-1. Except for MCP-1, no signal of these cytokines was detected in the different leukocyte populations. This no detection of cytokines is explained by the fact that leukocytes were not stimulated by ligands such as LPS or R848. Without such stimulation, the expression level of cytokines inside leukocytes is too low to be detected.

In our study, no non-classical monocytes ($CD14^{low}$ and $CD16^{high}$) were found in treated HIV-infected patients, neither before nor after the cell merging process. Indeed, all monocytes identified in this study were $CD14^{high}$ and $CD16^{neg/low}$. However, we found that all monocytes up-regulated the expression of CD11a, CD11b, CD11c, CD32, CD38, TLR2, and MCP-1. Thus, these results suggested that both classical and non-classical monocytes were impacted.

Classical myeloid dendritic cells from HIV-infected patients exhibit altered functions including a weak capacity of maturation and inefficient antigen presentation to $CD4^+$ T cells (40). Here, we observed a strong up-regulation of CD86 on monocyte and mDC populations, which is a protein essential for antigen presentation. The upregulation of this molecule on mDCs could compensate the dysregulations related to antigen presentation.

Furthermore, we found that the expression of CD83 was higher on monocytes and mDCs from HIV-infected patients compared to healthy subjects. CD83 is a costimulatory molecule and is upregulated after cell activation (41) and maturation (42). CD83-stimulated monocytes suppress T cell immune responses through the production of prostaglandin E2 (43). Upregulation of CD83 also highlights chronic activation of the immune system in ART-treated HIV-infected patients (42).

As pDCs are among the main cells producing IFN-I, they play a main role in the antiviral responses. In HIV-infected patients, the number of pDCs is known to be decreased compared to healthy patients (44). Moreover, the production of cytokines is also impacted by the infection, even in treated HIV-infected subjects (15). In our study, pDCs displayed a hyperactivation phenotype through an up-regulation of CD11b. Thus, we can suppose that pDCs chronically produce IFN-α, which can participate in the increase of myeloid-derived suppressor cells (MDSCs) counts.

Higher transcription of genes encoding TLR2, TLR3, TLR4, TLR6, TLR7, and TLR8 has been described in PBMCs from HIV infected individuals (45, 46). Here, we observed an overexpression of TLR2 in monocytes and PMNs from treated HIV-infected patients. As HIV is able to inhibit signaling pathways induced following the TLRs engagement, the upregulation of these receptors could compensate these inhibitions. In addition, the overexpression of TLRs could have a deleterious effect on the spread of HIV. Indeed, HIV is able to use TLR-dependent signaling pathways to facilitate its replication and propagation (47, 48). Importantly, as the microbial translocation is favored in HIV-infected patients, the multiplication of TLR2 activation could participate in the disease progression. Indeed, commensal bacteria (such as *Lactobacillus acidophilus, Prevotella melaninogenica, Prevotella bivia, and Mycobacterium smegmatis*) enhance the spread of HIV by activating TLR2-dependent signaling (49). Finally, the TLR2 activation is also associated with reactivation of latent viruses (50).

NK cells are critical antiviral effectors of the innate immune system, and deficiencies of this cell population are associated with an increased probability of HIV infection (51, 52). NK cells contribute to the elimination of HIV-infected cells during the acute phase. Indeed, NK cells can release cytotoxic granules, cytokines, and chemokines through the activation of the KIR receptors, the natural cytotoxicity receptors, the C-type lectin receptors, signaling lymphocyte activation family receptors, and Fc receptors.

Although the ADCC is mostly performed by NK cells (51, 52), monocytes and PMNs are also able to do it. Here, we did not observe upregulations of CD32 and CD64 in NK cells from HIV-infected individuals, unlike in monocytes and PMNs. Thus, the capacity of monocytes and PMNs to perform ADCC could be increased in HIV-infected patients.

Here, alterations observed in NK cells from HIV-infected patients characterize a hyperactivation state, which leads to the persistence of chronic inflammation. This inflammation leads to alterations of the NK cells distribution and their functional capacities. Moreover, the chronic inflammation enhances the generation of anergic NK cells, reduces the ADCC activity, and contributes to a poor immunologic reconstitution of CD4 T cells in HIV-infected individuals (53). Finally, we showed that NK cells overexpressed CD38, which is related to progression to AIDS (54).

CD27 is a protein constitutively expressed by naive T cells. This protein plays a main role in proliferation, survival, and differentiation of T cells. Especially, CD27 promotes immune activation and enhances primary, secondary, memory, and recall responses toward viral infections (55). Following the activation of CD4 or CD8 T cells via the TCR/CD3 pathway, the expression of CD27 is increased in T cells. However, after prolonged activation, CD27 becomes gradually switched off (56). Therefore, a high level of CD27 on T cells is often considered as a marker of early activation. Herein, we demonstrated that the expressions of CD27 on CD4 and CD8 T cells were higher in HIV-1 donors compared to healthy donors. These results again describe a persistence of inflammation in HIV-infected patients, which could be associated either to the residual replication HIV or to HIV-dependent inflammatory mechanisms (such as higher microbial translocation). CD27 also plays a key role in the generation and long-term maintenance of T cell responses. The long-term expression of CD27 is associated with impaired maturation of T cells (55). Finally, as the constitutive engagement of CD27/CD70 promotes T cell exhaustion, high levels of CD27 observed in HIV patients could contribute to the loss of T cells effector functions (57).

We found that the expression of CD83 on T cells and B cells from HIV-infected patients was also upregulated compared to healthy donors. The expression of CD83 on $CD4^+/CD25^+$ T cells confers immunosuppressive functions (58), whereas the upregulation of CD83 on murine B cells has a regulatory role in humoral responses (59). Finally, an up-regulation of CD38 was observed on T cells and B cells from HIV-ART patients relative to control individuals, which is associated with HIV disease progression (54). Together, these results support that chronic inflammation could induce important dysfunctions in adaptive immune responses.

NK cells and CD8 T cells naturally express high levels of Granzymes or Perforin. High expressions of Granzyme B and Perforin in CD8 T cells and NK cells are a signature of immune activation, which could be associated here to the persistence of HIV. Indeed, HIV replication is known to induce the production of these cytotoxic proteins in these two cell populations. Importantly, an increase in the number of T cells secreting Granzyme B is associated with reduced viral reservoirs in HIV infection. Thus, HIV infection could limit the secretion of Granzymes and Perforin, and could lead to an accumulation of granules in NK or CD8 T cells. Therefore, the accumulation of granules could lead to the loss of cytolytic activity for NK and CD8 T cells. Finally, the high level of granzymes or perforin observed in HIV-infected patients could be associated with Cytomegalovirus (CMV). Indeed, nearly 90% of HIV-infected patients are CMV positive contrasting with about 60% in healthy donors.

Because HIV-1 infected patients were ART-treated, we suppose that the replication of HIV is not involved in the reported alterations. However, the virus could still play a role, as increasing pieces of evidence point to the persistence of HIV in tissues despite undetectable viral load in plasma (60, 61). Here, we suppose that the phenotypical modifications observed in treated HIV-infected patients are linked to the persistence of inflammation. Indeed, chronic inflammation is associated with a hyperactivation and exhaustion of innate immune cells. This inflammation could be induced by a residual replication of HIV, the presence of HIV in reservoir cells, and an increasing microbial translocation.

Although our combined cytometry panel is composed of 72 cells markers, several important markers for phenotypical annotation of cell subsets are unfortunately absent. Indeed, markers such as CD10, CXCL13, CD278 (follicular T cells), NKG2A, NKp44 (NK cells), T-bet, GATA, RORγt, IL-17 (ILC), or FoxP3 (T regs) were not included in our antibodies panels. Thus, further research must be conducted to extend this approach to characterize all cutting-edge subpopulations involved in HIV.

In the viSNE analysis, monocytes were partly $CD64^{bright}$ and $TLR2^{neg}$ in the single-tube experiment. However, we did not observe this result in the heatmap from the multi-tube 72-marker experiment. The multi-tube 72-marker experiment was performed with three HIV-ART patients (named PAT-1 to PAT-3), whereas the single-tube experiment was performed with six HIV-ART patients (including PAT-1 to PAT-3, but also PAT-4 to PAT-6). After deeper analysis, we found this $CD64^{bright}$ and $TLR2^{neg}$ monocyte population to be detectable in patients PAT-2, PAT-4, PAT-5, and PAT-6. Thus, it was normal to not observe this population on the 72 cell-marker heatmap, as monocytes from patients PAT-1 to PAT-3 were mostly $CD64^{bright}$ and $TLR2^{high}$.

Overall, these analyses lead to the same conclusions: the effect of HIV infection on most innate and adaptive immune cell types are still largely present in the six HIV-infected patients, with a prolonged undetectable viral load and, for most, CD4 T cell counts $>500/mm^3$. These results are in agreement with several publications showing persistent chronic immune activation in patients on prolonged ART for whom increased levels of soluble biomarkers (such as sCD14 and IP10) were detected (62, 63).

ETHICS STATEMENT

This experiment was approved by the Comité de Protection des Personnes (CPP) Ile de France VII, under protocol number PP 14-003. All subjects gave written informed consent to participate in this study.

AUTHOR CONTRIBUTIONS

AL, NT, and AC: conceptualization and methodology, investigation. AL, NT, AC, RL, and OL: validation and writing—review and editing. AL and NT: formal analysis and writing—original draft. AL and OL: resources. AC and RL: funding acquisition. AC, RL, and OL: supervision.

ACKNOWLEDGMENTS

We warmly thank the HIV-infected patients and healthy donors. We are grateful to the physicians at the hospitals.

REFERENCES

1. Bendall SC, Nolan GP, Roederer M, Chattopadhyay PK. A deep profiler's guide to cytometry. *Trends Immunol.* (2012) 33:323–32. doi: 10.1016/j.it.2012.02.010
2. O'Neill K, Aghaeepour N, Parker J, Hogge D, Karsan A, Dalal B, Brinkman RR. Deep profiling of multitube flow cytometry data. *Bioinformatics.* (2015) 31:1623–31. doi: 10.1093/bioinformatics/btv008
3. Pedreira CE, Costa ES, Barrena S, Lecrevisse Q, Almeida J, Van Dongen JJM, et al. Generation of flow cytometry data files with a potentially infinite number of dimensions. *Cytometry Part A.* (2008) 73:834–46. doi: 10.1002/cyto.a.20608
4. Lee G, Finn W, Scott C. Statistical file matching of flow cytometry data. *J Biomed Inform.* (2011) 44:663–76. doi: 10.1016/j.jbi.2011.03.004
5. Leite Pereira A, Lambotte O, Le Grand R, Cosma A, Tchitchek N. CytoBackBone: an algorithm for merging of phenotypic information from different cytometric profiles. *Bioinformatics.* (2019). doi: 10.1093/bioinformatics/btz212. [Epub ahead of print].
6. Berger EA, Murphy PM, Farber JM. Chemokine receptors as HIV-1 coreceptors: roles in viral entry, tropism, and disease. *Ann Rev Immunol.* (2002) 17:657–700. doi: 10.1146/annurev.immunol.17.1.657
7. Simon V, Ho D, Karim Q. HIV/AIDS epidemiology, pathogenesis, prevention and treatment. *Lancet.* (2010) 368:489–504. doi: 10.1016/S0140-6736(06)69157-5
8. Campbell JH, Hearps AC, Martin GE, Williams KC, Crowe SM. The importance of monocytes and macrophages in HIV pathogenesis,treatment,and cure. *AIDS.* (2014) 28:2175–87. doi: 10.1097/QAD.0000000000000408
9. Simmons RP, Scully EP, Groden EE, Arnold KB, Chang JJ, Lane K, et al. HIV-1 infection induces strong production of IP-10 through TLR7/9-dependent pathways. *AIDS.* (2013) 27:2505–17. doi: 10.1097/01.aids.0000432455.06476.bc
10. Dutertre CA, Amraoui S, DeRosa A, Jourdain JP, Vimeux L, Goguet M, et al. Pivotal role of M-DC8(+) monocytes from viremic HIV-infected patients in TNFalpha overproduction in response to microbial products. *Blood.* (2012) 120:2259–68. doi: 10.1182/blood-2012-03-418681
11. Guo H, Gao J, Taxman DJ, Ting JPY, Su L. HIV-1 infection induces interleukin-1β production via TLR8 protein-dependent and NLRP3 inflammasome mechanisms in human monocytes. *J Biol Chem.* (2014) 289:21716–26. doi: 10.1074/jbc.M114.566620
12. Boasso A, Hardy AW, Landay AL, Martinson JL, Anderson SA, Dolan MJ, et al. PDL-1 upregulation on monocytes and T cells by HIV via type I interferon: Restricted expression of type I interferon receptor by CCR5-expressing leukocytes. *Clin Immunol.* (2008) 129:132–44. doi: 10.1016/j.clim.2008.05.009
13. Morlat P, Roussillon C, Henard S, Salmon D, Bonnet F, Cacoub P, et al. Causes of death among HIV-infected patients in France in 2010 (national survey). *AIDS.* (2014) 28:1181–91. doi: 10.1097/QAD.0000000000000222
14. Brenchley JM, Price DA, Schacker TW, Asher TE, Silvestri G, Rao S, et al. Microbial translocation is a cause of systemic immune activation in chronic HIV infection. *Nat Med.* (2007) 12:1365–71. doi: 10.1038/nm1511
15. Leite Pereira A, Tchitchek N, Marcos Lopez E, Lambotte O, Le Grand R, Cosma A. A high-resolution mass cytometry analysis reveals a delay of cytokines production after TLR4 or TLR7/8 engagements in HIV-1 infected humans. *Cytokine.* (2018) 111:97–105. doi: 10.1016/j.cyto.2018.08.018
16. Velu V, Shetty RD, Larsson M, Shankar EM. Role of PD-1 co-inhibitory pathway in HIV infection and potential therapeutic options. *Retrovirology.* (2015) 12:1–17. doi: 10.1186/s12977-015-0144-x
17. Porichis F, Hart MG, Zupkosky J, Barblu L, Kwon DS, McMullen A, et al. Differential Impact of PD-1 and/or interleukin-10 blockade on HIV-1-specific CD4 T cell and antigen-presenting cell functions. *J Virol.* (2014) 88:2508–18. doi: 10.1128/JVI.02034-13
18. Trono D, Van Lint C, Rouzioux C, Verdin E, Barre-Sinoussi F, Chun T-W, et al. HIV Persistence and the prospect of long-term drug-free remissions for HIV-infected individuals. *Science.* (2010) 329:174–80. doi: 10.1126/science.1191047
19. Kuller LH, Tracy R, Belloso W, De Wit S, Drummond F, Lane HC, et al. Inflammatory and coagulation biomarkers and mortality in patients with HIV infection. *PLoS Med.* (2008) 5:1496–508. doi: 10.1371/journal.pmed.0050203
20. Rodger AJ, Fox Z, Lundgren JD, Kuller L, Boesecke C, Skoutelis A, et al. Activation and coagulation biomarkers are independent predictors of the development of opportunistic disease in patients with HIV infection. *J Infect Dis.* (2009) 200:973–83. doi: 10.1086/605447
21. Elhmouzi-Younes J, Palgen JL, Tchitchek N, Delandre S, Namet I, Bodinham CL, et al. In depth comparative phenotyping of blood innate myeloid leukocytes from healthy humans and macaques using mass cytometry. *Cytometry Part A.* (2017) 91:969–82. doi: 10.1002/cyto.a.23107
22. Rahman AH, Tordesillas L, Berin MC. Heparin reduces nonspecific eosinophil staining artifacts in mass cytometry experiments. *Cytometry Part A.* (2016) 89:601–7. doi: 10.1002/cyto.a.22826
23. Gautreau G, Pejoski D, Cosma A, Le Grand R, Beignon AS, Tchitchek N. SPADEVizR: an R package for visualization, analysis and integration of SPADE results. *Bioinformatics.* (2016) 33:779–81. doi: 10.1093/bioinformatics/btw708
24. Amir ED, Davis KL, Tadmor MD, Simonds EF, Jacob H. viSNE enables visualization of high dimensional single-cell data and reveals phenotypic heterogeneity of leukemia. *Nat Biotechnol.* (2014) 31:545–52. doi: 10.1038/nbt.2594
25. Kawai T, Akira S. The roles of TLRs, RLRs and NLRs in pathogen recognition. *Int Immunol.* (2009) 21:317–37. doi: 10.1093/intimm/dxp017
26. Uematsu S, Akira S. Toll-like receptors and innate immunity. *Adv Immunol.* (2006) 78:1–56. doi: 10.2222/jsv.56.1

27. Aziz KE, Wakefield D. Modulation of endothelial cell expression of ICAM-1, E-selectin, and VCAM-1 by beta-estradiol, progesterone, and dexamethasone. *Cell Immunol.* (1996) 167:79–85. doi: 10.1006/cimm.1996.0010
28. Zhang H, Park Y, Wu J, Chen X, Lee S, Yang J, Dellsperger KC, Zhang C. Role of TNF-alpha in vascular dysfunction. *Clin Sci.* (2009) 116:219–30. doi: 10.1042/CS20080196
29. Donati KDG, Rabagliati R, Iacoviello L, Cauda R. Review HIV infection, HAART, and endothelial adhesion molecules: current perspectives. *Lancet Infect Dis.* (2004) 4:213–22. doi: 10.1016/S1473-3099(04)00971-5
30. Stacey AR, Norris PJ, Qin L, Haygreen EA, Taylor E, Heitman J, et al. Induction of a striking systemic cytokine cascade prior to peak viremia in acute human immunodeficiency virus type 1 infection, in contrast to more modest and delayed responses in acute hepatitis B and C virus infections. *J Virol.* (2009) 83:3719–33. doi: 10.1128/JVI.01844-08
31. Shi X, Sims MD, Hanna MM, Xie M, Gulick PG, Zheng Y, Basson MD, et al. Neutropenia during HIV infection: adverse consequences and remedies. *Int Rev Immunol.* (2014) 33:511–36. doi: 10.3109/08830185.2014.893301
32. Hensley-McBain T, Klatt NR. The dual role of neutrophils in HIV infection. *Curr HIV/AIDS Rep.* (2018) 15:206–21. doi: 10.1007/s11904-018-0370-7
33. Mazzolini J, Herit F, Niedergang F. Inhibition of phagocytosis in HIV-1 – infected macrophages relies on Nef-dependent alteration of focal delivery of recycling compartments. *Blood.* (2017) 115:4226–37. doi: 10.1182/blood-2009-12-259473
34. Debaisieux S, Lachambre S, Gross A, Mettling C, Besteiro S, Yezid H, et al. HIV-1 Tat inhibits phagocytosis by preventing the recruitment of Cdc42 to the phagocytic cup. *Nat Commun.* (2015) 6:6211. doi: 10.1038/ncomms7211
35. Garagiola DM, Huard TK, Lobuglio AF. Comparison of monocyte and alveolar macrophage dependent cellular cytotoxicity and fc-receptor activity. *Cell Immunol.* (1981) 370:359–70. doi: 10.1016/0008-8749(81)90487-1
36. Yeap WH, Wong KL, Shimasaki N, Chi E, Teo Y. CD16 is indispensable for antibody- dependent cellular cytotoxicity by human monocytes. *Nat Publish Group.* (2016) 6:34310. doi: 10.1038/srep34310
37. Young NJ De, Gill PG. Monocyte antibody-dependent cellular cytotoxicity in cancer patients. *Cancer Immunol Immunother.* (1984) 18:54–8. doi: 10.1007/BF00205400
38. Lehmann MH, Masanetz S, Kramer S, Erfle V. HIV-1 Nef upregulates CCL2/MCP-1 expression in astrocytes in a myristoylation- and calmodulin-dependent manner. *J Cell Sci.* (2006) 119:4520–30. doi: 10.1242/jcs.03231
39. Marban C, Forouzanfar F, Ait-Ammar A, Fahmi F, El Mekdad H, Daouad F, et al. Targeting the brain reservoirs: Toward an HIV cure. *Front Immunol.* (2016) 7:00397. doi: 10.3389/fimmu.2016.00397
40. Miller E, Bhardwaj N, Sinai M. Dendritic cell dysregulation during HIV-1 infection. *Immunol Rev.* (2017) 254:170–89. doi: 10.1111/imr.12082
41. Aerts-Toegaert C, Heirman C, Tuyaerts S, Corthals J, Aerts JL, Bonehill A, et al. CD83 expression on dendritic cells and T cells: correlation with effective immune responses. *Eur J Immunol.* (2007) 37:686–95. doi: 10.1002/eji.200636535
42. Harman AN, Wilkinson J, Bye CR, Stern JL, Nicholle M, Lai J, et al. HIV Induces maturation of monocyte-derived dendritic cells and langerhans cells. *J Immunol.* (2006) 177:7103–113. doi: 10.4049/jimmunol.177.10.7103
43. Chen L, Zhu Y, Zhang G, Gao C, Zhong W, Zhang X. CD83-stimulated monocytes suppress T-cell immune responses through production of prostaglandin E2. *Proc Natl Acad Sci USA.* (2011) 108:18778–83. doi: 10.1073/pnas.1018994108
44. Barblu L, MacHmach K, Gras C, Delfraissy JF, Boufassa F, Leal M, et al. Plasmacytoid dendritic cells (pDCs) from HIV controllers produce interferon-and differentiate into functional killer pDCs under HIV activation. *J Infect Dis.* (2012) 206:790–801. doi: 10.1093/infdis/jis384
45. Hernández JC, Stevenson M, Latz E, Urcuqui-Inchima S. HIV type 1 infection up-regulates TLR2 and TLR4 expression and function *in vivo* and *in vitro. AIDS Res Hum Retroviruses.* (2012) 28:1313–28. doi: 10.1089/aid.2011.0297
46. Lester RT, Yao XD, Ball TB, McKinnon LR, Kaul R, Wachihi C, et al. Toll-like receptor expression and responsiveness are increased in viraemic HIV-1 infection. *AIDS.* (2008) 22:685–94. doi: 10.1097/QAD.0b013e3282f4de35
47. Martinelli E, Cicala C, Van Ryk D, Goode DJ, Macleod K, Arthos J, Fauci AS. HIV-1 gp120 inhibits TLR9-mediated activation and IFN-{alpha} secretion in plasmacytoid dendritic cells. *Proc Natl Acad Sci USA.* (2007) 104:3396–401. doi: 10.1073/pnas.0611353104
48. Reuven EM, Ali M, Rotem E, Schwarzter R, Gramatica A, Futerman AH, et al. The HIV-1 envelope transmembrane domain binds TLR2 through a distinct dimerization motif and inhibits TLR2-mediated responses. *PLoS Pathog.* (2014) 10:e1004248. doi: 10.1371/journal.ppat.1004248
49. Ahmed N, Hayashi T, Hasegawa A, Furukawa H, Okamura N, Chida T, et al. Suppression of human immunodeficiency virus type 1 replication in macrophages by commensal bacteria preferentially stimulating Toll-like receptor 4. *J General Virol.* (2010) 91:2804–13. doi: 10.1099/vir.0.022442-0
50. Novis CL, Archin NM, Buzon MJ, Verdin E, Round JL, Lichterfeld M, et al. Reactivation of latent HIV-1 in central memory CD4+ T cells through TLR-1/2 stimulation. *Retrovirology.* (2013) 10:119. doi: 10.1186/1742-4690-10-119
51. Mikulak J, Oriolo F, Zaghi E, Di Vito C, Mavilio D. Natural killer cells in HIV-1 infection and therapy. *AIDS.* (2017) 31:2317–30. doi: 10.1097/QAD.0000000000001645
52. Scully E, Alter G. NK Cells in HIV disease. *Curr HIV/AIDS Rep.* (2016) 13:85–94. doi: 10.1007/s11904-016-0310-3
53. Schafer JL, Li H, Evans TI, Estes JD, Reeves RK. Accumulation of Cytotoxic CD16 + NK cells in simian immunodeficiency virus-infected lymph nodes associated with *in situ* differentiation and functional anergy. *J Virol.* (2015) 89:6887–94. doi: 10.1128/JVI.00660-15
54. Langford SE, Ananworanich J, Cooper DA. Predictors of disease progression in HIV infection: a review. *AIDS Res Ther.* (2007) 4:11. doi: 10.1186/1742-6405-4-11
55. Grant EJ, Nüssing S, Sant S, Clemens EB, Kedzierska K. The role of CD27 in anti-viral T-cell immunity. *Curr Opin Virol.* (2017) 22:77–88. doi: 10.1016/j.coviro.2016.12.001
56. Hintzen RQ, de Jong R, Lens SM, Brouwer M, Baars P, van Lier RA. Regulation of CD27 expression on subsets of mature T-lymphocytes. *J Immunol.* (1993) 151:2426–35.
57. Borst J. Targeting the T-cell co-stimulatory CD27 / CD70 pathway in cancer immunotherapy : rationale and potential. *Immunotherapy.* (2015) 7:655–67. doi: 10.2217/imt.15.32
58. Reinwald S, Wiethe C, Westendorf AM, Breloer M, Probst-Kepper M, Fleischer B, et al. CD83 Expression in CD4+ T cells modulates inflammation and autoimmunity. *J Immunol.* (2008) 180:5890–7. doi: 10.4049/jimmunol.180.9.5890
59. Breloer M, Kretschmer B, Lüthje K, Ehrlich S, Ritter U, Bickert T, et al. CD83 is a regulator of murine B cell function *in vivo. Eur J Immunol.* (2007) 37:634–48. doi: 10.1002/eji.200636852
60. Damouche A, Lazure T, Avettand-f V, Huot N, Dejucq-rainsford N, Satie A, et al. Adipose tissue is a neglected viral reservoir and an inflammatory site during chronic HIV and SIV infection. *PLoS Pathog.* (2015) 11:1–28. doi: 10.1371/journal.ppat.1005153
61. Estes JD, Kityo C, Ssali F, Swainson L, Makamdop KN, Del Prete GQ, et al. Defining total body AIDS virus burden: implications for curative strategies. *Nat Med.* (2018) 23:1271–6. doi: 10.1038/nm.4411
62. Hattab S, Guiguet M, Carcelain G, Fourati S, Guihot A, Autran B, et al. Soluble biomarkers of immune activation and inflammation in HIV infection : impact of 2 years of effective first-line combination antiretroviral therapy. *HIV Med.* (2015) 16:553–62. doi: 10.1111/hiv.12257
63. Noel N, Boufassa F, Lécuroux C, Saez-Cirion A, Bourgeois C, Dunyach-Remy C, et al. Elevated IP10 levels are associated with immune activation and low CD4+ T-cell counts in HIV controller patients. *AIDS.* (2014) 28:467–76. doi: 10.1097/QAD.0000000000000174

15

Differential Dynamics of the Maternal Immune System in Healthy Pregnancy and Preeclampsia

Xiaoyuan Han [1†], Mohammad S. Ghaemi [1†], Kazuo Ando [1], Laura S. Peterson [2], Edward A. Ganio [1], Amy S. Tsai [1], Dyani K. Gaudilliere [3], Ina A. Stelzer [1], Jakob Einhaus [1], Basile Bertrand [1], Natalie Stanley [1], Anthony Culos [1], Athena Tanada [1], Julien Hedou [1], Eileen S. Tsai [1], Ramin Fallahzadeh [1], Ronald J. Wong [2,4], Amy E. Judy [5], Virginia D. Winn [5], Maurice L. Druzin [5], Yair J. Blumenfeld [5], Mark A. Hlatky [6], Cecele C. Quaintance [4], Ronald S. Gibbs [5], Brendan Carvalho [1], Gary M. Shaw [2,4], David K. Stevenson [2,4], Martin S. Angst [1†], Nima Aghaeepour [1†] and Brice Gaudilliere [1†]*

[1] Department of Anesthesiology, Perioperative and Pain Medicine, School of Medicine, Stanford University, Palo Alto, CA, United States, [2] Department of Pediatrics, School of Medicine, Stanford University, Palo Alto, CA, United States, [3] Department of Surgery, School of Medicine, Stanford University, Palo Alto, CA, United States, [4] March of Dimes Prematurity Research Center, School of Medicine, Stanford University, Palo Alto, CA, United States, [5] Department of Obstetrics and Gynecology, School of Medicine, Stanford University, Palo Alto, CA, United States, [6] Department of Health Research and Policy, School of Medicine, Stanford University, Palo Alto, CA, United States

***Correspondence:**
Brice Gaudilliere
gbrice@stanford.edu

[†] These authors have contributed equally to this work

Preeclampsia is one of the most severe pregnancy complications and a leading cause of maternal death. However, early diagnosis of preeclampsia remains a clinical challenge. Alterations in the normal immune adaptations necessary for the maintenance of a healthy pregnancy are central features of preeclampsia. However, prior analyses primarily focused on the static assessment of select immune cell subsets have provided limited information for the prediction of preeclampsia. Here, we used a high-dimensional mass cytometry immunoassay to characterize the dynamic changes of over 370 immune cell features (including cell distribution and functional responses) in maternal blood during healthy and preeclamptic pregnancies. We found a set of eight cell-specific immune features that accurately identified patients well before the clinical diagnosis of preeclampsia (median area under the curve (AUC) 0.91, interquartile range [0.82–0.92]). Several features recapitulated previously known immune dysfunctions in preeclampsia, such as elevated pro-inflammatory innate immune responses early in pregnancy and impaired regulatory T (Treg) cell signaling. The analysis revealed additional novel immune responses that were strongly associated with, and preceded the onset of preeclampsia, notably abnormal STAT5ab signaling dynamics in $CD4^{+}T$ cell subsets (AUC 0.92, $p = 8.0E\text{-}5$). These results provide a global readout of the dynamics of the maternal immune system early in pregnancy and lay the groundwork for identifying clinically-relevant immune dysfunctions for the prediction and prevention of preeclampsia.

Keywords: preeclampsia, immunology, mass cytometry, PBMC, pregnancy

INTRODUCTION

Preeclampsia is a severe complication of pregnancy defined by the new onset of hypertension and signs of maternal organ dysfunction after the 20th week of gestation (1). Preeclampsia affects between 2 and 8% of all pregnant women—over 8 million women per year worldwide—and is a leading cause of maternal deaths (9–26%) (2). Preeclampsia also accounts for significant neonatal morbidity and mortality due to intrauterine growth restriction, intrauterine fetal demise, and preterm delivery (2). However, no diagnostic test reliably detects preeclampsia early in its development, so treatment can be started only after the onset of signs and symptoms, at which point irreparable harm to the mother and fetus may already have occurred.

Preeclampsia is a multisystem disorder characterized by placental and endothelial dysfunction, leading to hypertension and other end-organ damage such as impaired kidney, liver, neurological, or hematological function (3). Well-described placental abnormalities, including in trophoblast invasion and uterine spiral artery formation, suggest that the roots of preeclampsia are established in the first weeks of pregnancy, before the development of signs and symptoms (4). While markers of placental and endothelial dysfunction—such as increases in soluble FMS-like tyrosine kinase 1 (sFLT-1) levels, and decreases in vascular endothelial growth factor (VEGF) and placental growth factor (PLGF) levels—can be valuable clinically in ruling out suspected preeclampsia (5), early diagnosis of preeclampsia remains clinically challenging.

Systemic inflammation and alterations in the normal immune adaptations necessary for the maintenance of a healthy pregnancy are central features in the pathophysiology of preeclampsia (6–11). Accumulating evidence suggests that preeclampsia is associated with a breakdown of tolerogenic cellular adaptations, including a shift in T cell distributions toward Th1 and Th17 and away from Th2 and regulatory $CD4^{+}$T cell (Treg) populations (12–14). The potential role of the maternal immune system in the pathogenesis of preeclampsia was underscored by a recent multi-omic study of placental, coagulation, complement and vascular factors, highlighting that a majority of plasma proteins associated with preeclampsia were linked to immune functions (15).

Immune dysfunction may be detected well before the clinical onset of preeclampsia, as early as during the first trimester of pregnancy (16–18). For this reason, identifying immunological attributes in maternal blood that predict and help prevent preeclampsia at a preclinical state is of considerable clinical interest (3, 18–20). However, due to limitations in assay technology, prior studies of immune responses associated with preeclampsia have been restricted to a select number of cell subsets and may not have captured immune cell behaviors in the context of the entire peripheral immune system. In particular, the limited number of parameters available for the phenotypic and functional characterization of immune cell subsets may have hampered the detection of important cellular and functional signatures.

Recently developed, highly multiplex single-cell technologies such as mass cytometry—a flow cytometry platform that allows assessment of over 40 parameters on a cell-by-cell basis—offer unprecedented opportunities for comprehensive functional studies of the human immune system (21, 22). Combined with appropriate statistical tools that account for the high-dimensionality of the data, mass cytometry is uniquely capable of identifying alterations of the human immune system associated with normal physiological perturbations and disease pathogenesis (23–25).

In a recent study, we employed a high-parameter mass cytometry assay to characterize the dynamic changes in maternal immune cell distribution and signaling responses during an uncomplicated pregnancy (26). Here, we report on an in-depth profiling of the dynamics of the maternal immune system in healthy (normotensive) pregnancies and preeclampsia. Our primary goal was to detect characteristic immune dysfunctions in the maternal blood prior to the clinical onset of preeclampsia.

MATERIALS AND METHODS

Study Design

Pregnant women participating in a cohort study sponsored by the March of Dimes Prematurity Research Center were prospectively

TABLE 1 | Demographics of study participants.

	Control ($n = 12$)	Preeclampsia ($n = 11$)
DEMOGRAPHICS		
Age (years, mean ± SD)	33.4 ± 4.7	30.6 ± 5.4
BMI (kg/m^2, mean ± SD)	24.5 ± 5.6	29.4 ± 4.6 *
BMI at delivery (kg/m^2, mean ± SD)	28.2 ± 4.7	33.4 ± 4.5 *
GA at delivery (weeks, mean ± SD)	39.3 ± 1.2	37.6 ± 3.0
Gravida (mean ± SD)	3.0 ± 1.5	2.5 ± 2.5
Para (mean ± SD)	1.5 ± 1.5	0.7 ± 1.5
Twin pregnancy	0	1
RACE/ETHNICITY		
Asian	0	3
Black	0	1
White	10	4
Other	2	3
Hispanic	3	3
Non-hispanic	9	8
MODE OF DELIVERY		
Normal spontaneous vaginal delivery	8	5
Cesarean delivery	4	6
PREECLAMPSIA CHARACTERISTICS		
Preeclampsia with severe feature		7
Early-onset preeclampsia		2
COMORBIDITY		
Gestational diabetes	1	1
Type II diabetes	0	2
Autoimmune disease	0	3
Chronic hypertension	0	2

*$p < 0.05$, by using unpaired student t-test.

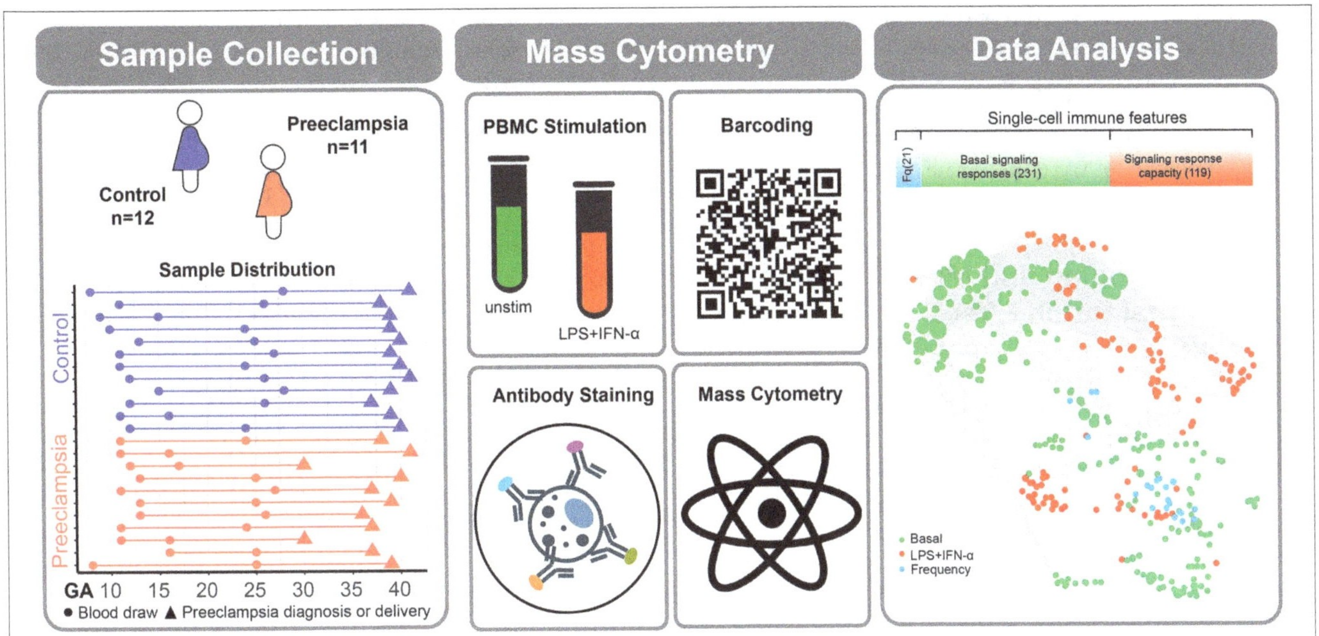

FIGURE 1 | Experimental workflow for the deep profiling of immune system dynamics in preeclampsia. Eleven women with preeclampsia and 12 healthy (normotensive) women were studied. PBMCs were obtained at two time points during the first 28 weeks of pregnancy. Sample collection time (dots), preeclampsia diagnosis (orange triangles), or delivery (purple triangles) are indicated for individual preeclamptic patients (orange lines) and controls (purple lines). PBMCs were either left unstimulated or stimulated with a cocktail of LPS and IFN-α. Immune cells were barcoded, stained with surface and intracellular antibodies and analyzed with mass cytometry. The assay produced three categories of immune features, providing information about cell frequency (Fq) measured in 21 immune cell subsets (blue bar), basal intracellular signaling activity (green bar), and cell type-specific signaling capacity in response to stimulation with LPS and IFN-α (red bar). The number of immune features contained within each data category is indicated in parentheses. Correlation network reveals the relationships between immune features within and across mass cytometry data categories. A correlation network highlights the relationship between measured immune features (Spearman's coefficient)

examined for an array of environmental and biological factors associated with uncomplicated and pathological pregnancies (27, 28). Participants all received routine antepartum care at the Lucile Packard Children's Hospital at Stanford University and were eligible for the study if they were 18 years of age or older and in their first trimester of pregnancy. Peripheral blood samples were obtained at least at 2 time points during pregnancy. The study was approved by the Institutional Review Board of Stanford University, and all participants signed an informed consent.

An in-depth mass cytometry analysis of peripheral immune cell responses was performed using the first (median 11 ± 1.9 weeks) and last samples (median 25 ± 4.1 weeks) collected from two subsets of study participants (11 women who developed preeclampsia and 12 women with a normotensive pregnancy). Sample selection criteria for analysis included a cell viability of over 60% and a cell count of over 10^6 cells. Samples from the 11 women in the preeclampsia group were selected based on a diagnosis of preeclampsia made (and verified by a senior obstetrician) according to the American College of Obstetricians and Gynecologists criteria (1). Early-onset preeclampsia was defined as preeclampsia developing before 34 weeks of gestation (1). Samples from the 12 women in the control group were selected if study participants had a normotensive pregnancy leading to the delivery of a healthy neonate at term (gestational age > 37 weeks), and to ensure matching of gestational age at time of sampling with the preeclampsia group. One patient in the control group had well-managed gestational diabetes mellitus (GDM) with an otherwise uncomplicated pregnancy.

Demographics and pregnancy characteristics for the 23 participants included in the analysis are summarized in **Table 1**.

Sample Collection and PBMC Stimulation

Peripheral blood mononuclear cells (PBMCs) were prepared and cryopreserved according to standard protocols. On the day of sample stimulation, PBMCs at indicated time points (**Figure 1**) were thawed and rested in culture media containing 10% fetal bovine serum (Gibco) at 37°C for 2 h. PBMCs were counted and checked for viability.

PBMC samples were stimulated with either lipopolysaccharide (LPS) (1 μg/mL) and interferon-α (IFN-α) (100 ng/mL), or left unstimulated at 37°C for 15 min, then fixed for further analysis with mass cytometry. The rationale for choosing the combined stimulation condition LPS+IFN-α in this study was driven by results from the multivariate model of normal pregnancy (26) and by experimental constraints. Of the 4 stimulation conditions used in our previous study, the basal (unstimulated), LPS and IFN-α stimulated conditions provided the most information to the multivariate model of normal pregnancy (basal, LPS, and IFN-α and IL-2+IL-6 stimulations accounted for 25, 46, 17, and 12% of the model features, respectively). To maximize the information obtained from stimulated samples, LPS and IFN-α were utilized together after ensuring that little overlap was detected in our immunoassay between immune signaling responses to LPS (restricted to pERK1/2, pP38, pMAPKAPK2, pS6, pCREB, pNF-κB in innate immune cells) and to IFN-α (restricted to pSTAT1, pSTAT3, pSTAT5, pSTAT6 in innate and adaptive immune cells) (**Figure S2**).

Sample Barcoding and Minimization of Experimental Batch Effect

To minimize the effect of experimental variability on mass cytometry measurements between samples from different time points and between samples from the control and preeclampsia groups, samples corresponding from the entire time series collected from one woman with preeclampsia and one control were processed, barcoded, pooled, stained and run simultaneously on the mass cytometry instrument (29, 30). There was no difference in total cell count, live cell count, viability, and storage time at time point 1 or 2 between the two groups.

Antibody Staining and Mass Cytometry

The mass cytometry antibody panel included 22 antibodies that were used for phenotyping of immune cell subsets and 11 antibodies for the functional characterization of immune cell responses (**Table S1**). Antibodies were either obtained pre-conjugated (Fluidigm, Inc.) or were obtained as purified, carrier-free (no BSA, gelatin) versions, which were then conjugated in-house with trivalent metal isotopes utilizing the MaxPAR antibody conjugation kit (Fluidigm, Inc.). After incubation with Fc block (Biolegend), pooled barcoded cells were stained with surface antibodies then permeabilized with methanol and stained with intracellular antibodies. All antibodies used in the analysis were titrated and validated on samples that were processed identically to the samples used in the study. Barcoded and antibody-stained cells were analyzed on a Helios mass cytometer (Fluidigm, Inc.).

Derivation of Immune Features

The mass cytometry data was normalized using Normalizer v0.1 MATLAB Compiler Runtime (MathWorks) (31). Files were then de-barcoded with a single-cell MATLAB de-barcoding tool (30). Manual gating was performed using CellEngine (https://immuneatlas.org/#/) (Primity Bio, Fremont, CA) according to our previous gating strategy (**Figure S1**) (26). The following 21 cell types were included in the analysis: B cells, Natural Killer cells (NK), $CD56^{hi}CD16^-$ NK cells, $CD56^{lo}CD16^+$ NK cells, $CD4^+$T cells, $CD4^+CD45RA^-$T cells ($CD4^+$Tmem), $CD4^+CD45RA^+$T cells ($CD4^+$Tnaive), $CD4^+Tbet^+$T cells (Th1), $CD25^+FoxP3^+CD4^+$T cells (Tregs), $CD8^+$T cells, $CD8^+CD45RA^-$T cells ($CD8^+$Tmem), $CD8^+CD45RA^+$T cells ($CD8^+$Tnaive), $CD8^+Tbet^+CD45RA^-$ cells, $CD8^+Tbet^+CD45RA^+$T cells, $TCR_{\gamma\delta}$T cells, $CD14^+CD16^-$ classical monocytes (cMCs), $CD14^-CD16^+$ non-classical MCs (ncMCs), $CD14^+CD16^+$ intermediate MCs (intMCs), monocytic myeloid-derived suppressor cells (M-MDSCs), myeloid dendritic cells (mDCs), and plasmacytoid dendritic cells (pDCs).

Cell frequency features

Cell frequencies were expressed as a percentage of gated singlet live mononuclear cells ($cPARP^-CD45^+CD66^-$).

Basal signaling immune features

Basal intracellular signaling activities were derived from the analysis of unstimulated samples. The phospho-signal intensity of the following functional markers was simultaneously quantified per single cells: pSTAT1, pSTAT3, pSTAT5, pSTAT6, pNFκB, pMAPKAPK2, pP38, prpS6, pERK1/2, pCREB. Total IκB was measured to assess IκB degradation. For each cell type, signaling immune features were calculated as the mean signal intensity (arcsinh transformed value) of each signaling protein.

Intracellular signaling response features

For each cell type, the arcsinh difference (arcsinh ratio) in signal intensity between the stimulated and unstimulated conditions was calculated for each functional marker. Stimulation conditions that yielded little or no responses in optimization experiments (**Figure S2**) were excluded from the analysis.

Correlation Network

Spearman correlation analyses were performed between pairs of immune features measured at each time point. The graphical representation of the correlation network shows edges for significant correlations between data pairs (p < 1.0E-12). Edge length is proportional to –log10 (p-value). The graph layout was calculated using the t-SNE algorithm and visualized using the i-graph R package (32). Communities of correlated immune features were detected by multi-level modularity optimization algorithm using the "cluster_louvain" function from i-graph R package (33, 34).

Parametrization of Immune Feature Dynamics

Parametrization of immune feature dynamics: For each immune feature, the rate of change between the two sampling time points was estimated as:

$$\rho = \frac{immune\,feature_{T2} - immune\,feature_{T1}}{GA_{T2} - GA_{T1}}$$

Statistical Analyses

A multivariate LASSO (least absolute shrinkage and selection operator) linear logistic regression method was utilized for this study (35). This method was chosen as it uses an L_1 penalization over the classifier's coefficients to develop a "sparse" model that is suitable for the modular and correlated structure of the immune dataset (35). In addition, the LASSO method utilizes few free-parameters, which enables effective optimization using cross-validation.

The feature matrix was constructed using the rate of change of immune feature (ρ) as follows: For a design matrix P of immune feature rates (ρ), and a binary response vector of preeclampsia Y, a multivariate linear logistic LASSO regression model was developed to calculate the coefficients β for each entity in P to maximize the overall log-likelihood using the conditional likelihood of C given P,

$$l(\beta) = \sum_{i=1}^{n} \log p_{yi}(\rho_i ; \beta)$$

where

$$p_{yi}(\rho_i ; \beta) = \Pr\left(C = y_i \middle| P = \rho_i ; \beta\right)$$

With this convention, log-likelihood can be rewritten as

$$l(\beta) = \sum_{i=1}^{n} [y_i \beta^T \rho_i - \log(1 + \exp\left(\beta^T \rho_i\right))]$$

An L_1 regularization was applied on the β coefficient to reduce the model complexity, such that

$$l(\beta) = \sum_{i=1}^{n} [y_i \beta^T \rho_i - \log(1 + \exp\left(\beta^T \rho_i\right))] + \lambda \sum_{j=1}^{p} |\beta_j|$$

where lambda λ is selected by cross-validation. This produces a sparse model in which only a limited number of features are used (35).

The model was trained on 20 randomly-selected patients and tested on the remaining three. After 100 iterations, the mean of all predictions for a given patient in the test set was used as the final blinded prediction. This strategy minimizes the risk of overfitting by ensuring the models are always tested on samples that were not previously seen by the algorithm.

Model Reduction

The relative weights of immune features selected by the LASSO method were determined using the frequency at which individual immune features were selected through all cross-validation iterations. The top ten features were chosen by a piecewise regression model, a statistical technique used to specify an abrupt shift over the response variable corresponding to the explanatory variable.

We used student t-test to compare individual immune features between control and preeclampsia groups if the data is normal distributed test by Shapiro-Wilk test, otherwise, a Mann-Whitney nonparametric test was used.

Confounder Analysis

We analyzed 14 demographic and comorbid conditions, including age, race, ethnicity, Body Mass Index (BMI), GA at delivery, total number of pregnancies, multiparity, parity, gestational diabetes, type 2 diabetes, preeclampsia history, autoimmune disease, and chronic hypertension. Women with preeclampsia had higher BMI (p = 2.0E-3) than the controls (student t-test). Higher rates of type 2 diabetes (p = 4.5E-2), chronic hypertension (p = 4.5E-2) and autoimmune diseases (p = 8.0E-3) were found in the patients with preeclampsia, which were significant by Fisher's exact test. To test whether these four comorbidities had an effect on immune features associated with preeclampsia, multiple linear regression analyses were performed to determine whether preeclampsia is a significant predictor of each immune feature when accounting for the four relevant comorbidities. This confounder analysis was performed using SPSS version 12.0 (SPSS Inc., Chicago, IL, USA).

RESULTS

Study Cohort

The 11 study participants with preeclampsia were slightly younger and heavier than the 12 study participants from the control group (**Table 1**). Seven of the women with preeclampsia had severe features, and two had early-onset preeclampsia (including one patient with severe features). Participants with preeclampsia had more comorbidities, including arterial hypertension, diabetes, and autoimmune diseases, including systemic lupus erythematosus (SLE) (**Table 1**). Samples were collected well before clinical diagnosis of preeclampsia: a median of 13 weeks (interquartile range (IQR), 12 to 14). The gestational age (GA) at time of sampling did not differ between the two groups (median at the first time point (T1): 11 ± 1.8 weeks vs. 11 ± 2.0 weeks, $p = 0.48$; median at the second time point (T2): 25.5 ± 4.2 weeks vs. 25 ± 4.2 weeks, $p = 0.36$).

Deep Profiling of Maternal Immune Responses in Healthy and Preeclamptic Pregnancies

PBMCs collected longitudinally during pregnancy were analyzed using a 41-parameter immunoassay for an in-depth profiling of peripheral immune cell adaptations. For each patient sample, 371 immune features were quantified on a per cell basis in 21 distinct innate and adaptive immune cell subsets (**Figure 1**). Immune features included cell frequencies and the activity (e.g., phosphorylation state) of 11 intracellular signaling proteins measured at baseline (basal signaling activity) as well as in response to extracellular stimulations with IFN-α and LPS (**Figure 1**; **Figure S2**). Stimulation conditions were chosen to activate receptor-specific signaling responses (Toll-Like Receptor (TLR) 4-dependent signaling for LPS, Janus kinase (JAK)-Signal Transducer and Activator of Transcription (STAT) signaling for IFN-α) that were most informative in characterizing immune cell dynamics in our previous mass cytometry analyses of healthy pregnancies (26).

The high-parameter immunological dataset yielded a correlation network that emphasized the interconnectivity of immune responses during pregnancy (**Figure 1**). The correlation network segregated into 6 major communities of closely interconnected immune features, which were identified using a multi-level modularity optimization algorithm (33, 34). These statistically defined communities were annotated on the basis of immune feature characteristics (signaling property, stimulation, or cell subset) most commonly represented within each community (**Figure 2A**).

In the control group, a targeted examination of select communities revealed peripheral immune cell adaptations that

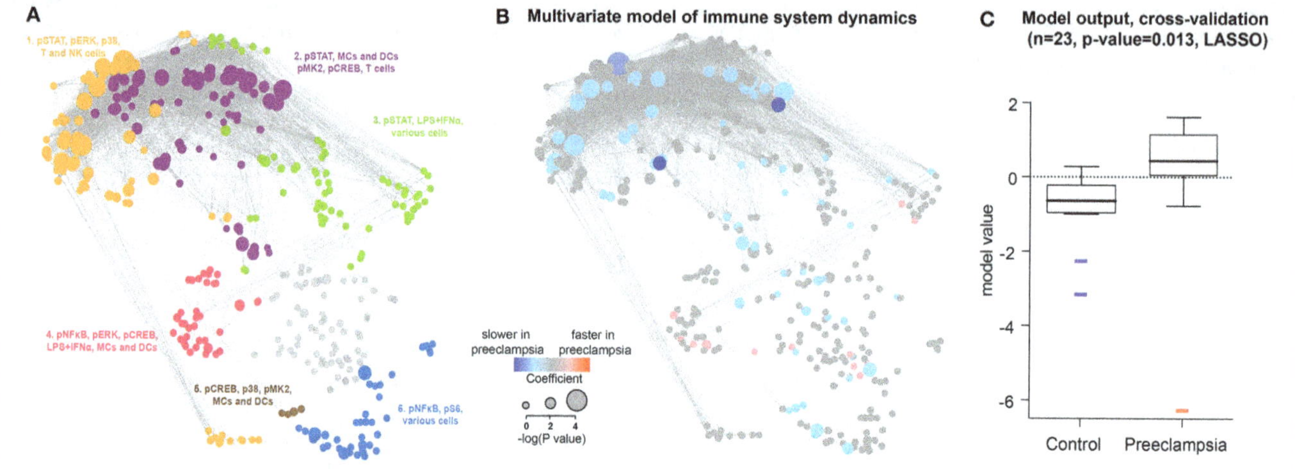

FIGURE 2 | Predictive modeling of immune response dynamics associated with preeclampsia. **(A)** The correlation network segregates into 6 major communities of correlated immune features. Communities were detected using the Louvain multi-level modularity optimization method (33, 34) and annotated on the basis of immune feature characteristics (signaling property, stimulation, or cell subset) most commonly represented within each community. **(B)** A predictive multivariate model built on immune feature dynamics (rate of change between the first and second time points). LASSO identified patients that develop preeclampsia within 12–14 weeks after the last sampling time. Red/blue dots highlight immune features that evolve faster/slower in preeclampsia compared to Control. Dot size indicates the $-log_{10}$ of *p*-value of model components compared between preeclamptic women and controls (Student *t*-test). **(C)** Boxplots showing model prediction for controls and preeclamptic women (AUC 0.803, cross-validation *p*-value = 0.013).

dovetailed with prior immune profiling studies of normal pregnancy (26, 36, 37). For instance, one of the communities (Community 1) was primarily defined by the basal activity of the transcription factor STAT5ab (phospho, pSTAT5 signal) in $CD4^{+}$T cells (**Figure S3A**), which increased during pregnancy as previously reported (26). Another community (Community 3) contained features that pointed at increasing pSTAT1 responses to stimulation in NK cells during pregnancy (**Figure S3B**), consistent with prior *in vitro* and *in vivo* studies showing that NK cell-mediated pathogen responses are exacerbated during pregnancy (26, 36, 38). In addition, Treg cell frequency increased between the first and second trimesters of pregnancy (**Figure S3C**), consistent with prior reports of Treg dynamics during pregnancy (26, 39). Thus, the immunoassay utilized in this study was sensitive to detect established hallmarks of maternal immune adaptations during a normal pregnancy.

Immune System-Wide Dynamics Are Disrupted in Preeclampsia

A number of observations in humans support the assessment of immune cell responses over time, rather than a cross-sectional assessment at a given time point, to understand how the human immune system adapts to a physiological or a pathological perturbation (40). We reasoned that an analysis focused on immune response dynamics would be particularly adapted to detect immune dysfunctions preceding the onset of preeclampsia.

To parameterize the dynamic changes in the peripheral immune system during pregnancy, the rate of change between the first and second sampling time points was calculated for each immune feature. The least absolute shrinkage and selection operator (LASSO) method (35) was applied to the dataset of immune feature dynamics. The predictive analysis identified a multivariate model that accurately differentiated women who developed preeclampsia from controls (**Figures 2B,C**). Components of the LASSO model were visualized on the correlation network as red or blue nodes highlighting immune features with accelerated or decelerated, respectively, dynamics in women who will develop preeclampsia (**Figure 2B**). The generalizability of the model was established using a stringent cross-validation method that accounts for the high-dimensionality of the dataset. No significant association was found between the LASSO model prediction and the presence of comorbid conditions, including autoimmune diseases, gestational diabetes, chronic hypertension and body mass index (BMI). When excluding patients with autoimmune disease and gestational diabetes, the LASSO model remained highly significant (cross-validated *p*-value = 0.016) and robust (AUC = 0.83). The results suggest that specific aspects of peripheral immune system dynamics, detectable 12–14 weeks before the clinical diagnosis of preeclampsia, are disrupted in preeclamptic pregnancies.

Pro-inflammatory Immune Responses Early in Pregnancy Contribute to Abnormal Immune System Dynamics in Preeclampsia

The LASSO method allowed a system-level analysis of immune dysfunction in preeclampsia anchored by a statistically-stringent multivariate model. To highlight the most informative features of the multivariate model and facilitate biological interpretation, we applied a piecewise regression method that reduced the model to 10 components (**Figure 3A**) that were highly discriminating between control and preeclamptic pregnancies: the median area under the curve (AUC) was 0.90, within an IQR of 0.81 to 0.92. Most (90%) of the informative immune features were intracellular signaling responses (AUC 0.80-0.92), while the cell frequency features had a much weaker predictive performance for preeclampsia (AUC = 0.65). Eight out of these ten immune features remained highly significant as predictors of preeclampsia after controlling for demographic and clinical variables (BMI, presence of autoimmune disease, hypertension, and type 2 diabetes) in a multivariate linear regression analysis (**Table S2**).

These eight informative immune features appeared within 3 of the 6 communities, consistent with dysregulated immune dynamics that spanned multiple immune compartments (**Figure 3B**). The most informative feature was the pSTAT5 signal (basal) in $CD4^+Tbet^+$Th1 cells (AUC = 0.92, $p = 8.0E\text{-}5$, **Figure 4A**). The pSTAT5 signal increased consistently in Th1 cells between the first and second trimesters in the control group but decreased consistently in women who developed preeclampsia (**Figure 4A**). Further examination of individual time points revealed that the pSTAT5 signal in Th1 cells was higher in women with preeclampsia compared with controls in the first trimester and then gradually decreased during the second trimester (**Figure 4A**, inset). These results are consistent with the prevailing theory of the presence of a predominance of Th1 in preeclampsia (41), given that STAT5 can potentiate Th1 differentiation (42).

Because the JAK/STAT5 signaling pathway is implicated in multiple aspects of $CD4^+$T cell differentiation, notably in the differentiation and stability of peripheral Tregs (43–45), we tested whether observed pSTAT5 dynamics were restricted only to Th1 cells. In Community 1 (defined by the STAT5 signaling response) the abnormal pSTAT5 dynamics were shared among several T cell subsets including $CD4^+$ Tnaive cells and $CD25^+FoxP3^+$ Tregs (**Figure S4**). The pSTAT5 signal in Tregs increased between the first and second trimesters in the control group, but did not change in the preeclamptic women. The results highlight an important role for STAT5-dependent responses across multiple $CD4^+$T cell subsets that are disrupted prior to the clinical onset of preeclampsia.

The remaining immune features of the reduced model suggested that, overall, strong pro-inflammatory cell responses early during pregnancy altered the immunologic trajectory of women who went on to develop preeclampsia. In innate immune compartments, the pSTAT1, pSTAT5, and pNFκB signals (basal) were elevated in intermediate monocytes (intMCs) (AUC = 0.93, p = 4.0E-4), myeloid dendritic cells (mDCs) (AUC = 0.92, p = 0.0026), and classical monocytes (cMCs) (pSTAT1: AUC = 0.90, p = 4.1E-4; pNFκB: AUC = 0.82, p = 4.0E-3), respectively, during the first trimester in preeclamptic women compared with controls (**Figures 4B–E**). These responses gradually decreased during preeclamptic pregnancies, but increased in the control group. In adaptive immune compartments, elevated pro-inflammatory signaling responses in Th1 cells (pSTAT5) during the first trimester of pregnancy were coupled with abnormal signaling dynamics in $CD4^+$Tnaïve cells (pMAPKAPK2, AUC = 0.91, p = 3.2E-3), $TCR_{\gamma\delta}$ (pP38, AUC = 0.9, p = 2.0E-4) and $CD25^+FoxP3^+$Tregs (pP38, AUC = 0.82, p = 0.032) (**Figures 4F–H**). Of note, the pP38 signal, which is required for Treg suppressive function (46), increased in Tregs during pregnancy in controls but not in women with preeclampsia.

DISCUSSION

We employed a high-parameter mass cytometry immunoassay for an in-depth assessment of the dynamics of the peripheral immune system during normal and preeclamptic pregnancies. Analysis of the high-dimensional immunological dataset identified immune system dysfunction detectable in the maternal blood 12–14 weeks before the clinical signs of preeclampsia were evident. Individual components of the multivariate model highlighted profound dysregulation of intracellular signaling dynamics that were strongly associated with the subsequent development of preeclampsia (median AUC 0.91, IQR [0.82, 0.92]).

High-parameter flow cytometry technologies such as mass cytometry have transformed the ability to profile the human immune system. However, the high dimensionality of the resulting data presents a major analytical challenge to conventional statistical analysis (47). Application of regularized regression algorithms (such as LASSO) combined with a cross-validation method to ensure generalizability of the model outputs provided a robust statistical solution to this analytic challenge (48). In this study, the LASSO analysis provided a statistically stringent multivariate model that distinguished healthy pregnancies from those with preeclampsia, while simultaneously assessing over 370 immune features. The performance of individual model components in stratifying women who develop preeclampsia was also remarkable. Using the AUC as a metric, the individual performances of the top five model components to predict preeclampsia were each above 0.9, which signifies excellent predictive performance. These results may be due to several aspects of our analysis that differ from prior studies reporting on immunological biomarkers of preeclampsia (6, 7, 18–20, 49). The functional interrogation of signaling responses, rather than cell distribution may have been more informative; the simultaneous survey of multiple innate and adaptive immune cell subsets allowed for agnostic identification of the most informative immune features; and the analysis, which focused on immune cell dynamics rather than static immunologic events, may have allowed a more sensitive detection of pregnancy-related immune dysfunctions.

The most informative features of our analysis were the basal pSTAT5 signals in $CD4^+$T cell subsets (AUC = 0.92, p = 8.0E-5). Notably, the pSTAT5 signal in $CD4^+$T cells was also the most informative component of a multivariate model predictive of the age of gestation in a prior study of normal pregnancy (26, 27). These findings, derived from two independent studies, suggest that assessing pSTAT5 dynamics in $CD4^+$T cell subsets early in pregnancy may be a key feature of an immuno-assay predicting the risk for developing preeclampsia.

The JAK/STAT5 pathway has been implicated in multiple, and seemingly conflicting, aspects of $CD4^+$T cell development. Downstream of IL-2, *in vivo* and *in vitro* studies show that the IL-2/STAT5 pathway controls Th2 differentiation [by inducing the

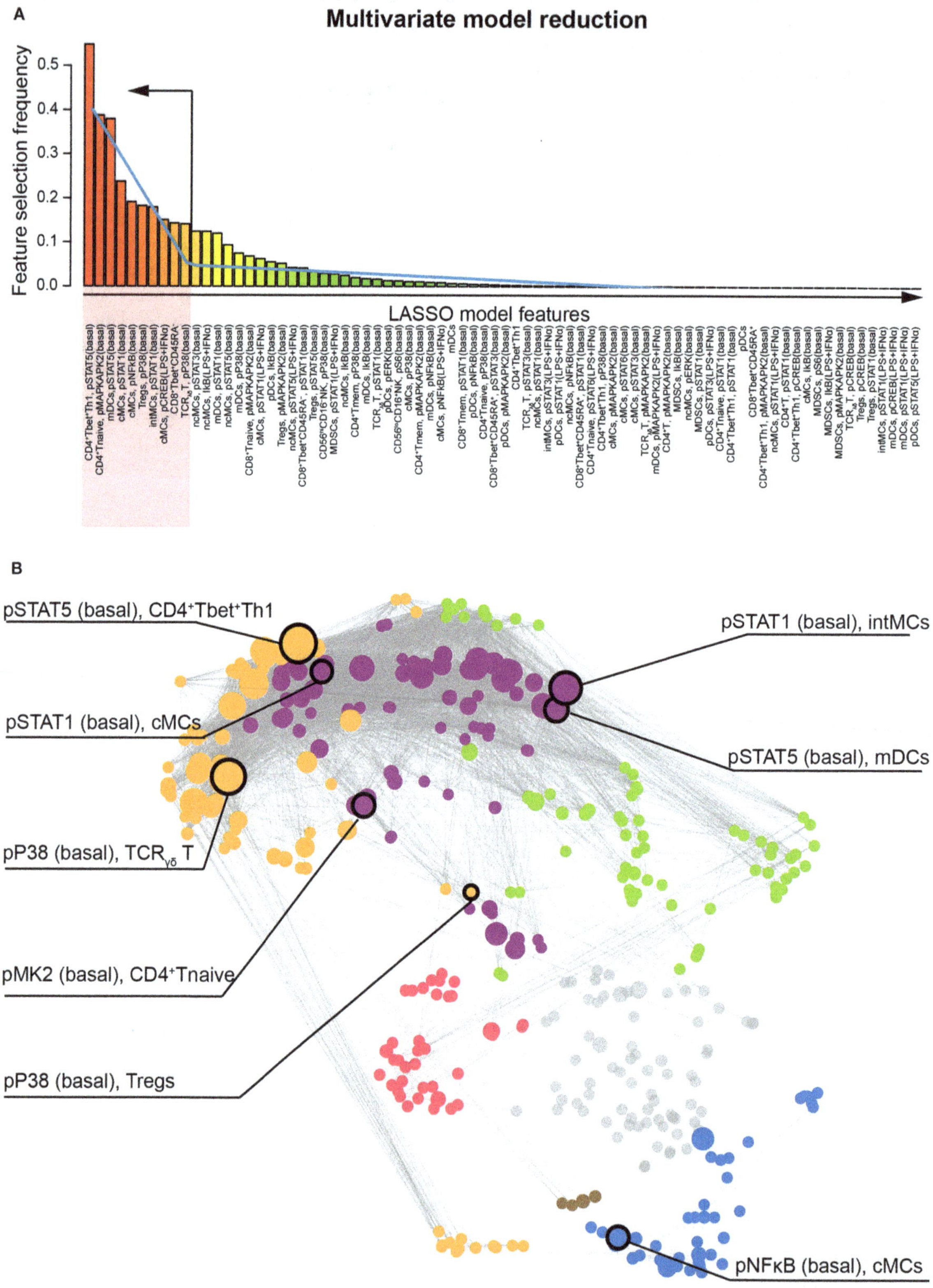

FIGURE 3 | Identification of the most informative features classifying patients who develop preeclampsia. **(A)** The bar graph depicts the frequency of immune feature selection across all cross-validation iterations. Blue line indicates piecewise regression fit for identification of a breakpoint indicating ten immune features that are most informative to the multivariate LASSO model. **(B)** The most informative immune features and their respective immunological communities are highlighted on the correlation network.

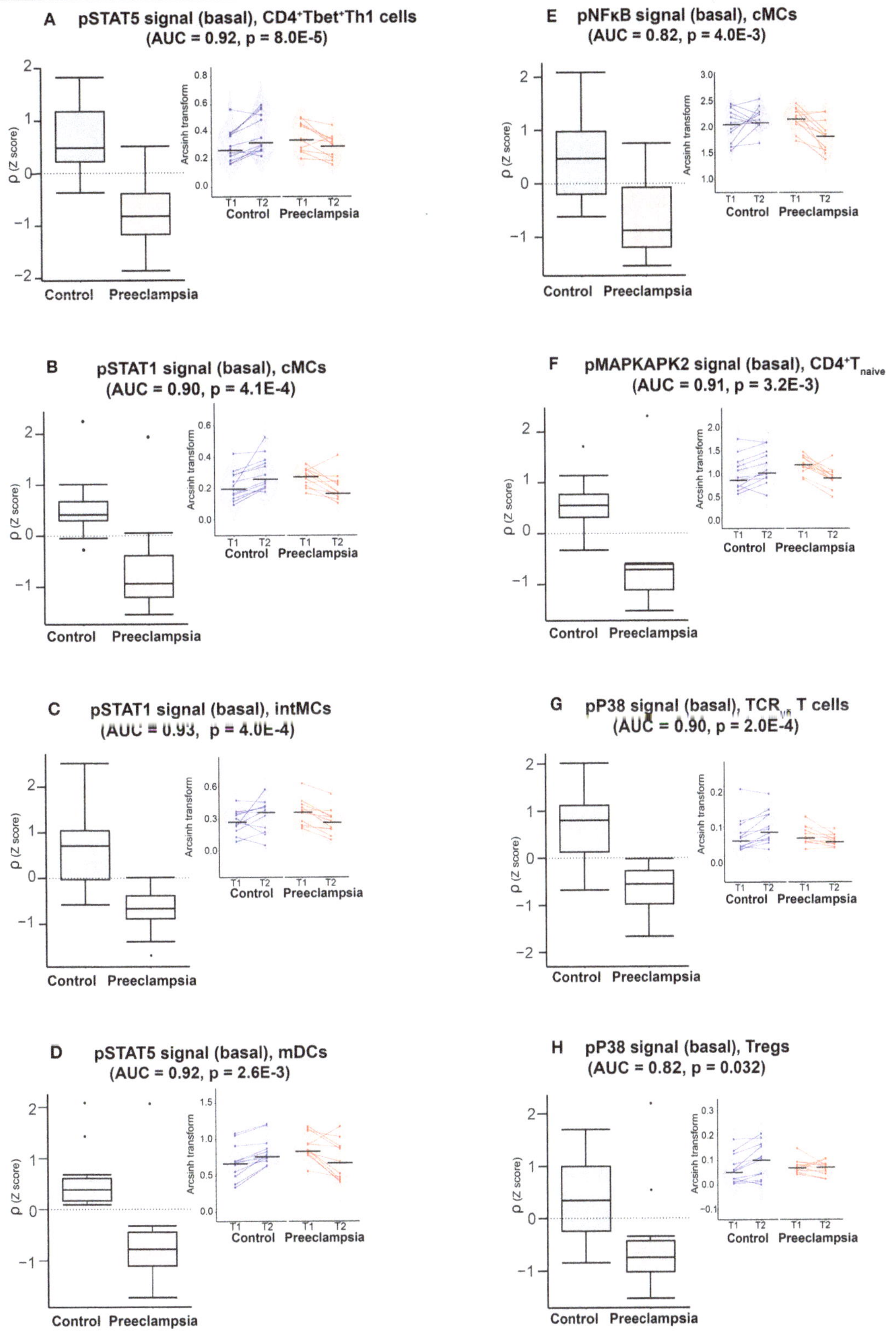

FIGURE 4 | Model components reveals disrupted innate and adaptive immune cell dynamics in preeclampsia. Boxplots (**left panels**) depict the rate of change (ρ) of indicated immune feature for the eigth most informative model components. AUC and p-values are indicated on each graph (ROC analysis). Insets (**right panels**) depict immune feature values (arcsinh transform of the mass cytometry intracellular signal mean intensity) at individual time points (T1, T2) and for each patient. Color code: purple = controls, orange = preeclampsia.

expression of the IL-4 receptor (50)] as well as Th1 differentiation [by inducing the expression of Tbet and the IL-12 receptor (42)]. The IL-2/STAT5 pathway is also critical for promoting peripheral Tregs (44) and inhibiting Th17 differentiation (51). Therefore, the decreasing pSTAT5 signal—which was higher during the first trimester in the preeclamptic group than in the control group—observed in CD4$^+$T cell subsets early in preeclamptic pregnancies likely reflects multiple dysfunctional processes affecting T cell differentiation, including increased Th1 over Th2 differentiation during the first trimester as well as decreased Treg differentiation between the first and second trimesters.

However, IL-2 is not the only factor regulating the JAK/STAT5 signaling pathway. In fact, multiple inflammatory, but also hormonal, and placental factors implicated in pregnancy converge onto the JAK/STAT5 pathway, including prolactin, chorionic somatomammotropin hormone (CSH)-1, IFN-γ and IL-3 (52, 53). Leptin, which has consistently been associated with preeclampsia in multiple large-scale proteomics studies can also activate the JAK/STAT5 pathway (54). Assessment of JAK/STAT5 signaling dynamics may therefore provide a sensitive cellular readout of immune dysfunction that reflects the integration of multiple signals ultimately driving abnormal CD4$^+$T cell responses early in the pathogenesis of preeclampsia.

Several other results of our analysis resonated well with prior knowledge of immune system dysfunction associated with preeclampsia, notably among innate immune cell subsets. In general, observed differences in the rate of change of innate immune responses (decelerated in the preeclampsia group compared to the control group) were driven in part by higher signaling responses during the first trimester of pregnancy in the preeclampsia group. In cMCs, the basal pNFκB signals was increased in the preeclampsia group in the first trimester compared to the control group (**Figure 4E**). A similar finding was observed for the pSTAT1 signal in the pro-inflammatory intMCs monocyte subtype (**Figure 4C**). An elevated signaling activity in innate immune cells early during pregnancy is consistent with previous studies suggesting exaggerated activation of proinflammatory innate immune responses in patients who develop preeclampsia (55, 56).

Interestingly, the majority of dysregulated immune responses were signaling responses rather than frequency changes. In this regard, some of our findings differ from previous analyses of peripheral immune responses associated with preeclampsia. For instance, neither the frequency of Tregs or of Th1 cells (13, 14, 41)—which have previously been shown to differ between normal and preeclamptic pregnancies—were selected as informative features of the multivariate model. Instead, measurement over time of signaling responses in Tregs (pP38 and pSTAT5) and in CD4$^+$Tbet$^+$Th1 cells (pSTAT5) were among the strongest individual classifiers for preeclampsia. These results suggest that a functional read-out of proximal signaling responses may be more informative than the assessment of cell distribution alone in identifying immune dysfunction associated with preeclampsia.

This study has several limitations. The recruitment of study participants at a single hospital limits the generalizability of the results. Larger, multicenter studies will be required to generalize our findings to women from various demographic, ethnic, and socioeconomic backgrounds. The sample size was also too small to allow us to distinguish between early (GA $<$ 34 weeks, $n = 2$) and late ($n = 9$) onset preeclampsia. Determining whether immune system dynamics differ between subtypes of preeclampsia will be important, since different pathophysiological mechanisms may underlie the clinical spectrum of preeclampsia. The study did not exclude patients with autoimmune diseases, such as SLE, which are known risk factors for preeclampsia (57–59). In particular, the pathogenesis of SLE involves an imbalance between Tregs and Th17 cells (60), which is also associated with immunological dysregulation in preeclampsia (13, 61, 62). Interestingly, our LASSO model and its major individual components remained strongly associated with preeclampsia when excluding patients with autoimmune diseases from our analysis. These results are in line with previous observations showing differential transcriptomic immune profiles in pregnant women with SLE who do or do not develop preeclampsia, suggesting that certain immune responses associated with preeclampsia are independent of SLE (63). While our study is underpowered to detect immune responses associated with SLE and other comorbidities (such as gestational diabetes), our results suggest that reported differences between the two study groups are not driven by the presence of these known immunological confounders.

In addition, while mass cytometry offers unprecedented informational content at the single-cell level, the technology remains limited to the measurement of ~50 pre-selected phenotypic and functional parameters per immune cell. For instance, selected antibody panel did not allow for the analysis of intracellular cytokines, which would be helpful for further characterization of Th1, Th2, and Th17 cell subsets. We cannot exclude that additional phenotypic markers not included in the current analysis will allow detecting more informative and predictive cell frequency features. Similarly, the choice of stimulation conditions was limited by sample availability. Finally, the analysis was limited to immune cell dynamics that vary linearly with time, and did not capture non-linear immunological adaptations which are known to occur during pregnancy. However, the approach provides an analytical and statistical framework for future studies aimed at exhaustive characterizations of immune cell dynamics in normal and preeclamptic pregnancies.

In summary, our study reveals significant alterations in the dynamics of maternal immune system adaptations months before the clinical onset of preeclampsia. The data and analytical approaches presented here suggest that measures of maternal immune system dynamics early in pregnancy hold significant promise for identifying women at risk for developing preeclampsia later during pregnancy.

ETHICS STATEMENT

This study was carried out in accordance with the recommendations of the Lucile Packard Children's Hospital at Stanford University Institutional Review Board with written informed consent from all subjects. All subjects gave written informed consent in accordance with the Declaration of Helsinki. The protocol was approved by the Stanford Institutional Review Board.

AUTHOR CONTRIBUTIONS

BG conceived and supervised the execution of the study and wrote the manuscript. BG supervised all mass cytometry data collection and curation. NA supervised all statistical analysis. MA assisted in interpreting data and writing the manuscript. XH conduct the sample process, cytometry data collection and analysis. MG performed statistical analysis. XH, MG, IAS, and LP wrote the manuscript. KA, RW, AJ, and DG assisted in clinical data collection and interpretation. EG and AST assisted in the fabrication of reagents and sample processing for mass cytometry analysis. JE, BB, ET, NS, AC, AT, JH, and RF assisted in data visualization. RW, VW, MD, YB, MH, CQ, RG, BC, GS, and DS assisted in interpreting mass cytometry data and writing the manuscript.

ACKNOWLEDGMENTS

The authors thank Adrian G. Yabut, Ana Campos, Olivia Tigre, Hector Romero from the March of Dimes Prematurity Research Center at Stanford University, and Girija Dhamdhere, Ph.D. (Basic Life Science Research Associate in David B. Lewis's Lab, Department of Pediatrics, Stanford University) for assistance with the PBMC stimulation experiment.

REFERENCES

1. American College of Obstetricians and Gynecologists, Task Force on Hypertension in Pregnancy, Roberts JM, August PA, Bakris G, Barton JR, et al. Report of the American college of obstetricians and gynecologists' task force on hypertension in Pregnancy. *Obstet Gynecol.* (2013) 122:1122–31. doi: 10.1097/01.AOG.0000437382.03963.88
2. Steegers EA, von Dadelszen P, Duvekot JJ, Pijnenborg R. Pre-eclampsia. *Lancet.* (2010) 376:631–44. doi: 10.1016/S0140-6736(10)60279-6
3. Chaiworapongsa T, Chaemsaithong P, Korzeniewski SJ, Yeo L, Romero R. Pre-eclampsia part 2: prediction, prevention and management. *Nat Rev Nephrol.* (2014) 10:531–40. doi: 10.1038/nrneph.2014.103
4. Redman CW, Sargent IL. Latest advances in understanding preeclampsia. *Science.* (2005) 308:1592–4. doi: 10.1126/science.1111726
5. Zeisler H, Hund M, Verlohren S. The sFlt-1:PlGF ratio in women with suspected preeclampsia. *N Engl J Med.* (2016) 374:1785–6. doi: 10.1056/NEJMc1602338
6. Freeman DJ, McManus F, Brown EA, Cherry L, Norrie J, Ramsay JE, et al. Short- and long-term changes in plasma inflammatory markers associated with preeclampsia. *Hypertension.* (2004) 44:708–14. doi: 10.1161/01.HYP.0000143849.67254.ca
7. Redman CW, Sargent IL. Immunology of pre-eclampsia. *Am J Reprod Immunol.* (2010) 63:534–43. doi: 10.1111/j.1600-0897.2010.00831.x
8. Laresgoiti-Servitje E. A leading role for the immune system in the pathophysiology of preeclampsia. *J Leukoc Biol.* (2013) 94:247–57. doi: 10.1189/jlb.1112603
9. Chaiworapongsa T, Chaemsaithong P, Yeo L, Romero R. Pre-eclampsia part 1: current understanding of its pathophysiology. *Nat Rev Nephrol.* (2014) 10:466–80. doi: 10.1038/nrneph.2014.102
10. Arck PC, Hecher K. Fetomaternal immune cross-talk and its consequences for maternal and offspring's health. *Nat Med.* (2013) 19:548–56. doi: 10.1038/nm.3160
11. PrabhuDas M, Bonney E, Caron K, Dey S, Erlebacher A, Fazleabas A, et al. Immune mechanisms at the maternal-fetal interface: perspectives and challenges. *Nat Immunol.* (2015) 16:328–34. doi: 10.1038/ni.3131
12. Saito S, Shiozaki A, Nakashima A, Sakai M, Sasaki Y. The role of the immune system in preeclampsia. *Mol Aspects Med.* (2007) 28:192–209. doi: 10.1016/j.mam.2007.02.006
13. Darmochwal-Kolarz D, Kludka-Sternik M, Tabarkiewicz J, Kolarz B, Rolinski J, Leszczynska-Gorzelak B, et al. The predominance of Th17 lymphocytes and decreased number and function of Treg cells in preeclampsia. *J Reprod Immunol.* (2012) 93:75–81. doi: 10.1016/j.jri.2012.01.006
14. Steinborn A, Schmitt E, Kisielewicz A, Rechenberg S, Seissler N, Mahnke K, et al. Pregnancy-associated diseases are characterized by the composition of the systemic regulatory T cell (Treg) pool with distinct subsets of Tregs. *Clin Exp Immunol.* (2012) 167:84–98. doi: 10.1111/j.1365-2249.2011.04493.x
15. Than NG, Romero R, Tarca AL, Kekesi KA, Xu Y, Xu Z, et al. Integrated systems biology approach identifies novel maternal and placental pathways of preeclampsia. *Front Immunol.* (2018) 9:1661. doi: 10.3389/fimmu.2018.01661
16. Kashanian M, Aghbali F, Mahali N. Evaluation of the diagnostic value of the first-trimester maternal serum high-sensitivity C-reactive protein level for prediction of pre-eclampsia. *J Obstetr Gynaecol Res.* (2013) 39:1549–54. doi: 10.1111/jog.12105
17. Tangeras LH, Austdal M, Skrastad RB, Salvesen KA, Austgulen R, Bathen TF, et al. Distinct first trimester cytokine profiles for gestational hypertension and preeclampsia. *Arterioscler Thrombosis Vasc Biol.* (2015) 35:2478–85. doi: 10.1161/ATVBAHA.115.305817
18. Salazar Garcia MD, Mobley Y, Henson J, Davies M, Skariah A, Dambaeva S, et al. Early pregnancy immune biomarkers in peripheral blood may predict preeclampsia. *J Reprod Immunol.* (2018) 125:25–31. doi: 10.1016/j.jri.2017.10.048
19. Raymond D, Peterson E. A critical review of early-onset and late-onset preeclampsia. *Obstet Gynecol Surv.* (2011) 66:497–506. doi: 10.1097/OGX.0b013e3182331028
20. Bastek JA, Elovitz MA. The role and challenges of biomarkers in spontaneous preterm birth and preeclampsia. *Fertil Steril.* (2013) 99:1117–23. doi: 10.1016/j.fertnstert.2013.01.104
21. Bendall SC, Simonds EF, Qiu P, Amir el AD, Krutzik PO, Finck R, et al. Single-cell mass cytometry of differential immune and drug responses across a human hematopoietic continuum. *Science.* (2011) 332:687–96. doi: 10.1126/science.1198704
22. Spitzer MH, Nolan GP. Mass cytometry: single cells, many features. *Cell.* (2016) 165:780–91. doi: 10.1016/j.cell.2016.04.019
23. Olin A, Henckel E, Chen Y, Lakshmikanth T, Pou C, Mikes J, et al. Stereotypic immune system development in newborn children. *Cell.* (2018) 174:1277–92 e14. doi: 10.1016/j.cell.2018.06.045
24. Good Z, Sarno J, Jager A, Samusik N, Aghaeepour N, Simonds EF, et al. Single-cell developmental classification of B cell precursor acute lymphoblastic leukemia at diagnosis reveals predictors of relapse. *Nat Med.* (2018) 24:474–83. doi: 10.1038/nm.4505

25. Simoni Y, Chng MHY, Li S, Fehlings M, Newell EW. Mass cytometry: a powerful tool for dissecting the immune landscape. *Curr Opin Immunol.* (2018) 51:187–96. doi: 10.1016/j.coi.2018.03.023
26. Aghaeepour N, Ganio EA, McIlwain D, Tsai AS, Tingle M, Van Gassen S, et al. An immune clock of human pregnancy. *Sci Immunol.* (2017) 2:2946. doi: 10.1126/sciimmunol.aan2946
27. Ghaemi MS, DiGiulio DB, Contrepois K, Callahan B, Ngo TTM, Lee-McMullen B, et al. Multiomics modeling of the immunome, transcriptome, microbiome, proteome and metabolome adaptations during human pregnancy. *Bioinformatics.* (2018) 2018:bty537-bty. doi: 10.1093/bioinformatics/bty537
28. Wise PH, Shaw GM, Druzin ML, Darmstadt GL, Quaintance C, Makinen E, et al. Risky business: meeting the structural needs of transdisciplinary science. *J Pediatr.* (2017) 191:255–8. doi: 10.1016/j.jpeds.2017.08.072
29. Zivanovic N, Jacobs A, Bodenmiller B. A practical guide to multiplexed mass cytometry. *Curr Topics Microbiol Immunol.* (2014) 377:95–109. doi: 10.1007/82_2013_335
30. Zunder ER, Finck R, Behbehani GK, Amir el AD, Krishnaswamy S, Gonzalez VD, et al. Palladium-based mass tag cell barcoding with a doublet-filtering scheme and single-cell deconvolution algorithm. *Nat Protoc.* (2015) 10:316–33. doi: 10.1038/nprot.2015.020
31. Finck R, Simonds EF, Jager A, Krishnaswamy S, Sachs K, Fantl W, et al. Normalization of mass cytometry data with bead standards. *Cytometry Part A J Int Soc Anal Cytol.* (2013) 83:483–94. doi: 10.1002/cyto.a.22271
32. van der Maaten L, Hinton G. Visualizing data using t-SNE. *J Mach Learn Res.* (2008) 9:2579–605. Available online at: http://www.jmlr.org/papers/v9/vandermaaten08a.html
33. Csardi G, Nepusz T. The igraph software package for complex network research. *Inter J Complex Syst.* (2006) 1695:1–9. Available online at: https://cran.r-project.org/web/packages/igraph/citation.html
34. Blondel VD, Guillaume JL, Lambiotte R, Lefebvre E. Fast unfolding of communities in large networks. *J Stat Mech-Theory E.* (2008) 10:1–12. doi: 10.1088/1742-5468/2008/10/P10008
35. Tibshirani R. Regression Shrinkage and Selection via the Lasso. *J R Stat Soc Series B.* (1996) 58:267–88. doi: 10.1111/j.2517-6161.1996.tb02080.x
36. Le Gars M, Kay AW, Bayless NL, Aziz N, Dekker CL, Swan GE, et al. Increased proinflammatory responses of monocytes and plasmacytoid dendritic cells to influenza A virus infection during pregnancy. *J Infect Dis.* (2016) 214:1666–71. doi: 10.1093/infdis/jiw448
37. Ruocco MG, Chaouat G, Florez L, Bensussan A, Klatzmann D. Regulatory T-cells in pregnancy: historical perspective, state of the art, and burning questions. *Front Immunol.* (2014) 5:389. doi: 10.3389/fimmu.2014.00389
38. Kay AW, Fukuyama J, Aziz N, Dekker CL, Mackey S, Swan GE, et al. Enhanced natural killer-cell and T-cell responses to influenza A virus during pregnancy. *Proc Natl Acad Sci USA.* (2014) 111:14506–11. doi: 10.1073/pnas.1416569111
39. Somerset DA, Zheng Y, Kilby MD, Sansom DM, Drayson MT. Normal human pregnancy is associated with an elevation in the immune suppressive CD25+ CD4+ regulatory T-cell subset. *Immunology.* (2004) 112:38–43. doi: 10.1111/j.1365-2567.2004.01869.x
40. Pradeu T, Jaeger S, Vivier E. The speed of change: towards a discontinuity theory of immunity? *Nat Rev Immunol.* (2013) 13:764–9. doi: 10.1038/nri3521
41. Saito S, Sakai M. Th1/Th2 balance in preeclampsia. *J Reprod Immunol.* (2003) 59:161–73. doi: 10.1016/S0165-0378(03)00045-7
42. Liao W, Lin JX, Wang L, Li P, Leonard WJ. Modulation of cytokine receptors by IL-2 broadly regulates differentiation into helper T cell lineages. *Nat Immunol.* (2011) 12:551–U247. doi: 10.1038/ni.2030
43. Burchill MA, Yang JY, Vogtenhuber C, Blazar BR, Farrar MA. IL-2 receptor beta-dependent STAT5 activation is required for the development of Foxp3(+) regulatory T cells. *J Immunol.* (2007) 178:280–90. doi: 10.4049/jimmunol.178.1.280
44. Cohen AC, Nadeau KC, Tu W, Hwa V, Dionis K, Bezrodnik L, et al. Cutting edge: decreased accumulation and regulatory function of CD4+ CD25(high) T cells in human STAT5b deficiency. *J Immunol.* (2006) 177:2770–4. doi: 10.4049/jimmunol.177.5.2770
45. Fainboim L, Arruvito L. Mechanisms involved in the expansion of Tregs during pregnancy: role of IL-2/STAT5 signalling. *J Reprod Immunol.* (2011) 88:93–8. doi: 10.1016/j.jri.2010.12.007
46. Adler HS, Kubsch S, Graulich E, Ludwig S, Knop J, Steinbrink K. Activation of MAP kinase p38 is critical for the cell-cycle-controlled suppressor function of regulatory T cells. *Blood.* (2007) 109:4351–9. doi: 10.1182/blood-2006-09-047563
47. Newell EW, Cheng Y. Mass cytometry: blessed with the curse of dimensionality. *Nat Immunol.* (2016) 17:890–5. doi: 10.1038/ni.3485
48. Hastie T, Tibshirani R, Friedman J. *The Elements of Statistical Learning: Data Mining, Inference and Prediction.* 2 edn. New York, NY: Springer (2009).
49. Taylor BD, Ness RB, Klebanoff MA, Zoh R, Bass D, Hougaard DM, et al. First and second trimester immune biomarkers in preeclamptic and normotensive women. *Pregnancy Hypertens.* (2016) 6:388–93. doi: 10.1016/j.preghy.2016.09.002
50. Zhu J, Cote-Sierra J, Guo L, Paul WE. Stat5 activation plays a critical role in Th2 differentiation. *Immunity.* (2003) 19:739–48. doi: 10.1016/S1074-7613(03)00292-9
51. Laurence A, Tato CM, Davidson TS, Kanno Y, Chen Z, Yao Z, et al. Interleukin-2 signaling via STAT5 constrains T helper 17 cell generation. *Immunity.* (2007) 26:371–81. doi: 10.1016/j.immuni.2007.02.009
52. O'Shea JJ, Plenge R. JAK and STAT signaling molecules in immunoregulation and immune-mediated disease. *Immunity.* (2012) 36:542–50. doi: 10.1016/j.immuni.2012.03.014
53. Murray PJ. The JAK-STAT signaling pathway: input and output integration. *J Immunol.* (2007) 178:2623–9. doi: 10.4049/jimmunol.178.5.2623
54. Gong Y, Ishida-Takahashi R, Villanueva EC, Fingar DC, Munzberg H, Myers MG Jr. The long form of the leptin receptor regulates STAT5 and ribosomal protein S6 via alternate mechanisms. *J Biol Chem.* (2007) 282:31019–27. doi: 10.1074/jbc.M702838200
55. Kim YM, Romero R, Oh SY, Kim CJ, Kilburn BA, Armant DR, et al. Toll-like receptor 4: a potential link between "danger signals," the innate immune system, and preeclampsia? *Am J Obstet Gynecol.* (2005) 193(3, Supplement):921.e1–.e8. doi: 10.1016/j.ajog.2005.07.076
56. Luppi P, Tse H, Lain KY, Markovic N, Piganelli JD, DeLoia JA. Preeclampsia activates circulating immune cells with engagement of the NF-kappaB pathway. *Am J Reprod Immunol.* (2006) 56:135–44. doi: 10.1111/j.1600-0897.2006.00386.x
57. Lin HC, Chen SF, Chen YH. Increased risk of adverse pregnancy outcomes in women with rheumatoid arthritis: a nationwide population-based study. *Ann Rheumatic Dis.* (2010) 69:715–7. doi: 10.1136/ard.2008.105262
58. Do SC, Druzin ML. Systemic lupus erythematosus in pregnancy: high risk, high reward. *Curr Opin Obstetr Gynecol.* (2019) 31:120–6. doi: 10.1097/GCO.0000000000000528
59. Chakravarty EF, Khanna D, Chung L. Pregnancy outcomes in systemic sclerosis, primary pulmonary hypertension, and sickle cell disease. *Obstet Gynecol.* (2008) 111:927–34. doi: 10.1097/01.AOG.0000308710.86880.a6
60. Tower C, Mathen S, Crocker I, Bruce IN. Regulatory T cells in systemic lupus erythematosus and pregnancy. *Am J Reprod Immunol.* (2013) 69:588–95. doi: 10.1111/aji.12081
61. Dhillion P, Wallace K, Herse F, Scott J, Wallukat G, Heath J, et al. IL-17-mediated oxidative stress is an important stimulator of AT1-AA and hypertension during pregnancy. *Am J Physiol Regulatory Integr Compar Physiol.* (2012) 303:R353–8. doi: 10.1152/ajpregu.00051.2012
62. Cornelius DC, Hogg JP, Scott J, Wallace K, Herse F, Moseley J, et al. Administration of interleukin-17 soluble receptor C suppresses TH17 cells, oxidative stress, and hypertension in response to placental ischemia during pregnancy. *Hypertension.* (2013) 62:1068–73. doi: 10.1161/HYPERTENSIONAHA.113.01514
63. Hong S, Banchereau R, Maslow BL, Guerra MM, Cardenas J, Baisch J, et al. Longitudinal profiling of human blood transcriptome in healthy and lupus pregnancy. *J Exp Med.* (2019) 216:1154–69. doi: 10.1084/jem.20190185
64. Maecker HT, McCoy JP, Nussenblatt R. Standardizing immunophenotyping for the Human Immunology Project. *Nat Rev Immunol.* (2012) 12:191–200. doi: 10.1038/nri3158

16

Early-Life Compartmentalization of Immune Cells in Human Fetal Tissues Revealed by High-Dimensional Mass Cytometry

Na Li[1], Vincent van Unen[1], Nannan Guo[1], Tamim Abdelaal[2,3], Antonios Somarakis[4], Jeroen Eggermont[4], Ahmed Mahfouz[4], Susana M. Chuva de Sousa Lopes[5], Boudewijn P. F. Lelieveldt[3,4] and Frits Koning[1]*

[1] Department of Immunohematology and Blood Transfusion, Leiden University Medical Center, Leiden, Netherlands, [2] Leiden Computational Biology Center, Leiden University Medical Center, Leiden, Netherlands, [3] Department of Pattern Recognition and Bioinformatics Group, Delft University of Technology, Delft, Netherlands, [4] Department of Radiology, Leiden University Medical Center, Leiden, Netherlands, [5] Department of Anatomy and Embryology, Leiden University Medical Center, Leiden, Netherlands

***Correspondence:**
Frits Koning
f.koning@lumc.nl

The human fetal immune system must protect the infant against the sudden exposure to a large variety of pathogens upon birth. While it is known that the fetal immune system develops in sequential waves, relatively little is known about the composition of the innate and adaptive immune system in the tissues. Here, we applied high-dimensional mass cytometry to profile the immune system in human fetal liver, spleen, and intestine. With Hierarchical Stochastic Neighbor Embedding (HSNE) we distinguished 177 distinct immune cell clusters, including both previously identified and novel cell clusters. PCA analysis indicated substantial differences between the compositions of the immune system in the different organs. Through dual t-SNE we identified tissue-specific cell clusters, which were found both in the innate and adaptive compartment. To determine the spatial location of tissue-specific subsets we developed a 31-antibody panel to reveal both the immune compartment and surrounding stromal elements through analysis of snap-frozen tissue samples with imaging mass cytometry. Imaging mass cytometry reconstructed the tissue architecture and allowed both the characterization and determination of the location of the various immune cell clusters within the tissue context. Moreover, it further underpinned the distinctness of the immune system in the tissues. Thus, our results provide evidence for early compartmentalization of the adaptive and innate immune compartment in fetal spleen, liver, and intestine. Together, our data provide a unique and comprehensive overview of the composition and organization of the human fetal immune system in several tissues.

Keywords: imaging mass cytometry (IMC), immune composition, fetal intestine, fetal spleen, fetal liver, high-dimensional analysis, mass cytometry (CyTOF)

INTRODUCTION

The notion of phenotypical and functional differences between the fetal and adult immune system has been widely accepted. The human fetal immune system has to maintain tolerance toward the semi-allogeneic environment *in utero* while being prepared for the massive exposure to foreign antigens directly after birth (1, 2). The ontogeny of the immune system occurs in sequential waves during gestation. Fetal hematopoiesis is initiated in the yolk sac around day 16 of the development, then transits to the fetal liver at 6 weeks until 22 weeks gestational age, where the progenitors give rise to both lymphoid and myeloid cells (3). T cells have been identified as early as 10 weeks of gestation while Foxp3^{+}CD4^{+} regulatory T (Treg) cells, whose generation is mainly driven by maternal alloantigens, have also been observed in different fetal tissues (4). Furthermore, it has been shown that human fetal dendritic cells in spleen, skin, thymus, and lung promote prenatal T-cell immune suppression (5). Interestingly, several studies have provided evidence for the existence of memory-like T (Tm) cells in fetal spleen (6), skin (7), intestine (8, 9), and cord blood (10), which produce pro-inflammatory cytokines such as IFN-γ and TNF-α, suggesting functional maturation of T cells *in utero*. In line with the discovery of pro-inflammatory T cells, mucosa-associated invariant T cells as well as natural killer (NK) cells and innate lymphoid cells (ILCs) have also been found to be present in the fetal intestine (11, 12). A potential link between the composition of the prenatal immune system and disease later in life has been proposed (9, 13). Thus, the fetal immune system has both pro-inflammatory and immune suppressive capacity.

Most investigations of the human fetal immune system are based on umbilical cord blood collected at birth. However, the representation of cord blood has recently been questioned as cord blood samples were heterogeneous without clearly shared patterns in cell and plasma protein composition (14). Although in recent years several reports (5, 8) have studied the fetal immune system in tissues, due to the scarcity of human fetal tissues and technique limitations, a system-wide and detailed characterization of the human fetal immune system is currently lacking. Mass cytometry (cytometry by time-of-flight; CyTOF) now offers the opportunity to analyze the heterogeneity of the human immune system in an unbiased and data-driven fashion by the simultaneous measurement of over 40 unique cellular markers at the single-cell level with unprecedented resolution (15). As traditional analysis approaches for flow cytometry are not compatible with high-dimensional mass cytometry datasets, dimensionality reduction-based approaches such as t-stochastic neighbor embedding (t-SNE) (16) have been widely used as they allow users to analyze all the markers concurrently in an unbiased manner. Moreover, hierarchical SNE (HSNE) has removed the scalability limitation of t-SNE, allowing the analysis of tens of millions of cells at single-cell resolution (17).

Here, we applied suspension mass cytometry to study the complexity and heterogeneity of the immune system in the human fetal intestine, liver, and spleen and confirmed the existence of previously identified subsets through the unsupervised HSNE analysis. In addition, we provide evidence for the existence of previously unrecognized distinct cell clusters. Besides the heterogeneity within each tissue, our data further reveals clear tissue-specific signatures in both the innate and adaptive immune compartment as early as week 16 of gestation. Finally, we employed imaging mass cytometry to reconstruct the tissue architecture and characterize and determine the location of the immune cell clusters within the tissue context, results that underpinned the compartmentalization of the immune system in the tissues. Together these data provide a comprehensive and valuable resource for understanding the fetal immune development and linking prenatal immunity with immunity after birth.

MATERIALS AND METHODS

Human Fetal Tissues and Cell Isolation

Human fetal tissues from elective abortions were obtained from healthy pregnancy after informed consent. The gestational age ranged from 16 to 21 weeks. In total, 10 fetuses were included in the current study. Single-cell suspensions from different tissues were prepared as previously described (18). Briefly, the mesentery and meconium were removed from the fetal intestine. The intestines were then cut into small fragments and treated with 1 mM dithiothreitol (Fluka) in 15 mL of HBSS (Sigma-Aldrich) for 2 × 10 min (replacing buffer) at room temperature to dissolve the mucus and subsequently with 1 mM ethylenediaminetetraacetic acid (Merck) in 15 mL of Hank's balanced salt solution (ThermoFisher Scientific), under rotation for 2 × 1 h (replacing buffer) at 37°C to separate the epithelium from the lamina propria fraction. To obtain single-cell suspensions from the lamina propria, the intestines were rinsed with HBSS and incubated with 15 mL Iscove's Modified Dulbecco's Medium (IMDM; Lonza) supplemented with 10% fetal calf serum (FCS), 10 U/mL collagenase IV (Worthington), 200 μg/mL DNAse I grade II (Roche Diagnostics), at 37°C overnight, after which cell suspensions were filtered through a 70 μm nylon cell strainer. Finally, the immune cells were isolated with a Percoll (GE Healthcare) gradient. Fetal liver and spleen tissues were cut into small pieces then filtered through a 70 μm nylon cell strainer and the immune cells were isolated with Ficoll-Paque^{TM} density gradient (provided by the pharmacy of Leiden University Medical Center). All isolated cells were stored in liquid nitrogen. Study approval was granted by the Medical Ethics Commission of Leiden University Medical Center (protocol P08.087). All experiments were conducted in accordance with local ethical guidelines and the principles of the Declaration of Helsinki.

Mass Antibodies and Antibody Conjugation

Antibodies used for suspension and imaging mass cytometry are listed in **Tables S1**, **S3**, separately. Conjugation of the purified antibodies lacking carrier protein with metal reporters was performed with the MaxPar X8 antibody labeling kit (Fluidigm Sciences) according to the manufacturer's instruction.

Suspension Mass Cytometry Staining and Data Acquisition

Procedures for suspension mass cytometry antibody staining and data acquisition were carried out as previously described (18). Briefly, cells from different fetal tissues were incubated with 1 mL 500x diluted 500 μM Cell-ID intercalator-103Rh (Fluidigm Sciences) for 15 min at room temperature to identify dead cells. Cells were then stained with metal-conjugated antibodies for 45 min at room temperature. After staining, cells were labeled with 1 mL 1,000x diluted 125 μM Cell-ID intercalator-Ir (Fluidigm Sciences) to stain all cells in MaxPar Fix and Perm Buffer (Fluidigm Sciences) overnight at 4°C. Finally, cells were acquired by CyTOF 2^{TM} mass cytometer (Fluidigm Sciences). Data were normalized by using EQ Four Element Calibration Beads (Fluidigm Sciences) with the reference EQ passport P13H2302 during the course of each experiment.

Imaging Mass Cytometry Staining and Data Acquisition

Snap-frozen human fetal splenic, intestinal and liver biopsies were sectioned at a thickness of 5 μm. All sections were fixed by incubating with 1% paraformaldehyde for 5 min at room temperature followed by 100% methanol for 5 min at −20 °C. After fixation, tissue sections were washed in Dulbecco's phosphate-buffered saline (ThermoFisher Scientific) containing 0.5% bovine serum albumin and 0.05% Tween, rehydrated in additive-free Dulbecco's phosphate-buffered saline. After washing again, tissue sections were blocked with Superblock Solution (ThermoFisher Scientific) for 30 min in a humid chamber. Tissue sections were then stained with a metal-conjugated antibody master mix overnight at 4°C, washed and incubated with 125 nM Cell-ID Intercalator-Ir for 30 min at room temperature. After a further wash, tissue sections were dipped in Milli-Q water (Merck Millipore) for 1 min and dried for 20 min at room temperature. The acquisition was performed using a Hyperion imaging mass cytometer (Fluidigm Sciences) at a resolution of 1 μm, with settings aligned to company guidelines. The ablation frequency was 200 Hz, and the energy was 6 dB. Regions of interest were acquired at a size of 1 × 1 mm^2. All data were stored as MCD files and txt files.

Data Analysis

Data for single, live CD45$^{+/dim}$ cells gated from each sample individually using Cytobank as shown in **Figure S1**, were sample tagged and hyperbolic arcsinh transformed with a cofactor of 5 within Cytosplore^{+HSNE} (17). The major immune lineages in **Figure 1** were then identified by performing hierarchical stochastic neighbor embedding (HSNE) in Cytosplore^{+HSNE} software (17). HSNE was carried out with default parameters (perplexity: 30; iterations: 1,000). For the cluster identification, each cluster contains at least 100 cells. All HSNE plots were generated in Cytosplore (19). Cellular signatures of immune cells for each sample individually were generated in Cytosplore. Due to homogeneity and abundance of B cells in the fetal spleen, B cells from each spleen were downsampled to 50,000 cells to deduce the cellular signatures. The similarity between two paired t-SNE maps was quantified by Jensen-Shannon (JS) divergence by measuring the similarity between corresponding probability density distribution after converting t-SNE maps to two-dimensional probability density functions in Matlab R2015b. Hierarchical clustering of the phenotype heatmap was created with Euclidean correction and average linkage clustering while the cell frequency heatmap with Spearman correction and average linkage clustering in Matlab R2015b. Principal component analysis (PCA) was computed with the cluster frequencies of CD45$^{+/dim}$ cells in the individual samples using "prcomp" function, and the result was visualized using "ggbiplot" function in R software. The cluster t-SNE map in **Figure 5B** was performed as our previous study (20). Briefly, the data matrix with cluster frequencies of CD45$^{+/dim}$ cells in the individual samples as input variance was normalized and computed to select the top ten highest variance principal components as input to the t-SNE analysis. Hence, the cluster with similar profiles clustered together in the t-SNE map. Images in **Figure 6** and **Figure S4** were generated using MCD Viewer software v1.0.560 (Fluidigm Sciences).

RESULTS

Identification of Major Immune Lineages Across Human Fetal Tissues

To explore the immune system in the human fetus, we employed a previously described CyTOF panel (**Table S1**) consisting of 35-metal isotope tagged monoclonal antibodies (18) designed to identify the major immune lineages (B cells, CD4$^+$ T, CD8$^+$ T, γδ T cells, ILCs, and myeloid cells) and determine the heterogeneity within these lineages. For this purpose, the panel consisted of lineage markers, markers specific for cell differentiation, activation, trafficking, and function. With this panel, single-cell suspensions from fetal intestines ($N = 7$), fetal spleens ($N = 3$), and fetal livers ($N = 3$) **Table S2**) were analyzed. Single, live CD45$^+$ cells were distinguished by event length, DNA stains, and CD45 antibody stains (**Figure S1A**). In the liver, but not in the spleen and intestine, three distinct subpopulations were observed based on different CD45 and DNA stainings (**Figure S1B**). Here, CD45^{hi}DNA^{low} cells represent lymphoid cells, while CD45^{hi}DNA^{hi} and CD45^{low}DNA^{hi} cells correspond to myeloid and CD34$^+$ precursor cells, respectively (**Figure S1B**). All antibodies displayed a clear separation between antibody-negative and -positive cells as described previously (18).

To determine the major immune lineages, we pooled the data (1.6 × 10^6 CD45$^+$ cells) derived from seven fetal intestines (39,357 ± 17,836 cells), three fetal spleens (365,653 ± 148.098 cells) and three fetal livers (69,928 ± 18,146 cells) (**Figure S1C**) and performed a 3-level HSNE analysis in Cytosplore^{+HSNE} (17) from a global overview down to the single cell level. Here, HSNE landmarks depicted the global composition of the immune system (**Figure 1**). Based on the marker expression profiles (**Figure 1A**) and density features of the embedded cells (**Figure 1B**), we identified 6 phenotypically distinct major lineage clusters at the overview level, namely CD20$^+$ B cells, CD3$^+$CD4$^+$ T cells, CD3$^+$CD8$^+$ T cells

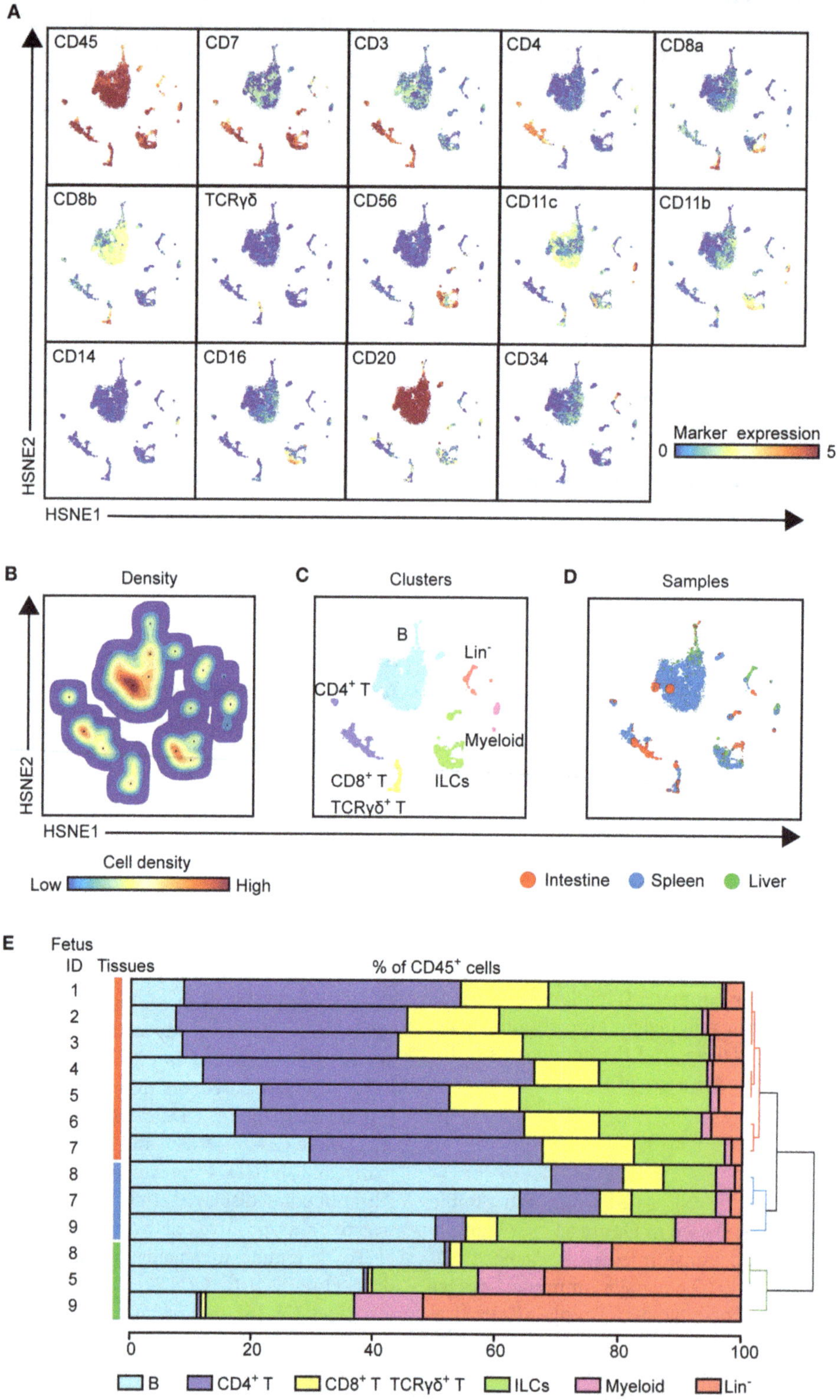

FIGURE 1 | HSNE analysis distinguishes major immune lineages across human fetal tissues. **(A)** HSNE embedding of 1.6 million immune cells derived from fetal intestines ($N = 7$, 0.3×10^6 cells), fetal spleens ($N = 3$, 1.1×10^6 cells), and fetal livers ($N = 3$, 0.2×10^6 cells) at the overview level. Each dot represents a HSNE landmark and the size of the landmark is proportional to the number of cells that each landmark represents. Colors of the landmarks represent ArcSinh5-transformed expression values of the indicated markers. **(B)** A density map showing the local probability density of the embedded cells where black dots display the centroids of identified clusters using GMS clustering. **(C)** A HSNE plot showing main immune lineage cluster partitions in different colors. **(D)** HSNE embedding as shown in **(A)**. Colors represent different tissues. **(E)** The composition of major immune lineage clusters for CD45$^+$ cells in the individual fetal tissues is represented in horizontal

(Continued)

FIGURE 1 | bars where the colored segment lengths represent the proportion of cells as a percentage of $CD45^+$ cells in the sample. The dendrogram shows the hierarchical clustering of samples. Colors represent the different tissues as shown in **(D)**. Numbers indicate fetus ID.

and $CD3^+TCR\gamma\delta^+$ T cells, $CD3^-CD20^-CD11c^-CD7^+$ ILCs, $CD11c^+$ myeloid cells and a $CD3^-CD20^-CD11c^-CD7^{+/-}$ lineage-negative (Lin^-) cell cluster (**Figure 1C**). In addition, the global differences in immune composition across tissues were revealed by visualizing the tissue-origin of the cells (**Figure 1D**). Next, we quantified the relative frequencies of major immune lineage clusters in each fetal tissue sample, showing that B cells were more abundant in the fetal spleen and fetal liver while Lin^- cells were most profound in the fetal liver. $CD4^+$ T, $CD8^+$ T, and $\gamma\delta$ T cells together comprised more than 50% of immune cells in the fetal intestine but were typically lower in the fetal liver. There was no significant difference in the distribution of ILCs across fetal tissues. The frequencies of myeloid cells were low in all fetal tissues, however, these cells were relatively more abundant in fetal liver (**Figure 1E**). Importantly, unbiased hierarchical clustering of cell frequencies grouped the tissue samples in a tissue-specific manner (**Figure 1E**), indicating that despite differences between the samples the composition of the major immune lineage of each fetal tissue was relatively constant and tissue-specific.

Together, these global analyses revealed that the major immune lineages could be readily identified in each fetal tissue, and that the composition of these lineages differs between the examined human fetal tissues.

Visualization of Cellular Signatures Across Human Fetal Tissues

To compare immune cells between all samples and between the tissues, we next selected the major immune lineage clusters individually and embedded the clusters at the single-cell level to deduce the cellular signatures (**Figure 2**) (20). The results demonstrate that the intestine, spleen, and liver displayed a distinct cellular signature for most of the seven major immune lineages. We observed especially highly distinct differences between the intestinal samples compared to the spleen and liver samples (**Figure 2A**). Also, the results underscore that samples from the same tissue type have a highly similar cellular signature (**Figure 2A**). We next applied the Jensen-Shannon (JS) divergence method to quantify the similarities and differences between pairs of t-SNE maps (**Figure 2B**). For all major immune lineages, the JS divergence was highest between the intestinal samples and the spleen and liver samples, while considerable differences in JS divergence were also found between the spleen and the liver samples, except for the ILC compartment. In general, the composition of the B cells, $CD4^+$ T cells and ILCs was more similar within a tissue group while more variation was present among $CD8^+$ T cells, $\gamma\delta$ T cells, and myeloid cells (**Figure 2B**). Together, the visualization of cellular signatures provided further evidence for the distinct composition of immune system in the fetal tissues.

High-Dimensional Analysis Reveals Unprecedented Immune Heterogeneity in Human Fetal Tissues

To extend the analysis we next selected every main immune lineage individually and embedded them at the second level (B cells) or single-cell data level to identify the phenotypically distinct clusters, here illustrated for the $CD8^+$ T cell compartment (**Figure 3**). First, the cluster including $CD8^+$ T and $\gamma\delta$ T cells (105,211 cells) were selected at the overview level and embedded in the second level of the HSNE analysis (**Figures 3A,B**), followed by selection of the $CD8^+$ T cells (69,269 cells) to zoom-in further (**Figure 3B**), revealing more single-cell details (**Figure 3C**). Based on the density features of the t-SNE-embedded cells, we identified 20 distinct $CD8^+$ T cell clusters (**Figure 3C**), each defined by a unique maker expression profile (**Figure 3D**). After hierarchical clustering of the heatmap, these clusters grouped into five main metaclusters (**Figures 3D,E**). $CD45RA^+CCR7^+$ naive T (Tn) cells were classified into two groups based on CD161 expression while $CD45RA^-CCR7^+$ central memory T (Tcm) and $CD45RA^+CCR7^-$ terminally differentiated T (Temra) cells were detected in the $CD127^{dim/-}$ compartment. In addition, a group of $CD127^+CD161^{high}CCR6^+KLRG\text{-}1^+$ Temra cells clustered separately from the other groups. We next quantified the cell frequencies of each cluster per sample and performed the hierarchical clustering of different samples based on the cell frequencies. In line with previous studies (21), several clusters including Tn cells (CD8_01-05, 15) and Tem cells (CD8_08, CD8_10) were present in all tissues (**Figure 3E**). $CD127^-CD161^{+/-}$ Temra (CD8_07, CD8_11, CD8_13, and CD8_20) mainly existed in the spleen and liver whereas $PD\text{-}1^-$ Tem (CD8_09) were mainly abundant in the intestine. Hierarchical clustering revealed that all the intestinal samples clustered together whereas the spleen and liver samples clustered intermixed with each other.

By applying this approach to all 7 major immune lineage clusters, we identified 177 phenotypically distinct clusters (8 B cell clusters, 24 $CD4^+$ T cell clusters, 20 $CD8^+$ T cell cluster, 38 $\gamma\delta$ T cell cluster (**Figures S2A–C** and **Figure 4A**), 39 ILC clusters, 26 myeloid cell clusters and 22 Lin^- clusters (**Figures S3A,B** and **Figure 4B**). Consistent with previous reports (2), $IgM^+HLA\text{-}DR^+$ B cells were identified in all three tissues while the plasmacytoid dendritic cells (pDC)-like cells and monocytes were mainly identified in the intestine and non-intestine, respectively. In addition to Tn cells, we also identified several clusters of Tm cells, which were more prominent in the $CD4^+$ T cell compartment in the fetal intestine, as reported (9). Strikingly, some of these Tm cells expressed a higher level of CD127, CD161, CCR6 and c-KIT, the latter a marker typically associated with progenitor cell types. Similarly, we identified a rare $c\text{-}KIT^+$ ($CD117^+$) $CD8^+$ T cell population (CD8_16, <1%

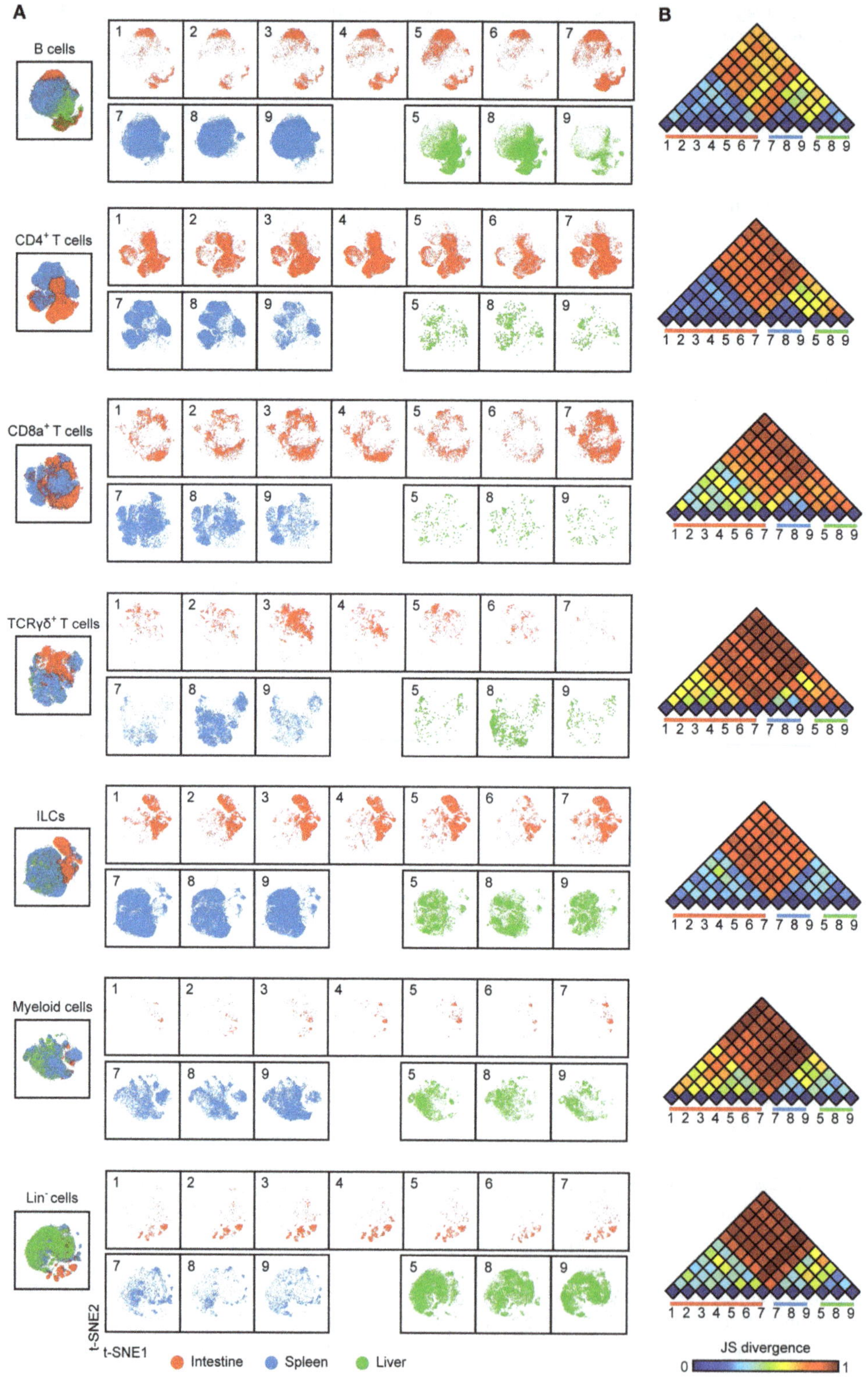

FIGURE 2 | Cellular signatures reveal the immune cell compartmentalization across human fetal tissues. **(A)** A collective t-SNE was performed on each major immune lineage individually and stratified for samples. The plots are showing in total 1.5×10^5 B cells, 2.3×10^5 $CD4^+$ T cells, 6.9×10^4 $CD8^+$ T cells, 3.6×10^4 $\gamma\delta$ T cells, 2.6×10^5 ILCs, 6.4×10^4 myeloid cells and 8.7×10^4 Lin^- cells. Colors represent different tissues. Numbers indicate fetus ID. **(B)** The similarity of a pair of t-SNE plots is shown by Jensen-Shannon (JS) divergence within the major immune lineage. A higher JS divergence value indicates higher dissimilarity between pairwise t-SNE plots.

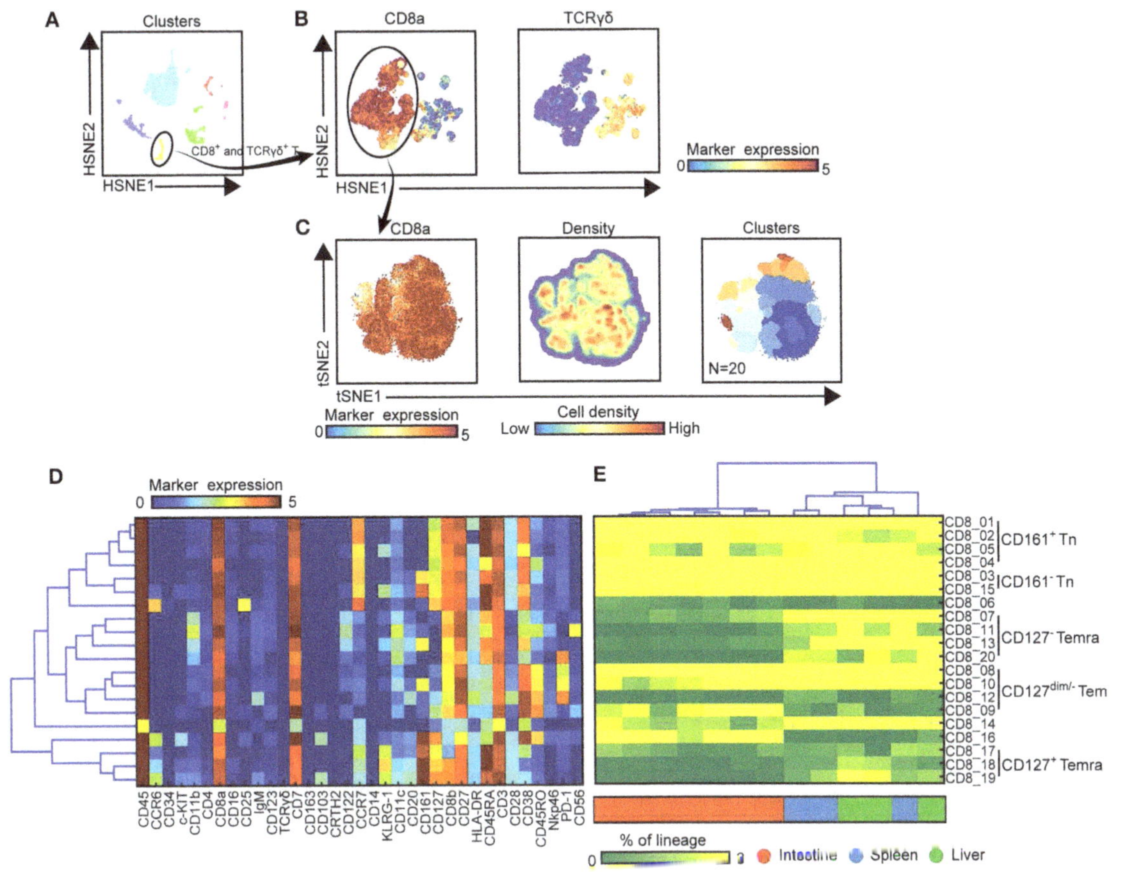

FIGURE 3 | Identification of phenotypically distinct clusters in the CD8$^+$ T cell compartment across human fetal tissues. **(A)** Global level of HSNE embedding of 1.6 million immune cells as shown in **Figure 1C** showing major immune lineage cluster partitions in different colors. **(B)** Second level of HSNE embedding of CD8$^+$ T and γδ T cells (1.1 × 10^5 cells) derived from fetal intestines (N =7), fetal spleens (N = 3), and fetal livers (N = 3). Colors represent the ArcSinh5-transformed expression values of CD8a and TCR γδ. **(C)** A t-SNE embedding of collective CD8$^+$ T cells (6.9 × 10^4 cells) derived from fetal intestines (N = 7), fetal spleens (N = 3), and fetal livers (N = 3). Colors represent the ArcSinh5-transformed expression values of CD8a (left panel). A density map showing the local probability density of the embedded cells (middle panel). Colors represent cluster partitions (right panel). **(D)** Heatmap (blue-to-red scale) showing the median marker expression values of the clusters identified in **(C)** and hierarchical clustering thereof. **(E)** Heatmap (green-to-yellow scale) showing the corresponding cell frequencies of identified clusters of total CD8$^+$ T cells in each sample. The dendrogram shows the hierarchical clustering of samples. Colors represent different fetal tissues. Tn, naive T cells; Tem, effector memory T cells; Temra, terminally differentiated T cells.

of CD45$^+$ cells) that is almost exclusively present in the intestine. As reported (22), helper-ILCs were more dominant in the fetal intestine than the fetal spleen and liver, where the majority of ILCs were different types of NK cells such as CD27$^-$CD11b$^+$, CD27$^+$CD11b$^+$ NK clusters. Moreover, CD34$^+$CD38$^+$, CD34$^+$CD38^{dim}, CD34$^+$CD38$^-$ precursor cell clusters and several previously unknown precursor-like cell clusters were mainly identified in the fetal liver (e.g., Lin$^-$_02, Lin$^-$_03, Lin$^-$_15, Lin$^-$_17) (**Figure 4**), an important organ for fetal hematopoiesis. Unbiased hierarchical clustering of cell frequencies for each sample revealed a clear distinction between the fetal intestine and the other two tissues in both the adaptive and innate immune compartment (**Figure 4**). The separation between fetal spleen and liver was readily observed in the innate immune compartment, due to the differential abundance of CD34$^+$ cells and certain types of ILCs, such as ILC2 and CD7^{dim} ILC3-like cells (**Figure 4B**), but not in the adaptive immune compartment.

Altogether, our data reveal that there is far greater heterogeneity of the immune system in human fetal tissues than previously appreciated and provide evidence for the existence of previously unknown immune cell types.

An Integrated System-Wide Analysis of the Immune System Reveals Early Immune Compartmentation Across Fetal Tissues

In order to investigate the entire immune profiles across fetal tissues, a PCA was performed on the samples based on the cluster frequency values of CD45$^{+/dim}$ cells. The samples were clearly separated from each other based on the tissue origin, especially the intestines and the other two organs by principal component 1 (explaining 39.1% variance) (**Figure 5A**). In consistency with the cellular signatures (**Figure 2**), the variance of immune composition within spleens was higher than that within intestines and livers (**Figure 5A**).

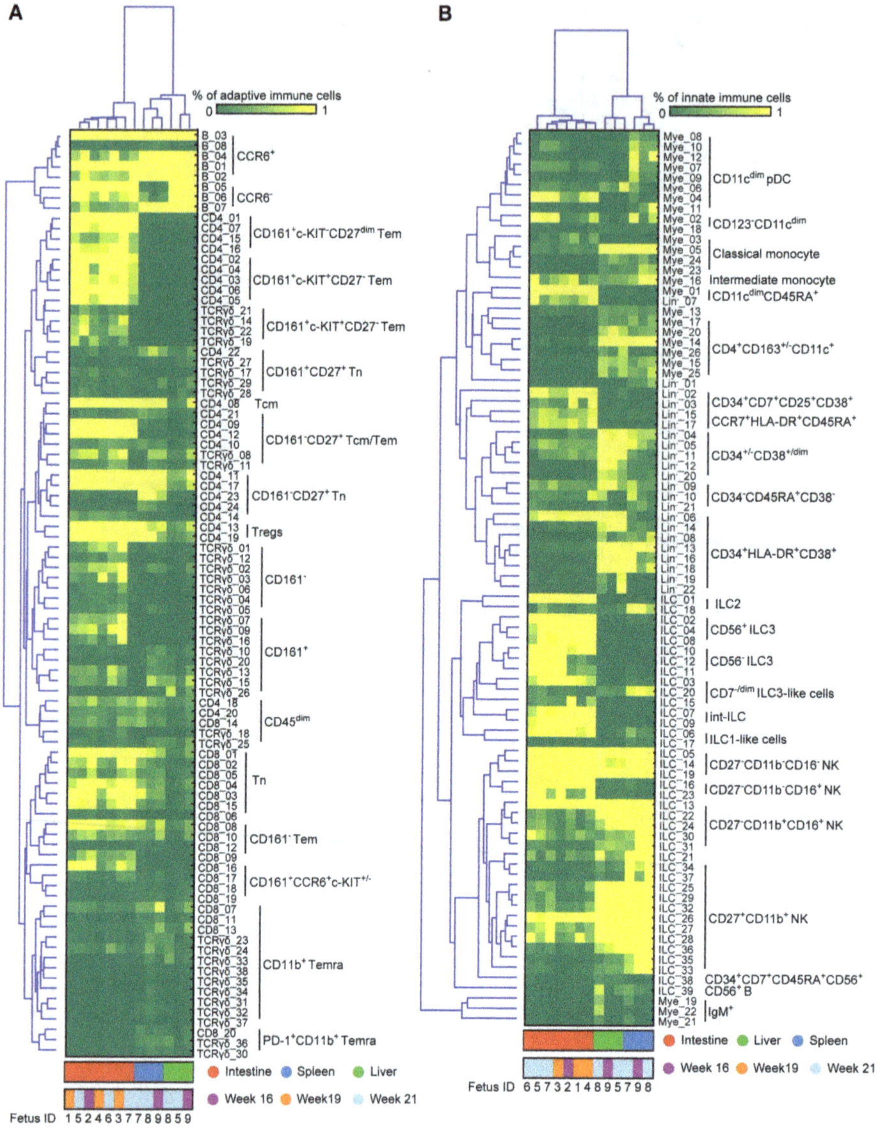

FIGURE 4 | Immune system landscapes visualize cell cluster composition across human fetal tissues. **(A,B)** Heatmap showing the cell frequencies of 90 adaptive and 87 innate immune clusters identified in **Figures S2, S3** combined with hierarchical clustering of samples (Top) and phenotype of clusters (Left). Colors represent different fetal tissues as indicated. Tem, effector memory T cells; Tcm, central memory T cells; Temra, terminally differentiated T cells; pDC, plasmacytoid dendritic cells.

To reveal which cell clusters were most strongly associated with the tissue-specificity, we performed a t-SNE analysis on 177 clusters based on the frequency values, visualizing networks of cell clusters, which determined the tissue-associated patterns (**Figure 5B**). Moreover, the dual-tSNE identified the top ten ranked clusters that contributed to the sample clustering patterns (**Figure 5C**). This analysis yielded three distinct networks of cell clusters corresponding to the three tissue types (**Figure 5B**). Several distinct hematopoietic progenitor clusters (Lin$^-$_16, ILC_38, Lin$^-$_04, Lin$^-$_18, Lin$^-$_20, and Lin$^-$_12) and four myeloid populations (Mye_13, Mye_14, Mye_15, and Mye_25) were specifically found in the fetal liver. For the fetal intestines, the main types of contributing cells were lymphoid precursors (Lin$^-$_15 and Lin$^-$_17) and CD4$^+$ Tm clusters (CD4_01, CD4_08, CD4_09, CD4_06, CD4_04, CD4_05), including three previously unidentified c-KIT$^+$ clusters, while for the spleen a diverse pool of CD8$^+$ T cells, B cells and myeloid cells contributed to the tissue-specific signature (**Figure 5C**). Together, the integrated system-wide analysis of the immune system reveals a unique immune cell landscape and early-life immune compartmentation across human fetal tissues, suggesting different immune responses *in situ* during human fetal development.

Imaging Mass Cytometry Reveals the Tissue-Specific Signatures *in situ*

To extend the understanding of the fetal immune system, we applied an imaging mass cytometry panel comprising

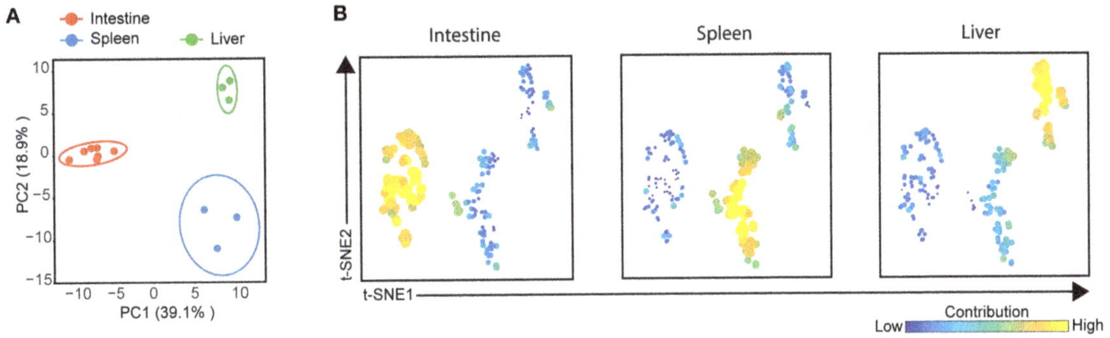

C

Top ten ranked clusters cotributing to the tissue-specific t-SNE sample signatures

Nr	Intestine	Spleen	Liver
1	CD4_01 CD161^{+}c-KIT^{-} Tem	Mye_12 IgM^{+}CD11c^{dim} pDC	Lin^{-}_16 CD34^{+}CD7^{-}HLA-DR^{+}CD38^{dim}
2	CD4_08 CD161^{+} Tcm	B_04 CCR7^{-}CCR6^{+} B	ILC_38 CD34^{+}CD7^{+}CD38^{+}CD45RA^{+}CD56^{+}
3	CD4_14 CCR6^{+}CD161^{-}CD27^{+} Tn	CD8_19 CD103^{+}CCR6^{+}c-KIT^{-} Tn	Lin^{-}_04 CD34^{-}c-KIT^{+}
4	CD4_06 CD27^{dim}CD161^{+}c-KIT^{+} Tem	Lin^{-}_01 CD34^{+}CD56^{+}CD38^{dim}HLA-DR^{+}	Mye_13 CD11c^{dim}CD45RA^{-}
5	CD4_09 CD161^{-}CD27^{+} Tcm	B_03 CCR7^{dim}CCR6^{+} B	Mye_14 CD4^{+} M2 macrophage
6	CD4_04 CD161^{+}c-KIT^{+}CD103^{+} Tem	CD8_20 PD-1^{+}CD11b^{+} Temra	Lin^{-}_18 CD34^{+}CD7^{-}c-KIT^{+}HLA-DR^{+}CD38^{dim}
7	CD4_05 CD161^{+}c-KIT^{+} DN	CD8_11 CD56^{+}PD-1^{-}CD11b^{+} Temra	Mye_15 CD4^{+} pDC
8	Mye_01 CD45RA^{dim}CD123^{dim}CD11c^{dim}	ILC_34 CD16^{+}CD11b^{+}CD11c^{+}CD27^{+} NK	Lin^{-}_20 CD34^{+}CD38^{dim}c-KIT^{+}HLA-DR^{-}
9	Lin^{-}_15 CD34^{+}CD7^{+}CCR7^{+}CD45RA^{+}CD38^{dim}	CD8_12 PD-1^{+}CD161^{-} Tem	Mye_25 CD4^{+}CD123^{dim}CD45RA^{+}
10	Lin^{-}_17 CD34^{+}CD7^{+}CCR7^{dim}CD45RA^{+}CD38^{+}	B_07 CCR6^{-}CD38^{dim} B	Lin^{-}_12 CD34^{dim}CD38^{+}CD7^{dim}HLA-DR^{-}

FIGURE 5 | Integrated analysis of immune cluster composition reveals highly discriminatory tissue-specific signatures. **(A)** Principal component analysis (PCA) of 13 fetal samples. PCA was computed on the cell frequencies of 177 immune clusters per sample (as the percentage of CD45^{+} cells) and top 2 principal components are shown describing 58% of total variance. One dot represents a single sample. Colors represent different fetal tissues. **(B)** t-SNE embedding of 177 immune clusters derived from 13 samples showing the tissue-specific signatures. Every dot represents a single immune cluster. The size of the dot is proportional to the value of cell frequency, which is more similar across tissues when the clusters are together closer. **(C)** Table depicting top ten ranked clusters contributing to tissue-specific t-SNE sample signatures with biological annotation. Tem, effector memory T cells; Tcm, central memory T cells; Temra, terminally differentiated T cells; pDC, plasmacytoid dendritic cells; NK, natural killer cell.

31 antibodies to determine the spatial distribution of the immune and stromal cells in the tissues *in situ* from one individual. This panel contained markers for visualizing the tissue architecture such as E-cadherin (epithelium), D2-40 (lymphatic endothelium), vimentin (intermediate filament), smooth muscle actin (SMA) and collagen I (extracelluar matrix), markers to identify various immune cell subsets such as T cells (CD3, CD8, CD4, CD45RA, CD45RO), NK cells (CD7 and CD56), myeloid cells (CD163) and antigen presenting cells/activated cells (HLA-DR), as well as markers expressed by both stromal and immune cells such as CD31. In addition, the proliferation marker Ki-67 was included (**Table S3**). With this panel, tissue sections derived from the fetal intestine, spleen and liver were analyzed. All antibodies showed clear positive signals as illustrated in one of the regions of interest (ROIs) derived from the fetal intestine (**Figure S4**).

To obtain further information on the phenotype and localization of immune cell subsets within the tissue context, we visualized combinations of specific markers (**Figure 6**). Staining with E-cadherin, SMA and DNA were used to show the tissue structure, reflecting the overall morphological differences between the tissues and the distribution of the immune cells was revealed by CD45 staining. Most CD45^{+} immune cells were in the E-cadherin^{-} lamina propria in the intestine whereas these cells were scattered in the fetal spleen and liver (**Figure 6A**). While the majority of CD45^{+} immune cells lacked expression of Ki-67 in all three tissues, many non-immune cells in the fetal liver and to a lesser extent in the fetal spleen were stained by the Ki-67-specific antibody, indicative of cell division and likely linked to the development of these organs at this stage (**Figure 6B**). In agreement with earlier work, Ki-67^{+} cells in the intestines resided in the crypt (**Figure 6B**), where stem cells and progenitor cells are enriched (23). Consistent with findings using suspension mass cytometry, both CD45RA^{+} Tn and CD45RA^{-} Tm cells were identified in all three tissues. Compared with the spleen and liver, the CD45RA^{-} Tm cells were most abundant in the intestine, especially CD161^{+}CD45RA^{-} T cells (**Figure 6C**). CD161^{-}CD45RA^{-} T cells and CD161^{+}CD45RA^{+} T cells were more predominate in the spleen and liver as compared with the other two tissues, respectively (**Figure 6C**). Finally, simultaneous visualization of CD3, CD7, and CD127 reveals that $CD3^+$ T cells and $CD3^-CD7^+CD127^+$ ILCs (**Figure 6D**, white and purple arrows) were located in close proximity of each other in the lamina propria of the intestine.

Together, these data confirmed the existence of tissue-specific subsets *in situ* and underpinned the distinctness of the immune system in the tissues at the second trimester during pregnancy.

DISCUSSION

While recent studies have investigated the heterogeneity and functionality of the developing immune system in prenatal life (5, 9, 10), knowledge of the immune system development remains sparse due to the relative scarcity of fetal tissues. In the current study, we applied high-dimensional mass cytometry to dissect both the innate and adaptive immune compartment in the human fetal intestine, spleen, and liver in an unbiased and data-driven manner. For data analysis, we used HSNE (17), an in-house developed software, which allows the identification of phenotypically distinct clusters in datasets consisting of millions of cells. In line with previous work (5, 6, 9, 10, 22), we were able to readily define the major cell lineages and substantial heterogeneity therein, and reveal the identity of previously unrecognized cell clusters. Moreover, our results provide evidence for tissue-specific compartmentalization of both the innate and adaptive immune compartment early in the second trimester of pregnancy. Altogether, our results confirm and extend previous studies that have analyzed the immune subsets in mucosal and lymphoid tissues from human fetus with immunohistochemical analysis (8, 24) or traditional multi-color flow cytometry (5, 25). Our comprehensive analysis provides a valuable resource that may aid future studies into the development of the human immune system during gestation.

Consistent with previous reports, our analysis confirmed the distinctness of the human fetal liver, with enrichment of myeloid and $CD34^+$ precursor cell clusters. Six out of the top ten ranked clusters contributing to liver-specific signatures were $CD34^+$ precursor cells. Also, we observed extensive diversity within the $CD34^+$ cell population due to differential expression of several markers including c-KIT and HLA-DR, possibly reflecting differentiation pathways and linked to the crucial role of the fetal liver in haematopoiesis in prenatal life.

In addition, several other features distinguished the immune systems found in the tissues examined. Here, $CD27^-CD11b^-$ NK cells exhibiting dominant inhibitory signals (26) were found primarily in the intestine while $CD27^-CD11b^+$ NK and $CD27^+CD11b^+$ NK cells with dominant activating signals (26) predominate in the spleen and liver and contribute to the tissue partitions and demarcate different functions in the tissues examined. Also, helper-ILCs were mainly present in the fetal intestine, as reported (22). Moreover, we have previously reported that memory-like T cells are located in the fetal intestine (9) but to a much lower degree in fetal spleen and liver indicative of *in situ* immune priming and maturation of T cells in the developing intestine. Intriguingly, previously unidentified $CCR6^+$c-$KIT^+CD45RO^+$ subpopulations of T cells were identified in all lineages in the fetal intestine, but not in other organs. Expression of c-KIT, a receptor for stem cell factor, has been shown to demarcate a subset of human $CD8^+$ Tm cells with self-renewal properties (27). Moreover, flow-sorted c-KIT^+ Tm cells cocultured with OP9 stromal cells in the presence of stem cell factor and IL-7 proliferated *in vitro* (data not shown). These observations suggest a potential role for $CCR6^+$c-KIT^+ Tm cells in the conservation of mucosal T cell memory.

CD161 has previously been shown to define a transcriptional and functional phenotype across human T cell lineages with an innate-like ability to respond to cytokines (28) while another study has described that CD161 mediates prenatal immune suppression (29). In our study, CD161-expressing T cells are more pronounced in the human fetal intestine as compared to fetal spleen and liver, consistent with a unique function of $CD161^+$ cells within the fetal intestine. HLA-DR^+ myeloid cells and B cells were found in all three organs, however, all B cells lacked expression of CD27, a classical memory B cell marker.

We have used imaging mass cytometry to gain insight into the localization of specific immune subsets within the tissue context. The results reiterate the highly distinct organization of the immune compartment in the three tissues investigated and allow the simultaneous analysis of cellular activity, i.e., cell proliferation. We demonstrate that this can be used to confirm results obtained by single-cell suspension mass cytometry while simultaneously obtaining information on the co-localization of specific immune subsets. For example, we obtained evidence that in the intestinal lamina propria $CD3^+$ T cells are found in close proximity of $CD3^-CD7^+CD127^+$ ILC, possibly pointing toward "crosstalk" between these cell subsets. This will be the topic of future studies.

While this study is one of the first to study the immune landscape in human fetal tissues with high-dimensional analysis at the single-cell level, our study has limitations. First, we did not observe much heterogeneity in the B population as our antibody panel lacked several markers required for this. It would thus be important to include other antibodies such as IgD, CD10 and CD5 to dissect the B compartment further. Second, we had only access to fetal material from the second trimester (16–21 gestational weeks) and obtained only a limited number of fetal tissues. In future studies, it would thus be valuable also to include samples from the first and third trimester and increase the number of fetal tissues. Third, while we identified 177 known and unknown cell clusters, the functional properties of these subsets need to be clarified in future studies. Also, as we did notice some minor differences in the composition of the myeloid compartment when comparing tissue samples of different gestational age, future studies should address this in more detail. Finally, due to the cell isolation procedure the dataset does not provide information on granulocytes and red blood cells. It will be valuable to investigate this in future studies. It should be noted that while the analysis provides comprehensive insight into the organization of the tissue sample investigated, a single specimen biopsy cannot reflect the structural complexity of these organs, this will be the subject of future studies.

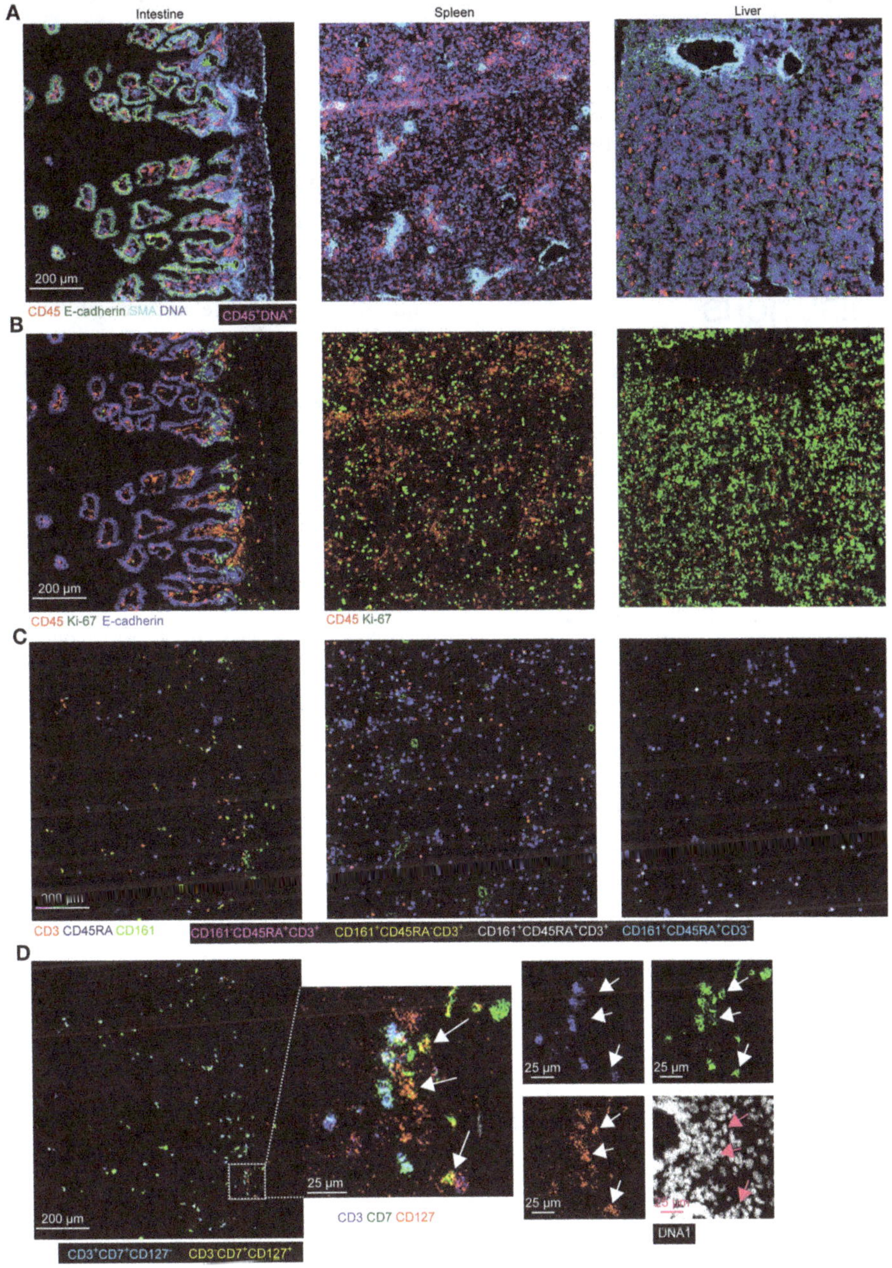

FIGURE 6 | Spatial localization of immune and stromal cell subsets across tissues. **(A–D)** Representative mass cytometry images of one region of interest (ROI) of the fetal intestine, spleen, and liver derived from one individual, displaying the overlay of the indicated makers. Scale bar: 200 μm. Colors and scale bars are identical in **(A–C)**. The numbers of ROIs for intestine, spleen, and liver are 6, 2 and 4, respectively. **(A)** CD45 in red, E-cadherin in green, SMA in cyan and DNA in blue. **(B)** CD45 in red, Ki-67 in green and E-cadherin in blue. **(C)** CD3 in red, CD45RA in blue and CD161 in green. **(D)** CD3 in blue, CD7 in green, CD127 in red and DNA in white. White and purple arrows indicate the $CD3^{-}CD7^{+}CD127^{+}$ ILCs.

Nevertheless, our mass cytometric analysis provides the first global, comprehensive, and detailed description of the immune landscape in the developing fetus in several tissues, reveals tissue-specific signatures, and demonstrates a clear immune compartmentalization in the tissues in prenatal life. Recent studies have indicated that events shaping the immune system *in utero* and in early life can have a significant impact on the development of diseases in adult life (30–32). Detailed understanding of the early development of the immune system is crucial for the development of strategies to prevent such diseases and our study may help to achieve that goal.

ETHICS STATEMENT

Human fetal tissues from elective abortions were obtained after informed consent. Study approval was granted by the Medical Ethics Commission of Leiden University Medical Center (protocol P08.087). All experiments were conducted in accordance with local ethical guidelines and the principles of the Declaration of Helsinki.

AUTHOR CONTRIBUTIONS

NL and FK conceived the study and wrote the manuscript. NL performed most experiments with the help of NG. NL performed most of the analyses with the help of VvU, TA, AS, JE, AM, and BL. SC provided human fetal tissues. All authors discussed the results and commented on the manuscript.

ACKNOWLEDGMENTS

We thank the Center for Contraception, Abortion and Sexuality (CASA) in Leiden and The Hague for their efforts in collecting and providing the fetal material, Dr. M. Bialecka and M. Nieveen for the dissection of the fetal tissues and ME Ijsselsteijn and NFCC de Miranda for optimizing the imaging mass cytometry panel.

REFERENCES

1. Frascoli M, Coniglio L, Witt R, Jeanty C, Fleck-Derderian S, Myers DE, et al. Alloreactive fetal T cells promote uterine contractility in preterm labor via IFN-γ and TNF-α. *Sci Transl Med.* (2018) 10:eaan2263. doi: 10.1126/scitranslmed.aan2263
2. Steiniger B, Ulfig N, Risse M, Barth PJ. Fetal and early post-natal development of the human spleen: from primordial arterial B cell lobules to a non-segmented organ. *Histochem Cell Biol.* (2007) 128:205–15. doi: 10.1007/s00418-007-0296-4
3. Zhang X, Zhivaki D, Lo-Man R. Unique aspects of the perinatal immune system. *Nat Rev Immunol.* (2017) 17:495–507. doi: 10.1038/nri.2017.54
4. Mold JE, Michaëlsson J, Burt TD, Muench MO, Beckerman KP, Busch MP, et al. Maternal alloantigens promote the development of tolerogenic fetal regulatory T cells *in utero*. *Science.* (2008) 322:1562–5. doi: 10.1126/science.1164511
5. McGovern N, Shin A, Low G, Low D, Duan K, Yao LJ, et al. Human fetal dendritic cells promote prenatal T-cell immune suppression through arginase-2. *Nature.* (2017) 546:662–6. doi: 10.1038/nature22795
6. Michaëlsson J, Mold JE, McCune JM, Nixon DF. Regulation of T cell responses in the developing human fetus. *J Immunol.* (2006) 176:5741–8. doi: 10.4049/jimmunol.176.10.5741
7. Schuster C, Vaculik C, Prior M, Fiala C, Mildner M, Eppel W, et al. Phenotypic characterization of leukocytes in prenatal human dermis. *J Invest Dermatol.* (2012) 132:2581–92. doi: 10.1038/jid.2012.187
8. Bunders MJ, van der Loos CM, Klarenbeek PL, van Hamme JL, Boer K, Wilde JC, et al. Memory CD4(+)CCR5(+) T cells are abundantly present in the gut of newborn infants to facilitate mother-to-child transmission of HIV-1. *Blood.* (2012) 120:4383–90. doi: 10.1182/blood-2012-06-437566
9. Li N, van Unen V, Abdelaal T, Guo N, Kasatskaya SA, Ladell K, et al. Memory CD4(+) T cells are generated in the human fetal intestine. *Nat Immunol.* (2019) 20:301–12. doi: 10.1038/s41590-018-0294-9
10. Zhang X, Mozeleski B, Lemoine S, Dériaud E, Lim A, Zhivaki D, et al. CD4 T cells with effector memory phenotype and function develop in the sterile environment of the fetus. *Sci Transl Med.* (2014) 6:238ra272. doi: 10.1126/scitranslmed.3008748
11. Leeansyah E, Loh L, Nixon DF, Sandberg JK. Acquisition of innate-like microbial reactivity in mucosal tissues during human fetal MAIT-cell development. *Nat Commun.* (2014) 5:3143. doi: 10.1038/ncomms4143
12. Hazenberg MD, Spits H. Human innate lymphoid cells. *Blood.* (2014) 124:700–9. doi: 10.1182/blood-2013-11-427781
13. Williams TJ, Jones CA, Miles EA, Warner JO, Warner JA. Fetal and neonatal IL-13 production during pregnancy and at birth and subsequent development of atopic symptoms. *J Allergy Clin Immunol.* (2000) 105:951–9. doi: 10.1067/mai.2000.106211
14. Olin A, Henckel E, Chen Y, Lakshmikanth T, Pou C, Mikes J, et al. Stereotypic immune system development in newborn children. *Cell.* (2018) 174:1277–92.e1214. doi: 10.1016/j.cell.2018.06.045
15. Bandura DR, Baranov VI, Ornatsky OI, Antonov A, Kinach R, Lou X, et al. Mass cytometry: technique for real time single cell multitarget immunoassay based on inductively coupled plasma time-of-flight mass spectrometry. *Anal Chem.* (2009) 81:6813–22. doi: 10.1021/ac901049w
16. van der Maaten L, Hinton G. Visualizing data using t-SNE. *J Mach Learn Res.* (2008) 9:2579–605.
17. van Unen V, Höllt T, Pezzotti N, Li N, Reinders MJT, Eisemann E, et al. Visual analysis of mass cytometry data by hierarchical stochastic neighbour embedding reveals rare cell types. *Nat Commun.* (2017) 8:1740. doi: 10.1038/s41467-017-01689-9
18. Li N, van Unen V, Höllt T, Thompson A, van Bergen J, Pezzotti N, et al. Mass cytometry reveals innate lymphoid cell differentiation pathways in the human fetal intestine. *J Exp Med.* (2018) 215:1383–96. doi: 10.1084/jem.20171934
19. Hollt T, Pezzotti N, van Unen V, Koning F, Eisemann E, Lelieveldt BPF, et al. Cytosplore: interactive immune cell phenotyping for large single-cell datasets. *Comput Graph Forum.* (2016) 35:171–80. doi: 10.1111/cgf.12893
20. van Unen V, Li N, Molendijk I, Temurhan M, Höllt T, van der Meulen-de Jong AE, et al. Mass cytometry of the human mucosal immune system identifies tissue- and disease-associated immune subsets. *Immunity.* (2016) 44:1227–39. doi: 10.1016/j.immuni.2016.04.014
21. Howie D, Spencer J, DeLord D, Pitzalis C, Wathen NC, Dogan A, et al. Extrathymic T cell differentiation in the human intestine early in life. *J Immunol.* (1998) 161:5862–72.
22. Artis D, Spits H. The biology of innate lymphoid cells. *Nature.* (2015) 517:293–301. doi: 10.1038/nature14189
23. Howell JC, Wells JM. Generating intestinal tissue from stem cells: potential for research and therapy. *Regen Med.* (2011) 6:743–55. doi: 10.2217/rme.11.90
24. Hwang SE, Kim JH, Yu HC, Murakami G, Cho BH. Lymphocyte subpopulations in the liver, spleen, intestines, and mesenteric nodes: an immunohistochemical study using human fetuses at 15-16 weeks. *Anat Rec.* (2014) 297:1478–89. doi: 10.1002/ar.22940
25. Gunther U, Holloway JA, Gordon JN, Knight A, Chance V, Hanley NA, et al. Phenotypic characterization of CD3-7+ cells in developing human intestine and an analysis of their ability to differentiate into T cells. *J Immunol.* (2005) 174:5414–22. doi: 10.4049/jimmunol.174.9.5414
26. Fu B, Tian Z, Wei H. Subsets of human natural killer cells and their regulatory effects. *Immunology.* (2014) 141:483–9. doi: 10.1111/imm.12224
27. Turtle CJ, Swanson HM, Fujii N, Estey EH, Riddell SR. A distinct subset of self-renewing human memory CD8+ T cells survives cytotoxic chemotherapy.

Immunity. (2009) 31:834–44. doi: 10.1016/j.immuni.2009.09.015

28. Fergusson JR, Smith KE, Fleming VM, Rajoriya N, Newell EW, Simmons R, et al. CD161 defines a transcriptional and functional phenotype across distinct human T cell lineages. *Cell Rep*. (2014) 9:1075–88. doi: 10.1016/j.celrep.2014.09.045
29. Halkias J, Rackaityte E, Hillman SL, Aran D, Mendoza VF, Marshall LR, et al. CD161 contributes to prenatal immune suppression of IFN-γ-producing PLZF+ T cells. *J. Clin. Invest*. (2019). doi: 10.1172/jci125957. [Epub ahead of print].
30. Chen JC, Chan CC, Wu CJ, Ou LS, Yu HY, Chang HL, et al. Fetal phagocytes take up allergens to initiate T-helper cell type 2 immunity and facilitate allergic airway responses. *Am J Respir Crit Care Med*. (2016) 194:934–47. doi: 10.1164/rccm.201508-1703OC
31. Prescott SL, Macaubas C, Holt BJ, Smallacombe TB, Loh R, Sly PD, et al. Transplacental priming of the human immune system to environmental allergens: universal skewing of initial T cell responses toward the Th2 cytokine profile. *J Immunol*. (1998) 160:4730–7.
32. Renz H, Adkins BD, Bartfeld S, Blumberg RS, Farber DL, Garssen J, et al. The neonatal window of opportunity-early priming for life. *J Allergy Clin Immunol*. (2018) 141:1212–4. doi: 10.1016/j.jaci.2017.11.019

17

Increased T Cell Differentiation and Cytolytic Function in Bangladeshi Compared to American Children

Lisa E. Wagar[1], Christopher R. Bolen[1], Natalia Sigal[2], Cesar J. Lopez Angel[1], Leying Guan[3], Beth D. Kirkpatrick[4], Rashidul Haque[5], Robert J. Tibshirani[3], Julie Parsonnet[6], William A. Petri Jr.[7] and Mark M. Davis[1,2,8]*

[1] Department of Microbiology and Immunology, Stanford University, Stanford, CA, United States, [2] Institute for Immunity, Transplantation, and Infection, Stanford University, Stanford, CA, United States, [3] Data Sciences and Statistics, Stanford University, Stanford, CA, United States, [4] Department of Microbiology and Molecular Genetics, University of Vermont College of Medicine and Vaccine Testing Center, Burlington, VT, United States, [5] International Centre for Diarrhoeal Disease Research, Bangladesh, Dhaka, Bangladesh, [6] Departments of Medicine and of Health Research and Policy, Stanford University, Stanford, CA, United States, [7] Department of Medicine, Pathology, and Microbiology, Immunology and Cancer Biology, University of Virginia, Charlottesville, VA, United States, [8] Howard Hughes Medical Institute, Stanford University School of Medicine, Stanford, CA, United States

***Correspondence:**
Mark M. Davis
mmdavis@stanford.edu

During the first 5 years of life, children are especially vulnerable to infection-related morbidity and mortality. Conversely, the Hygiene Hypothesis suggests that a lack of exposure to infectious agents early in life could explain the increasing incidence of allergies and autoimmunity in high-income countries. Understanding these phenomena, however, is hampered by a lack of comprehensive, direct immune monitoring in children with differing degrees of microbial exposure. Using mass cytometry, we provide an in-depth profile of the peripheral blood mononuclear cells (PBMCs) of children in regions at the extremes of exposure: the San Francisco Bay Area, USA and an economically poor district of Dhaka, Bangladesh. Despite variability in clinical health, functional characteristics of PBMCs were similar in Bangladeshi and American children at 1 year of age. However, by 2–3 years of age, Bangladeshi children's immune cells often demonstrated altered activation and cytokine production profiles upon stimulation with PMA-ionomycin, with an overall immune trajectory more in line with American adults. Conversely, immune responses in children from the US remained steady. Using principal component analysis, donor location, ethnic background, and cytomegalovirus infection status were found to account for some of the variation identified among samples. Within Bangladeshi 1-year-olds, stunting (as measured by height-for-age z-scores) was found to be associated with IL-8 and TGFβ expression in PMA-ionomycin stimulated samples. Combined, these findings provide important insights into the immune systems of children in high vs. low microbial exposure environments and suggest an important role for IL-8 and TGFβ in mitigating the microbial challenges faced by the Bangladeshi children.

Keywords: pediatric immunity, CyTOF, environment, immune development, immune profiling

INTRODUCTION

Infants and young children are particularly vulnerable to infectious diseases (1–3). Before the widespread availability of vaccines, ~40% of children died before reaching 5 years old, mostly due to infections (4, 5). Although vaccines and modern medicine have mitigated this vulnerability significantly, in poorer areas of the world where pathogen exposure is elevated, many children are at risk for either infection-related mortality or, more commonly, lifelong disability such as stunting and poor cognitive development. This latter condition is often accompanied by environmental enteropathy (EE), a subclinical condition common in developing countries, characterized by intestinal inflammation, lymphocyte infiltration, and damage to the gut epithelium (6–8). Observational and mouse model studies have pointed to repeated enteric pathogen exposure as a potential driver of the condition (9, 10). It is reported that EE contributes to poor nutrient absorption, malnutrition, developmental delay, and potentially oral vaccine underperformance in children (7, 8, 11, 12).

The pediatric immune system undergoes many changes during the first 5 years of life (13–15). It is important to understand differences in pediatric immune responses in high- and low-income countries, as these differences can affect the success of interventional strategies such as immunization (16). For example, oral rotavirus vaccine was remarkably effective in Finland and the United States (98%) but only 50–80% effective in Nicaragua, Malawi, and South Africa (17–19). Numerous studies have investigated human population-level differences in immune responses, with a focus on either genetic or environmental influences. Innate cells from adults and infants have been well-characterized and both genetic- and environment-driven effects appear to play a role in how these responses are shaped (20–27). Investigations of pediatric populations support the idea that these alterations occur early in life (28). The diversity and level of pathogen burden have been shown to broadly alter Th1/Th2 cytokine bias (23, 29, 30). Antigen-specific responses have also been studied for infectious diseases with higher incidence in low-income countries, such as tuberculosis (31, 32). However, relatively little is known about the effect of environment more broadly on the early events of developing adaptive immunity and to our knowledge, no studies have directly compared deeply-profiled peripheral blood mononuclear cells (PBMCs) from children in high vs. low pathogen environments.

It has been proposed that some degree of diverse microbial exposure is beneficial to developing immune systems, tuning them in some way to avoid childhood allergies and early onset autoimmunity; this is known as the "Hygiene Hypothesis," proposed by Strachan (33). Given the long-term consequences of a highly immunostimulatory environment on early-life innate immunity, we posited that a pathogen-rich setting would profoundly alter adaptive immune development and function early in life.

To gain further insights into how environment influences immunologic development in children, immune profiles of PBMCs from children in two cohorts, Performance of Rotavirus and Oral Polio Vaccines in Developing Countries (PROVIDE) and Stanford's Outcomes Research in Kids (STORK), were examined. The PROVIDE study was designed to explore the effects of environmental enteropathy and enteric infections on development and immunity by tracking infants born in Mirpur, a poor district of Dhaka, Bangladesh from birth through 4 years of age (34). The STORK study tracked childhood development in 1–3 year old children located in the San Francisco Bay Area, USA (35). We analyzed samples from an overlapping age range of 1–3 years of age in both cohorts using time-of-flight mass cytometry (CyTOF) for deep immune profiling with a focus on T cell differentiation and their responses to stimulation. Longitudinal samples were available for a subset of the participants. At the initiation of this study, it was unknown what cell populations would be of interest in dissecting the role of environment on immunity. Thus, we developed a panel that would cover all of the major immune populations found in pediatric PBMCs (mostly T cells, B cells, NK cells, and to a lesser extent, monocytes). In addition, we measured the functional capacity of these cell types with a broad array of cytokines and activation markers. We compared the phenotype and function of unstimulated and *ex vivo* phorbol-12-myristate-13-acetate (PMA)-ionomycin-stimulated PBMCs to determine how environment shapes immune development and function early in life, and whether immune changes correlate with clinical measures of health.

RESULTS

Clinical Features of PROVIDE (Bangladeshi) and STORK (American) Cohorts

The PROVIDE cohort subjects were monitored for evidence of enteric infections and diarrheal disease for the first 2 years of life. Stool samples were collected and tested for a panel of infectious agents, including protozoa (*cryptosporidium*, *Entamoeba histolytica*, *giardia*) and common enteroviruses (polioviruses, rotavirus, and other non-polio enteroviruses). At least one of these agents was detected in all of the PROVIDE subjects tested in this study (**Figure 1A**). Non-polio enteroviruses were the most common infection, with 83% of donors testing positive at least once. A third of donors tested rotavirus positive in their stool at least once during the surveillance period. Protozoa were also prevalent, with *giardia* being the most common (59% of participants). The presence of poliovirus is most likely due to immunization with oral polio vaccine or from vaccine-strain polioviruses in the environment. Most donors tested positive for cytomegalovirus (CMV) antibodies, indicating early infection in the Bangladeshi cohort was common. We examined PBMC samples for CyTOF analysis from weeks 53 ($n = 18$ unstimulated; $n = 19$ stimulated), 104 ($n = 9$), and 156 ($n = 6$).

The STORK cohort is an ethnically and socioeconomically diverse cohort of infants living in the San Francisco Bay Area of the United States (**Figure 1B**). No protozoan infections were detected or suspected in this cohort and the rotavirus vaccine, which has high effectiveness in the United States (36),

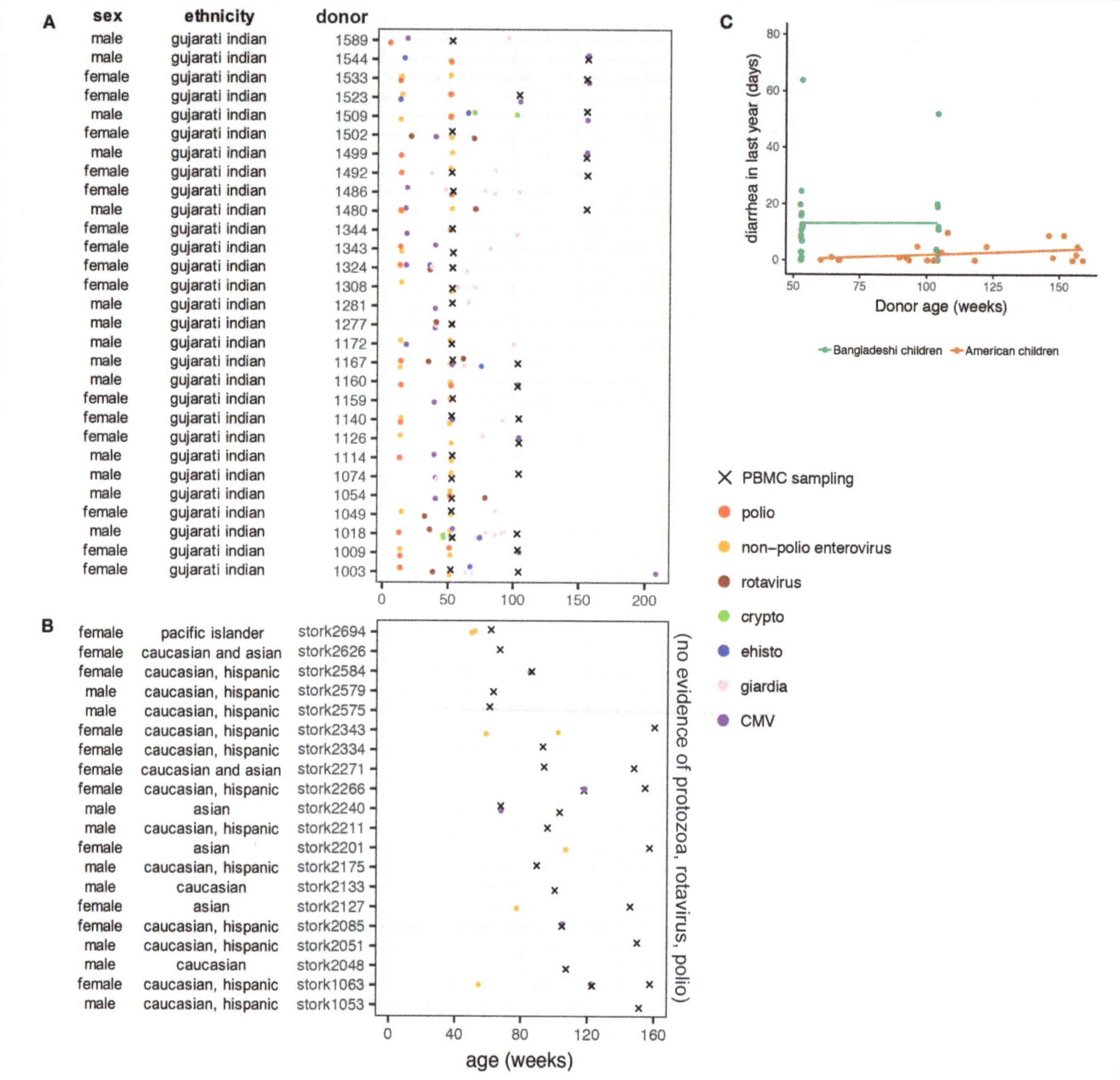

FIGURE 1 | Basic characteristics and clinical data on donor populations. Ethnicity from the PROVIDE cohort is based on genome-wide association study data showing the cohort is genetically homogeneous and most closely resembles the Gujarati Indians from Houston from the HapMap project. Ethnicity data from the STORK cohort is self-reported by the mothers of the infants. **(A)** Stool samples from the Bangladeshi cohort (PROVIDE) were tested for cryptosporidium, giardia, and E histolytica when infants presented with diarrhea and surveilled for shedding of polioviruses (including vaccine strains) and non-polio enteroviruses on weeks 14 and 52. **(B)** PBMC sampling periods for the STORK cohort of American children. Note that no infection data were available for the American children included in the study but based on medical chart review and vaccination status, parasitic, rotavirus, and poliovirus infections are unlikely. **(C)** Diarrheal surveillance data in Bangladeshi and American children. Diarrheal incidence data were available for the first 2 years of life in the Bangladeshi cohort and throughout the entire study period in the American cohort. Rates were found to be significantly different ($p = 0.015$) using a linear mixed effects model that accounts for repeat samples from the same donor.

is part of the standard immunization schedule in California. Waterborne disease outbreaks are not common in California (37, 38). Inactivated polio vaccine is used in the United States, thus poliovirus infections are not likely. Some subjects (25%) were diagnosed with viral gastroenteritis at least once during the study (**Figure 1B**). A small number ($n = 5$) of the STORK donors tested positive for CMV. Other common diagnoses included upper respiratory infection, rash, fever with no etiology specified, dermatitis, and evaluation for allergy. For analysis purposes, we binned PBMC samples from the

STORK cohort to the nearest equivalent sampling period as the PROVIDE cohort: weeks 53 ($n = 5$), 104 ($n = 11$), and 156 ($n = 8$).

Children in the PROVIDE cohort had significantly more diarrheal disease than American children, independent of age (**Figure 1C**; $p = 0.015$ using a mixed linear effects model to account for repeat donors). The available infection surveillance and diarrheal disease data show that enteropathogen exposure and diversity differ between the Bangladeshi and American cohorts. These findings are consistent with previous studies that found a high enteropathogen burden in children growing up in urban slum regions of Bangladesh (12, 39–42).

Automated Clustering Effectively Delineates Complex Cell Types With Minimal User Direction

To investigate the high-dimensional CyTOF data in a minimally directed way, we employed a dimensionality reduction algorithm coupled with semi-automated clustering to characterize and simplify the complex expression patterns of 23 (unstimulated) or 32 (PMA-ionomycin) of the parameters measured. We used the t-stochastic neighborhood embedding (tSNE) technique utilized in other CyTOF applications to reduce the dimensionality of our data on unstimulated and PMA-ionomycin stimulated samples as separate analyses. Like other tSNE-based algorithms (43–46), cells with similar marker expression patterns cluster more closely in 2-dimensional space and the data can be visualized with a clustering map. Then, using a custom designed clustering algorithm, referred to as AdjClust hereafter, we defined groups of similar cells based on both the 2-dimensional maps and the original N-dimensional dataset. AdjClust allows the user to manually assign relative weighting to the markers to be used in the clustering, thus providing more control over which markers are considered useful for clustering and characterization. We performed a preliminary test of the clustering with a mixture of unstimulated and PMA-ionomycin stimulated cells. AdjClust appropriately separated cells with distinctive activation and functional profiles into different clusters (**Supplementary Figure 1**).

Increased Effector and Senescent-Phenotype T Cells in Bangladeshi 2- and 3-Year-Olds

We first investigated the phenotypes of unstimulated PBMCs from Bangladeshi and American children. We identified 28 clusters (see **Supplementary Table 1** for cluster assignment quick-reference) that accurately separated biologically meaningful populations and reflected their diverse phenotypes (**Figure 2A**). Even small populations, such as effector memory RA (EMRA) and CD57$^+$ CD4, CD8, and $\gamma\delta$ T cells were effectively clustered using AdjClust (**Figure 2B**). We stratified the data by donor age and study location to investigate cohort-based differences in immune phenotypes. A "cluster occupancy" value was determined for each sample; the occupancy value refers to the fraction of total cells from a sample that falls within a given cluster. We then calculated the relative contribution ("estimated occupancy") of cells coming from age-matched Bangladeshi and American children's samples to understand differences in the distribution of their cell types.

There were surprisingly few significant differences in immune phenotypes in Bangladeshi vs. American 1-year-olds (**Figure 2C**; Mann-Whitney test with BH correction; FDR = 0.07 for cluster 11, EMRA CD8 T cells). However, there were several trends indicating differences between the two locations at 1 year of age that became more robust with increasing age. Bangladeshi 2-year-olds had fewer monocytes (FDR = 0.03 and 0.04; clusters 26 and 28), naive CD8 T cells (FDR = 0.07; cluster 12), and early-differentiated (i.e., CD27$^+$) memory CD4 T cells (FDR = 0.02; cluster 19) relative to American children. They also showed a decrease in three small populations of EMRA phenotype T cells (CD8 T cells FDR = 0.07, cluster 24; $\gamma\delta$ T cells FDR = 0.04 and 0.08, clusters 6 and 2). Bangladeshi 2-year-olds had increased naive and memory B cells (FDR = 0.03, 0.04, and 0.09; clusters 25, 17, and 18) and highly differentiated T cells (CD57$^+$ CD4 T cells FDR = 0.02, cluster 1; EMRA $\gamma\delta$ T cells FDR = 0.02, cluster 14; EMRA CD8 T cells FDR = 0.03, cluster 11; CD27$^-$ CD4 T cells FDR = 0.03, cluster 22). The reduced monocyte (FDR = 0.03, 0.05, 0.03; clusters 26, 27, 28) and increased effector and cytolytic phenotypes (NK cells FDR = 0.06, cluster 7; CD8 T cells FDR = 0.03, 0.05, 0.06, clusters 11, 8, 21; $\gamma\delta$ T cells FDR = 0.05, cluster 4; CD4 T cells FDR = 0.05, 0.08, clusters 1, 22) also persisted in Bangladeshi 3-year-olds. Overall, these findings suggest that Bangladeshi children have fewer peripherally-circulating monocytes and more differentiated T cell subsets compared to American children and that these effects become more pronounced with increasing age.

We then validated the automated clustering findings using manual gating with standard markers for main cell populations and T cell subsets (see **Supplementary Figure 2** for representative gating). We confirmed via manual gating that monocytes (and transiently at age two, total T cells) were reduced among Bangladeshi children while total B cells and $\gamma\delta$ T cells were elevated at select time points (**Figure 3A**; significance determined by Mann-Whitney with BH correction for multiple testing). These findings closely matched those identified using AdjClust. Given the strong signal for T cell differentiation in the automated analysis, we further investigated the frequency of naive, central memory, effector memory, and EMRA T cell phenotypes (using CD45RA, CD45RO, and CCR7) and other differentiation indicators (CD27, CD57, PD-1, regulatory T cells). Compared to age-matched American children, Bangladeshi children's CD4 and CD8 T cells were indeed more differentiated (**Figure 3B**). At many time points, Bangladeshi children had fewer CD27$^+$ T cells and more CD57$^+$ cells, suggesting differentiation toward a more effector-like and potentially senescent (47) phenotype. In nearly all instances where Bangladeshi children's T cells differed from those of American children, they more closely resembled an adult phenotype. Based on these findings, we determined that the T cells of Bangladeshi children, though more similar to their American counterparts at 1 year of age, are more differentiated at ages two and three and increasingly resemble the proportions of differentiated T cells from adults.

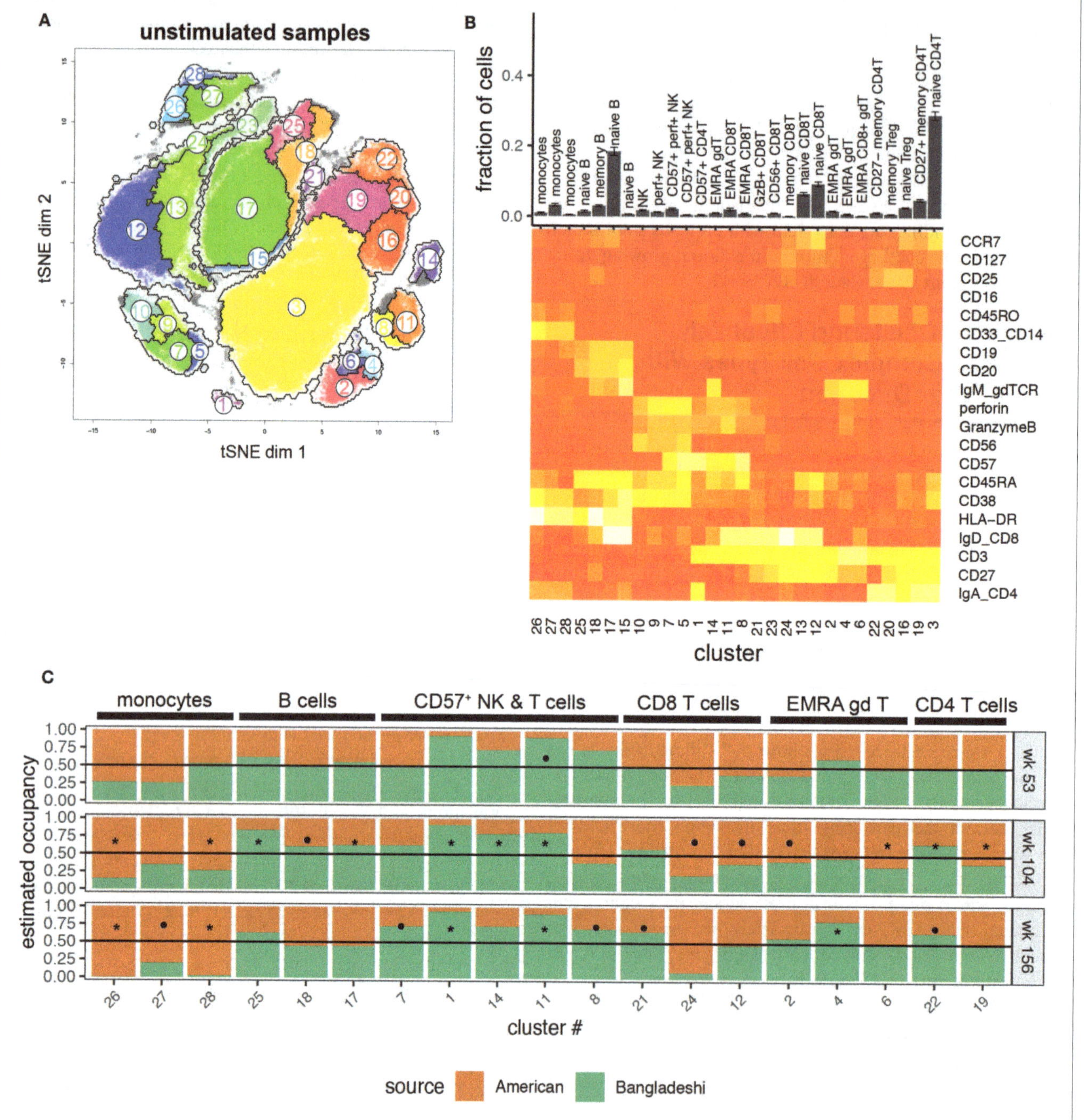

FIGURE 2 | Location-based differences in immunophenotypes identified with automated clustering. Markers used for the tSNE and clustering processes were selected based on relevence to cell identification under unstimulated conditions. Samples include 24 from American children (week 53 $n = 5$, week 104 $n = 11$, week 156 $n = 8$), 33 from Bangladeshi children (week 53 $n = 18$, week 104 $n = 9$, week 156 $n = 6$), and 30,000 randomly sampled cells from 3 American adults. **(A)** tSNE map with overlaid AdjClust clusters on aggregate of all samples included in the analysis. Using AdjClust, 28 unique clusters were identified that delineated cell phenotypes of interest. Minimum cluster size was set to 1,500 cells. **(B)** Distribution of cells among AdjClust clusters in unstimulated samples from combined Bangladeshi and American children's PBMC samples and their phenotypic characteristics. Values plotted are means ± SEM. **(C)** Ratio of cluster occupancy between age-matched Bangladeshi vs. American children. Only clusters with FDR < 0.01 are shown. For each time point, Mann-Whitney tests were performed for each of the 28 clusters. p-values were then corrected for multiple testing using the Benjamini and Hochberg method. Significance levels of the cluster occupancy differences between Bangladeshi and American children are indicated by FDR < 0.1 (•), FDR < 0.05 (*).

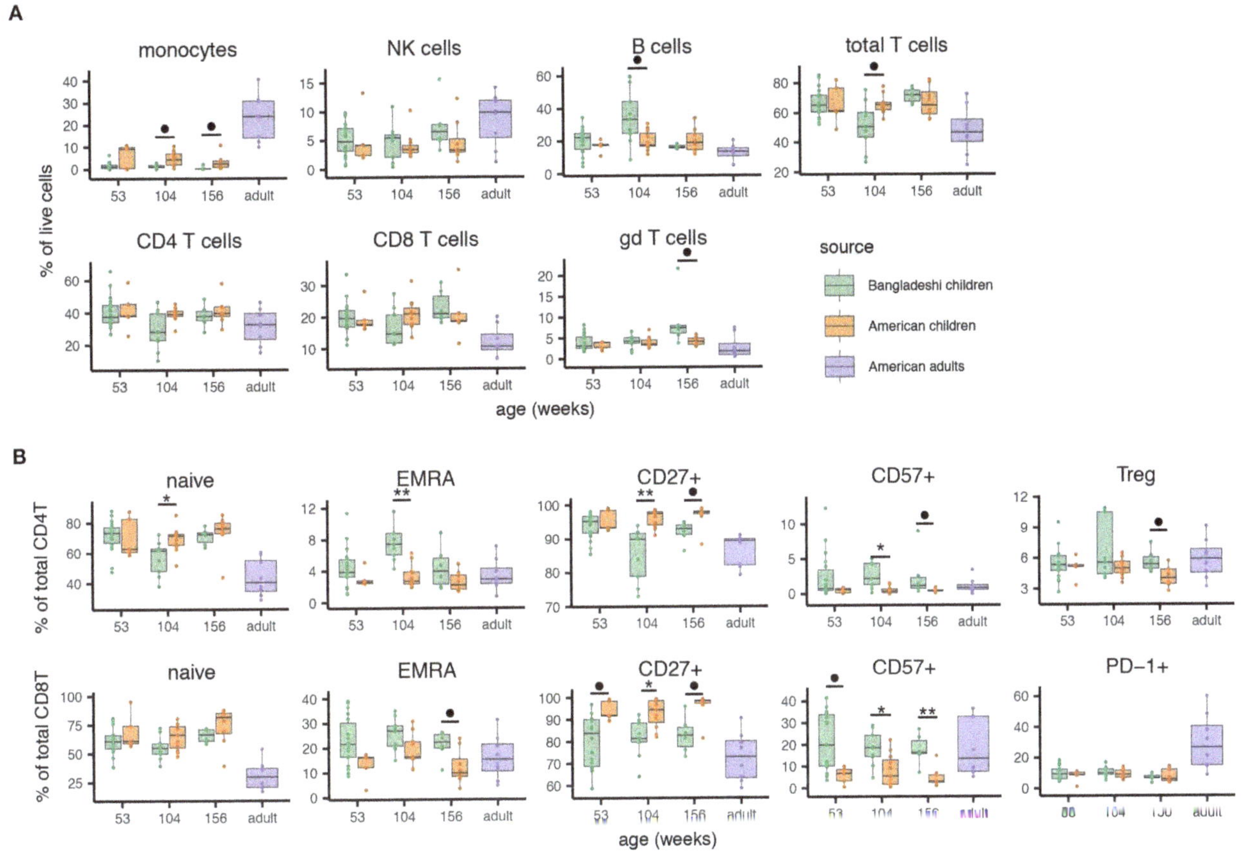

FIGURE 3 | Manual gating validation of altered immune phenotypes associated with location. After identifying cell subsets that differed between Bangladeshi and American cohorts with automated analyses, main cell populations and phenotypes of interest were manually gated. Samples include 24 from American children (week 53 $n = 5$, week 104 $n = 11$, week 156 $n = 8$) and 33 from Bangladeshi children (week 53 $n = 18$, week 104 $n = 9$, week 156 $n = 6$). Cell phenotypes from 8 American adults are shown as a reference for typical values derived from the CyTOF panel and gating scheme utilized here and were not used for statistical analyses. **(A)** Minor differences in main cell populations are detectable between equivalent-aged Bangladeshi and American children. Bangladeshi children show reduced monocyte and total T cell populations and increased B cell and gamma delta T cell populations compared to American children at select ages. **(B)** Bangladeshi children show more T cell differentiation and senescence phenotypes but not exhaustion compared to equivalent-aged American children. To compare Bangladeshi and American children's cell populations from manual gating, Mann-Whitney tests were performed for each population and time point shown. *p*-values were then corrected for multiple testing using the Benjamini and Hochberg method. Significance levels of the cell population differences between Bangladeshi and American children are indicated by FDR < 0.1 (•), FDR < 0.05 (*), FDR < 0.01 (**). Values plotted are means ± SEM.

Cytokine Suppression and Shift to Cytotoxicity in T Cells From Bangladeshi 2-Year-Olds

To investigate the functional potential of immune cells from the two cohorts, we studied the clustered cell populations from PMA-ionomycin stimulated samples (**Figures 4A,B**). Thirty clusters of immune cells at varying levels of activation, based on expression of activation markers in combination with zero to four or more cytokines, were created using AdjClust. Similar to the unstimulated cell population analysis, Bangladeshi and American children's stimulated PBMC samples had similar functional profiles at 1 year of age (**Figure 4C**). Bangladeshi 1-year-olds had a small but detectable population of cytolytic (MIP-1β^+ granzyme B$^+$ perforin$^+$ TNF$^+$) CD4 T cells that were virtually absent in American children (FDR = 0.01; cluster 16). They also showed a reduced frequency of a large population of CD4 T cells that express CD40L and produce both IL-2 and TGFβ (FDR = 0.04; cluster 21).

At age two, Bangladeshi children's T cells appeared to be broadly defective in their ability to respond to stimulation, with significant increases in non-activated CD8 T cells (FDR = 0.02; cluster 19) and large decreases in numerous activated and cytokine-producing CD4 and CD8 T cells (FDR < 0.001 for all three significant activated CD8 T cell clusters, 3, 7, and 20; FDR < 0.001 for all three significant activated CD4 T cell clusters, 21, 8, 4) compared to American children. Interestingly, by age three this defective response to stimulation was replaced with a shift toward a cytotoxic profile. Compared to American 3-year-olds, Bangladeshi children's $\gamma\delta$, NK, CD4, and CD8 T cells were more likely to produce cytokines such as perforin, granzyme B, TNF, and MIP-1β (FDR = 0.07, 0.08, 0.07, and 0.02, respectively; clusters 11, 27, 16, and 26), in response

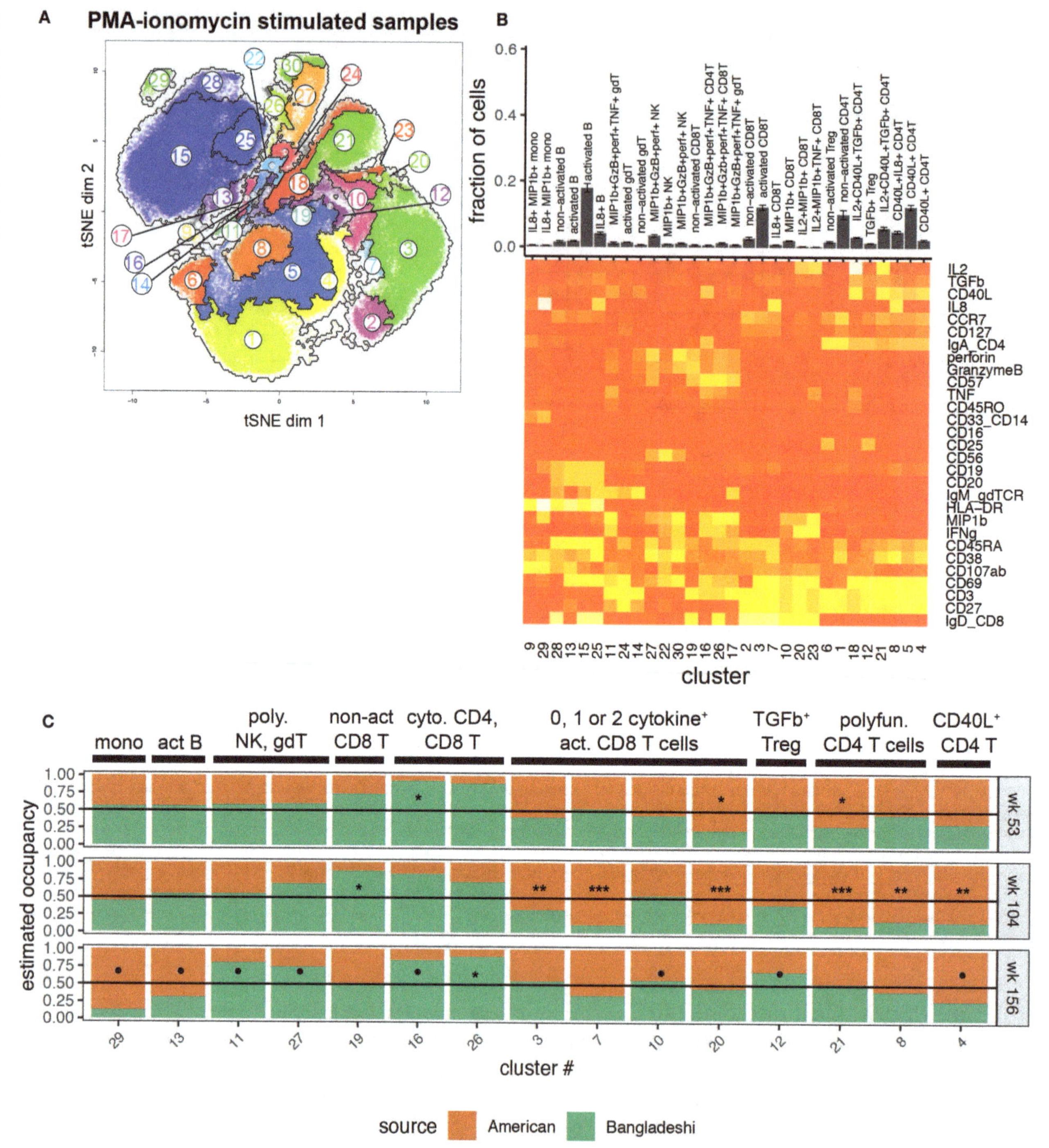

FIGURE 4 | Location-based differences in functional responses to stimulation. Markers used for the tSNE and clustering processes were selected based on relevance to cell phenotypes and functional characterization. Samples include 24 from American children (week 53 $n = 5$, week 104 $n = 11$, week 156 $n = 8$), 34 from Bangladeshi children (week 53 $n = 19$, week 104 $n = 9$, week 156 $n = 6$), and 30,000 randomly sampled cells from 3 American adults. **(A)** tSNE map with overlaid AdjClust clusters on aggregate of all samples included in the analysis. Using AdjClust, 30 unique clusters were identified that delineated cell differentiation and function/activation. Minimum cluster size was set to 1,500 cells. **(B)** Cell phenotypes and functions identified with AdjClust on PMA-ionomycin stimulated samples. Labels were manually assigned based on marker expression. The fraction of cells in each cluster represents aggregate data from Bangladeshi and American children's stimulated samples. **(C)** Ratio of cluster occupancy between age-matched Bangladeshi vs. American children. Only clusters with FDR < 0.01 are shown. For each time point, Mann-Whitney tests were performed for each of the 28 clusters. p-values were then corrected for multiple testing using the Benjamini and Hochberg method. Significance levels of the cluster occupancy differences between Bangladeshi and American children are indicated by FDR < 0.1 (•), FDR < 0.05 (*), FDR < 0.01 (**), FDR < 0.001(***).

to stimulation. Bangladeshi children also had an increased population of TGFβ-producing Tregs (FDR = 0.1). Overall, this automated analysis showed that there are a small number of highly active cytolytic (i.e., perforin, granzyme, TNF, MIP-1β) cells in many subsets (NK, γδ T, CD8 T, and even CD4 T cells) in Bangladeshi kids and fewer cells with CD40L, IL-8, and IL-2 phenotypes across many T cell subsets, particularly in 2-year-olds and somewhat at 3 years.

Due to the number of cytokines and activation markers included in this CyTOF panel, manual gating for every functional combination was not practical. Therefore, we focused on a few cytokines that were of interest either for their broad immune cell relevance (IL-8, TGFβ) or identified across multiple populations from the clustering analysis (perforin, granzyme B, MIP-1β). The manual gating validated the findings from AdjClust, with overall increased cytolytic functions in Bangladeshi compared to American children at all ages in a number of T cell and NK cell subsets and suppressed T cell cytokine production (IL-8, TGFβ) at 2 years of age (**Supplementary Figure 3**). Combined, automated and manual analyses of stimulated PBMC samples point to a significant but transient reduction in the ability of lymphocytes to respond to stimulation (IL-8, TGFβ) in Bangladeshi 2-year-old children and overall development of a cytotoxic (perforin, granzyme B, TNF) functional profile.

Location Is the Strongest Demographic Feature of Immune Variance

The manual gating analyses (**Figure 3**, **Supplementary Figure 3**) suggested that American children's immune profiles were generally more stable throughout the time period studied here, while more variance was observed among Bangladeshi children. The primary goal of this study was to identify environmental, clinical, or other factors that might contribute to pediatric immune development. To accomplish this in an unbiased way, we applied principal component analysis to the AdjClust cluster frequencies from the unstimulated and PMA-ionomycin stimulated analyses (**Figure 5A**). The principal components were then modeled as a function of available demographic variables (donor location, age, sex, CMV status, and ethnicity) using a linear multivariate multiple regression model. In this study, location serves as a proxy for differences in immune challenges, such as the disparity in exposure to non-polio enteroviruses and CMV (**Figure 1**). See **Supplementary Figure 4** for plots comparing each of the first four principal components against one another. After accounting for batch effects ("set"), we found the strongest biological source of variation out of the features examined was donor location (**Figure 5B**; partial variance explained 81 and 89% for unstimulated and stimulated samples, respectively; $p = 0.018$ and 0.0014, mixed linear model, type II MANOVA test with p-values from Pillai statistic). No other feature tested in the PCA significantly accounted for variance detected in unstimulated cells. In PMA-ionomycin stimulated samples, ethnicity and CMV seroconversion status explained a small amount of the variation but were not strongly significant (73 and 69%, respectively; $p = 0.09$ and 0.096). These data suggest that location, and to a lesser extent, ethnic background and specific infections such as CMV, contribute to immune cell function during pediatric immune development.

Functional Responses to Stimulation Are Associated With Clinical Stunting in Bangladeshi Children

Given the observation that immune cells from children in Bangladesh were undergoing substantial changes over time, we considered whether immune functions correlated with clinical surrogates of infection and overall health. CMV infection is known to shape much of the immune system (48), particularly CD8 T cells, over time (49) and PCA suggested that CMV infection may explain some of the functional changes observed. Therefore, we asked whether there were any phenotypic or functional differences between Bangladeshi CMV negative (n = 4 for unstimulated; n = 3 for stimulated) and CMV positive (n = 14 for unstimulated; n = 16 for stimulated) 1-year-olds' CD8 T cells. Though there was an overall trend toward more differentiation and effector-like functions in CMV positive donors, the sample size for CMV negative Bangladeshi subjects was too small to achieve statistical significance for any particular variable (**Figure 6A**; statistical analysis by Mann-Whitney test with BH correction). Only a single donor from the STORK cohort was CMV positive at 1 year of age (n = 1 CMV positive; n = 4 CMV negative), therefore this cohort was not analyzed for the effect of CMV on CD8 T cell phenotypes.

As stunting is a major problem in Bangladeshi children, we were particularly interested in any immunological correlates of this in the PROVIDE cohort, as defined by the height-for-age z score (HAZ). Here we identified a chemokine, a cytokine, and an activation marker associated with HAZ score in Bangladeshi 1-year-olds. We performed permutation testing to identify immune cell features that may be involved in the stunting process. Using a cut-off of $p = 0.05$ and FDR = 0.2, we identified seven candidate cell populations that correlated with stunting (statistical analysis details are provided in the methods section). Stunted children made more IL-8 (in B cells, CD4 T cells, γδ T cells, and NK cells) and TGFβ (in CD4 T cells and γδ T cells) after PMA-ionomycin stimulation compared to their less stunted counterparts (**Figure 6B**). The seventh candidate was a weak association observed for the B cell costimulation molecule CD40L post-stimulation on CD4 T cells. These findings were then validated in a separate set of Bangladeshi 1-year-olds by flow cytometry, where IL-8 ($p = 0.037$; combined $p = 0.009$) and TGFβ ($p = 0.043$; combined $p = 0.002$) were both produced at higher levels in stimulated samples from stunted children (**Figure 6C**; $n = 9$). Combined, these findings suggest that stunting in Bangladeshi 1-year-olds is correlated with higher functional responses to stimulation, as measured by IL-8 and TGFβ.

DISCUSSION

The findings of this study indicate that environment plays an important role in shaping the early pediatric immune system. By performing a high dimensional analysis of PBMCs,

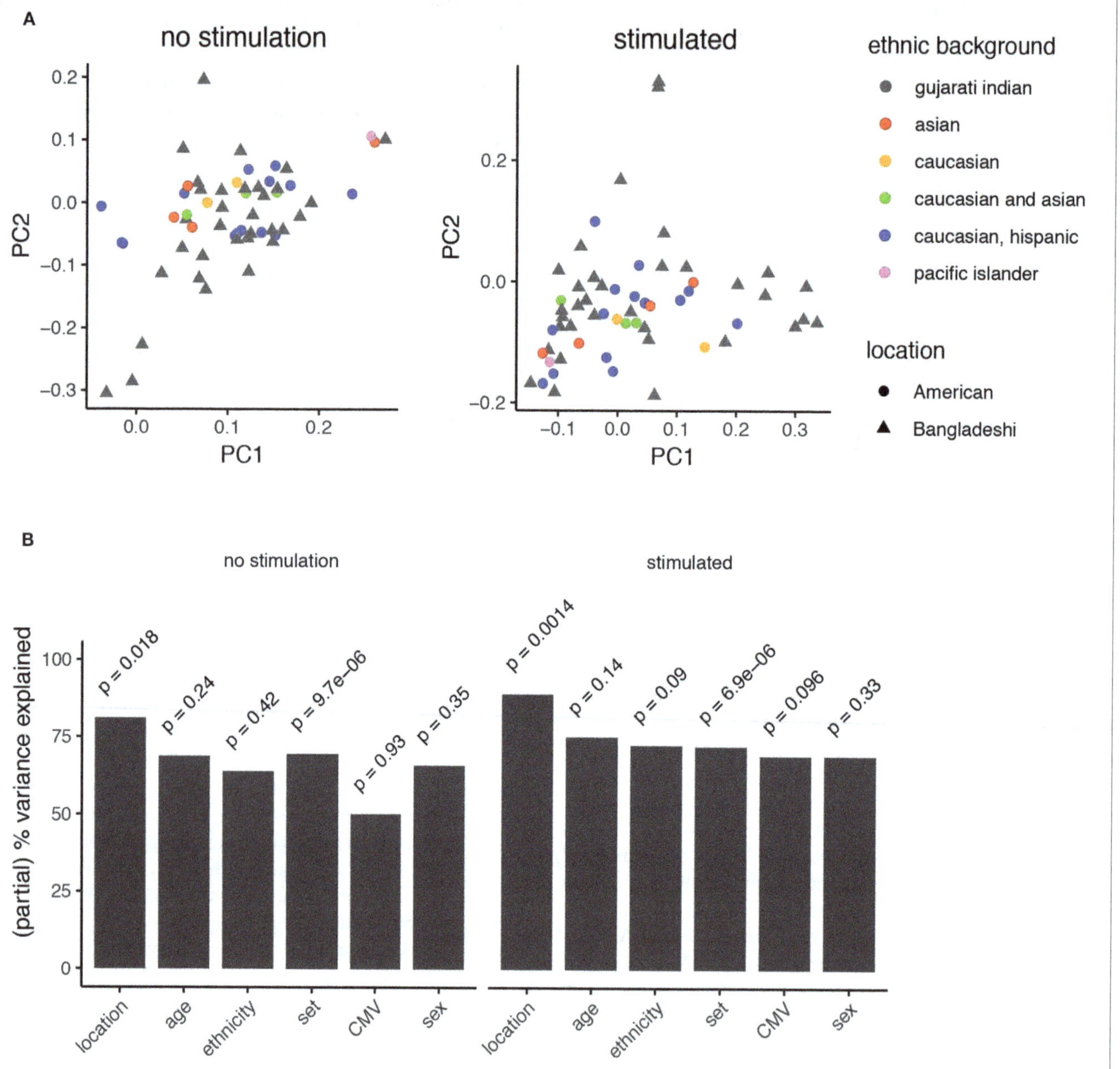

FIGURE 5 | Principal component analysis identifies features explaining immune variation in PBMCs from children. **(A)** Principal component analysis of automated clustering output from PBMCs either left unstimulated (left) or stimulated with PMA-ionomycin (right). Point shapes represent data from American (circles) and Bangladeshi (triangle) cohorts. Points are filled based on reported ethnic background. **(B)** Variance explained by known clinical features. A mixed linear model was used to describe the partial variance explained in PBMC samples from unstimulated (left) and stimulated (right) analyses. Partial percent variance explained (partial eta^2) calculates the percent variance explained for each variable from the Pillai statistic. A type-II MANOVA test was performed on the linear model and *p*-values for the contribution of each variable were calculated from the Pillai test statistic.

we found numerous differences in immune function between Bangladeshi and American children at key developmental milestones. Principal component analysis indicated that, of the clinical features we were able to examine, location explained the most variance. This corresponds with what we know about the relative genetic diversity of our cohorts. The American STORK cohort is a more genetically diverse group (**Figure 1**) yet immunologically similar to one another, whereas the PROVIDE study participants were more genetically homogenous yet immunologically variable. Natural selection events have certainly shaped innate immune-related genes among geographically disparate human populations (20, 27, 50–52), which could have consequences on the subsequent adaptive response. Indeed, we find that ethnic background does explain some of the variance detected among samples stimulated with PMA-ionomycin (**Figure 5**). However, genetic studies of European and Asian

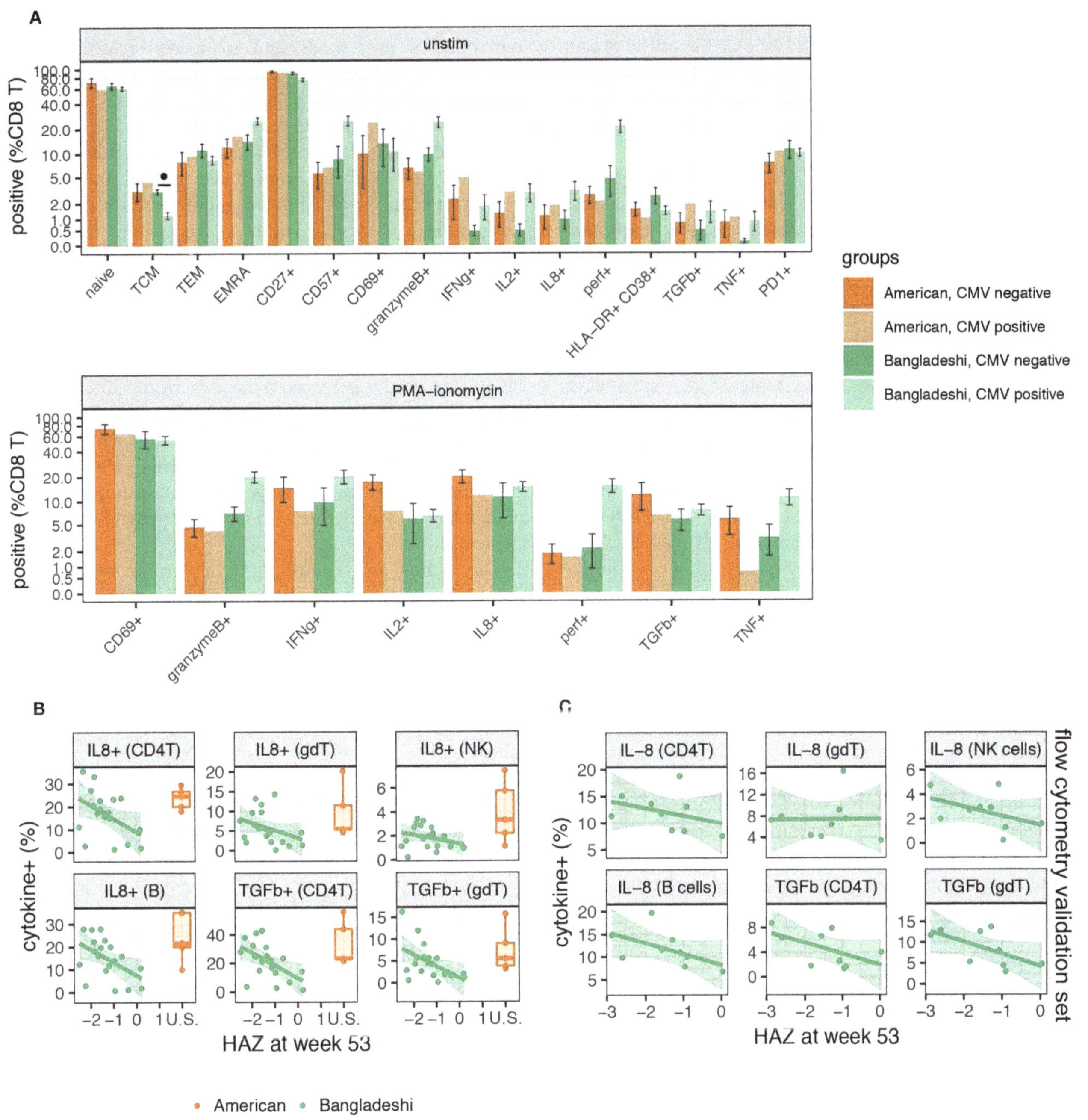

FIGURE 6 | Higher functional responses to stimulation are associated with stunting in Bangladeshi 1-year-olds. **(A)** Frequencies of CD8 T cells with and without stimulation in CMV positive and negative 1-year-olds. Mann-Whitney tests were performed for each population shown. p-values were then corrected for multiple testing using the Benjamini and Hochberg method. Significant differences in cell population frequencies between Bangladeshi CMV positive and negative subjects are indicated by FDR < 0.1 (•). Values plotted are means ± SEM. The number of donors in each group were $n = 4$ and 14 Bangladeshi CMV negative and positive, respectively, in unstimulated samples; $n = 3$ and 16 Bangladeshi CMV negative and positive, respectively, in stimulated samples; $n = 4$ American CMV negative for unstimulated and stimulated samples; $n = 1$ CMV positive American child for unstimulated and stimulated samples. **(B)** Relationship between stunting (as measured by height for age z-score, HAZ) and IL-8 or TGFβ cytokine production in unstimulated or PMA-ionomycin stimulated PBMCs from Bangladeshi 1-year-olds ($n = 8$ less stunted; $n = 8$ more stunted). After permuting HAZ scores 5,000 times and setting a cut-off of $p = 0.05$ and FDR = 0.2, we identified IL-8 and TGFβ in stimulated PBMCs as significantly associated with HAZ across multiple populations. No significance was found in unstimulated populations. After PCA and a validation **(C)** set analysis ($n = 9$), the combined p-values from training and validation sets were $p = 0.009$ (IL-8) and $p = 0.002$ (TGFβ) using the first principal component. Values from American children ($n = 5$) are presented for comparison purposes.

populations, which represent the majority of study participants, find these groups have undergone similar genetic selection events compared to African populations (53–56). This might explain why we see a stronger correlation with location rather than genetic factors. Together, these data suggest that non-genetic influences are strong contributors to the immune variance observed here.

What might these non-genetic influences be? We propose that microbial exposure, maternal health during pregnancy, breastfeeding duration, immunization, chronic infection, hygiene, and diet could all be possible contributors. The socioeconomic disparity between these cohorts also links a number of these factors together, making it difficult to disentangle individual contributors. Though we were unable to consider all non-genetic influences individually in the cohorts described here, we discuss below some of the most likely contributions to the immune variation observed.

The immunization schedules up to 1 year of age are quite similar between the PROVIDE cohort and the standard California vaccine schedule. The main differences are in live vaccines: Bangladeshi children receive BCG vaccine at birth, are immunized against polioviruses with mostly oral polio vaccine in this study, and did not receive varicella vaccine. It is possible that immunization with live vaccines has long-term consequences on immune development, though we did not find any correlation between oral vaccine responses and the immune cell subsets examined in the PROVIDE cohort (data not shown). Hepatitis B, diphtheria, tetanus, pertussis, *Haemophilus influenzae* type B, pneumococcal, measles, and rubella vaccines were similar in number and timing. Therefore, it is unlikely that vaccination schedules alone explain the immune differences observed between the cohorts. However, based on infection surveillance data (**Figure 1**) as well as literature, Bangladeshi children are exposed to a more diverse enteropathogen environment, experience diarrheal illness more frequently, and most show evidence of environmental enteropathy by 12 weeks (57).

Given these early microbial differences, it was surprising to find Bangladeshi and American 1-year-olds' peripheral immune profiles to be quite similar. Several studies of infants in low- and middle-income countries have shown that innate immunity is shaped early in life and can differ substantially depending on location (21–25, 28). Previous data also suggest that innate responses to stimulation decrease over the first year of life (22). We see an interesting parallel in the adaptive response at 2 years, where lymphocytes appeared to be largely refractory to stimulation in Bangladeshi children. At 1 year of age, some Bangladeshi children's PBMC phenotypes and functional responses look more like the changes observed at 2 years, suggesting some degree of variance in terms of the timing of acquiring these immune changes. It may take more time for early innate immune changes to have functional consequences on adaptive immune cells' phenotypes and functions.

There are other environmental factors that might explain why immune differences among these cohorts increase with increasing age. Passive immunity to some antigens is conferred by maternal and breast milk antibodies early in life. Bangladeshi babies were exclusively breastfed for a median of 142 days and partial breastfeeding continued for at least the first year of life. However, as the children are weaned, begin eating potentially contaminated solid foods, and are increasingly mobile, their exposure to antigen dramatically increases, while passive immunity wanes. These developmental milestones are coincident with the period in which we see the strongest differences between Bangladeshi and American children. Dampened functional responses and enhanced immune maturation, as exhibited by reduced cytokine production and more T cell differentiation in Bangladeshi 2-year-olds (**Figure 4**), may be a way to protect against pathological inflammatory damage in a high pathogen environment. These data are consistent with the Hygiene Hypothesis, as immune phenotypes of American children remained virtually unchanged throughout the 2-year time course we analyzed, while the Bangladeshi children were much more variable, especially at 1 year. While American children certainly acquire many childhood diseases, the effect these have on their immune system seems negligible compared to the major shifts we see in Bangladeshi children. Perhaps American children later go through a phase of reduced response to stimulation as well when antigen exposure is high (e.g., at daycare or school) and immune memory forms.

The timing and contribution of chronic infections may also play an important role in shaping adaptive immunity. Though we identified human cytomegalovirus infection as a source of immune variation by PCA (**Figure 5B**), the study was underpowered to identify a specific cell phenotype or function associated with CMV infection. In our cohort of American 1-year-olds, only one subject was CMV positive. In the PROVIDE cohort, early CMV infection was the norm; 83% of participants were CMV positive before 1 year of age. Although it is known that CMV can alter the function of antigen-specific CD4 T cells in children (58), we mostly observed trends (FDR = 0.1 to 0.2) pointing to increased effector T cell phenotypes (granzyme B, perforin, and CD57 expression) in CMV positive individuals. These trends should be validated in future studies via quantification and characterization of CMV-specific T cell subsets. CMV is a unique human virus that has correlates with profound changes in the immune systems of infected organisms, as shown earlier in CD8 T cells in humans and rhesus macaques (59–61). Brodin et al. also showed that monozygotic twins discordant for CMV seropositivity displayed divergences in almost 60% of over two hundred immunological variables (48). Particularly interesting in terms of the biological implications of CMV infection are the data of Furman and colleagues who found that CMV positive young adults had reproducibly superior antibody responses to influenza vaccination compared to CMV negative individuals (62). The implication that CMV infection can boost the immune response of humans was reinforced by the finding in this same report that mice infected by murine CMV were substantially protected from a subsequent influenza infection (62). Taken together these data suggest that for healthy individuals, CMV infection could be beneficial, though the virus is clearly life threatening for immunocompromised individuals. A question from these studies is whether this boost in immunity is only advantageous for individuals in high income countries like the United States. The fact that we see a trend toward more robust

CD8 T cell activity in the CMV positive vs. negative children in this study suggests that CMV infection is generally beneficial regardless of the pathogen environment. This could explain why CMV infection is so common across the globe.

We found that stronger IL-8 and TGFβ production across multiple immune cell types was associated with stunting in Bangladeshi 1-year-olds. Even taking false discovery rate into account, it is not likely that IL-8 and TGFβ are false signals since they were found across numerous cell types. Stunting is thought to be a consequence of poor nutrition combined with other causative factors, as malnutrition alone is not sufficient to induce stunting (63) and previous studies have found no clear association with immune cell composition (64). Interestingly, both IL-8 and TGFβ can play important immunological roles that are relevant to a high enteropathogen environment. TGFβ's effects can vary by cell type, differentiation status, and cytokine milieu (65, 66). However, TGFβ production can provide a protective benefit in the intestine (and peripherally) by regulating the inflammatory function of various immune and non-immune cells (67). IL-8 is a potent neutrophil chemoattractant (68) and there is ample evidence that circulating IL-8 is nearly undetectable in healthy children (69) but elevated during infection (70–72). It was recently shown that IL-8 is abundantly produced by newborn but not adult *in vitro* stimulated T cells (73). The authors proposed that IL-8 performs a neonatal inflammatory function, compensating for low levels of other inflammatory cytokines in babies. Consistent with this previous study, we found T cells (and also B cells) from American children produced a strong IL-8 response upon stimulation (**Supplementary Figure 3**). In the context of the PROVIDE cohort, where enteropathogen exposure and intestinal alterations like environmental enteropathy are common, IL-8 and TGFβ likely play a critical role in gut health and wound healing. *In vitro* studies have shown that intestinal epithelial cells, in addition to making IL-8 in response to inflammatory stimuli, can also be stimulated by IL-8 through a CXCR-1 dependent mechanism (74). IL-8 and TGFβ both enhance migration of intestinal epithelial cells, a function required for efficient repair after physical damage to the barrier surface (74–76).

We hypothesize that the combination of enteric infection, subclinical environmental enteropathy, and the subsequent alterations to the intestinal barrier may explain the association (**Figure 6B**) observed between IL-8 and TGFβ production post-stimulation and stunting in Bangladeshi children. This hypothesis is consistent with two key pieces of evidence from prior work: (1) that markers of enhanced neutrophil recruitment and inflammation precede clinical malnutrition and stunting in the cohort (57), and (2) that malnourishment in Bangladeshi children is associated with an immature gut microbiome (77), possibly as a consequence of diarrhea as well as other factors (78). However, we note that our study was designed to identify associations with clinical stunting, not causes. Further work examining both IL-8 and TGFβ peripherally (from both PBMCs and serum cytokine analysis) as well as locally at the intestine along with the microbiome are needed to determine whether the stunting association observed reflects specific microbial alterations and host responses.

Another limitation of our study was that we were restricted to analyzing immune responses in peripheral blood. Oral vaccine failure is prevalent in low-income countries (7), while parenteral vaccines show no such defect. We were unable to identify any PBMC population that correlated with oral vaccine failure, suggesting that mucosa-specific responses are likely more important. Indeed, Naylor and colleagues determined that enteric rather than systemic inflammatory markers were better indicators of oral vaccine failure and stunting in the PROVIDE cohort (57). Since rates of environmental enteropathy are very different between high- and low-income countries, it would be of great interest to profile immune alterations at the gut interface. A point of future exploration is whether interventional strategies, such as improved sanitation and additional early immunization for enteroviruses, would have an effect on clinical factors like chronic infection and stunting, and whether there is a corresponding effect on pediatric immune development. One would expect that these strategies would reduce the rate of enteric infection, which might alter immune profiles to be more in line with those seen in more developed countries. Whether this would provide a benefit in terms of oral vaccine efficacy, immune, and overall health of children in countries like Bangladesh remains to be determined.

In summary, we present here a comparative study of early immune development in Bangladeshi vs. American children. While very similar at 1 year of age, marked differences are evident at 2 years of age and beyond, when Bangladeshi children show marked increases in effector T cells and other indicators of pathogen engagement. We also note a loss of IL-8 and TGFβ in healthier Bangladeshi 1-year-olds, perhaps associated with a reduced requirement for wound healing responses in the gut. Overall the results have implications for both the phenomenon of stunting, a major problem in poorer countries and are consistent with the Hygiene Hypothesis, with far more immune activity and accelerated immune maturation evident in Bangladeshi children than their American counterparts.

MATERIALS AND METHODS

Study Enrollment and Sample Preparation

Samples were collected with ethics approval from all regulatory bodies involved. The PROVIDE study was performed in the Mirpur area of Dhaka, Bangladesh. A detailed explanation of the study design is published (34). Dhaka is densely populated with over a million inhabitants. Participants were selected from predominantly lower socioeconomic households living in slum conditions. A door-to-door community census was done to identify pregnant women; within seven days of birth, eligible infants were enrolled (eligibility criteria included no obvious congenital abnormalities or birth defects, no abnormal stools since birth, and no history of seizures or neurologic disorders) (34). Children were visited in their homes twice a week and a structured questionnaire administered that included diarrheal illness, fever, and use of antibiotics or oral rehydration solution. Nutritional status was measured at every study visit using a calibrated baby scale and supine length measurement equipment, with two complete measurements made at each time and the average reported. Subjects were tested for protozoa and rotavirus in stool samples when infants had diarrheal disease. For poliovirus and non-polio enterovirus surveillance, stool samples were tested on weeks 6, 14, and 52 of life. Children from the Bay Area in California, USA were enrolled at birth in the STORK study. English- or Spanish-speaking women with low-risk pregnancies and without non-gestational diabetes or other serious chronic illness were recruited prior to 36 weeks' gestation from several Bay Area clinics. Following the babies' births, mothers in STORK were interviewed weekly via automated phone call or email regarding disease symptoms in their babies. Infection surveillance was performed based on medical chart review. Whole blood samples from babies were obtained by venipuncture annually through age three (35). Adult control samples were collected from the Stanford Blood Bank (6 CMV negative, 1 CMV positive, and 1 CMV status unknown; mean age 50 years old; diverse ethnic backgrounds). Whole blood was collected into heparin or EDTA coated vacutainer tubes by standard venipuncture. For both studies, blood samples were maintained as close as possible to 21°C prior to processing and processing was performed within 4 h of draw. Peripheral blood mononuclear cells (PBMCs) were isolated by standard Ficoll density gradient centrifugation and cryopreserved until use. Samples from both study sites were maintained in long-term storage in liquid nitrogen and samples from Bangladesh were shipped in a nitrogen-charged dry shipper for transport to the United States to minimize study-specific storage and handling differences. Both studies enrolled participants on a rolling enrollment basis, from 2011 to 2014 for the PROVIDE study (with samples examined here collected from 2011 to 2016) and 2011 to 2015 for the STORK study (with samples from 2014 to 2015). In both cohorts, CMV seropositivity was determined by detecting CMV-specific IgG in serum or plasma by ELISA.

CyTOF Antibody Reagents

Metal-conjugated antibodies were either purchased from Fluidigm or coupled in-house with DN3 or X8 polymers using the MaxPar antibody labeling kit (Fluidigm). For palladium coupling, metal was added to anti-CD45 antibodies with amine-reactive isothiocyanobenzyl-EDTA chelator, as described by Mei and colleagues (79). See **Supplementary Table 2** for staining panel and clone details.

Stimulation and Cell Staining

Cryopreserved PBMCs were thawed and washed in warmed, complete (R10) media (RPMI media with glutamax and HEPES (Gibco), 10% fetal bovine serum (Sigma), 1X penicillin/streptomycin, 1X non-essential amino acids, 1X sodium pyruvate). Cells were rested for 1 h at 37°C in R10 with benzonase (Sigma), then enumerated and assessed for viability by trypan blue exclusion; any samples with <70% live cells after the 1 h resting period were excluded from data analysis. Samples were split in half (up to five million live PBMCs) for use in stimulation assays. Five million live PBMCs (or half of the total if <10 million cells were available) were washed and resuspended either in 500 μl of R10 (for non-stimulated controls), or R10 with 1X cell stimulation cocktail (containing PMA-ionomycin, eBioscience) and maintained in 24-well plates (BD Biosciences). Anti-CD107a and anti-CD107b metal-coupled antibodies were added to all samples at a final concentration of 0.5 μg/ml each. PBMCs were incubated for 1 h at 37°C. Then, 1X protein transport inhibitor cocktail (containing monensin and brefeldin, eBioscience) was added to all samples. PBMCs were further incubated for 5 h at 37°C.

After a total of 6 h of stimulation, PBMCs were harvested for staining. Cells were washed two times with CyFACS buffer (PBS with 0.1% w/v bovine serum albumin, 2 mM EDTA, and 0.05% v/v sodium azide), then barcoded with anti-CD45 antibodies coupled to Pd104, Pd106, Pd108, and In113 as previously described (79), using combinations of two or three metals to define one barcode. Barcode staining was completed on ice for 30 min, then samples were washed three times with CyFACS buffer and compatible barcoded samples were pooled (up to 10 samples per pool). Each barcoded pool included a control PBMC sample from a local adult blood bank donor to control for potential differences in staining between pools. Samples were surface stained with primary antibodies for 30 min on ice. After further washing, dead cells were detected with cisplatin (Fluidigm) diluted 1/1,000 in PBS for 5 min at room temperature. Samples were washed two times with CyFACS buffer, then fixed overnight at 4°C with 2% paraformaldehyde (Electron Microscopy Sciences) diluted in PBS. The following day, samples were washed and permeabilized with 1X permeabilization buffer (eBioscience), then stained with intracellular antibodies for 30 min on ice. After further washes, samples were resuspended in 1X iridium DNA intercalator (Fluidigm) diluted in PBS containing 2% paraformaldehyde. Intercalator staining was done on ice for 30 min. Finally, PBMCs were washed once with perm buffer, twice with PBS, and three times with water. Prior to acquisition, samples were diluted to $\sim 7.5 \times 10^5$ cells/ml in water with 10% v/v four-element calibration bead solution (Fluidigm). Data were collected on a CyTOF2 instrument (Fluidigm). Signal normalization using calibration beads was done with the built-in CyTOF2 software.

Manual Gating

Manual gating was done using Flowjo (TreeStar) software. First, normalized fcs files were gated on event length, DNA intercalator staining to discriminate singlets from doublets, then on live cells. Barcodes were deconvoluted and individual samples were exported as separate fcs files for manual gating and automated clustering analysis. Samples with <3,000 live intact singlet cells were discarded from the analysis. See **Supplementary Figure 2** for sample gating strategy.

Dimensionality Reduction and Automated Gating

In order to accommodate the large size of the dataset, computational down-sampling was used to draw 6,000 live cells from each data file (donor, time point, and stimulation), as well as an additional 30,000 cells from the healthy adult controls. We opted to include some cells from healthy adults so that we could identify cell types that were infrequent in both PROVIDE and STORK cohorts, presumably as a consequence of age. In total, about 375,000 cell events were included for each clustering analysis. A subset of phenotypic markers ($n = 23$ markers for unstimulated; $n = 32$ markers for stimulated) was selected from the total CyTOF panel (**Supplementary Table 2**), and dimensionality reduction was performed using t-Distributed Stochastic Neighbor Embedding (t-SNE) (80, 81), with a perplexity of 60, theta of 0.5, and 2,000 iterations.

After dimensionality reduction, a novel clustering algorithm (referred to as AdjClust) was developed to define individual subsets of cells. Briefly, AdjClust uses hierarchical clustering of the original n-dimensional cell data, with the added stipulation that the cells must be "adjacent" in 2-dimensional space. The 2-dimensional t-SNE map was first partitioned into equal-sized hexagonal bins (~10,000 in total), and the marker values of all cells within a bin were averaged to get a "bin expression" value. Bins that did not contain any cells were dropped from the analysis. Pairwise distances between two bins, p and q, were calculated using the following formula:

$$d(p,q) = \sqrt{\sum_{i=1}^{n} w_i(p_i - q_i)^2}$$

where w_i is a manually-defined weighting value for marker *i*. A complete list of manually-assigned weights for the markers in the AdjClust analyses can be found in **Supplementary Table 3**.

Using the resulting distance matrix, complete-linkage hierarchical clustering was performed, with the added stipulation that, at each combination step, two clusters can only be combined if at least one hexagonal bin within each cluster is directly "adjacent" to a bin in the other cluster. Hexagons were defined as adjacent if either: (A) they shared a border with each other, or (B) if a bin had no non-empty neighbors, then the closest bins were defined as neighbors. Adjacency clustering was performed until no "adjacent" clusters remained; at which point the final clustering steps were completed using standard complete-linkage hierarchical clustering. The resulting tree was cut to the desired number of clusters, and then cells within each hexagonal bin were assigned to the same cluster as the bin. A minimum cluster size of 1,500 cells was manually assigned.

Statistical Analysis

All statistical analyses except the multivariable clinical correlation analysis were done using R (82). To evaluate diarrheal disease burden between the PROVIDE and STORK cohorts, a linear mixed model was used to correct for multiple measurements from repeat subjects. For analyses where cell clusters or manually gated populations were compared between Bangladeshi and American children of similar ages, Mann-Whitney non-parametric tests were used and the resulting *p*-values were adjusted for multiple hypothesis testing using the Benjamini and Hochberg (BH) false discovery rate method, with a cutoff of FDR<0.1 used for consideration.

For evaluating variance associated with clinical features, PCA was applied to the automated clustering cell count datasets for dimensionality reduction and all but the final dimension were retained. The principal components were then modeled as a function of demographic and other variables (batch number, age, location, ethnic background, sex, CMV status) using a linear multivariate multiple regression model. Partial percent variance explained (partial eta^2) was calculated using the "etasq" function in the "heplots" package (version 1.3-4), which calculates the percent variance explained for each variable from the Pillai statistic. A type-II MANOVA test was performed on the linear model using the "Anova" function from the "car" R package (version 2.1-5), and *p*-values for the contribution of each variable were calculated from the Pillai test statistic.

To explore the potential relationship between immune cell functions and stunting, we performed several filtering steps followed by a permutation analysis. First, outliers were removed based on k-means clustering on the CyTOF data acquired from stimulated and unstimulated samples. Only samples that clustered with the appropriate stimulation condition were included in the analysis to eliminate possible complications from donors actively responding to an acute infection. Next, we divided the qualifying samples into three groups: five samples from American children (group 0; HAZ values were estimated to be 0), eight samples from non-stunted (HAZ > −1.5) Bangladeshi children (group 1), and eight samples from more stunted (HAZ <= −1.5) Bangladeshi children (group 2). We then considered the following event:

$$\frac{\mu_{i0} - \mu_{i1}}{s_{i,0}} \geq \theta, \frac{\mu_{i2} - \mu_{i1}}{s_{i,2}} \geq \theta$$

where μ_{ij} is the group mean for group *j* and feature *j*, and $_{i,j}$ is the pooled standard deviation for group *j* and group 1. The cell populations were filtered based on whether they satisfy the above criterion. For different cut-offs θ, we estimate the -value and FDR for selected features based on permutation testing. To account for cytokine and cell population correlations within a single individual, HAZ scores were permuted 5,000 times and a cutoff of $p = 0.05$ and FDR = 0.2 was established. Since both IL-8 and TGFβ were identified across multiple cell populations with this cutoff, we first validated these two markers on the training data. Using the first component from a principal component analysis to perform a linear regression with one-sided -tests, we calculated *p*-values for IL-8 ($p = 0.24$; first principal component explains 75% of total variation) and TGFβ ($p = 0.04$; first principal component explains 86% of total variation). Nine independent samples from the PROVIDE study were run to serve as a validation set for IL-8 and TGFβ; we observe $p = 0.037$ and = 0.043, respectively, with a one-sided test. The combined *p*-values from both training and validation data are $p = 0.009$ (IL-8) and $p = 0.002$ (TGFβ).

ETHICS STATEMENT

This study was carried out in accordance with the recommendations of the World Health Organization and National Institutes of Health guidelines by Research Review Committee and Ethics Review Committee at the ICDDRB,B and at Institutional Review Boards at the University of Virginia, University of Vermont, and Stanford University with written informed consent from all literate subjects. The consent process for illiterate subjects was approved by the same review committees and is described in detail in Kirkpatrick et al. (34). All literate subjects gave written informed consent in accordance with the Declaration of Helsinki. The protocol was approved by the Research Review Committee and Ethics Review Committee at the ICDDRB,B and at Institutional Review Boards at the University of Virginia, University of Vermont, and Stanford University.

AUTHOR CONTRIBUTIONS

LW, NS, and CL designed and performed experiments, collected, and analyzed data. CB designed the clustering algorithm and analyzed data. LW and CB did statistical analysis. LG and RT performed the stunting clinical correlation analysis. BK, RH, JP, and WP led study design, sample and clinical data collection and logistics, and oversaw clinical assays. LW, WP, and MD conceived of the study and guided it throughout. LW, CB, CL, JP, WP, and MD wrote the manuscript.

ACKNOWLEDGMENTS

The authors thank Cristina Tato and Michael Leipold for critical feedback and the children and families of the PROVIDE and STORK studies for their participation.

REFERENCES

1. Basha S, Surendran N, Pichichero M. Immune responses in neonates. *Expert Rev Clin Immunol.* (2014) 10:1171–84. doi: 10.1586/1744666X.2014.942288
2. MacGillivray DM, Kollmann TR. The role of environmental factors in modulating immune responses in early life. *Front Immunol.* (2014) 5:434. doi: 10.3389/fimmu.2014.00434
3. Simon AK, Hollander GA, McMichael A. Evolution of the immune system in humans from infancy to old age. *Proc Biol Sci.* (2015) 282:20143085. doi: 10.1098/rspb.2014.3085
4. Casanova JL, Abel L. Inborn errors of immunity to infection: the rule rather than the exception. *J Exp Med.* (2005) 202:197–201. doi: 10.1084/jem.20050854
5. Su LF, Davis MM. Antiviral memory phenotype T cells in unexposed adults. *Immunol Rev.* (2013) 255:95–109. doi: 10.1111/imr.12095
6. Veitch AM, Kelly P, Zulu IS, Segal I, Farthing MJ. Tropical enteropathy: a T-cell-mediated crypt hyperplastic enteropathy. *Eur J Gastroenterol Hepatol.* (2001) 13:1175–81. doi: 10.1097/00042737-200110000-00009
7. Korpe PS, Petri WA Jr. Environmental enteropathy: critical implications of a poorly understood condition. *Trends Mol Med.* (2012) 18:328–36. doi: 10.1016/j.molmed.2012.04.007
8. Guerrant RL, DeBoer MD, Moore SR, Scharf RJ, Lima AA. The impoverished gut–a triple burden of diarrhoea, stunting and chronic disease. *Nat Rev Gastroenterol Hepatol.* (2013) 10:220–9. doi: 10.1038/nrgastro.2012.239
9. Lindenbaum J, Kent TH, Sprinz H. Malabsorption and jejunitis in American Peace Corps volunteers in Pakistan. *Ann Intern Med.* (1966) 65:1201–9. doi: 10.7326/0003-4819-65-6-1201
10. Brown EM, Wlodarska M, Willing BP, Vonaesch P, Han J, Reynolds LA, et al. Diet and specific microbial exposure trigger features of environmental enteropathy in a novel murine model. *Nat Commun.* (2015) 6:7806. doi: 10.1038/ncomms8806
11. Campbell DI, Murch SH, Elia M, Sullivan PB, Sanyang MS, Jobarteh B, et al. Chronic T cell-mediated enteropathy in rural west African children: relationship with nutritional status and small bowel function. *Pediatr Res.* (2003) 54:306–11. doi: 10.1203/01.PDR.0000076666.16021.5E
12. Mondal D, Minak J, Alam M, Liu Y, Dai J, Korpe P, et al. Contribution of enteric infection, altered intestinal barrier function, and maternal malnutrition to infant malnutrition in Bangladesh. *Clin Infect Dis.* (2012) 54:185–92. doi: 10.1093/cid/cir807
13. Hayward AR. The human fetus and newborn: development of the immune response. *Birth Defects Orig Artic Ser.* (1983) 19:289–94.
14. Levy O. Innate immunity of the newborn: basic mechanisms and clinical correlates. *Nat Rev Immunol.* (2007) 7:379–90. doi: 10.1038/nri2075
15. Ygberg S, Nilsson A. The developing immune system - from foetus to toddler. *Acta Paediatr.* (2012) 101:120–7. doi: 10.1111/j.1651-2227.2011.02494.x
16. Rook GA, Dheda K, Zumla A. Immune systems in developed and developing countries; implications for the design of vaccines that will work where BCG does not. *Tuberculosis.* (2006) 86:152–62. doi: 10.1016/j.tube.2006.01.018
17. Vesikari T, Matson DO, Dennehy P, Van Damme P, Santosham M, Rodriguez Z, et al. Safety and efficacy of a pentavalent human-bovine (WC3) reassortant rotavirus vaccine. *N Engl J Med.* (2006) 354:23–33. doi: 10.1056/NEJMoa052664
18. Patel M, Pedreira C, De Oliveira LH, Tate J, Orozco M, Mercado J, et al. Association between pentavalent rotavirus vaccine and severe rotavirus diarrhea among children in Nicaragua. *JAMA.* (2009) 301:2243–51. doi: 10.1001/jama.2009.756
19. Madhi SA, Cunliffe NA, Steele D, Witte D, Kirsten M, Louw C, et al. Effect of human rotavirus vaccine on severe diarrhea in African infants. *N Engl J Med.* (2010) 362:289–98. doi: 10.1056/NEJMoa0904797
20. Barreiro LB, Quintana-Murci L. From evolutionary genetics to human immunology: how selection shapes host defence genes. *Nat Rev Genet.* (2010) 11:17–30. doi: 10.1038/nrg2698
21. Nguyen M, Leuridan E, Zhang T, De Wit D, Willems F, Van Damme P, et al. Acquisition of adult-like TLR4 and TLR9 responses during the first year of life. *PLoS ONE.* (2010) 5:e10407. doi: 10.1371/journal.pone.0010407
22. Burl S, Townend J, Njie-Jobe J, Cox M, Adetifa UJ, Touray E, et al. Age-dependent maturation of Toll-like receptor-mediated cytokine responses in Gambian infants. *PLoS ONE.* (2011) 6:e18185. doi: 10.1371/journal.pone.0018185
23. Teran R, Mitre E, Vaca M, Erazo S, Oviedo G, Hubner MP, et al. Immune system development during early childhood in tropical Latin America: evidence for the age-dependent down regulation of the innate immune response. *Clin Immunol.* (2011) 138:299–310. doi: 10.1016/j.clim.2010.12.011
24. Lisciandro JG, Prescott SL, Nadal-Sims MG, Devitt CJ, Pomat W, Siba PM, et al. Ontogeny of Toll-like and NOD-like receptor-mediated innate immune responses in Papua New Guinean infants. *PLoS ONE.* (2012) 7:e36793. doi: 10.1371/journal.pone.0036793

25. Reikie BA, Adams RC, Ruck CE, Ho K, Leligdowicz A, Pillay S, et al. Ontogeny of Toll-like receptor mediated cytokine responses of South African infants throughout the first year of life. *PLoS ONE.* (2012) 7:e44763. doi: 10.1371/journal.pone.0044763
26. Kollmann TR. Variation between populations in the innate immune response to vaccine adjuvants. *Front Immunol.* (2013) 4:81. doi: 10.3389/fimmu.2013.00081
27. Nedelec Y, Sanz J, Baharian G, Szpiech ZA, Pacis A, Dumain, A, et al. Genetic ancestry and natural selection drive population differences in immune responses to pathogens. *Cell.* (2016) 167:657–69 e621. doi: 10.1016/j.cell.2016.09.025
28. Corbett NP, Blimkie D, Ho KC, Cai B, Sutherland DP, Kallos A, et al. Ontogeny of Toll-like receptor mediated cytokine responses of human blood mononuclear cells. *PLoS ONE.* (2010) 5:e15041. doi: 10.1371/journal.pone.0015041
29. Djuardi Y, Wammes LJ, Supali T, Sartono E, Yazdanbakhsh M. Immunological footprint: the development of a child's immune system in environments rich in microorganisms and parasites. *Parasitology.* (2011) 138:1508–18. doi: 10.1017/S0031182011000588
30. Cooper PJ, Amorim LD, Figueiredo CA, Esquivel R, Tupiza F, Erazo S, et al. Effects of environment on human cytokine responses during childhood in the tropics: role of urban versus rural residence. *World Allergy Organ J.* (2015) 8:22. doi: 10.1186/s40413-015-0071-2
31. Hussey GD, Watkins ML, Goddard EA, Gottschalk S, Hughes EJ, Iloni K, et al. Neonatal mycobacterial specific cytotoxic T-lymphocyte and cytokine profiles in response to distinct BCG vaccination strategies. *Immunology.* (2002) 105:314–24. doi: 10.1046/j.1365-2567.2002.01366.x
32. Rook GA, Dheda K, Zumla A. Immune responses to tuberculosis in developing countries: implications for new vaccines. *Nat Rev Immunol.* (2005) 5:661–7. doi: 10.1038/nri1666
33. Strachan DP. Hay fever, hygiene, and household size. *BMJ.* (1989) 299:1259–60. doi: 10.1136/bmj.299.6710.1259
34. Kirkpatrick BD, Colgate ER, Mychaleckyj JC, Haque R, Dickson DM, Carmolli MP, et al. The performance of rotavirus and oral Polio Vaccines in Developing Countries (PROVIDE) study: description of methods of an interventional study designed to explore complex biologic problems. *Am J Trop Med Hyg.* (2015) 92:744–51. doi: 10.4269/ajtmh.14-0518
35. Ley C, Sanchez Mde L, Mathur A, Yang S, Sundaram V, Parsonnet J. Stanford's Outcomes Research in Kids (STORK): a prospective study of healthy pregnant women and their babies in Northern California. *BMJ Open.* (2016) 6:e010810. doi: 10.1136/bmjopen-2015-010810
36. Pindyck T, Tate JE, Parashar UD. A decade of experience with rotavirus vaccination in the United States - vaccine uptake, effectiveness, and impact. *Expert Rev Vaccines.* (2018) 17:593–606. doi: 10.1080/14760584.2018.1489724
37. Beer KD, Gargano JW, Roberts VA, Hill VR, Garrison LE, Kutty PK, et al. Surveillance for waterborne disease outbreaks associated with drinking water - United States, 2011-2012. *Morb Mortal Wkly Rep.* (2015) 64:842–8. doi: 10.15585/mmwr.mm6431a2
38. McClung RP, Roth DM, Vigar M, Roberts VA, Kahler AM, Cooley LA, et al. Waterborne disease outbreaks associated with environmental and undetermined exposures to water - United States, 2013-2014. *Morb Mortal Wkly Rep.* (2017) 66:1222–5. doi: 10.15585/mmwr.mm6644a4
39. Haque R, Mondal D, Duggal P, Kabir M, Roy S, Farr BM, et al. Entamoeba histolytica infection in children and protection from subsequent amebiasis. *Infect Immun.* (2006) 74:904–9. doi: 10.1128/IAI.74.2.904-909.2006
40. Kotloff KL, Nataro JP, Blackwelder WC, Nasrin D, Farag TH, Panchalingam S, et al. Burden and aetiology of diarrhoeal disease in infants and young children in developing countries (the Global Enteric Multicenter Study, GEMS): a prospective, case-control study. *Lancet.* (2013) 382:209–22. doi: 10.1016/S0140-6736(13)60844-2
41. Taniuchi M, Sobuz SU, Begum S, Platts-Mills JA, Liu J, Yang Z, et al. Etiology of diarrhea in Bangladeshi infants in the first year of life analyzed using molecular methods. *J Infect Dis.* (2013) 208:1794–802. doi: 10.1093/infdis/jit507
42. Gilchrist CA, Petri SE, Schneider BN, Reichman DJ, Jiang N, Begum S, et al. Role of the gut microbiota of children in diarrhea due to the protozoan parasite *Entamoeba histolytica. J Infect Dis.* (2015) 213:1579–85. doi: 10.1093/infdis/jiv772
43. Amir el AD, Davis KL, Tadmor MD, Simonds EF, Levine JH, Bendall SC, et al. viSNE enables visualization of high dimensional single-cell data and reveals phenotypic heterogeneity of leukemia. *Nat Biotechnol.* (2013) 31:545–52. doi: 10.1038/nbt.2594
44. Becher B, Schlitzer A, Chen J, Mair F, Sumatoh HR, Teng KW, et al. High-dimensional analysis of the murine myeloid cell system. *Nat Immunol.* (2014) 15:1181–9. doi: 10.1038/ni.3006
45. Shekhar K, Brodin P, Davis MM, Chakraborty AK. Automatic Classification of Cellular Expression by Nonlinear Stochastic Embedding (ACCENSE). *Proc Natl Acad Sci USA.* (2014) 111:202–7. doi: 10.1073/pnas.1321405111
46. Chester C, Maecker HT. Algorithmic Tools for Mining High-Dimensional Cytometry Data. *J Immunol.* (2015) 195:773–9. doi: 10.4049/jimmunol.1500633
47. Brenchley JM, Karandikar NJ, Betts MR, Ambrozak DR, Hill BJ, Crotty LE, et al. Expression of CD57 defines replicative senescence and antigen-induced apoptotic death of CD8+ T cells. *Blood.* (2003) 101:2711–20. doi: 10.1182/blood-2002-07-2103
48. Brodin P, Jojic V, Gao T, Bhattacharya S, Angel CJ, Furman D, et al. Variation in the human immune system is largely driven by non-heritable influences. *Cell.* (2015) 160:37–47. doi: 10.1016/j.cell.2014.12.020
49. Klenerman P, Oxenius A. T cell responses to cytomegalovirus. *Nat Rev Immunol.* (2016) 16:367–77. doi: 10.1038/nri.2016.38
50. Barreiro LB, Laval G, Quach H, Patin E, Quintana-Murci L. Natural selection has driven population differentiation in modern humans. *Nat Genet.* (2008) 40:340–5. doi: 10.1038/ng.78
51. Vasseur E, Boniotto M, Patin E, Laval G, Quach H, Manry J, et al. The evolutionary landscape of cytosolic microbial sensors in humans. *Am J Hum Genet.* (2012) 91:27–37. doi: 10.1016/j.ajhg.2012.05.008
52. Quach H, Rotival M, Pothlichet J, Loh YE, Dannemann M, Zidane N, et al. Genetic adaptation and neandertal admixture shaped the immune system of human populations. *Cell.* (2016) 167:643–56 e617. doi: 10.1016/j.cell.2016.09.024
53. Barreiro LB, Ben-Ali M, Quach H, Laval G, Patin E, Pickrell JK, et al. Evolutionary dynamics of human Toll-like receptors and their different contributions to host defense. *PLoS Genet.* (2009) 5:e1000562. doi: 10.1371/journal.pgen.1000562
54. Wlasiuk G, Khan S, Switzer WM, Nachman MW. A history of recurrent positive selection at the toll-like receptor 5 in primates. *Mol Biol Evol.* (2009) 26:937–49. doi: 10.1093/molbev/msp018
55. Fumagalli M, Cagliani R, Riva S, Pozzoli U, Biasin M, Piacentini L, et al. Population genetics of IFIH1: ancient population structure, local selection, and implications for susceptibility to type 1 diabetes. *Mol Biol Evol.* (2010) 27:2555–66. doi: 10.1093/molbev/msq141
56. Quintana-Murci L, Clark AG. Population genetic tools for dissecting innate immunity in humans. *Nat Rev Immunol.* (2013) 13:280–93. doi: 10.1038/nri3421
57. Naylor C, Lu M, Haque R, Mondal D, Buonomo E, Nayak U, et al. Environmental enteropathy, oral vaccine failure and growth faltering in infants in Bangladesh. *EBio Med.* (2015) 2:1759–66. doi: 10.1016/j.ebiom.2015.09.036
58. Tu W, Chen S, Sharp M, Dekker C, Manganello AM, Tongson EC, et al. Persistent and selective deficiency of CD4+ T cell immunity to cytomegalovirus in immunocompetent young children. *J Immunol.* (2004) 172:3260–7. doi: 10.4049/jimmunol.172.5.3260
59. Appay V, Dunbar PR, Callan M, Klenerman P, Gillespie GM, Papagno L, et al. Memory CD8+ T cells vary in differentiation phenotype in different persistent virus infections. *Nat Med.* (2002) 8:379–85. doi: 10.1038/nm0402-379
60. Pitcher CJ, Hagen SI, Walker JM, Lum R, Mitchell BL, Maino VC, et al. Development and homeostasis of T cell memory in rhesus macaque. *J Immunol.* (2002) 168:29–43. doi: 10.4049/jimmunol.168.1.29

61. Sylwester AW, Mitchell BL, Edgar JB, Taormina C, Pelte C, Ruchti F, et al. Broadly targeted human cytomegalovirus-specific CD4+ and CD8+ T cells dominate the memory compartments of exposed subjects. *J Exp Med.* (2005) 202:673–85. doi: 10.1084/jem.20050882
62. Furman D, Jojic V, Sharma S, Shen-Orr SS, Angel CJ, Onengut-Gumuscu S, et al. Cytomegalovirus infection enhances the immune response to influenza. *Sci Transl Med.* (2015) 7:281ra243. doi: 10.1126/scitranslmed.aaa2293
63. Bhutta ZA, Ahmed T, Black RE, Cousens S, Dewey K, Giugliani E, et al. What works? Interventions for maternal and child undernutrition and survival. *Lancet.* (2008) 371:417–40. doi: 10.1016/S0140-6736(07)61693-6
64. Najera O, Gonzalez C, Toledo G, Lopez L, Ortiz R. Flow cytometry study of lymphocyte subsets in malnourished and well-nourished children with bacterial infections. *Clin Diagn Lab Immunol.* (2004) 11:577–80. doi: 10.1128/CDLI.11.3.577-580.2004
65. Gorelik L, Flavell RA. Transforming growth factor-beta in T-cell biology. *Nat Rev Immunol.* (2002) 2:46–53. doi: 10.1038/nri704
66. Li MO, Wan YY, Sanjabi S, Robertson AK, Flavell RA. Transforming growth factor-beta regulation of immune responses. *Annu Rev Immunol.* (2006) 24:99–146. doi: 10.1146/annurev.immunol.24.021605.090737
67. Smith PD, Smythies LE, Shen R, Greenwell-Wild T, Gliozzi M, Wahl SM. Intestinal macrophages and response to microbial encroachment. *Mucosal Immunol.* (2011) 4:31–42. doi: 10.1038/mi.2010.66
68. Huber AR, Kunkel SL, Todd RF III, Weiss SJ. Regulation of transendothelial neutrophil migration by endogenous interleukin-8. *Science.* (1991) 254:99–102. doi: 10.1126/science.1718038
69. Sack U, Burkhardt U, Borte M, Schadlich H, Berg K, Emmrich F. Age-dependent levels of select immunological mediators in sera of healthy children. *Clin Diagn Lab Immunol.* (1998) 5:28–32.
70. Franz AR, Steinbach G, Kron M, Pohlandt F. Interleukin-8: a valuable tool to restrict antibiotic therapy in newborn infants. *Acta Paediatr.* (2001) 90:1025–32. doi: 10.1111/j.1651-2227.2001.tb01359.x
71. Mehr SS, Doyle LW, Rice GE, Vervaart P, Henschke P. Interleukin-6 and interleukin-8 in newborn bacterial infection. *Am J Perinatol.* (2001) 18:313–24. doi: 10.1055/s-2001-17857
72. Simonsen KA, Anderson-Berry AL, Delair SF, Davies HD. Early-onset neonatal sepsis. *Clin Microbiol Rev.* (2014) 27:21–47. doi: 10.1128/CMR.00031-13
73. Gibbons D, Fleming P, Virasami A, Michel ML, Sebire NJ, Costeloe K, et al. Interleukin-8 (CXCL8) production is a signatory T cell effector function of human newborn infants. *Nat Med.* (2014) 20:1206–10. doi: 10.1038/nm.3670
74. Sturm A, Baumgart DC, d'Heureuse JH, Hotz A, Wiedenmann B, Dignass AU. CXCL8 modulates human intestinal epithelial cells through a CXCR1 dependent pathway. *Cytokine.* (2005) 29:42–8. doi: 10.1016/j.cyto.2004.09.007
75. Dignass AU, Podolsky DK. Cytokine modulation of intestinal epithelial cell restitution: central role of transforming growth factor beta. *Gastroenterology.* (1993) 105:1323–32. doi: 10.1016/0016-5085(93)90136-Z
76. Dignass AU. Mechanisms and modulation of intestinal epithelial repair. *Inflamm Bowel Dis.* (2001) 7:68–77. doi: 10.1097/00054725-200102000-00014
77. Subramanian S, Huq S, Yatsunenko T, Haque R, Mahfuz M, Alam MA, et al. Persistent gut microbiota immaturity in malnourished Bangladeshi children. *Nature.* (2014) 510:417–21. doi: 10.1038/nature13421
78. David LA, Weil A, Ryan ET, Calderwood SB, Harris JB, Chowdhury F, et al. Gut microbial succession follows acute secretory diarrhea in humans. *MBio.* (2015) 6:e00381-00315. doi: 10.1128/mBio.00381-15
79. Mei HE, Leipold MD, Schulz AR, Chester C, Maecker HT. Barcoding of live human peripheral blood mononuclear cells for multiplexed mass cytometry. *J Immunol.* (2015) 194:2022–31. doi: 10.4049/jimmunol.1402661
80. van der Maaten LHG. Visualizing Data using t-SNE. *J Mach Learn Res.* (2008) 9:2579–605.
81. van der Maaten L. Accelerating t-SNE using Tree-Based Algorithms. *J Mach Learn Res.* (2014) 15:3221–45.
82. R Core Team (2015). *R: A Language and Environment for Statistical Computing.* R Foundation for Statistical Computing. Available online at: http://www.R-project.org/ (accessed December 1, 2018).

Permissions

All chapters in this book were first published by Frontiers; hereby published with permission under the Creative Commons Attribution License or equivalent. Every chapter published in this book has been scrutinized by our experts. Their significance has been extensively debated. The topics covered herein carry significant findings which will fuel the growth of the discipline. They may even be implemented as practical applications or may be referred to as a beginning point for another development.

The contributors of this book come from diverse backgrounds, making this book a truly international effort. This book will bring forth new frontiers with its revolutionizing research information and detailed analysis of the nascent developments around the world.

We would like to thank all the contributing authors for lending their expertise to make the book truly unique. They have played a crucial role in the development of this book. Without their invaluable contributions this book wouldn't have been possible. They have made vital efforts to compile up to date information on the varied aspects of this subject to make this book a valuable addition to the collection of many professionals and students.

This book was conceptualized with the vision of imparting up-to-date information and advanced data in this field. To ensure the same, a matchless editorial board was set up. Every individual on the board went through rigorous rounds of assessment to prove their worth. After which they invested a large part of their time researching and compiling the most relevant data for our readers.

The editorial board has been involved in producing this book since its inception. They have spent rigorous hours researching and exploring the diverse topics which have resulted in the successful publishing of this book. They have passed on their knowledge of decades through this book. To expedite this challenging task, the publisher supported the team at every step. A small team of assistant editors was also appointed to further simplify the editing procedure and attain best results for the readers.

Apart from the editorial board, the designing team has also invested a significant amount of their time in understanding the subject and creating the most relevant covers. They scrutinized every image to scout for the most suitable representation of the subject and create an appropriate cover for the book.

The publishing team has been an ardent support to the editorial, designing and production team. Their endless efforts to recruit the best for this project, has resulted in the accomplishment of this book. They are a veteran in the field of academics and their pool of knowledge is as vast as their experience in printing. Their expertise and guidance has proved useful at every step. Their uncompromising quality standards have made this book an exceptional effort. Their encouragement from time to time has been an inspiration for everyone.

The publisher and the editorial board hope that this book will prove to be a valuable piece of knowledge for researchers, students, practitioners and scholars across the globe.

List of Contributors

Ronald P. Schuyler, Conner Jackson, Josselyn E. Garcia-Perez, Ryan M. Baxter, Sidney Ogolla and Rosemary Rochford
Department of Immunology and Microbiology, University of Colorado School of Medicine, Aurora, CO, United States

Debashis Ghosh
Department of Biostatistics and Informatics, Colorado School of Public Health, Aurora, CO, United States

Pratyaydipta Rudra
Department of Statistics, Oklahoma State University, Stillwater, OK, United States

Elena W. Y. Hsieh
Division of Allergy and Immunology, Department of Pediatrics, University of Colorado School of Medicine, Children's Hospital Colorado, Aurora, CO, United States

Mehdi R. Pirozyan, Abdullah Al Emran, Hsin-Yi Tseng and Jessamy C. Tiffen
Melanoma Immunology and Oncology, Centenary Institute, Sydney, NSW, Australia
Central Clinical School, The University of Sydney, Camperdown, NSW, Australia
Melanoma Institute Australia, The University of Sydney, Sydney, NSW, Australia

Peter Hersey
Melanoma Immunology and Oncology, Centenary Institute, Sydney, NSW, Australia
Melanoma Institute Australia, The University of Sydney, Sydney, NSW, Australia

Barbara Fazekas de St Groth
Ramaciotti Facility for Human Systems Biology, The University of Sydney, Sydney, NSW, Australia
Discipline of Pathology, Sydney Medical School, The University of Sydney, Sydney, NSW, Australia
Charles Perkins Centre, The University of Sydney, Sydney, NSW, Australia

Helen M. McGuire
Ramaciotti Facility for Human Systems Biology, The University of Sydney, Sydney, NSW, Australia
Discipline of Pathology, Sydney Medical School, The University of Sydney, Sydney, NSW, Australia
Charles Perkins Centre, The University of Sydney, Sydney, NSW, Australia
Discipline of Pathology, Faculty of Medicine and Health, The University of Sydney, Sydney, NSW, Australia

Jenny H. Lee
Melanoma Institute Australia, The University of Sydney, Sydney, NSW, Australia
Biomedical Sciences, Faculty of Medicine and Health Sciences, Macquarie University, Sydney, NSW, Australia

Matteo S. Carlino
Melanoma Institute Australia, The University of Sydney, Sydney, NSW, Australia
Westmead and Blacktown Hospitals, Sydney, NSW, Australia

Alexander M. Menzies and Georgina V. Long
Melanoma Institute Australia, The University of Sydney, Sydney, NSW, Australia
Royal North Shore Hospital, St Leonards, NSW, Australia

Richard A. Scolyer
Melanoma Institute Australia, The University of Sydney, Sydney, NSW, Australia
Charles Perkins Centre, The University of Sydney, Sydney, NSW, Australia
Royal Prince Alfred Hospital, Camperdown, NSW, Australia
New South Wales Health Pathology, NSW, Australia

Purvesh Khatri
Department of Medicine, Stanford University, Palo Alto, CA, United States

Nicholas L. Bayless
Department of Stanford Immunology Program, Stanford University, Palo Alto, CA, United States

Mathieu Le Gars
Department of Medicine, Stanford University, Palo Alto, CA, United States
Department of Stanford Immunology Program, Stanford University, Palo Alto, CA, United States

Christof Seiler and Cornelia L. Dekker
Department of Statistics, Stanford University, Palo Alto, CA, United States

Susan Holmes and Alexander W. Kay
Department of Pediatrics, Stanford University, Palo Alto, CA, United States

Elina Starosvetsky, Lindsay Moore and Shai S. Shen-Orr
Faculty of Medicine, Technion - Israel Institute of Technology, Haifa, Israel

Natali Aziz and Gary E. Swan
Department of Obstetrics and Gynecology, Stanford Prevention Research Center, Stanford University School of Medicine, Stanford University, Palo Alto, CA, United States

Mark M. Davis
Department of Microbiology and Immunology, Stanford University, Palo Alto, CA, United States
Howard Hughes Medical Institute, Stanford University School of Medicine, Stanford, CA, United States

Catherine A. Blish
Department of Medicine, Stanford University, Palo Alto, CA, United States
Department of Stanford Immunology Program, Stanford University, Palo Alto, CA, United States
Chan Zuckerberg Biohub, San Francisco, CA, United States

Diana Shinko and Kellie A. Charles
Discipline of Pharmacology, Faculty of Medicine and Health, The University of Sydney, Sydney, NSW, Australia

Connie I. Diakos, Nick Pavlakis and Stephen J. Clarke
Northern Sydney Cancer Centre, Royal North Shore Hospital, St Leonards, NSW, Australia
Faculty of Medicine and Health, Northern Clinical School, The University of Sydney, Sydney, NSW, Australia
Bill Walsh Translational Research Laboratories, Kolling Institute of Medical Research, St Leonards, NSW, Australia

Scott N. Byrne
Westmead Institute for Medical Research, Centre for Immunology and Allergy Research, Westmead, NSW, Australia
Discipline of Infectious Diseases and Immunology, Faculty of Medicine and Health, Central Clinical School, The University of Sydney, Sydney, NSW, Australia

Ramy Gadalla, Babak Noamani, Bethany L. MacLeod, Russell J. Dickson, Wenxi Xu, Sabelo Lukhele, Heidi J. Elsaesser, Albiruni R. Abdul Razak, Ben Wang, Marcus Butler and Lillian L. Siu
Tumor Immunology Program, Princess Margaret Cancer Center, University Health Network, Toronto, ON, Canada

Mengdi Guo
Department of Immunology, University of Toronto, Toronto, ON, Canada

Naoto Hirano, Tracy L. McGaha, Pam S. Ohashi and David G. Brooks
Tumor Immunology Program, Princess Margaret Cancer Center, University Health Network, Toronto, ON, Canada
Department of Immunology, University of Toronto, Toronto, ON, Canada

Cynthia J. Guidos
Department of Immunology, University of Toronto, Toronto, ON, Canada
Program in Developmental and Stem Cell Biology, Hospital for Sick Children Research Institute, Toronto, ON, Canada

Ellis Patrick
The Westmead Institute for Medical Research, University of Sydney, Westmead, NSW, Australia
School of Mathematics and Statistics, University of Sydney, NSW, Australia

Heeva Baharlou, Nicolas P. Canete, Anthony L. Cunningham and Andrew N. Harman
The Westmead Institute for Medical Research, University of Sydney, Westmead, NSW, Australia
Centre for Virus Research, The Westmead Institute for Medical Research, Westmead, NSW, Australia

Coindre, Lamine Alaoui, Bruno Vaslin, Christine Bourgeois, Camille Lecuroux, Anne-Sophie Beignon and Benoit Favier
CEA-Université Paris Sud-INSERM U1184, IDMIT Department, IBFJ, DRF, Fontenay-aux-Roses, France

Cecile Goujard
Service de médecine interne et d'immunologie clinique, Hôpital Bicêtre, APHP, Le Kremlin Bicêtre, France
INSERM U1018-Université Paris Sud, CESP (Centre for Research in Epidemiology and Population Health), Le Kremlin Bicêtre, France

Pierre Bruhns
Unit of Antibodies in Therapy and Pathology, Institut Pasteur, UMR1222 INSERM, Paris, France

Martina Bertolo and Philipp Enghard
Department of Nephrology, Charité Universitätsmedizin Berlin, Berlin, Germany

Sabine Baumgart, Pawel Durek, Anette Peddinghaus, Henrik Mei and Andreas Grützkau
Deutsches Rheuma-Forschungszentrum Berlin (DRFZ), a Leibniz-Institute, Berlin, Germany

Thomas Rose
Department of Rheumatology and Clinical Immunology, Charité Universitätsmedizin Berlin, Berlin, Germany

Frances Winkler
Department of Medicine II, Gastroenterology, Hepatology, Endocrinology, and Infectious Diseases, Faculty of Medicine, University Medical Center Freiburg, Freiburg, Germany
Faculty of Biology, University of Freiburg, Freiburg, Germany

Bertram Bengsch
Department of Medicine II, Gastroenterology, Hepatology, Endocrinology, and Infectious Diseases, Faculty of Medicine, University Medical Center Freiburg, Freiburg, Germany
Signalling Research Centres BIOSS and CIBSS, University of Freiburg, Freiburg, Germany

Shadi Toghi Eshghi, Amelia Au-Yeung, Chikara Takahashi, Maclean N. Nyachienga, Sean P. Lear, Cherie Green, W. Rodney Mathews and William E. O'Gorman
OMNI Biomarker Development, Genentech Inc., South San Francisco, CA, United States

Christopher R. Bolen
Bioinformatics, Genentech Inc., South San Francisco, CA, United States
Department of Microbiology and Immunology, Stanford University, Stanford, CA, United States

Lucius Bader and Clara Gram Gjesdal
Bergen Group of Epidemiology and Biomarkers in Rheumatic Disease, Department of Rheumatology, Haukeland University Hospital, Bergen, Norway
Department of Clinical Science, University of Bergen, Bergen, Norway

Stein-Erik Gullaksen
Center of Cancer Biomarkers, University of Bergen, Bergen, Norway
Department of Internal Medicine, Hematology Section, Haukeland University Hospital, Bergen, Norway

Nello Blaser and Morten Brun
Department of Mathematics, University of Bergen, Bergen, Norway

Gerd Haga Bringeland and Christian Vedeler
Department of Neurology, Haukeland University Hospital, Bergen, Norway
Department of Clinical Medicine, University of Bergen, Bergen, Norway

André Sulen
Bergen Group of Epidemiology and Biomarkers in Rheumatic Disease, Department of Rheumatology, Haukeland University Hospital, Bergen, Norway
Department of Neurology, Haukeland University Hospital, Bergen, Norway

Sonia Gavasso
Bergen Group of Epidemiology and Biomarkers in Rheumatic Disease, Department of Rheumatology, Haukeland University Hospital, Bergen, Norway
Department of Neurology, Haukeland University Hospital, Bergen, Norway
Department of Clinical Medicine, University of Bergen, Bergen, Norway

Felix Marsh-Wakefield
Discipline of Infectious Diseases and Immunology, Faculty of Medicine and Health, Central Clinical School, The University of Sydney, Sydney, NSW, Australia
Discipline of Pathology, Faculty of Medicine and Health, School of Medical Science, The University of Sydney, Sydney, NSW, Australia

Annabel Kruzins and Najah Nassif
School of Life Sciences, University of Technology Sydney, Sydney, NSW, Australia

Shihong Yang and Christian Bryant
Royal Prince Alfred Hospital, Institute of Haematology, Sydney, NSW, Australia

John Gibson, Christina Brown, Stephen Larsen, Douglas Joshua, Phoebe Joy Ho and Derek McCulloch
Royal Prince Alfred Hospital, Institute of Haematology, Sydney, NSW, Australia
Sydney Medical School, The University of Sydney, Sydney, NSW, Australia

Richard Boyle
Orthopaedics Department, Royal Prince Alfred Hospital, Sydney, NSW, Australia

Georgina Clark
Concord Repatriation General Hospital, ANZAC Research Institute, Concord, NSW, Australia

Slavica Vuckovic
Royal Prince Alfred Hospital, Institute of Haematology, Sydney, NSW, Australia
Faculty of Medicine, University of Queensland, Brisbane, QLD, Australia

Ting Zhang, Junwei Lv, Ziyang Tan, Boqian Wang, Antony R. Warden, Hui Jiang, Yiyang Li and Xianting Ding
State Key Laboratory of Oncogenes and Related Genes, School of Biomedical Engineering, Institute for Personalized Medicine, Shanghai Jiao Tong University, Shanghai, China

Hao Li
Department of General Surgery, Affiliated First People's Hospital, Shanghai Jiao Tong University, Shanghai, China

Adrien Leite Pereira, Nicolas Tchitchek, Roger Le Grand and Antonio Cosma
CEA-Université Paris Sud 11-INSERM U1184, Immunology of Viral Infections and Autoimmune Diseases, IDMIT Infrastructure, Fontenay-aux-Roses, France

Olivier Lambotte
CEA-Université Paris Sud 11-INSERM U1184, Immunology of Viral Infections and Autoimmune Diseases, IDMIT Infrastructure, Fontenay-aux-Roses, France
APHP, Service de Médecine Interne-Immunologie Clinique, Hôpitaux Universitaires Paris Sud, Le Kremlin-Bicêtre, France
Université Paris Sud, Le Kremlin-Bicêtre, France

Xiaoyuan Han, Mohammad S. Ghaemi, Kazuo Ando, Edward A. Ganio, Amy S. Tsai, Ina A. Stelzer, Jakob Einhaus, Basile Bertrand, Natalie Stanley, Anthony Culos, Athena Tanada, Julien Hedou, Eileen S. Tsai, Ramin Fallahzadeh, Brendan Carvalho, Martin S. Angst, Nima Aghaeepour and Brice Gaudilliere
Department of Anesthesiology, Perioperative and Pain Medicine, School of Medicine, Stanford University, Palo Alto, CA, United States

Laura S. Peterson
Department of Pediatrics, School of Medicine, Stanford University, Palo Alto, CA, United States

Dyani K. Gaudilliere
Department of Surgery, School of Medicine, Stanford University, Palo Alto, CA, United States

Ronald J. Wong, Gary M. Shaw and David K. Stevenson
Department of Pediatrics, School of Medicine, Stanford University, Palo Alto, CA, United States
March of Dimes Prematurity Research Center, School of Medicine, Stanford University, Palo Alto, CA, United States

Cecele C. Quaintance
March of Dimes Prematurity Research Center, School of Medicine, Stanford University, Palo Alto, CA, United States

Amy E. Judy, Virginia D. Winn, Maurice L. Druzin, Yair J. Blumenfeld and Ronald S. Gibbs
Department of Obstetrics and Gynecology, School of Medicine, Stanford University, Palo Alto, CA, United States

Mark A. Hlatky
Department of Health Research and Policy, School of Medicine, Stanford University, Palo Alto, CA, United States

Na Li, Vincent van Unen, Nannan Guo and Frits Koning
Department of Immunohematology and Blood Transfusion, Leiden University Medical Center, Leiden, Netherlands

Tamim Abdelaal
Leiden Computational Biology Center, Leiden University Medical Center, Leiden, Netherlands
Department of Pattern Recognition and Bioinformatics Group, Delft University of Technology, Delft, Netherlands

Antonios Somarakis, Jeroen Eggermont and Ahmed Mahfouz
Department of Radiology, Leiden University Medical Center, Leiden, Netherlands

Boudewijn P. F. Lelieveldt
Department of Pattern Recognition and Bioinformatics Group, Delft University of Technology, Delft, Netherlands
Department of Radiology, Leiden University Medical Center, Leiden, Netherlands

Susana M. Chuva de Sousa Lopes
Department of Anatomy and Embryology, Leiden University Medical Center, Leiden, Netherlands

Lisa E. Wagar and Cesar J. Lopez Angel
Department of Microbiology and Immunology, Stanford University, Stanford, CA, United States

Natalia Sigal
Institute for Immunity, Transplantation, and Infection, Stanford University, Stanford, CA, United States

Leying Guan and Robert J. Tibshirani
Data Sciences and Statistics, Stanford University, Stanford, CA, United States

Beth D. Kirkpatrick
Department of Microbiology and Molecular Genetics, University of Vermont College of Medicine and Vaccine Testing Center, Burlington, VT, United States

Rashidul Haque
International Centre for Diarrhoeal Disease Research, Bangladesh, Dhaka, Bangladesh

Julie Parsonnet
Departments of Medicine and of Health Research and Policy, Stanford University, Stanford, CA, United States

William A. Petri Jr.
Department of Medicine, Pathology, and Microbiology, Immunology and Cancer Biology, University of Virginia, Charlottesville, VA, United States

Mark M. Davis
Department of Microbiology and Immunology, Stanford University, Stanford, CA, United States
Institute for Immunity, Transplantation, and Infection, Stanford University, Stanford, CA, United States
Howard Hughes Medical Institute, Stanford University School of Medicine, Stanford, CA, United States

Index

A

Acquired Resistance Groups, 19-20, 22-24, 27

Antibody Conjugation, 146, 186, 196

Antiretroviral Therapies, 168, 171

Astrocytes, 72, 74, 179, 182

Autoimmune Disorders, 71-72

B

Batch Adjustment, 1-5, 7-10, 12, 14

Bovine Serum Albumin, 46, 197, 220

C

Cancer Cells, 31, 33, 37, 40, 72, 86, 165-167

Cancer Clinical Trials, 55-56, 63

Cancer Immunotherapy, 18, 29, 58, 60, 115, 121, 166, 238

Cell Clusters, 92-97, 99-100, 107-109, 119, 135, 171, 173-176, 195, 199, 201-202, 204, 213, 221

Cell Frequency, 125, 185-186, 188, 192, 197, 203

Cell Membrane, 79

Cell Phenotype, 31, 33, 37, 40, 44, 83, 85, 116, 218

Cell Segmentation, 76, 78-80, 89

Cell Subpopulations, 1, 3, 24, 93, 97, 101, 107, 111, 119, 129, 143, 150, 161

Cell Surface, 37, 40, 60, 239

Cell-cell Interactions, 74, 78, 84-85, 89

Chemokines, 49, 54, 118, 160, 165, 177, 179

Chemotherapy, 43-45, 48-53, 88, 157, 206

Clinical Studies, 1, 14, 85, 112

Cohorts, 32-33, 35, 37, 40, 85, 112, 116, 141, 147, 149, 152, 209, 213, 216, 218, 220-221

Colorectal Cancer, 43-44, 52-54, 88, 156, 166

D

Dimensionality Reduction, 24, 60, 83, 122, 125-127, 129, 132, 134, 146, 196, 211, 220-221

Disease Progression, 43, 70, 81-82, 85-86, 90-91, 101, 112, 115, 120, 123, 153-155, 179-180

E

Elite Controllers, 90-92, 97-98, 101

Endothelial Dysfunction, 184

F

Fetal Intestine, 86, 195-196, 199, 201, 203-206

Fetal Liver, 195-196, 199, 201, 203-204

Fetal Spleen, 195-196, 201, 203-204

Flow Cytometry, 3, 15, 18, 33, 35, 44, 53, 55-64, 66-67, 79, 104, 106, 116, 119, 121, 126-127, 129, 134-135, 137, 140-141, 143-147, 154, 156-158, 160, 181, 184, 189, 204, 215, 224

Functional Markers, 9, 11, 60, 75, 83, 136-141, 186

G

Gestation, 184-185, 189, 196, 204, 220

H

Healthy Donors, 32, 53, 56, 60, 63-64, 88, 93-94, 96-98, 127, 134, 136-137, 139-142, 145, 168-177, 180-181

Healthy Pregnancy, 183, 196

Hematopoiesis, 91, 101, 196, 201, 239

High Dimensional Analysis, 48, 55, 66, 97, 215

Human Immunology, 1-2, 194

I

Imaging Cytometry, 68, 85

Imaging Mass Cytometry, 68-69, 86-87, 156, 159, 195-197, 202, 204

Immune Cell, 2, 11, 14, 22-23, 25, 30-31, 43-44, 48-49, 56, 59, 62-63, 65, 67, 72, 74, 79, 81-82, 84, 89, 103, 107, 113, 115-116, 121, 125, 127-129, 131-132, 134, 136-137, 139, 141-143, 168-169, 180, 183-189, 191-192, 195-196, 200-201, 203, 206, 215, 218-219, 221

Immune Cell Pro iling, 71, 103, 106, 115, 142, 147, 159, 186, 211, 228

Immune Checkpoints, 90, 115-116, 156, 163

Immune Compartment, 195-196, 201, 204

Immune Composition, 195, 197, 199

Immune Correlates, 55, 73

Immune Development, 204, 208-209, 215, 218-219

Immune Dysfunction, 119, 124, 184, 192

Immune Infiltration, 81, 84

Immune Monitoring, 60, 63, 115-116, 143, 208, 225-226, 237-238

Immune Profiling, 55-56, 116-117, 120, 122, 188, 208-209

Immune Responses, 19, 37, 40, 55, 90-91, 97-98, 101, 152, 179-180, 182-184, 187-188, 192, 202, 208-209, 219, 222-224

Immune System, 13, 29, 31, 37, 41, 43-44, 52, 55, 60, 63, 66, 68, 72, 86, 89, 127, 136, 143, 145, 154, 157, 166, 169, 179, 183-185, 188-189, 192-197, 199, 201-202, 204-207, 209, 215, 218, 222-223

Immunofluorescence, 70-71, 86, 156, 159, 162

Immunotherapy, 2, 17-19, 21, 23-25, 27, 29-30, 44, 53, 55, 58, 60, 87, 115, 121, 123, 143, 156-157, 163, 165-167, 182

Influenza Virus, 31-33, 35, 37, 40-42

Innate Immunity, 41, 178, 181, 218, 222-223

Ion Beam, 68-69, 75, 86-87

L

Liquid Biopsies, 71-74, 86

Lupus Nephritis, 103-105, 113-114

Lymphoid Tissue, 74, 87

M
Manual Gating, 7-11, 21, 24-25, 35, 46, 48-49, 58, 64, 66, 80, 91, 99-100, 107-108, 111, 125-128, 130-132, 134-135, 138, 161, 186, 211, 213, 215, 220
Manual Gating Strategy, 8, 46, 48, 91, 107, 127-128, 130, 134
Mass Cytometry, 1-2, 11-16, 19, 21-22, 24, 29-33, 35, 37, 39-41, 43-46, 49-50, 52-53, 107, 109, 112-113, 115-116, 118-125, 128, 134-137, 141-149, 151-154, 156-160, 164, 166, 168-172, 174, 176, 181, 183-187, 189, 191-197, 202-206, 208-209, 224
Melanoma, 14, 17-19, 24-25, 27-30, 52, 54, 56, 62, 65, 89, 120-124, 166
Meta-cluster, 48, 50, 139
Microbial Translocation, 91, 101, 179-181
Mononuclear Cells, 3, 18, 45, 56, 58-59, 66-67, 98, 104, 111, 127, 136-137, 143, 156-157, 185-186, 208-209, 220, 223-224
Multiple Myeloma, 144-145, 154-155
Multiple Sclerosis, 71-73, 82, 85, 87-88, 142, 153, 155
Multiplexed Imaging, 68, 70, 72, 86-87, 166
Myeloid Cells, 24, 51, 56, 74, 90-92, 95-96, 99-100, 110, 197, 199-200, 202-204

N
Non-polio Enterovirus, 220

P
Pathogenesis, 31-32, 37, 70, 74-75, 88-90, 111, 113-114, 122, 136-137, 141, 152, 181, 184, 192
Patient Stratification, 136-137
Perforin, 24, 26-27, 57-58, 60, 118, 144, 151-152, 155, 172, 180, 213, 215, 218
Phosphorylation, 38, 43-44, 49-50, 52, 138, 141, 166, 187
Post-partum Period, 33, 37, 40
Preeclampsia, 183-194
Progressive Disease, 19-20, 52, 72, 81, 121

R
Rheumatoid Arthritis, 136-137, 142, 194

S
Sequential Waves, 195-196
Signalling Pathways, 43, 49
Single Cell, 2, 18, 27, 41, 44, 56, 59, 62, 65, 67-68, 71, 75, 79-80, 89, 113, 122, 124, 134, 137, 143, 168-169, 197, 206
Subcellular Resolution, 68, 70, 86, 166
Suspension Mass Cytometry, 196-197, 203-204
Systems Biology, 17, 28, 43, 45, 53, 144, 146, 193
Systems Immunology, 1, 115, 120

T
Tumor Necrosis Factor, 136-137, 142-143

U
Urinary Leukocytes, 103-104, 107-109

www.ingramcontent.com/pod-product-compliance
Lightning Source LLC
LaVergne TN
LVHW082158200926
848484LV00008B/2177
* 9 7 9 8 8 8 7 4 0 2 4 1 3 *